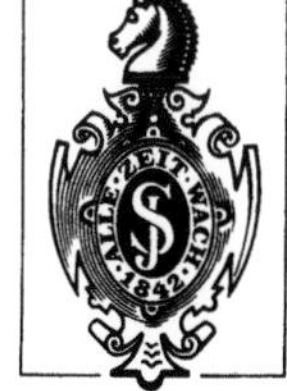

Geriatrics 1

Cardiology and Vascular System
Central Nervous System

Contributors

A. Baldinger   L. Blaha   H. T. Blumenthal   J.-U. Brückmann
A. Brun   F. I. Caird   D. R. Crapper McLachlan   U. De Boni
K. A. Flügel   H. Haimovici   R. Harris   S. Hoyer
R. D. Kennedy   C. Lang   E. G. McGeer   P. L. McGeer
W. Meier-Ruge   K. Nandy   M. S. J. Pathy   A. Pomerance
T. Strandell   A. E. Tàmmaro   H. H. Wieck

Edited by Dieter Platt

With 88 Figures

Springer-Verlag
Berlin   Heidelberg   New York   1982

Professor Dr. med. DIETER PLATT
Institut für Gerontologie
2. Medizinische Klinik
Universität Erlangen-Nürnberg
Flurstraße 17
D-8500 Nürnberg, FRG

ISBN-13:978-3-642-68216-2   e-ISBN-13:978-3-642-68214-8
DOI: 10.1007/978-3-642-68214-8

Library of Congress Cataloging in Publication Data. Main entry under title: Geriatrics I. Bibliography: p.
Includes index. 1. Geriatrics. 2. Geriatric cardiology. 3. Geriatrics neurology. I. Baldinger, A.
II. Platt, Dieter. III. Title: Geriatrics 1. [DNLM: 1. Cardiovascular diseases – In old age. 2. Central
nervous system diseases – In old age. WG 100 G369]   RC952.5.G4435   618.97′61   81-18481 AACR2

2122/3130-543210

List of Contributors

BALDINGER, A., Ph.D.
Research Associate in Gerontology, Aging and Development
Program, Department of Psychology, Washington University,
St. Louis, MO 63130, USA

BLAHA, L., Dr.
Leiter der Einheit für Klinische Pharmakologie,
Universitäts-Nervenklinik Erlangen-Nürnberg,
Schwabachanlage 6–10, D-8520 Erlangen, FRG

BLUMENTHAL, H. T., Ph.D., M.D.
Research Professor of Gerontology, Aging and Development
Program, Department of Psychology, Washington University,
St. Louis, MO 63130, USA

BRÜCKMANN, J.-U., Dr.
Universitäts-Nervenklinik mit Poliklinik Erlangen-Nürnberg,
Schwabachanlage 6–10, D-8520 Erlangen, FRG

BRUN, A., M.D.
Assistant Professor, Head of Department of Neuropathology,
Institute of Pathology, University Hospital of Lund,
S-221 85 Lund, Sweden

CAIRD, F. I., M.A., D.M., F.R.C.P.
Professor of Geriatric Medicine, Department of Geriatric Medicine,
University of Glasgow, Southern General Hospital
Glasgow G51 4TF, Great Britain

CRAPPER MCLACHLAN, D. R., Dr.
Department of Physiology, Medical Science Building,
University of Toronto, Toronto, Canada M5S 1A8

DE BONI, U., Ph.D.
Assistant Professor, Department of Physiology,
Medical Science Building, University of Toronto,
Toronto, Canada M5S 1A8

FLÜGEL, K. A., Professor Dr.
Nervenklinik mit Poliklinik der Universität Erlangen-Nürnberg,
Kopfklinikum, Schwabachanlage 6, D-8520 Erlangen, FRG

HAIMOVICI, H., M.D.
Clinical Professor, Emeritus of Surgery,
862 Park Avenue, New York, NY 10021, USA

HARRIS, R., M.D.
President, Center for the Study of Aging,
Associate Clinical Professor of Medicine, Albany Medical College,
706 Madison Avenue, Albany, NY 12208, USA

HOYER, S., Professor Dr.
Institut für Pathochemie und Allgemeine Neurochemie
im Zentrum Pathologie der Universität Heidelberg,
Im Neuenheimer Feld 220–221, D-6900 Heidelberg 1, FRG

KENNEDY, R. D., Dr.
Consultant Physician, Department of Geriatric Medicine,
Stobhill General Hospital, Glasgow G21 3UW, Great Britain

LANG, C., Dr.
Universitäts-Nervenklinik mit Poliklinik Erlangen-Nürnberg,
Schwabachanlage 6–10, D-8520 Erlangen, FRG

McGEER, EDITH G., Ph.D.
Professor and Acting Head, Faculty of Medicine,
Kinsmen Laboratory of Neurological Research,
The University of British Columbia, 2075 Wesbrook Mall,
Vancouver, B.C., Canada V6T 1W5

McGEER, PATRICK L., Ph.D., M.D.
Professor, Faculty of Medicine,
Kinsmen Laboratory of Neurological Research,
The University of British Columbia, 2075 Wesbrook Mall,
Vancouver, B.C., Canada V6T 1W5

MEIER-RUGE, W., Doz. Dr.
Präklinische Forschung, Pharmazeutisches Departement,
Sandoz AG, CH-4002 Basel, Switzerland

NANDY, K., M.D., Ph.D.
Associate Director, Geriatric Research,
Educational and Clinical Center,
Edith Nourse Rogers Memorial Veterans Hospital,
200 Springs Road, Bedford, MA 01730, USA

PATHY, M. S. J., F.R.C.P.
Professor of Geriatric Medicine,
Welsh National School of Medicine, University of Wales,
University Hospital of Wales, Heath Park,
Cardiff CF4 4XN, Great Britain

POMERANCE, ARIELA, M. D., M.R.C.P.
Consultant Histopathologist, Harefield and Mount Vernon
Pathology Laboratories, Harefield Hospital,
Harefield, Middlesex UB9 6JH, Great Britain

STRANDELL, T., M.D.
Assistant Professor, Head of Department of Clinical Physiology,
S:t Erik's Hospital, Box 12600, Fleminggatan 22,
S-11282 Stockholm, Sweden

TÀMMARO, A. E., Professor Dr.
Viale Monte Nero 11, I-20135 Milano, Italy

WIECK, H. H. †, Professor Dr.
former Universitäts-Nervenklinik Erlangen-Nürnberg, FRG

Preface

In 1909 a short contribution entitled "Geriatrics" was published in the *New York Medical Journal*. According to this article, old age represents a distinct period of life in which the physiologic changes caused by aging are accompanied by an increasing number of pathologic changes. We now know that the organs of the body age neither at the same rate nor to the same extent and that physiologic alterations are indeed superimposed by pathologic changes; as a result of the latter phenomenon the origins and course of illnesses in the elderly can present unusual characteristics. The frequency of concurrent disorders in the elderly entails the danger of polypragmatic pharmacotherapy, i.e., the use of various drugs to combat various disorders while neglecting the possibly adverse combined effects of these drugs. To obviate this danger, special knowledge in the field of geriatrics, the medical branch of gerontology, is necessary.

Geriatrics is constantly increasing in importance owing to the near doubling of life expectancy over the past 130 years and to the improved diagnostic and therapeutic techniques made available by medical progress. The rapid recent development of experimental gerontology has played an essential role in enabling us to understand the special features of geriatrics. This progress has, however, been accompanied by such a vast increase in the volume of literature on the subject that specialists in the field can scarcely maintain an overall perspective of new publications. Remarks such as "we, too, treat old people" are factually correct, but fail to reach the heart of the matter: rather they very strikingly emphasize the need for a comprehensive interdisciplinary presentation of geriatrics. This need is met at an international level for the first time by this three-volume series, which should facilitate the daily work of physicians in various specialties.

At this point I would like to thank all those who have collaborated on this series for their painstaking work. Special thanks are owed to Springer-Verlag, who by publishing this work in English have underlined the importance of geriatrics at an international level.

Winter 1981/82 DIETER PLATT

Contents

Cardiac Output. T. STRANDELL. With 7 Figures

Myocardium and Valves. A. POMERANCE. With 35 Figures

Valvular Disease of the Heart. F. I. CAIRD

Cardiac Arrhythmias. R. HARRIS. With 7 Figures

Heart Block. A. E. TÀMMARO. With 3 Figures

The Arterial and Venous System. H. HAIMOVICI. With 7 Figures

Central Nervous System

Cerebral Blood Flow, Electroencephalography and Behavior. S. HOYER

Functional Consequences of Neurofibrillary Degeneration of the Alzheimer Type. D. R. CRAPPER McLACHLAN and U. DE BONI

Neurochemistry of the Aging Brain. W. MEIER-RUGE

Neuronal Lipofuscin and Its Significance. K. NANDY

Neurotransmitters in Normal Aging. E. G. McGeer and
P. L. McGeer. With 6 Figures

Neuroimmunology of the Aging Brain. A. Baldinger and
H. T. Blumenthal. With 5 Figures

Senile Dementia. H. H. Wieck†, J. U. Brückmann, C. Lang and
L. Blaha. With 2 Figures

Alzheimer's Disease and its Clinical Implications. A. BRUN.
With 12 Figures

Stroke. K. A. FLÜGEL

Vertebrobasilar Syndrome. M. S. J. PATHY

Cardiology and Vascular System

Epidemiology of Heart Disease, High Blood Pressure and Cardiovascular Disease

R.D. KENNEDY

A. Mortality and Morbidity of Heart Disease in Old Age

Eighty years ago, the writing of a chapter concerned with cardiac disease in the elderly would have seemed at least indulgent, if not positively wasteful. At that time, the percentage of the population surviving to 65 years was less than 10% in industrialised countries. Acute and chronic infections were a major cause of death in old people, which was frequently ascribed to that non-specific entity, senescence. Even then, however, after infectious fevers, gastro-enteritis and tuberculosis, heart disease was the most frequent cause of death (McKEOWN 1965).

Heart disease is now the major cause of death amongst the elderly in industrialised countries (Table 1). Several reasons for this change have been advanced. Improved public health measures and the development of antimicrobial agents have diminished many previously major causes of mortality. Diagnosis has become more accurate, an example being the establishment of coronary thrombosis as a clinical entity, dating from 1912, following HERRICK's classic description of this condition in the medical literature (HERRICK 1912), although an earlier account had been published by LEYDEN in 1884.

Another factor to consider is the changing age structure of the population in industrialised nations. At the beginning of the twentieth century the average expectation of life was 34 years. This has more than doubled in these countries.

Life expectancy for a male child born in the United Kingdom is 69.6 years and for a female child 75.8 years. The expectation of life for a 65-year-old man today is a further 12 years and 16 years for a woman of the same age. Population projections suggest that the percentage of elderly people in the total population of industrialised countries will continue to increase into the next century. The projected in-

Table 1. Causes of death in ten industrialised countries in order of frequency. (WHO 1974)

	0–4	5–14	15–44	45–64	65+
1.	Accidents	Accidents	Accidents	New growths	HEART DISEASE
2.	Congenital	New growths	New growths	HEART DISEASE	Stroke
3.	New growths	Congenital	HEART DISEASE	Stroke	New growths
4.	Pneumonia	Pneumonia	Suicide	Accidents	Pneumonia
5.	Enteritis and diarrhoea	HEART DISEASE	Stroke	Chest infection	Chronic chest infections

Table 2. Estimated increases in the elderly population in the United Kingdom (1971–2011) and France (1970–2000)

United Kingdom		France	
Age group	Percentage increase	Age group	Percentage increase
60–74	3.13%	65 and over	29%
75–84	22.56%	80 and over	42%
85 and over	62.34%	85 and over	122%

Table 3. Percentage increase in the elderly population in various world regions. ANDERSON et al. 1981

Region and age	Percent change 1970–2000
Latin America	
All ages	+ 119.0
80 and over	+ 215.5
North America	
All ages	+ 30.8
80 and over	+ 96.2
East Asia	
All ages	+ 47.8
80 and over	+ 176.2
Europe	
All ages	+ 17.5
80 and over	+ 62.4
USSR	
All ages	+ 29.8
80 and over	+ 142.6

crease ranges from over 15% of the total population for Western European countries to just over 10% for the United States and Australia. Women predominate, particularly in the very old age groups. It should be appreciated that this increase will occur primarily among those aged 75 years or more (Table 2). In other parts of the world, including the non-industrialised regions, improved public health measures and control of infectious disease along with a high birth rate again suggest that there will be a dramatic increase in the total number of elderly by the year 2000 (Table 3). In these countries also, cardiac diseases will increasingly be diagnosed as the principal cause of death in old age.

Apart from cardiac abnormalities, the major physical disorders of old age are those affecting the musculoskeletal system, the nervous system and malignant conditions. While arteriosclerosis is often thought of as a natural and universal component of ageing, that may not be necessarily so. ROLLESTON (1922) observed that arteriosclerosis was an inconstant finding in the elderly, an observation which has been confirmed several times since. In recent years pathological studies have amply confirmed the major role of heart disease as the principal cause of death in old age. These have required the pathologist to differentiate between the effects of ageing and the effects of pathology in old age, just as the physician in geriatric medicine must unravel the symptoms and signs of disease superimposed on the ageing process from the ageing process itself. Aschoff (1938) stressed that arteriosclerosis was common in the population over 65. Groddeck (1939) found that cardiovascular pathology, including cerebrovascular accidents, accounted for 37% of all deaths in his series of patients aged 80 years or over, and commented that coronary artery disease was not inevitable in this age group. Monroe's monograph (1951) on the clinical and pathological findings in 7,941 elderly persons aged 60 and over noted that cardiovascular pathology was present in 72% of those subjects on whom a post-mortem was performed.

While the high incidence of cardiac pathology in later years is undoubted, it is often difficult at post-mortem to demonstrate the exact role of the cardiac abnormality in the causation of death. The older person is frequently found to have several diseases coexisting at the same time, and these may be interrelated, or entirely independent of each other in their clinical effects. Illness or death may occur from the summation of these varied causes and this should be remembered when ascribing death to one sole cause in old age.

I. Mortality

In those aged 65 or over, heart disease accounts for one-third of all deaths. Initially women have a lower incidence of cardiac mortality due to the lesser frequency of fatal coronary artery disease in younger women. With advancing years this difference is gradually abolished, and the death rate from heart disease for very old women approximates to that for men of the same age (Table 4). The proportion of deaths due to heart disease in women over the age of 65 is approximately 37% and varies little with further years. In men, however, heart disease as a cause of death occurs in 37% over the age of 65 years and falls slightly with age from 39% for those aged 65–69, to 34% over the age of 85 (Caird and Kennedy 1976). The death rates from heart disease increase twofold for men and threefold for women for every 10-year increase in age.

Table 4. Death rate from heart disease per 100,000 population. (Scottish Health Statistics 1978)

Age	Men	Women
25–34	12	5
35–44	83	31
45–54	383	107
55–64	974	378
65–74	2,209	1,134
75–84	4,367	2,708
85+	8,266	6,705

When the various cardiac causes of death are examined, the importance of ischaemic heart disease is immediately apparent. It is the major cause of cardiac death in old people in industrialised nations. In Scotland, it accounts for 80% of cardiac deaths in the elderly (Registrar General for Scotland 1978). The mortality from ischaemic heart disease in the 65–74 year old age group of females is only half that for men in the same age range, but this increases until it approximates to the

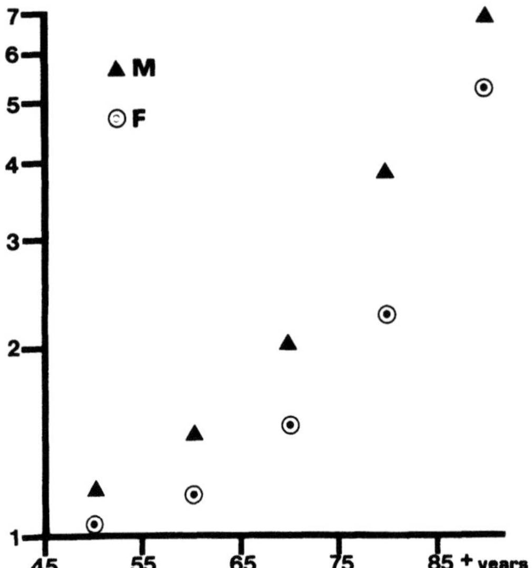

Fig. 1. Death rate from ischaemic heart disease per 100,000 population, Scotland, 1978. Note semi-logarithmic scale. (Scottish Health Statistics 1978)

Table 5. Deaths in the elderly from heart disease, 1978. Rate per 100,000 population. (Scottish Health Statistics 1978 and 8th review I.C.D.)

Age	Ischaemic I.C.D. 410–414		Hypertensive I.C.D. 400–404		Rheumatic I.C.D. 393–398		Other forms	
	M	F	M	F	M	F	M	F
55–64	908	316	16	14	25	32	25	17
65–74	2,030	988	51	37	37	44	91	66
75–84	3,684	2,246	88	105	56	58	360	299
85+	6,852	5,232	184	227	97	65	1,135	1,181

male rate at the age of 85 (Fig. 1). Hypertensive heart disease, rheumatic heart disease, and "other" forms of heart disease are much less frequent (Table 5). Where the classification of heart disease is "other," the death certificate usually states "myocardial insufficiency," "congestive heart failure" or "left ventricular failure." The annual reports of the Registrar General for Scotland have shown that the death rate from heart disease classified as "other" has fallen considerably in recent years. This decrease may well indicate a lessening in the uncertainties in reaching a definite diagnosis in the elderly, with a consequent improvement in identifying and diagnosing cardiac disease correctly.

II. Morbidity and Prevalence

As would be expected, the morbidity of heart disease in industrialised countries is high in old age. Pathological studies have confirmed the high incidence of abnormality in the elderly heart (McKeown 1965; Pomerance 1976). In the elderly at home, the high prevalence of heart disease has been confirmed by several observers

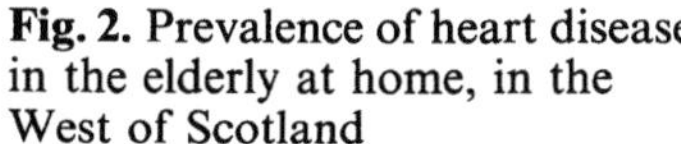

Fig. 2. Prevalence of heart disease in the elderly at home, in the West of Scotland

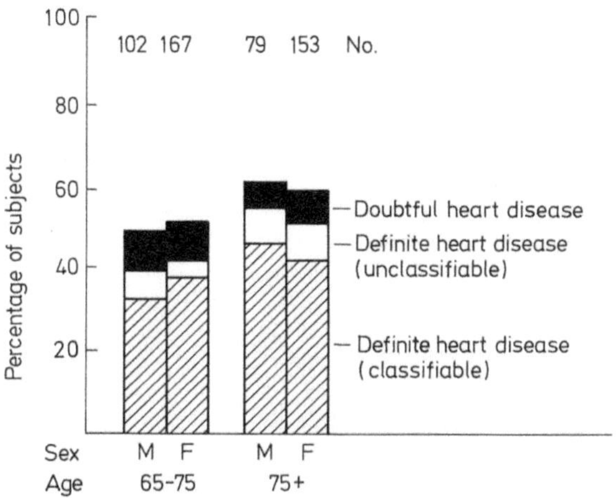

(DROLLER and PEMBERTON 1953; ACHESON and ACHESON 1958; KITCHIN et al. 1973; MARTIN and MILLARD 1973; CAIRD and KENNEDY 1976), though comparability between these series is affected by differing methods and diagnostic criteria.

KENNEDY and colleagues (unpublished work) investigated an elderly population, randomly selected and living at home. Heart disease was classified as "definite classifiable" where a complete cardiac diagnosis could be made; "unclassifiable" where this was not possible, though there was evidence of cardiac abnormality, as shown by chest radiograph or electrocardiogram; or "doubtful" where there was a minor electrocardiographic or radiological abnormality of uncertain significance. Only 50% of those under 75 had no evidence of cardiac abnormality, and the percentage free from cardiac disorders fell to 40% in those aged 75 and over. Moreover, this older group may well have contained patients with occult heart disease which was not manifest at the time of the survey, for example, cardiac amyloidosis, a diagnosis unlikely to be made in life but found with increasing frequency at autopsy in subjects aged 80 years or more.

The major proportion of cardiac disease detected in the elderly can be given a satisfactory diagnostic label. In the 65–74 year old age group, 32% of men and 38% of women were found to have definite classifiable heart disease rising to 46% in men and 42% in women in those aged 75 and over (Fig. 2). Definite unclassifiable heart disease occurred in 4%–8% of subjects aged 65–74, and between 8% and 10%, according to sex, in those over the age of 75. Doubtful heart disease occurred in a small percentage of elderly, being present in 8%–9% of those aged 65–74 and 6%–8% over the age of 75 (Table 6).

The effect of this high incidence of cardiac disease is reflected in the mortality statistics from many industrialised nations. What is more difficult is to determine the extent to which such cardiac disorders contribute to morbidity in the elderly. AKHTAR and colleagues (1973) investigated the causes of disability and dependency at home in a randomly selected group of people aged 65 years and over. Disability was defined as inability to exist at home without help and dependency as a further degree of impairment in self-care. Of those who were found to be unable to live at home without help, 22% had evidence of cardiac disease, and this was consid-

Table 6. Prevalence (percent) of heart disease in elderly people living at home. Caird and Kennedy 1976

Age	65–74		75+	
Sex	M	F	M	F
No.	102	167	79	153
Ischaemic heart disease	20	12	20	12
Hypertensive heart disease	8	16	13	12
Valvular heart disease[a]	1	5	4	8
Pulmonary heart disease	2	0	4	0
Mixed heart disease[b]	2	2	14	12
Total "Definite classifiable"	32	38	46	42
"Definite unclassifiable"[c]	8	4	10	8
Total "Definite" heart disease	40	42	56	51
"Doubtful" heart disease[c]	8	9	6	8
No heart disease	52	50	38	41

[a] Ten cases of mitral, twelve of aortic, valve disease
[b] Hypertensive and ischaemic
[c] See text for definition

ered to be at least a contributory factor to their disability. A further 18% had cardiorespiratory disorders contributing to their dependency. The effect of definable cardiac pathology on morbidity and mortality with advancing age has been amply demonstrated.

B. Prevalence of Heart Disease in Old Age

I. Ischaemic Heart Disease

1. Incidence

Ischaemic heart disease is the commonest form of cardiac disorder encountered in the elderly of both sexes. When defined as a history of angina pectoris or of a previous myocardial infarction and/or the presence of abnormal Q/QS patterns on the electrocardiogram, myocardial ischaemia was found in approximately 20% of men and 12% of women over the age of 65 (Kennedy 1974).

Pathological studies of the elderly have demonstrated an even higher incidence of ischaemic heart disease. In a series of 1,500 post-mortems on elderly patients, McKeown (1965) found that coronary atheroma increased with age even in the very late decades. She found a frequency of 72% in men and 68% in women aged 70–80 years, and 85% in men and 71% in women aged 80–90 years. She correctly stresses that coronary atheroma, however, is not an inevitable accompaniment of old age and demonstrated its absence in 15% of men and 29% of women in the 80–90 year old age group, and in four patients in the 10th decade. It should be remembered that in many of these patients the presence of coronary atheroma was a coincidental autopsy finding. In her autopsy series of patients aged over 70 years, 13% died from coronary heart disease and a further 6% showed the scars of a healed myocardial infarction. McKEOWN also found that the increase in the incidence of ischaemic heart disease at post-mortem fell in patients aged 80 or over.

In another autopsy series, POMERANCE (1965) found that 48% of patients over the age of 75 had evidence of ischaemic myocardial changes. Both authors stress that such changes are often a coincidental finding in those without clinical evidence of cardiac disease and this is supported by the incidence of myocardial ischaemia found in community surveys of the elderly who are not thought to be unwell. The hospital mortality of myocardial infarction increases with age (BJÖRCK 1962; NORRIS et al. 1969). However, this may reflect selective admission of the more severe and readily diagnosed cases, as routine electrocardiographic (KENNEDY and CAIRD 1972) and post-mortem studies (McKEOWN 1965) show a prevalence of unsuspected myocardial infarction of at least 5% in the elderly.

2. Complications

The complications of myocardial infarction also appear to increase with age. An increasing incidence of cardiac rupture secondary to infarction, especially in the elderly female, has been noted by ZEMAN and RODSTEIN (1960), and SIEVERS and colleagues (1961), but this was during the era of anticoagulant therapy. Rupture of the interventricular septum, a rare complication, again increases with age (EDMONSON and HOXIE 1942). However, cardiac aneurysm, as a result of myocardial infarction, does not appear to increase with old age (McKEOWN 1965; PARKINSON et al. 1938).

3. Risk Factors

The defined risk factors for coronary artery disease undergo changes in later years. Male sex is recognised as the most important risk factor in the young and middle-aged (JOINT WORKING PARTY 1976), but this is not so marked in the elderly, in whom the prevalence rate in men exceeds that in women by only 10%–20% (KITCHIN et al. 1973). Divergence of opinion as to the influence of the commonly accepted risk factors has arisen. The significant association between cigarette smoking and ischaemic heart disease as a risk factor is carried over into old age (KENNEDY et al. 1977), and this applies either to current or total cigarette consumption. This agrees with the data from the Framingham study (KANNEL 1976), but is not supported by a study from Edinburgh (KITCHIN et al. 1973) of elderly people staying at home. KENNEDY in Glasgow and KITCHIN in Edinburgh were unable to confirm the importance of high blood pressure as a significant risk factor for ischaemic heart disease in old age, and both of these studies included many subjects aged 75 and over. Neither blood glucose nor serum cholesterol was associated with the presence of ischaemic heart disease in these two surveys in contrast to the findings of KANNEL (1976). In the Glasgow survey, the presence of ischaemic heart disease was highest in those women whose serum cholesterol was in the middle tertile of the range. A similar finding was noted by CARLSTON and BOTTIGER (1972) in a prospective study. They found that the highest incidence of episodes of ischaemic heart disease occurred in elderly men whose serum cholesterol was in the middle frequency of distribution. Despite the predominance of coronary artery disease as the major cardiac cause of death and morbidity, the usually accepted risk factors appear much less dominant in old age, apart from cigarette smoking.

The long-term survival of old people with a myocardial infarction is better than that of younger patients relative to their natural expected mortality. CAMPBELL and colleagues (1974) found that, in an elderly population at home, the difference in mortality between those with an abnormal electrocardiogram and that expected for the whole group was similar to that for elderly patients discharged from hospital following an acute myocardial infarction (BJÖRCK et al. 1958; LIBRACH et al. 1976). The Swedish workers recorded that the ratio of actual to expected mortality in men discharged from hospital after a myocardial infarction was 4.6 in the 6th decade and 1.3 in the 9th. There is, thus, a factual basis for some optimism when considering the long-term prognosis of myocardial infarction in later years. It has been noted that an abnormal electrocardiogram carries an excess mortality in old age, rather than the symptoms of angina with a normal electrocardiogram (KENNEDY et al. 1977; CAMPBELL et al. 1974).

II. Hypertension

A rise of blood pressure is seen in all Western societies with advancing age. This is not paralleled in primitive or non-urbanised societies, nor in those with low dietary salt consumption. Obesity of 25% or more is related to an elevated blood pressure in the elderly (ANDERSON and COWAN 1959), and this is not entirely dependent on arm girth. There is evidence that the blood pressures of relatives of hypertensive patients are higher than those of non-hypertensive members of the general population. Monozygotic twins have a stronger correlation between blood pressure levels than dizygotic (STOCKS 1924).

HAMILTON, PICKERING and colleagues conclude that "arterial pressure is inherited as a graded character through the ranges hitherto described as normal blood pressure and hypertension" (HAMILTON et al. 1954). The quantifiable combination of environmental and hereditary influences remain in dispute.

Black populations in America and in the United Kingdom tend to have higher blood pressures than white populations of the same age group. But this may also be due to cultural and social differences. In Europe the Scots, and particularly those living in the west of Scotland, have the unenviable distinction of having a higher incidence of hypertension, strokes and heart attacks than other Europeans. In general, southern Europeans tend to have lower blood pressures than northerners. These features are carried over into immigrants, the first generation of Scots emigrating to Australia having a higher blood pressure than native-born Australians, and Italian immigrants to Australia having the lowest prevalence of hypertension of all groups.

Epidemiological surveys suggest that the height of the blood pressure represents a degree of risk appropriate to its level. Thus, there is difficulty in establishing a firm dividing line indication "hypertension" or "normotension." (KANNEL et al. 1976; MIALL and CHINN 1974).

Hypertension can be defined as a systolic pressure of 160 mm Hg or more and a diastolic pressure of 95 mm Hg or more. Epidemiological surveys have consistently shown that many elderly people, both in hospital and in the community,

Table 7. Blood pressure in people aged over 65 years. MASTER et al. (1958)

Range of blood pressure in people over 65 years

Age	No. examined	Systolic blood pressure (mm Hg) Mean ± SE	Upper 80% limit	Upper 95% limit	Diastolic blood pressure (mmHg) Mean ± SE	Upper 80% limit	Upper 95% limit
Men							
65– 69	911	143 ± 26	191	195	83 ± 10	101	103
70– 74	694	145 ± 26	193	198	82 ± 15	110	113
75– 79	534	146 ± 22	186	190	81 ± 13	105	107
80– 84	385	145 ± 26	192	196	82 ± 10	100	102
85– 89	325	145 ± 24	190	193	79 ± 15	106	109
90– 94	124	145 ± 23	188	192	78 ± 12	100	102
93–106	25	145 ± 28	196	198	78 ± 13	101	103
Women							
65– 69	856	154 ± 29	207	212	85 ± 14	110	113
70– 74	682	159 ± 26	207	211	85 ± 15	113	116
75– 79	464	158 ± 26	206	210	84 ± 13	108	110
80– 84	344	157 ± 28	208	213	83 ± 17	115	109
85– 89	263	154 ± 28	205	210	82 ± 12	104	107
90– 94	122	150 ± 24	197	198	79 ± 13	102	105
95–106	28	149 ± 24	192	197	81 ± 15	108	110

Table 8. Range of blood pressure in clinically healthy older people. (ANDERSON and COWAN 1959)

Number			Mean ± SE			
			Systolic (mm Hg)		Diastolic (mm Hg)	
Age	Male	Female	Male	Female	Male	Female
60–64	44	48	151 ± 2.8	158 ± 2.7	85 ± 1.2	86 ± 1.2
65–69	63	42	154 ± 2.8	163 ± 3.3	85 ± 0.9	86 ± 1.2
70–74	69	54	164 ± 2.4	168 ± 2.6	86 ± 0.9	87 ± 1.1
75–79	59	35	168 ± 2.7	179 ± 4.2	86 ± 1.2	88 ± 1.9
80–84	50	35	171 ± 2.9	187 ± 4.1	88 ± 1.2	89 ± 2.1
85–89	21	26	173 ± 5.6	189 ± 5.0	87 ± 2.9	92 ± 2.0

have pressures in excess of these levels. MASTER et al. (1958) showed that there is relatively little increase in blood pressure over the age of 65, but the range of values widens. The middle 80% of the range included diastolic pressures up to 100 mm Hg in both sexes and systolic pressures of up to 185 mm Hg in men and 190 mm Hg in women (Table 7). The blood pressures of a group of elderly people aged between 60 and 89 selected as healthy by strict criteria were investigated by ANDERSON and COWAN (1959). They confirmed that the mean systolic and diastolic blood pressures increase with age, the rise being greater for the systolic values. At all ages, females showed a higher mean value of blood pressure than men. With advancing years, the range of blood pressure, particularly systolic, widened (Table 8). ANDERSON and COWAN (1972) attempted to correlate the level of arterial pressure with detectable vascular abnormalities in their elderly population. When blood pressure was related to abnormal findings on ophthalmoscopy and on palpation of the radial artery, and also to the absence of foot pulses, it was noted that the upper limits of systolic pressure were 204 mm Hg for men and 211 mm Hg for women at 60 years, and 218 mm Hg for men and 255 mm Hg for women at 85 years, if all these vascular abnormalities were present. In the absence of such abnormalities, the upper limits of systolic pressure for both sexes were 185 mm Hg at 60 years and 200 mm Hg at 85 years. Diastolic pressures were uninfluenced by age in either sex, and only in women did the diastolic pressure appear to be related significantly to vascular abnormalities.

BECHGAARD (1946) followed up 1,000 hypertensive patients who had blood pressures in excess of 160/100 mm Hg at their first attendance at a general medical clinic in Copenhagen. Re-examination was carried out at 10-year intervals thereafter. Of those who survived to a third examination, 80% had lived beyond the age of 60. He noted that mortality in elderly women did not increase unless the systolic pressure was in excess of 200 mm Hg. There is also evidence to suggest that the absolute risk of raised blood pressure is worse for elderly men than women from studies carried out in South Wales and Framingham, United States (MIALL and CHINN 1974; KANNEL 1976).

That raised systolic blood pressure is associated with a definite effect on the cardiovascular systems of elderly people has been demonstrated (COLANDREA et al. 1970; KENNEDY et al., unpublished work). The former study showed that in the elderly population residing in a retirement community in the United States, isolated systolic hypertension occurred in almost 14% and was frequently labile, but was associated with an increasing risk of developing cardiovascular complications. KENNEDY and colleagues (unpublished work) found that 21% of an ambulant elderly population aged 65 years and over and living at home had pressures in excess of 180/110 mm Hg. Hypertensive heart disease was classified as electrocardiographic changes of "probable" left ventricular hypertrophy (KENNEDY and CAIRD 1972) in the setting of these pressure levels. It was present in 8% and 16% of men, and 13% and 12% of women, in the age groups 65–74 years and 75 years and over.

Atherothrombotic brain infarction was found by KANNEL et al. (1976) to be seven times more frequent in those aged 45–74 years with hypertension than without. In studying the role of raised blood pressure in stroke, SHEKELLE et al. (1974) found that 43% of the population studied had a systolic blood pressure equal to or in excess of 160 mm Hg and that 28% of the strokes in this age group (65–74) could be attributed to hypertension. In middle-aged adults, hypertensive patients with congestive heart failure have an extremely poor prognosis (KANNEL et al. 1972), with one in five of men and one in seven of women dying within 1 year of diagnosis. Whether this trend is confirmed in patients aged 75 or over remains to be seen.

In summary, blood pressure rises with age, particularly systolic blood pressure. In the elderly aged 65–74 this has been shown to be associated with increasing risk of atherothrombotic cerebrovascular occlusions, and an increasing frequency of myocardial infarction and of fatal congestive cardiac failure (MCKEE et al. 1971). The high incidence of morbid events associated with a graded increase in blood pressure in old age is a feature of the male more than the female sex.

Malignant hypertension is rare in those over 70 years (KINCAID-SMITH et al. 1958). Where it occurs, a vascular lesion affecting the kidney, or polyarteritis nodosa should be suspected. Renal hypertension of any kind is uncommon in old age and when found, chronic pyelonephritis or analgesic nephropathy may be incriminated (CAIRD and DALL 1979). Bacteruria on its own is not associated with raised blood pressure in the elderly (AKHTAR et al. 1972).

III. Hypotension

Orthostatic or postural hypotension is frequent in old age and symptoms are often ascribed to it (RODSTEIN and ZEMAN 1957; JOHNSON et al. 1965; CAIRD et al. 1973). On standing, 17% of elderly patients in hospital showed a systolic drop of 20 mm Hg or more and 5% a drop of 40 mm Hg (JOHNSON et al. 1965). Elderly people at home are also prone to orthostatic hypotension. CAIRD et al. (1973) investigated the postural drop in systolic pressure in 494 people aged 65 or more living at home, and noted a fall of 20 mm Hg or more in systolic pressure in 24%, of 30 mm Hg in 9% and of 40 mm Hg or more in 5%. The frequency of such a drop of pressure on standing increases with advancing age. No association with organic brain disease, heart disease, absent ankle jerks, varicose veins, anaemia, urinary infections, low serum sodium concentration or the taking of potentially hypotensive drugs was noted in those whose pressures fell on standing when compared with those whose pressures were unaffected (Fig. 3). Where two or more of these factors were present, however, there was a greater likelihood of a severe postural fall in pressure occurring. The elderly are more subject to disorders of the neurological mechanisms which normally control blood pressure on standing (JOHNSON et al.

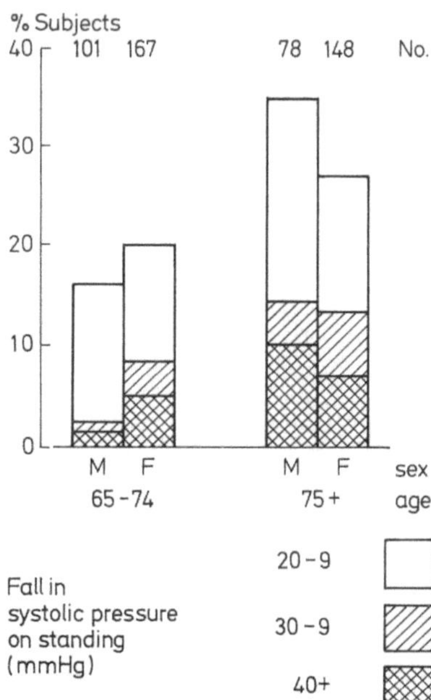

Fig. 3. Fall in systolic blood pressure in the elderly on standing. (CAIRD et al. 1973)

1965). Other factors which may be involved in causing postural hypotension in this age group include acute infections, reduction in blood volume or of cardiac output, varicose veins (RODSTEIN and ZEMAN 1957), hyponatraemia and a wide variety of commonly used drugs.

IV. Valvular Heart Disease

Pathological studies have increasingly emphasised the presence of valvular lesions in elderly patients. These reports have attempted to determine the site of the lesion, and where possible, the aetiology of the lesion. An incidence of 3.5% for valvular heart disease was found in the general elderly population, women being affected twice as frequently as men (KENNEDY et al., unpublished work).

1. Rheumatic Heart Disease

In an analysis of autopsies on over 1,200 patients whose ages ranged from 50 to 90 years, MEDALIA and WHITE (1952) found rheumatic heart disease in 5% of patients in the 6th decade, a similar incidence in the 7th, 3.5% in the 8th, and 2.5% in the 9th. HARGREAVES (1961), in a series of 2,086 autopsies on patients over 50 years of age, found mitral valve disease in 3.1% and McKEOWN (1965) and POMERANCE (1965) have suggested a figure of 4% for the post-mortem incidence of mitral stenosis.

In clinical practice, rheumatic heart disease was found in 4% of patients admitted to a geriatric unit in Oxford (BEDFORD and CAIRD 1960), and in 2.3% of the general elderly population. These authors comment that only about 40% of elderly patients with signs of rheumatic heart disease can recall an appropriate antecedent illness.

2. Aortic Valve Disease

Abnormality of the aortic valve is extremely common with old age. An aortic ejection systolic murmur is present in over two-thirds of patients aged 70 years or more (BRUNS and VAN DER HAWERT 1958) and this is frequently associated with calcific aortic stenosis. The high incidence of this condition has been confirmed by autopsy studies (POMERANCE 1972) and the prevalence in geriatric hospital patients is approximately 4% (BEDFORD and CAIRD 1960).

V. Pulmonary Heart Disease

Pulmonary heart disease varies in frequency according to the place of domicile of the population studied and their smoking habits. Currently, it occurs almost exclusively in men, with an incidence of 6%–7%. It is infrequent in older women, is very rarely seen over the age of 85 (KENNEDY et al., unpublished work) and in industrialised countries is associated with chronic obstructive airway disease. The incidence and sex preponderance may alter with the changing smoking habits of various populations.

Pulmonary embolism is common in old age. It has been found in 30% or more of routine autopsies in old people (TOWBIN 1954).

VI. Miscellaneous Forms of Heart Disease

Certain forms of cardiac disease show a changing age incidence, or are found almost exclusively in older patients.

1. Subacute Bacterial Endocarditis

The incidence of this condition, and the bacterial organisms involved, have been changing. In the immediate post-war years the highest incidence was in the 4th decade. Now, the peak incidence occurs in the 6th and 7th decades (SHINEBOURNE et al. 1969), and men are affected more than women. With this increase there has also been a rise in the number of sufferers who have no previously known heart disease. In these elderly patients the aortic valve is most often involved. Mortality is also higher in later years (Fig. 4) (LOWES et al. 1980).

2. Cardiac Amyloidosis

The finding of cardiac amyloidosis at post-mortem increases dramatically with age. POMERANCE (1976) reported that cardiac amyloid deposits were seen in 42% of over 300 geriatric autopsies. Series from other countries have shown a lower frequency of 2%–15% in their elderly population. Cardiac amyloidosis increases in the very old and is found more frequently in women than men.

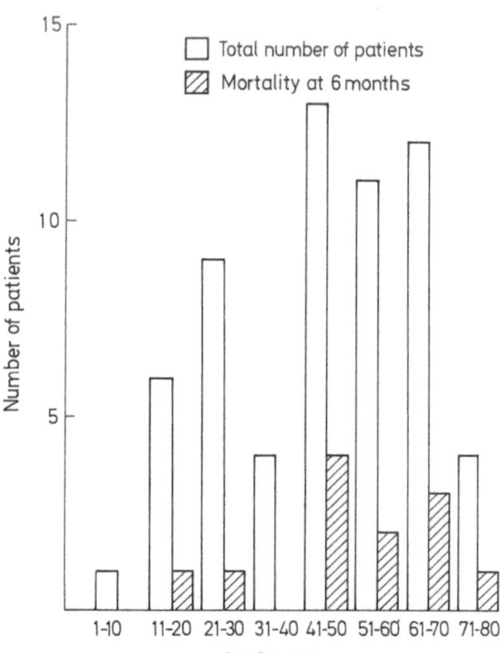

Fig. 4. Mortality in relation to age in patients with infective endocarditis

VII. Congestive Heart Failure

Mortality statistics reflect the basic underlying causes of death, rather than the symptom complex these initiate. Therefore, it is difficult to assess the true incidence of congestive heart failure although it is known to rise with age (KLAINER et al. 1965). It occurs more frequently in men than in women, and has a correspondingly higher mortality in men (MCKEE et al. 1971).

BEDFORD and CAIRD (1956) found that 14% of admissions to a geriatric unit had signs of congestive cardiac failure, although that condition was not necessarily the principal reason for admission. That appropriate management has much to offer the elderly is shown by their finding that only one-third of those admitted with congestive cardiac failure died from it, or with it present.

VIII. Electrocardiographic Abnormalities

The application of the Minnesota Code (BLACKBURN et al. 1960) to the electrocardiographic data from several series has allowed detailed comparison of the incidence of electrocardiographic abnormalities in the elderly. Earlier studies involved old people in hospital or residential institutions (WOSIKA et al. 1950; FISCH et al. 1957; TARAN and SZILAGYI 1958; MIHALICK and FISCH 1974), and demonstrated a high incidence of electrocardiographic abnormalities. Of more value are the findings from various community surveys which are summarised in Table 9 and are de-

Table 9. Percentage prevalence of electrocardiographic abnormalities in unselected old people

Sex	Men				Women			
Study No.[a]	1	2	3	4	1	2	3	4
Age	70+	62+	70+	65+	70+	62+	70+	65+
Number	127	214	213	872	162	268	190	1,382
Q/QS patterns	9.5	7.9	9.4	10.0	3.1	7.4	7.4	4.0
T wave changes	36.2	23.3	24.0	19.2	32.0	29.8	15.7	12.6
Left ventricular hypertrophy	8.7	3.7	12.6[b]	6.7[b]	12.9	14.5	10.5[b]	10.3[b]
Right ventricular hypertrophy	–	–	–	1.4	–	–	–	0.3
First degree heart block	10.2	3.7	5.2	1.5	7.4	3.0	4.7	0.6
Left bundle branch block	0	1.4	1.4	1.6	3.1	0	3.7	1.2
Right bundle branch block	4.7	2.3	3.3	2.7	1.9	2.2	2.1	1.2
Frequent ectopic beats (1 in 10)	11.8	–	4.2	4.0	3.1	–	2.6	2.5
Atrial fibrillation	3.1	2.3	5.2	2.1	4.3	2.6	3.2	2.4

[a] Study No. 1, OSTRANDER et al. (1965); 2, KITCHIN et al. (1973); CULLEN et al. (1974); 4, CAMPBELL et al. (1974)
[b] Includes Minnesota Codes 3.1 and 3.3; others include 3.1 only

rived from three continents (OSTRANDER et al. 1965; KITCHIN et al. 1973; CULLEN et al. 1974; CAMPBELL et al. 1974). Abnormal Q/QS patterns are found in approximately 10% of elderly men and 5% of similarly aged women. That there is reasonable correlation between these electrocardiographic abnormalities and a previous myocardial infarction has been demonstrated at autopsy by KURIHARA et al. (1967).

T wave changes, often of uncertain significance, show some variation in reported frequency. Patterns of left ventricular hypertrophy are common in men. The criteria for right ventricular hypertrophy are more difficult to define. Using those of GOODWIN and ABDIN (1959), KENNEDY and CAIRD (1972) found right ventricular hypertrophy in 2% of both men and women aged 65 and over in the community, while CAMPBELL and colleagues (1974) found it present in 1.4% of men and 0.3% of women.

The most common codable rhythm abnormality is frequent ectopic beats, though many more show only the occasional ectopic, a non-codable feature. Atrial fibrillation occurred in 3% of KENNEDY and CAIRD's subjects, and CAMPBELL and colleagues noted that it was more frequent over the age of 75 years, being present in 1.7% of subjects aged 65–74 and in 4.8% over 75 years. The incidence of atrial fibrillation in old people in hospital is much higher, being estimated at 10%–15% (WOSIKA et al. 1950).

First degree atrioventricular block is not uncommon, with an incidence of at least 2%–3% (KENNEDY and CAIRD 1972), but higher degrees of block are much less frequently encountered. SHAW and ERAUT (1970) have estimated the prevalence of second and third degree block together as 0.03% at 65–69, 0.04% at 70–74 and 0.11% over 75 years. Ventricular conduction defects are common. Left anterior hemiblock with or without right bundle branch block was found in 4% of men and 1% of women in the community studied by CAMPBELL and colleagues (1974) and is probably the most frequent conduction defect.

There is, therefore, electrocardiographic evidence of cardiac abnormality in many apparently fit elderly people. KENNEDY and CAIRD (1972) found that only 42% of their subjects had normal electrocardiograms, a fact confirmed by CAMPBELL et al. (1974), who demonstrated abnormal electrocardiograms in 40%–60% of elderly people living in the community.

Together with the clinical studies already mentioned, these findings stress the high prevalence of cardiac disease, known or unknown, in the elderly population.

References

Acheson RM, Acheson ED (1958) Coronary and other heart diseases in a group of Irish males aged 65–85. Br J Prev Soc Med 12:147
Akhtar AJ, Andrews GR, Caird FI, Fallon RJ (1972) Urinary tract infection in the elderly: A population study. Age Ageing 1:48–54
Akhtar AJ, Broe GA, Crombie A, McLean WMR, Andrews GR, Caird FI (1973) Disability and dependence in the elderly at home. Age Ageing 2:102–110
Anderson WF, Cowan NR (1959) The influence of adiposity and varicose veins on arterial pressure in older women. Clin Sci 18:103–135
Anderson WF, Cowan NR (1972) Arterial blood pressure in healthy old people. Geront Clin 14:129–136

Anderson WF, Caird FI, Kennedy RD, Schwartz D (in press 1981) Gerontology and geriatric nursing. Hodder and Stoughton, London

Aschoff L (1938) Zur normalen und pathologischen Anatomie des Greisenalters. Med Klin 34:635, 773

Bechgaard P (1946) Arterial hypertension: a follow up of 1,000 hypertonics. Acta Med Scand Suppl 172

Bedford PD, Caird FI (1956) Congestive heart failure in the elderly. QJ Med NS 25:407–426

Bedford PD, Caird FI (1960) Valvular disease of the heart in old age. J and A Churchill, London

Björck G (1962) Course and prognosis in some cardiac diseases. J Chronic Dis 15:9–28

Björck G, Sievers J, Blomqvist J (1958) Studies in myocardial infarction in Malmo (III). Acta Med Scand 162:81–97

Blackburn H, Keys A, Simonson E, Rautharju P, Punsar S (1960) The electrocardiogram in population studies – a classification system. Circulation 21:1160–1175

Bruns DL, van der Hawert LG (1958) The aortic systolic murmur developing with increasing age. Br Heart J 20:370–378

Caird FI, Dall JLC (1979) The cardiovascular system. In: Brocklehurst JC (ed) Textbook of geriatric medicine and gerontology. Churchill Livingstone, Edinburgh London, Chap 7, pp 125–157

Caird FI, Kennedy RD (1976) Epidemiology of heart disease in old age. In: Caird FI, Dall JLC, Kennedy RD (eds) Cardiology in old age. Plenum, New York London pp 1–10

Caird FI, Andrews GR, Kennedy RD (1973) Effect of posture on blood pressure in the elderly. Br Heart J 35:527–530

Campbell A, Caird FI, Jackson TFM (1974) Significance of abnormalities of electrocardiogram in old people. Br Heart J 36:1012–1018

Carlston LA, Bottiger LE (1972) Ischaemic heart disease in relation to fasting values of plasma triglycerides and cholesterol. Lancet 1:865–868

Colandrea MA, Friedman GD, Nichaman MZ, Lynd CN (1970) Systolic hypertension in the elderly: an epidemiological assessment. Circulation 41:239–245

Cullen KJ, Murphy BP, Cumpston GN (1974) Electrocardiograms in the Busselton population. Aust NZ J Med 4(4):325–330

Droller H, Pemberton J (1953) Cardiovascular disease in a random sample of elderly people. Br Heart J 15:199–204

Edmonson HA, Hoxie HJ (1942) Hypertension and cardiac rupture. Am Heart J 24:719

Fisch C, Genovese PD, Dyke RW, Laramore W, Marvel RJ (1957) The electrocardiogram in persons over seventy. Geriatrics 12:616–620

Goodwin JF, Abdin ZH (1959) The cardiogram of congenital and acquired right ventricular hypertrophy. Br Heart J 21:523–544

Groddeck H (1939) Sektionsbefunde bei Achtzigjährigen. Z Alternsforsch 1:238

Hamilton M, Pickering GW, Fraser-Roberts JA, Sowry GSG (1954) Aetiology of essential hypertension: role of inheritance. Clin Sci 13:273–304

Hargreaves T (1961) Rheumatic mitral valve disease in the elderly, incidence found at necropsy. Br Med J 2:342–345

Herrick JB (1912) Clinical features of sudden obstruction of the coronary arteries. JAMA 59:2015

Johnson RH, Smith AC, Spalding TMK, Wollner L (1965) Effect of posture on blood pressure in elderly patients. Lancet 1:731–733

Joint Working Party (1976) Prevention of coronary heart disease. J R Coll Physicians Lond 10:213–275

Kannel WB (1976) Blood pressure and cardiovascular disease in the aged. In: Caird FI, Dall JLC, Kennedy RD (eds) Cardiology in old age. Plenum, New York London, pp 143–175

Kannel WB, Castelli WP, McNamara PM, McKee PA, Feinleib M (1972) Role of blood pressure in the development of congestive cardiac failure. N Engl J Med 287:782–787

Kannel WB, Dawber TR, Sorlie P, Wolt PA (1976) Components of blood pressure and risk of athero-thrombotic brain infarction: the Framingham Study. Stroke 7:327–331

Kennedy RD (1974) Recent Advances in Cardiology. In: Anderson WF, Judge TG (eds) Geriatric Medicine. Academic Press London New York, p. 218

Kennedy RD, Caird FI (1972) Application of the Minnesota Code to population studies of the electrocardiogram in the elderly. Geront Clin 14:5–16

Kennedy RD, Andrews GR, Caird FI (1977) Ischaemic heart disease in the elderly. Br Heart J 39:1121–1127

Kincaid-Smith P, McMichael J, Murphy EA (1958) The clinical course and pathology of hypertension with papilloedema (Malignant hypertension). QJ Med NS 27:117–153

Kitchin AH, Lowther CP, Milne JS (1973) Prevalence of clinical and electrocardiographic evidence of ischaemic heart disease in the older population. Br Heart J 35:946–953

Klainer LM, Gibson TC, White KL (1965) The epidemiology of cardiac failure. J Chronic Dis 18:797–814

Kurihara H, Kuramota K, Teresawa F, Matsushita S, Seki M, Ikeda M (1967) Reliability of abnormal Q and QS patterns classified by the Minnesota Code for the diagnosis of myocardial infarction in old people. Jpn Heart J 8:514–521

Leyden E (1884/85) Über die Sclerose der Coronar-Arterien und die davon abhängigen Krankheitszustände. Z Klin Med 7:459, 539

Librach G, Schadel M, Seltzer M, Hart A, Tellis N (1976) Immediate and long-term prognosis of acute myocardial infarction in the aged. J Clin Dis 29:483–495

Lowes JA, Hamer J, Williams G, Houang E, Tabaqchali S, Shaw EJ, Hill IM, Rees GM (1980) Ten years of infective endocarditis at St. Bartholomew's Hospital: analysis of clinical features and treatment in relation to prognosis and mortality. Lancet 1:8160, 133–136

Martin A, Millard PH (1973) Cardiovascular assessment in the elderly. Age Ageing 2:211–217

Master AM, Lasser RP, Jaffe HL (1958) Blood pressure in white people over 65 years of age. Ann Intern Med 48:284–299

McKee PA, Castelli WP, McNamara PM, Kannel WB (1971) The natural history of congestive heart failure. The Framingham study. N Engl J Med 285:1441–1446

McKeown F (1965) Pathology of the aged. Butterworth, London, Chap I, pp 5, 44–45

Medalia LS, White PD (1952) Diseases of the aged: analysis of pathological observations in 1,251 autopsy protocols in old persons. JAMA 149:1433–1437

Miall WE, Chinn S (1974) Screening for hypertension: some epidemiological observations. Br Med J 3:595–600

Mihalick MJ, Fisch C (1974) Electrocardiographic findings in the aged. Am Heart J 87:117–127

Monroe RT (1951) Disease in old age. Harvard Univ Press, Cambridge Mass

Norris RM, Brandt PWT, Coughey DE, Lee AJ, Scott PJ (1969) A new coronary prognostic index. Lancet 2:690–694

Ostrander LO Jr, Brandt RC, Kjelsberg MO, Epstein FH (1965) Electrocardiographic findings among the adult population of a total natural community. Tecumseh, Michigan Circulation 31:888–898

Parkinson J, Bedford DE, Thomson WAR (1938) Cardiac aneurysm. Q J Med 7:455–478

Pomerance A (1965) Pathology of the heart with and without cardiac failure in the aged. Br Heart J 27:697–710

Pomerance A (1972) Pathogenesis of aortic stenosis and its relation to age. Br Heart J 34:569–574

Pomerance A (1976) Pathology of the myocardium and valves. In: Caird FI, Dall JLC, Kennedy RD (eds) Cardiology in old age. Plenum, New York London, p 17

Registrar General for Scotland (1978) Scottish health statistics. Her Majesty's Stationery Office, Edinburgh

Rodstein M, Zeman FD (1957) Postural blood pressure changes in the elderly. J Chronic Dis 6:581–588

Rolleston H (1922) Medical aspects of old age. McMillan, London

Scottish Health Statistics Edinburgh (1978) Her Majesty's Stationary Office

Shaw DB, Eraut D (1970) Prevalence and morbidity of heart block in Devon. Br Med J 1:144–147

Shekelle RB, Ostfeld AM, Klawans HL (1974) Hypertension and risk of stroke in an elderly
    population. Stroke 5:71–75
Shinebourne EA, Cripps CM, Hayward GW, Shooter RA (1969) Bacterial endocarditis
    1956–65: analysis of clinical features and treatment in relation to prognosis and mortal-
    ity. Br Heart J 31:536–542
Sievers J, Blonquist G, Björck G (1961) Studies in myocardial infarction in Malmo, 1935–54
    (VI). Acta Med Scand 169:95–103
Stocks P (1924) Blood pressure in early life: a statistical study. Draper's Co. Research Mem-
    oirs, No 11, Cambridge Univ. Press, London
Taran LM, Szilagyi H (1958) Electrocardiographic changes with advancing years. Geriatrics
    13:352–358
Towbin A (1954) Pulmonary embolism, incidence and significance. JAMA 156:209–215
Ten leading causes of death for selected countries in North America, Europe and Oceania.
    1969, 70, 71 – WHO 1974:27:No 9, p 563
Wosika PH, Feldman E, Chesrow EJ, Myers GJ (1950) Unipolar precordial and limb lead
    electrocardiograms in the aged. Geriatrics 5:131–141
Zeman FD, Rodstein M (1960) Cardiac rupture complicating myocardial infarction in the
    aged. Arch Int Med 105, 431

Conduction System

A. E..Tàmmaro

A. Introduction

In recent years improved means of research, especially in the electrophysiological field, have made possible thorough examination of the mechanisms underlying normal function and defects of intracardiac conduction. Thus, major pathogenetic and clinical aspects of conduction disorders have been clarified. However, as also emphasized recently (KULBERTUS and DEMOULIN 1977), the changes evoked by ageing in the conduction tissue have scarcely aroused physiologists' and pathologists' interest. Therefore only poor and fragmentary information exists on the anatomical and functional aspects of this system in elderly people.

B. Age-Related Anatomical Changes

In order to understand the pathogenesis of some dromotropic disorders, a knowledge of the normal anatomy of the conduction system is essential. For this purpose the structure and topography of the components of the conduction system will be briefly reviewed.

I. Sinus Node

The sinus node is situated in the conjunction point between the superior vena cava and the side edge of the right atrium. It has been shown (JAMES et al. 1966) that over 50% of the sinus node is composed of small pale scarcely striated cells, with well-colored nuclei, embedded in a network of elastic, collagenous, and reticular fibers.

These cells, named P or pacemaking cells, are supposed to act as a pacemaker. With advancing age a change in the relationships between the muscular and the connective components of the sinus node occurs. As early as 1954, LEV observed that starting from 40 years of age muscle cells tend to decrease in number while here is an increase in elastic and reticular and, to a lesser extent, in collagenous fibers as well as fatty infiltration inside the node and in the neighboring atrial area.

From a comparison between findings in people aged under 50 and over 75 years, DAVIES and POMERANCE (1972) observed that ageing is accompanied by a significant reduction in muscular tissue percentage, passing from 46% to 27% and by an increase in the fibrous component. These changes are thought by the authors to begin at about 60 years of age and then to become gradually more pronounced.

This study did not support the view that the fatty infiltration of the sinus node is a change peculiar to ageing (Balsaver et al. 1967). Sims (1972) observed a nonsignificant reduction in node cells as well as an increase in the fatty and elastic tissue.

A particularly marked sinuatrial node fibrosis after 75 years of age has been emphasized by Baldi et al. (1977) and a reduction in the number of muscular fibers has also been confirmed by other investigators (Lev 1968; Rossi 1969). Foci of hypertrophic muscle fibers were also found (Lev 1954), which were shown to be particularly evident at the periphery of the sinus node, with cells often presenting intermediate features between those of the specific tissue and those of the common atrial myocardium (Visioli and Botti 1956).

II. Internodal Myocardium

Electrophysiological studies have pointed to the presence of internodal junction pathways in the atrial myocardium. However, the morphological evidence of this is still under some debate (Osawa 1959; Janse and Anderson 1974).

A histological study of the interatrial septum and the atrial myocardium covering the areas crossed by the internodal tracts has demonstrated that in elderly subjects there is a significant increase in the fibrous component from 16.7% to 36%. The reduction in muscular fibers was shown to be moderate and appreciably less marked than that found in the sinuatrial node (Davies and Pomerance 1972). The fatty infiltration reported by Prior (1964) was not confirmed.

III. Atrioventricular Node

The atrioventricular (AV) node is situated beneath the endocardium of the right atrium, anterior to the opening of the coronary sinus, behind the posterior contour of the membranous interventricular septum, and above the insertion of the septal leaflet of the tricuspid valve (Titus 1973; Anderson et al. 1975). The latter authors believed the AV node to consist of a compact deep and a transitional superficial portion. Furthermore, on the basis of embryogenetic considerations other investigators (Kulbertus and Demoulin 1977) regard the node as consisting of three kinds of cells: small pale cells at the surface, small star-shaped cells with multiple anastomoses in the intermediary area, and larger cells arranged longitudinally at depth, parallel with each other and directed toward the bundle of His.

Erickson and Lev (1952) found that with ageing a considerable increase in collagenous and elastic fibers as well as a marked fatty infiltration occurs. The fibroadipose infiltration of the AV node and His system in elderly subjects was shown to be variable enough to persuade Rossi (1960) to regard it as not necessarily attributable to ageing. In the specific myocardium there was no lipofuscin storage even in the hearts where the common myocardium showed a marked pigment infiltration. Reticular fibers show no changes if the collagenous component does not prevail over the muscular one. Otherwise an increase is observed (Rossi 1960).

More recent investigations (Anderson et al. 1975) have demonstrated that there is progressive fibrosis in the deepest nodal portion as well as fat infiltration at the level of the transitional superficial zone which results in attenuation of the junctions between transitional cells and deep zone.

IV. His's Bundle and Branches

In agreement with ROSENBAUM et al. (1970) His's bundle may be regarded as composed of two segments, i.e., the penetrating and the branching portion. The former starts from the distal end of the AV node and penetrates the central fibrous body in close proximity to the mitral and tricuspid valve rings and the atrial portion of the membranous septum.

These anatomical relationships are of particular importance in geriatrics as they account for the genesis of AV blocks due to sclerocalcific alterations of these structures with consequent infiltration, disruption, and/or compression of the bundle of His. His's bundle emerges then from the central fibrous body at the level of the posterior third of the aortic noncoronary leaflet. At this point the most posterior left bundle branch fibers arise. The branching portion extends to the line which separates the noncoronary from the coronary aortic cusp, where the right bundle branch and the anterior fascicle of the left bundle branch originate.

The branching portion is in close relationship with the lower part of the membranous interventricular septum and the aortic valve ring. It is because of these anatomical relationships that the branching portion is the most vulnerable part in the conduction system. The sclerocalcific alterations of these structures, which are particularly frequent and marked in elderly people, underlie the conduction disorders localized in the right bundle branch and in the anterior fascicle of the left bundle branch.

According to ROSENBAUM et al. (1970) the conduction system has a trifascicular structure, consisting of the right bundle branch and of both (anterosuperior and posteroinferior) fascicles of the left bundle branch. According to more recent data there is also a third conduction fibers system lying in the middle portion of the septum, characterized by considerable individual variability (HECHT et al. 1973; DE-MOULIN and KULBERTUS 1972, 1973).

Collagenous and elastic fibers have been found to increase with ageing. A marked lipid infiltration has also been observed, which was found to be mainly localized at the proximal level (ERICKSON and LEV 1952). In the proximal portion of the left fascicles a constant loss of fibers was noted, which sometimes may even be over 50%. Distal portions, and in particular the left distal portions, may also show this process, albeit to a lesser extent (DEMOULIN and KULBERTUS 1972; DAVIES 1976).

As regards Purkinjes' network, investigations carried out on cattle have demonstrated that these cells increase gradually in volume with ageing. The long myofibrils continue to increase in number and in very advanced age invade the central sarcoplasma, which appears markedly hydrated. When myofibrils are very numerous the limits between the cells tend to disappear and cells join to form long streaks (BERTOLINI et al. 1962).

C. Age-Related Functional Changes

A survey of the cardiologic and geriatric literature gives but few indications on the functional changes provoked by ageing in the conduction system.

It has been shown that ageing results in a significant reduction in the spontaneous contraction frequency in rat atrial tissue (CAVOTO et al. 1974). It has been demonstrated in dogs and man that the positive chronotropic response to isoproterenol decreases significantly with advancing age (YIN et al. 1976). These authors think that this fact is due to the reduced number of atrial chronotropic beta-receptors.

By recording the transmembrane action potential, CAVOTO et al. (1974) found that a reduction in upstroke velocity, an increase in plateau duration, and a rise in the time required to reach 95% repolarization occur with increasing age. These changes were found to be statistically significant and independent of heart rate. The amplitude of the action potential and the resting potential level were unaltered. As the reduced upstroke velocity of the action potential is accompanied by depressed conductivity, a similar change at the level of the AV node and the His–Purkinje system could underlie an increase in the P-R interval as observed in the ECG tracing of many elderly subjects (MORPURGO 1961; CARDUS and SPENCER 1967; HARRIS 1976).

A prolonged repolarization gives no evidence of possible changes in refractoriness, which is thought by HARRIS (1976) to undergo no alterations with ageing.

The sinus node recovery time is a parameter generally used for studying the sinus node function. A mean recovery time of 1,100 ms was calculated from a group of subjects aged between 50 and 72 years (KULBERTUS et al. 1975). In older subjects (69–88 years) a mean value of 1,363 ms was obtained (OKIMOTO et al. 1976) while the mean value obtained by BREITHARDT et al. (1978 a) on young subjects was 1,026 ms and those recorded by other investigators did not differ substantially.

The value of the sinus node recovery time cannot therefore be regarded as essentially modified in advanced age. This is in agreement with the observations of BREITHARDT et al. (1978 a, b), who found a rising tendency in elderly subjects only in the presence of evident sinus node disfunction.

The study of sinoatrial conduction time on elderly subjects without signs of sinusal dysfunction has highlighted no substantial differences compared with values regarded as normal (UEDA et al. 1977), this being 97.5 ms in elderly subjects against 82 and 110 ms in young and adult persons (SEIPEL and BREITHARDT 1975; SCHEINMAN et al. 1973).

In my knowledge and in agreement with CAIRD's views (1976), the practical value of His-bundle electrography in geriatrics has not yet been clearly established. Also ROSEN et al. (1978) pointed to the paucity of studies on the electrophysiological alterations induced by ageing on myocardial cells. By studying the action potential of Purkinje cells in dogs of various ages these authors have demonstrated that in more advanced age classes there is a significant reduction in maximum upstroke velocity and in the action potential amplitude without changes in the duration of the action potential, as well as a slowing of repolarization. These changes, which could be due to alteration in calcium ion uptake inside the cell, need to be further investigated especially in order to discover any possible pathophysiological implications.

D. Age-Related Changes in the Blood Supply

The sinuatrial node is supplied by an artery which runs along its longitudinal axis and gives rise to numerous branches. The sinus node artery derives from the initial portion of the right coronary artery in about 60% and from the left circumflex artery in about 35% of subjects. In about 5% of cases, branches deriving from both these arteries join to develop an arterial ring around the node. VISIOLI and BOTTI (1956) observed that the sinus node artery appeared to be surprisingly intact from an anatomical point of view in elderly people, even in subjects with marked arteriosclerotic involvement of the main coronary branches. By comparing sinus node arteries in subjects under 50 and over 75 years old, DAVIES and POMERANCE (1972) found a reduced thickness of the intima and the media as well as an increase in the caliber of arterial lumen.

The AV node is supplied by the ramus septi fibrosi, starting from the posterior descending artery in about 90% of cases and from the left circumflex artery in remaining subjects. The His bundle and the proximal portion of the right bundle branch are usually supplied by the AV node artery and by the first septal branch of the anterior descending artery, while the distal portion of the right bundle branch is supplied by the anterior septal arteries (FRINK and JAMES 1973). The anterior and middle-septal fibers of the left branch are supplied by the anteroseptal branches of the left anterior descending artery; the posterior fascicle is supplied by the AV node artery and by perforating septal branches deriving from both the anterior and posterior coronary area (FRINK and JAMES 1973; KULBERTUS and DEMOULIN 1977).

With ageing, hyalinization and fibrosis of the media has been found to occur, with a slight caliber reduction of the first millimeters in the AV node artery. Beyond this site the artery appears either intact or only negligibly compromised and the blood supply is constant and abundant (KENNEL et al. 1973). This pattern does not vary considerably even in the presence of marked coronary arteriosclerosis.

In conclusion, ageing is not associated with an important reduction in the blood supply to the conduction system.

References

Anderson RH, Becker AE, Brechenmacher C, Davies MJ, Rossi L (1975) The human atrioventricular junctional area. Eur J Cardiol 3:11–25

Baldi N, Fonda F, Morgera T, Silvestri F, Camerini F (1977) La sindrome del seno malato. In: Furlanello F, Disertori M, Lanzetta T (eds) Le nuove frontiere delle aritmie. Piccin, Padova, p 304

Balsaver AM, Morales AR, Whitehouse FW (1967) Fat infiltration of myocardium as a cause of cardiac conduction defect. Am J Cardiol 19:261–265

Bertolini AM, Massari N, Quarto di Palo F (1962) Gerontologia. Aspetti metabolici. C.E.A., Milano, p 731

Breithardt G, Seipel L, Gramsch H, Wiebringhaus E, Lenner Ch (1978a) Die klinische Bedeutung der Sinusknotenerholungszeit. Z Kardiol 67:443–451

Breithardt G, Seipel L, Hildebrandt U, Lenner Ch, Wiebringhaus E (1978b) Methodische Aspekte bei der Bestimmung der Sinusknotenerholungszeit beim Menschen. Z Kardiol 67:395–404

Caird FI (1976) Clinical examination and investigation of the heart. In: Caird FI, Dall JLC, Kennedy RD (eds) Cardiology in old age. Plenum Press, London New York, p 136

Cardus D, Spencer WA (1967) Recovery time of heart frequency in healthy men: its relation to age and physical condition. Arch Phys Med Rehabil 48:71–77

Cavoto FV, Kelliher GJ, Roberts J (1974) Electrophysiological changes in rat atrium with age. Am J Physiol 226:1293–1297

Davies MJ (1976) Pathology of the conduction system. In: Caird FI, Dall JLC, Kennedy RD (eds) Cardiology in old age. Plenum Press, New York London, p 65

Davies MJ, Pomerance A (1972) Quantitative study of ageing changes in the human sinoatrial node and internodal tracts. Brit Heart J 34:150–152

Demoulin JC, Kulbertus HE (1972) Histopathological examination of left hemiblock. Brit Heart J 34:807–814

Demoulin JC, Kulbertus HE (1973) Left hemiblocks revisited from the histopathological viewpoint. Am Heart J 86:712–713

Erickson EE, Lev M (1952) Aging changes in the human atrioventricular node, bundle, and bundle branches. J Gerontol 7:1–12

Frink RJ, James TN (1973) Normal blood supply to the human His-bundle and proximal bundle branches. Circulation 47:8–18

Harris R (1976) Cardiac arrhythmias in the aged. In: Caird FI, Dall JLC, Kennedy RD (eds) Cardiology in old age. Plenum Press, London New York, p 317

Hecht HH, Kossmann CE, Childers RW, Langendorf R, Lev M, Rosen KM, Pruitt R, Truex RC, Uhley HN, Watt TB Jr (1973) Atrioventricular and intraventricular conduction. Revised nomenclature and concepts. Am J Cardiol 31:232–244

James TN, Sherf L, Fine G, Morales AR (1966) Comparative ultrastructure of the sinus node in man and dog. Circulation 34:139–163

Janse MJ, Anderson RH (1974) Specialized internodal atrial pathways. Fact or fiction? Eur J Cardiol 2:117–136

Kennel AJ, Titus JL, McCallister BD, Pruitt RD (1973) The vasculature of the atrioventricular conduction system in heart block. Am Heart J 85:593–600

Kulbertus HE, Demoulin JC (1977) Il sistema di conduzione: aspetti anatomici e patologici. In: Krikler DM, Goodwin JF (eds) Aritmie cardiache. Verduci, Roma, p 22

Kulbertus HE, De Levalrutten F, Mary L, Casters P (1975) Sinus node recovery time in the elderly. Br Heart J 37:420–425

Lev M (1954) Aging changes in the human sinoatrial node. J Gerontol 9:1–9

Lev M (1968) The conduction system. In: Gould SE (ed) Pathology of the heart and blood vessels, 3rd ed. Thomas, Springfield, p 182

Morpurgo M (1961) Il cuore senile. Minerva Medica, Torino, p 126

Okimoto T, Ueda K, Kamata C, Yoshida H, Ohkawa S, Hiraoka K, Kuwajima I, Sugiura M, Murakami M, Matsuo H (1976) Sinus node recovery time and abnormal post pacing phase in the aged patients with sick sinus syndrome. Jpn Heart J 17:290–301

Osawa M (1959) Histological study of the cardiac conducting system in the atrial portion of the dog's heart (II) (Japanese). Jpn Circ J 23:718–725

Prior JT (1964) Lipomatous hypertrophy of cardiac interatrial septum. Arch Pathol 78:11–15

Rosen MR, Reder RF, Hordorf AJ, Davies M, Danilo P Jr (1978)Age-related changes in Purkinje fiber action potential of adult dogs. Circ Res 43:931–938

Rosenbaum MB, Elizari MV, Lazzari JO (1970) The hemiblocks. Tampa Tracings, Oldsmar, pp 18–39

Rossi L (1960) La senescenza del sistema di conduzione atrioventricolare. Biol Latina 13:71–91

Rossi L (1969) Histopathological features of cardiac arrhythmias. C.E.A., Milano, p 126

Scheinman MM, Kunkel FW, Peters RW, Schoenfeld PL, Abbott JA (1973) Sinoatrial function and atrial refractoriness (abstr). Circulation 48 (suppl IV):215

Seipel L, Breithardt G (1975) Sinusknotenautomatie und sinuatriale Leitung. Z Kardiol 64:1014–1022

Sims BA (1972) Pathogenesis of atrial arrhythmias. Br Heart J 34:336–340

Titus JL (1973) Anatomy of the conduction system. Circulation 47:170–177

Ueda K, Kamata C, Matsuo H, Ohkawa S, Okimoto T, Sugiura M (1977) A study on sinoatrial conduction in the aged. Jpn Heart J 18:143–153

Visioli O, Botti G (1956) La morfologia del nodo senoatriale dell'uomo in rapporto all'età. G Clin Med 37:1478–1504

Yin FC, Spurgeon HA, Raizes GS, Leon Greene H, Weisfeldt ML, Shock NW (1976) Age associated decrease in chronotropic response to isoproterenol (abstr). Circulation 54 (suppl II):167

Cardiac Output

T. STRANDELL

A. Resting Conditions

Determinations of cardiac output at rest with the direct Fick principle, i.e., measurements of oxygen uptake and oxygen difference between arterial and mixed venous blood, were first made by COURNAND et al. (1945). After catheterization of the right auricle or ventricle, these workers measured the cardiac output in 17 normal males, 21–58 years old, and found a definite decrease with rising age.

The dye dilution technique was applied by BRANDFONBRENER et al. (1955), in a larger cross-sectional study. They used bolus injections of Evans blue dye through a short catheter in an antecubital vein and rapid sampling from a brachial artery. Their material consisted of 67 ambulatory male patients, 19–86 years old, all with normal electrocardiograms and none with signs or symptoms of cardiovascular disease. Some were convalescing from respiratory infections or awaiting discharge after admission for orthopedic conditions. A linear decrease in cardiac output and cardiac index with age, averaging 1.0% and 8.0% per year, respectively, was found at rest in the supine position (Fig. 1).

These findings by BRANDFONBRENER et al. were reinforced when GRANATH et al. (1961, 1964) studied 17 healthy male volunteers, 61–83 years old, with pulmonary artery catheterization and measurements of cardiac output according to the direct Fick principle. These values were compared with data similarly obtained from 25 young men (mean age 23 years) previously studied in the same laboratory by BEVEGÅRD et al. (1960) and HOLMGREN et al. (1960). The 17 elderly men (mean age 71 years) were invited from a previous health survey of the city of Stockholm, from the Labour Exchange, from old age homes, and from gymnastic groups for the aged, and were probably more physically fit than the average healthy subject of the same age. Their average cardiac output at rest in a recumbent position was 5.8 liters/min, which was 1.8 liters/min or about 25%, lower than the corresponding value in the 23-year-old males.

By the same technique slightly lower cardiac outputs were observed in 55 male patients, 60–86 years old, studied before prostatectomy (RENCK 1969). Not all these patients had normal hearts, however; some had heart or lung diseases, or both.

Other studies by the direct Fick, or dye dilution techniques – by FOSTER et al. (1964) on 16 normal males 16–51 years old, by MALMBORG (1965) on 11 males 39–55 years old, by JULIUS et al. (1967) on 54 sedentary males and females 18–68 years old, and by HANSSON et al. (1968) on 75 normal males 20–49 years old – have failed

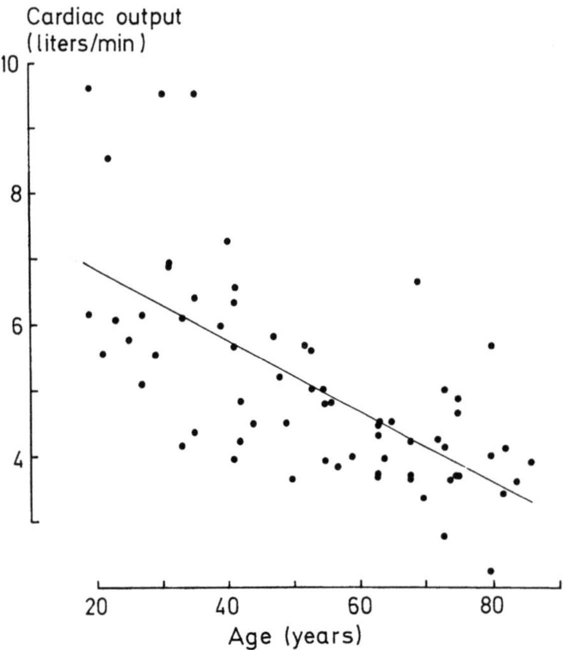

Fig. 1. Cardiac output at rest in supine position in relation to age in 67 "basal" males without circulatory disorder. BRANDFONBRENER et al. (1955)

to show any significant effect of age on resting cardiac output in the supine position.

The reason for this finding may be at least partly that the age ranges studied were too narrow. It is evident from Fig. 1 that the inter-individual variation in cardiac output is large, and that age accounts for only a minor part of this variation. Therefore, unless the number of subjects studied and their age ranges are large, this decrease with age will not be shown. Another possibility is that the decrease in cardiac output with age is not linear, as Fig. 1 would suggest, but that the most marked changes occur after, for example, 50 years of age.

There is no reason to believe that the decrease in cardiac output with age is different in women that in men, but sufficient data for proof are not available.

In the sitting position at rest no significant difference in cardiac output was observed between old and young men (GRANATH et al. 1961, 1964; JULIUS et al. 1967), and no age change was recorded in the standing position (HANSSON et al. 1968). This lack of differences with age is explained by the less marked decrease in cardiac output of elderly compared to young subjects when changing from the supine to the upright position, the decrease being 0.5 liters/min and 2.0 liters/min, respectively (GRANATH et al. 1961, 1964; BEVEGÅRD et al. 1960).

B. Physical Exercise

In the supine position, the increase in cardiac output with increasing work load and oxygen uptake has been found to be the same in old and young (Figs. 2 and 3). At a given oxygen uptake, the cardiac output was thus lower in the old men, both at

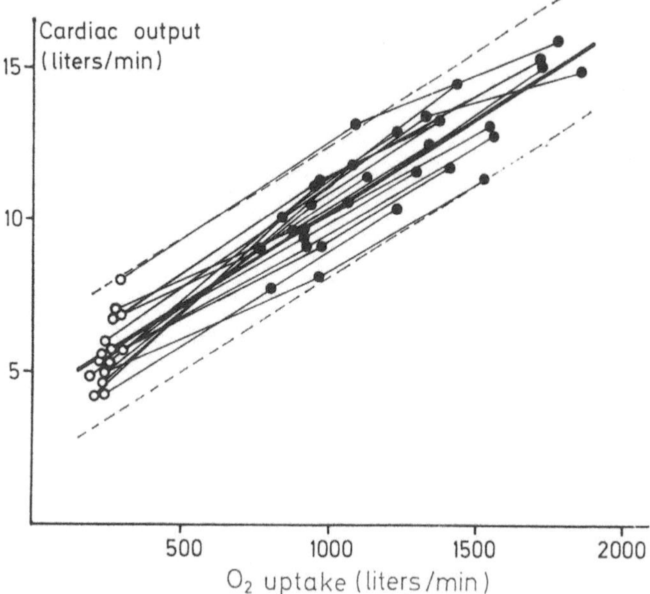

Fig. 2. Cardiac output at rest *(open circles)* and during exercise *(solid circles)* in supine position in relation to oxygen uptake in 16 men, 61–83 years old. GRANATH et al. (1964)

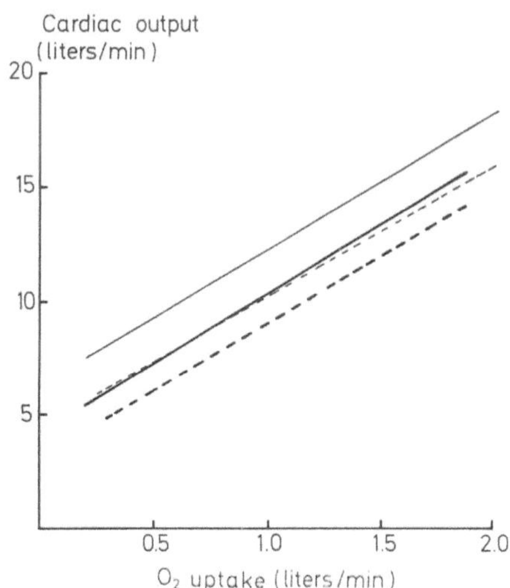

Fig. 3. Regression lines for cardiac output on oxygen uptake in 16 old men (mean age 71 years, heavy lines) and 25 young men (mean age 23 years, light lines) in supine *(solid lines)* and sitting *(dashed lines)* position. GRANATH et al. (1964), BEVEGÅRD et al. (1960), and HOLMGREN et al. (1960)

rest and during exercise, the average difference being 2.0 liters/min. With narrower age spans, no significant age differences in cardiac output during supine exercise were observed (FOSTER et al. 1964; MALMBORG 1965).

In the sitting position, the increase in cardiac output with increasing work load and oxygen uptake was also found to be the same in old and young (Fig. 3). At all levels of oxygen uptake the cardiac output, like that in the supine position, was lower in the old men, the average difference during exercise being 1.3 liters/min. Because the old men had lower maximal oxygen uptakes than the young men, the calculated maximal cardiac output with exercise was also lower in old age.

Less regular or insignificant effects of age have also been reported (HANSSON et al. 1968; JULIUS et al. 1967; HARTLEY et al. 1969). With the nitrous oxide method, higher cardiac outputs were observed with exercise in the elderly men and women studied (BECKLAKE et al. 1965); in view of the data derived from more direct methods previously mentioned, methodological errors or differences in material may be assumed to explain these findings.

From cross-sectional studies there is thus evidence that cardiac output in elderly men is lower than in young men, both at rest in the supine position and during exercise in both the sitting and supine positions.

C. Causes of Reduced Cardiac Output in Old Age

The exact mechanisms that lead to the decrease in cardiac output with age are not yet completely understood. In some way, however, this decrease is related to the structural changes that occur with advancing age. These changes include increase in thickness and rigidity of the walls of the larger arteries and veins due to an increased collagen-elastin ratio, cross-linking, degenerative, and sclerotic lesions in the endocardium, and increase of the elastic tissue in the myocardium (see BOURNE 1961). There is also a progressive increase of coronary artery sclerosis with age (LOBER 1953). These structural changes will not be discussed in detail, but it should be noted that it is impossible to distinguish clearly between degenerative changes and "normal" physiological alterations with age. Naturally, the reduced vascular distensibility affects the reflex mechanisms that regulate cardiovascular function by means of stretch receptors, but the influence of age on these functions is not yet sufficiently studied.

With increasing age, there is a decrease in lean body mass (SHOCK et al. 1953), with a reduction of the muscle mass and the number of cells in the parenchymatous organs. This change is reflected in a progressive decrease in basal metabolic rate with age, which reduces the need for circulatory transport of oxygen. This decrease, however, does not seem to account for more than about half the decrease in cardiac output with age, as judged by the estimates of LANDOWNE et al. (1955) and the observations by GRANATH et al. (1961, 1964).

I. Heart Rate

The hypokinetic circulation in elderly subjects with low values for cardiac output both at rest and during exercise could be due to reduction in heart rate or stroke volume, or in both. No significant changes with age, however, have been observed in heart rate at rest or during submaximal work loads, either in cross-sectional studies of subjects with similar degrees of physical activity (ROBINSON 1938; Åstrand 1960; König et al. 1961; HOLLMAN 1963; STRANDELL 1964a) or in longitudinal studies (DILL and CONSOLAZIO 1962).

Fig. 4. Maximal heart rate during upright exercise in relation to age in 81 normal nonathletic males. ROBINSON (1938)

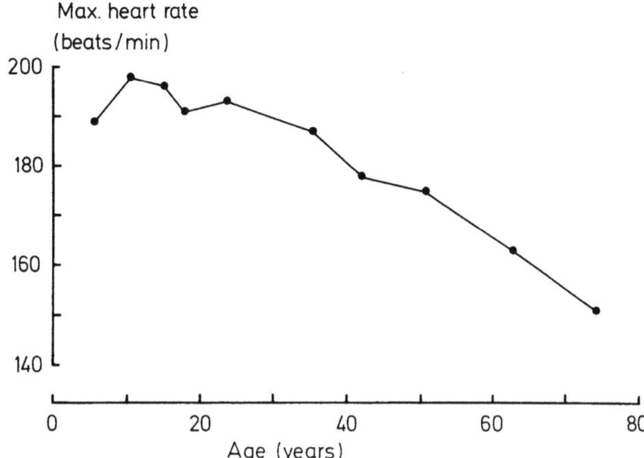

The maximal heart rate during exercise (Fig. 4) on the other hand, has always been found to decrease with age (ROBINSON 1938; Åstrand 1960; König et al. 1961; HOLLMAN 1963; STRANDELL 1964 b). In all these studies, the variability of the maximal heart rate was the same within the various age groups. Within a certain age group the level of the maximal heart rate was closely related to the level of heart rate at rest and during submaximal work (STRANDELL 1964 b); i.e., subjects who have low heart rates at rest and during exercise also have low maximal heart rates.

The reason for this inability to reach high heart rates during exercise in old age is not clear. It cannot be due to inability of the heart to beat fast, however, because heart rates far above the maximal can be recorded during exercise in some apparently healthy old subjects during short bursts of paroxysmal supraventricular tachycardia during and after exercise (STRANDELL 1963).

It has long been known that the heart in old subjects reacts with a smaller rate increase on standing than in younger subjects (NORRIS et al. 1953). This finding, however, does not necessarily mean a changed sensitivity of the heart to sympathetic stimulation. A decline with age of the sympathetic drive to the heart during exercise has been suggested, however, by CONWAY et al. (1971), who observed a smaller effect of propranolol on heart rate and cardiac output during exercise in older than in younger subjects. This age difference needs further study, however, because it seemed to be present only at the highest work loads and only in the male group.

II. Stroke Volume

The decrease in cardiac output with age at rest and during submaximal exercise is thus entirely due to a reduction of stroke volume (BRANDFONBRENER et al. 1955; GRANATH et al. 1961, 1964). On the other hand, the decrease in the maximal cardiac output with age is more marked, and also due to the decrease in maximal heart rate during exercise. The smaller increase in stroke volume in old compared to young men on changing from rest in the sitting position to rest in the supine position or to exercise is evident from Fig. 5.

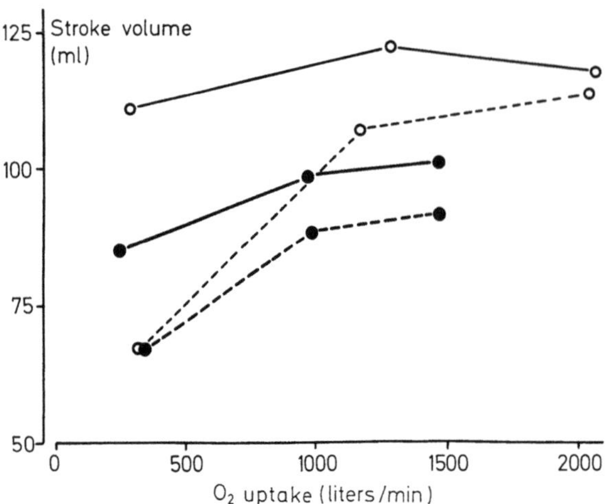

Fig. 5. Mean stroke volumes in relation to oxygen uptake at rest and during exercise in old *(solid circles)* and young men *(open circles)* in supine *(solid lines)* and sitting *(dashed lines)* position. GRANATH et al. (1964), BEVEGÅRD et al. (1960), and HOLMGREN et al. (1960)

The magnitude of the stroke volume is influenced both by factors related to diastolic filling and initial fiber length, such as filling pressures and ventricular distensibility, and by factors related to systolic ejection, such as arterial pressures and myocardial contractility.

The systolic pressure load of the left ventricle, the systolic arterial pressure, is the best studied of these variables. Due to the increase in the rigidity of the walls of the aorta and the larger arteries with age the function of these vessels as a compression chamber is reduced, and the arterial pulse pressure increases with age, as does the resistance of the systemic circulation (MASTER et al. 1950; LANDOWNE et al. 1955). The rise during exercise in systolic and mean arterial pressure has been found to be greater in old than in young subjects (ABBOUD and HUSTON 1961; KÖNIG et al. 1962; GRANATH et al. 1961, 1964). The higher systolic pressure load of the left ventricle in old compared to young subjects is therefore still more marked during exercise than at rest.

The distensibility of the pulmonary artery also decreases with increasing age (HARRIS et al. 1965). The pulse pressure at rest is accordingly increased with age; this increase, however, is due not to an increase in the pulmonary artery systolic pressure, but to a slight decrease in the diastolic pressure (GRANATH et al. 1961, 1964; GLOGER 1972). During exercise in both the supine and sitting positions, the systolic and mean pressures in the pulmonary artery increased about 10 mm Hg more in old than in young subjects (Table 1), indicating an increased flow resistance in the pulmonary vascular bed (GRANATH et al. 1961, 1964; EMIRGIL et al. 1967; GLOGER 1972).

In old age, there is thus evidence, both at rest and still more during exercise, of increased impedance to systolic ejection by both the left and the right ventricle, which could contribute to a decrease in stroke volume or an increase in filling pressure.

The filling pressures at rest of both the left and the right ventricle, as judged by the pulmonary capillary venous pressure and the right ventricle end-diastolic pressure, were found to be the same in old and young subjects (GRANATH et al. 1961, 1964). During exercise, however, these pressures increased significantly more in the

Table 1. Pressures (mm Hg) at rest and during supine bicycle exercise in 17 healthy elderly men compared to similar data in 25 young men

Group	Oxygen uptake (liters/min)	Heart rate (beats/min)	Pulmonary capillary venous	Pulmonary artery			Right ventricle		
				Systolic	Diastolic	Mean	Systolic	End diastolic	Initial diastolic
Old men[a]									
Rest	0.26	67	9.9	24.3	10.1	15.9	25.8	8.1	3.1
Work I	0.96	104	22.0	45.3	19.9	31.6	48.1	13.5	4.3
Work II	1.46	130	22.1	45.7	21.3	32.4	51.4	13.1	2.9
Young men[b]									
Rest	0.29	70	12.5	23.3	12.3	17.2	27.6	9.3	3.1
Work I	0.96	97	15.4	33.3	16.9	24.5	37.6	9.3	3.7
Work II	2.06	157	15.6	35.3	15.1	23.5	46.6	6.2	−2.4

[a] Mean age, 70.5 years (GRANATH et al. 1964)
[b] Mean age, 23.3 years (BEVEGÅRD et al. 1960; HOLMGREN et al. 1960)

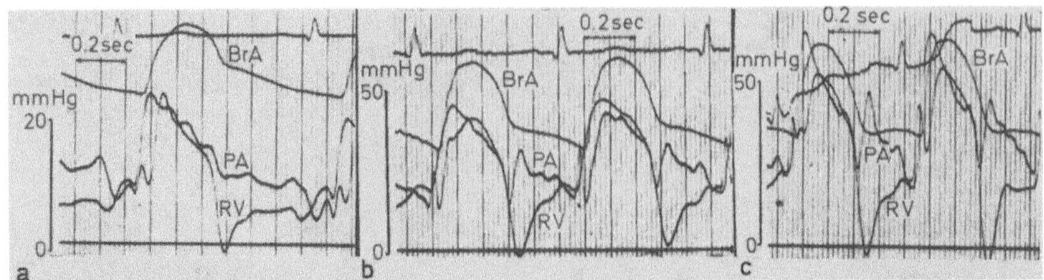

Fig. 6 a–c. Marked early-diastolic dip in pressure tracing from the right ventricle *(RV)*, during supine exercise in a 75-year-old healthy man. **a** At rest, heart rate 81 beats/min, stroke volume 71 ml. **b** At 300 kpm/min, heart rate 104 beats/min, stroke volume 88 ml. **c** At 600 kpm/min, heart rate 125 beats/min, stroke volume 103 ml. GRANATH et al. (1964)

60–83 year old males than in the young ones, with average values about 7 mm Hg higher in the group of old men (Table 1).

With a normal distensibility of the ventricular walls, these increased filling pressures during exercise in old age would cause a substantial increase in myocardial fiber length and stroke volume. There was evidence of reduced heart wall compliance, however, since in some cases the right ventricular pressure tracings during exercise showed very marked early diastolic dips (Fig. 6), as have been described in conditions with increased rigidity of the heart wall, such as constrictive pericarditis and endocardial or myocardial fibrosis.

The high filling pressures observed during exercise may therefore be related to increased rigidity of the heart wall in old age, rather than to myocardial insufficiency requiring an increased length and tension of the myocardial fibers (STRANDELL 1964c).

The increased incidence of myocardial fibrosis in old age might contribute to this heart wall rigidity. Thus, the old men with the highest filling pressures during exercise were those with the most marked left axis deviation in the frontal plane ECG (GRANATH and STRANDELL 1964) and signs of left anterior fascicular block, which is most often related to myocardial fibrosis (GRANT 1956). Another possibility might be the greater rigidity of the intercellular collagenous connective tissue that has been observed in old compared to young hearts (KOHN and ROLLERSON 1959). A stiffer heart wall would increase the internal friction during contraction, which would affect unfavorably the relationship between useful and total ventricular work.

The high filling pressures during exercise observed in old age thus seem to be an adjustment to a reduced distensibility of the heart wall, which probably also increases the internal frictional losses, and to an increased impedance to ejection (STRANDELL 1964c, 1976). The decrease in stroke volume with age may be related both to the changes mentioned above and to a decrease in the myocardial contractility. This last factor is difficult to measure exactly, but can be evaluated indirectly.

It can be argued that the finding of a hypokinetic circulation with low cardiac output and stroke volume in old age combined with high filling pressures during exercise indicates myocardial insufficiency. Many facts, however, contradict such a view. Within the group of healthy elderly men studied by cardiac catheterization thus far, there was no relationship between high filling pressures and large heart volumes or the degree of S–T depression in the exercise ECG (STRANDELL 1964c). Nor were the lowest values of stroke work observed in the subjects with the largest hearts and the most marked electrocardiographic abnormalities, as is the case in patients with arterial hypertension (VARNAUSKAS 1955). On the contrary, the healthy old men with the highest pulmonary capillary venous pressure during exercise had the most marked simultaneous increases in cardiac output in relation to oxygen uptake (GRANATH and STRANDELL 1964). They also had the most marked increases of stroke volume on exercise and the most marked simultaneous increases in pulse pressure in both the brachial and pulmonary arteries.

The high filling pressures during exercise in old compared to young men were thus related to a higher stroke work. In addition, those who were physically most active had the highest filling pressures during exercise.

These healthy elderly men were thus quite different from those patients with myocardial insufficiency due to previous infarction or angina pectoris studied with heart catheterization by MALMBORG (1965). His patients with the highest pulmonary capillary venous pressures during exercise had the lowest cardiac outputs, the smallest increases of cardiac output with increasing oxygen uptake, and the lowest exercise tolerance. Thus, high filling pressures seem to be a prerequisite for an effective response of the central circulation during exercise in physically fit healthy elderly men; in coronary artery disease and myocardial insufficiency, on the other hand, high filling pressures were a compensatory mechanism in the most disabled patients, who had poor responses of the central circulation to exercise.

Within the group of elderly men studied, there were also significant relationships between the filling pressures of the heart and pulmonary ventilation; the lowest pressures during exercise were observed in the subjects in whom the highest values for airway resistance could be expected (GRANATH and STRANDELL 1964).

D. Digitalization

In order to evaluate further the possibility of myocardial insufficiency in old age, five healthy men, 66–80 years old, were studied by right heart catheterization at rest and at two work loads in the supine position (STRANDELL 1970). Thereafter, they were digitalized with 1.6 mg deslanoside (Cedilanid) i.v., and the study was repeated 1 ½ h later.

At rest, the subjects had a slightly lower average stroke volume and a higher heart rate after digitalization, but unchanged cardiac output, and slightly lower filling pressures in both the left and the right ventricle. All these changes, however, could be related to the effect of the previous exercise.

During exercise, the heart rate, stroke volume, and cardiac output were the same before and after digitalization. The filling pressures of the left and right ventricles during exercise were somewhat lower at the first work load after digitalization, but less so at the second. It was not possible to state whether or not the slightly lower filling pressures during mild exercise with unchanged stroke volume were an effect of digitalization or of the previous exercise period. In some of the healthy elderly men, however, the high filling pressures during exercise did not decrease after digitalization.

Thus, although the pumping capacity of the heart decreases with age, there are no indications that in healthy subjects this decrease is related to subclinical coronary artery disease or myocardial insufficiency.

E. Effect of Physical Training

The effect of short-term physical training on the central circulation in old age is not well known. In the group of 61–83 year old men, the recent degree of physical activity, as recorded in the case history, was positively related to the ability to increase the stroke volume during an increase in work load in the supine position (GRANATH and STRANDELL 1964). A positive relationship was also observed between the degree of physical activity and the pulmonary capillary venous pressure during exercise in the supine position. Thus, the physically active men had the largest stroke volumes and the highest pulmonary capillary venous pressures during exercise.

Three of these men took part in intense physical training for 3–4 weeks; they increased their maximal oxygen uptake by 10% and reduced their heart rates at submaximal loads accordingly. When these men were again studied by right heart catheterization, no change in the relationship between cardiac output and oxygen uptake was observed, but the average stroke volume during sitting exercise and the stroke volume at the highest work load in the supine position were about 10% higher than before the training period. At the same time, the average pulmonary capillary venous pressures and pulmonary artery pressures were about 5 mm Hg higher at the work load in the supine position.

These changes after training are in agreement with the previous findings, and indicate that the effect of physical activity and training on the central circulation, with an increase in stroke volume during exercise and maximal cardiac output, is connected largely with regulation of the distribution of the blood volume, and presumably with the ability to increase the central blood volume during exercise. Simultaneously, the heart volume in the supine position increased after training by an average of about 10%.

The findings in these elderly men were thus similar to observations in young men, among whom active athletes have higher filling pressures during exercise than ordinarily trained men (BEVEGÅRD et al. 1963).

Dye dilution studies on the effect of short-term physical training in men 38–55 years old (HARTLEY et al. 1959) have shown, as in the group of elderly men studied, that the increase in maximal oxygen uptake was due solely to an increase in stroke volume, not to a simultaneous increase in the arteriovenous oxygen difference, as occurs in young men. They therefore suggested that changes in the distribution of blood flow by training are minimized by the aging process.

The effect of long-term intense physical training and aging on the cardiac output was studied by dye dilution in nine active athletes 44–55 years old by GRIMBY et al. (1966). Higher cardiac outputs in relation to oxygen uptake were observed at rest and during exercise, in comparison to young athletes and to untrained men.

Apart from somewhat low hemoglobin concentrations, which might have been compensated for by an increased cardiac output, no explanation of these high cardiac outputs has thus far been found.

From the cross-sectional studies mentioned and the longitudinal studies of HOLLMAN (1965) and DILL et al. (1967), it is quite clear that the maximal cardiac output and maximal oxygen uptake decrease less with increasing age in physically active than in sedentary subjects. Regular physical activity of suitable intensity and type should therefore be a good way of maintaining physical working capacity into old age.

F. Distribution of Cardiac Output

The distribution of cardiac output at rest and during exercise in young subjects has been extensively described by WADE and BISHOP (1962). Exactly how the reduction in cardiac output with age affects the various regional blood flows is less well known, but in all organs studied the regional flow resistance increases with age.

DAVIES and SHOCK (1950) observed a progressive decrease with age in *renal blood flow*, measured as iodopyracet (Diodrast) clearance. The decrease of flow between the 4th and 9th decades was about 55%, or 0.6 liters/min; it is most probably related to the decrease with age in the number of active nephrons.

The *cerebral blood flow* has also been found to decline with age. FAZEKAS et al. (1952), using a modification of Kety's nitrous oxide method, compared groups of men between the ages of 34 and 68, and observed a decrease of about 20% with a slightly greater decrease in cerebral oxygen uptake.

The effect of aging on the *splanchnic blood flow*, which is the major regional flow in the body, is not known in detail. No major decrease with age has been observed, but it is likely that the blood flow to the metabolically active liver decreases at least in proportion to the decrease with age in the basal metabolic rate, or about 15% between 25 and 65 years of age.

No reports on the effect of age on the *coronary blood flow* in healthy subjects are available because of the methodology involved. No major effects are to be expected, however, since HOLMBERG et al. (1971) showed no difference in the coronary blood flow at rest and during moderate exercise between patients with coronary heart disease and slightly younger control patients without coronary heart disease. Only during severe exercise were the coronary blood flow and the myocardial oxygen consumption lower than in the control group. When only such slight differences can be observed between patients with and without proven coronary artery stenosis, change with age in apparently healthy subjects is probably slight, except for the expected decrease of the maximal flow capacity.

Changes in total *skeletal muscle blood flow* are difficult to assess, but no significant decline with age in calf blood flow at rest was found by venous occlusion plethysmography by ALLWOOD (1958). In his groups of healthy males, aged 18–24 and 70–82, the average values were, however, lower in the calf in the older group, and the vascular resistance was significantly higher in the old compared to the young group.

Like the renal circulation, the *skin blood flow* has functions other than to satisfy the metabolic needs of the tissues, and the arteriovenous oxygen difference is high. Since the skin blood flow is an integrated part of the thermoregulatory system of the body, the range of normal flow levels is wide even during standard conditions. Although a somewhat lower average value of the foot blood flow at rest was obtained in men 70–82 years old, compared to men 18–24 years old, the difference was not significant (ALLWOOD 1958).

Low skin temperatures are a well-known clinical finding in old age even in healthy subjects, however, and this finding indicates a low skin blood flow. In some healthy elderly men with low cardiac outputs, the reduction in blood flow to the lips, nose, and hands can lead to clearly visible cyanosis, especially in the erect position, when sympathetic tone is high. Thus, cyanosis of these parts in old age can be a simple effect of the normal reduction in cardiac output, and need not signify cardiac decompensation.

The effect of age on the *distribution of cardiac output during exercise* has not yet been studied in detail. That the rise in cardiac output in relation to oxygen uptake was the same in old (GRANATH et al. 1961, 1964) and young men (BEVEGÅRD et al. 1960; HOLMGREN et al. 1960), in both the supine and the sitting position, favors the idea of a similar distribution in old and young.

Some studies are available of leg blood flow, which constitutes a major part of the increase in cardiac output during exercise. No differences in femoral venous oxygen saturation at rest or during bicycle exercise with one leg were observed by CARLSON and PERNOW (1961) between groups of healthy male volunteers 20–37 and 48–56 years old, indicating no significant change in leg blood flow with age.

In a group of seven healthy, well-trained, athletic men 52–59 years old, the same leg blood flow at rest was found by WAHREN et al. (1974) as in a group of eight physically fit, healthy men 25–30 years old (JORFELDT and WAHREN 1971). In both studies, the same constant-rate intraarterial indicator infusion technique was applied. During exercise, however, the increase in leg blood flow was less in the middle-aged athletes, and was largely compensated for by a larger arteriovenous oxygen difference. It cannot be stated at present whether this difference in leg blood flow during exercise is due to age or to the exceptionally high degree of physical fitness of the older group, which had more than 10 years participation in cross-country running and an average maximal oxygen uptake of 3.5 liters/min. Because muscle blood flow measured with the ^{133}Xe-clearance method has been found to be lower at a given work load in trained subjects than in untrained ones (GRIMBY et al. 1967), it is still an open question whether or not age per se reduces blood flow during exercise.

G. Limiting Factors for Physical Work Capacity in Old Age

Physical performance is reduced in old age in parallel with the decrease with age in the maximal heart rate and stroke volume during exercise, and thus in the maximal cardiac output. The decrease with age observed in cross-sectional studies of the maximal oxygen uptake (Fig. 7), however, is for various reasons less marked than the decrease in longitudinal studies (HOLLMAN 1965; DILL et al. 1967). It has

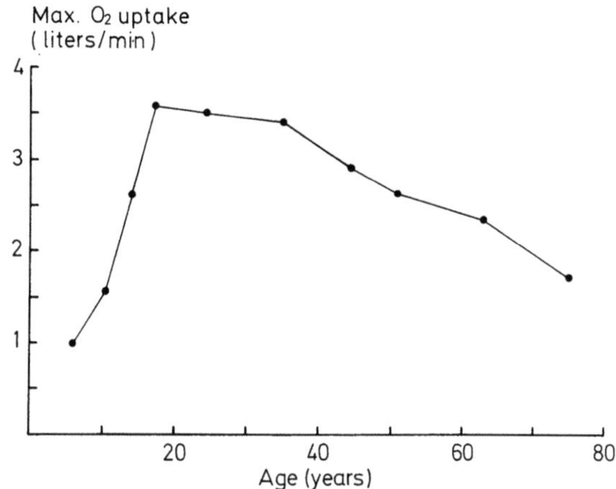

Fig. 7. Maximal oxygen uptake during upright exercise in relation to age in 81 normal nonathletic males. ROBINSON (1938)

also been shown that the decrease in maximal oxygen uptake is more marked in sedentary than in physically active subjects (HOLLMAN 1965; DILL et al. 1967).

The question then arises whether or not the reduced maximal cardiac output in old age is the main cause of the reduced physical work capacity. As age changes occur simultaneously in other organs, such as skeletal muscle and the lungs, the limitation might well be found outside the central circulation.

In young subjects, both the physical work capacity (KJELLBERG et al. 1949; ÅSTRAND et al. 1963) and the stroke volume during exercise (HOLMGREN et al. 1960) are closely related to cardiovascular dimensions such as heart volume, total hemoglobin, and blood volume, suggesting that the work capacity is limited mainly by central circulatory factors (SJÖSTRAND 1960).

Among 26 healthy men, 61–83 years old (STRANDELL 1964b), however, there was no correlation of even probable significance between maximal work capacity and circulatory dimensions. Within the group of 17 of these old men (GRANATH and STRANDELL 1964) who were studied by right heart catheterization, the maximal work capacity was not related to any data on pressure and flow, except slightly to stroke volume at the highest work load. This relationship was lost, however, when the influence of age on the maximal work capacity was eliminated.

Thus, there are no indications of a close relationship between maximal work capacity and central circulatory factors in old age. Nor were there any relationships in the group of 26 elderly men between maximal work capacity and lung volumes or measurements of pulmonary ventilatory function obtained by static and dynamic spirometry. Ventilatory factors, therefore, do not significantly limit the capacity for this type of physical exercise, but pulmonary limitation may be present in some subjects. In none of these subjects, however, were signs of pulmonary insufficiency present during maximal working intensity when arterial oxygen and carbon dioxide tensions were studied.

The closest relationship observed among the 26 elderly men was the negative one between the maximal work capacity and the lactate concentration in arterial blood at a given submaximal work load. The maximal work capacity representing the aerobic capacity thus varied with the ability of the subjects to avoid accumulation of metabolites from anaerobic metabolism, and this ability could be assessed at submaximal work loads. The maximal physical work capacity was accordingly related to peripheral factors (STRANDELL 1964c, 1976), as has been suggested earlier in young subjects (ÅSTRAND 1952; COBB and JOHNSSON 1963); it may have been associated with the muscular mass engaged in the exercise, the distribution of muscle blood flow, the diffusion of oxygen from the capillaries into the muscle cell, and cellular metabolic factors. The increased oxygen extraction by well-trained muscles has been related to the marked increase in the activity of oxidative mitochondrial enzymes and in the number and size of the mitochondria after physical training (MORGAN et al. 1969). To date, however, these factors have not been studied in detail in old age.

References

Abboud FM, Huston JH (1961) The effects of aging and degenerative vascular disease on the measurement of arterial rigidity in man. J Clin Invest 40:933–940

Allwood MJ (1958) Blood flow in the foot and calf in the elderly; a comparison with that in young adults. Clin Sci 17:331–338

Åstrand I (1960) Aerobic work capacity in men and women with special reference to age. Acta Physiol Scand 49, Suppl 49:1–171

Åstrand PO (1952) Experimental studies of physical working capacity in relation to sex and age. Munksgaard, Copenhagen

Åstrand PO, Engström L, Eriksson BO, Karlberg P, Nylander I, Saltin B, Thoren C (1963) Girl swimmers. With special reference to respiratory and circulatory adaptation and gynaecological and psychiatric aspects. Acta Paediatr Scand Suppl 147:1–75

Becklake MR, Frank H, Dagenais GR, Ostiguy GL, Guzman CA (1965) Influence of age and sex on exercise cardiac output. J Appl Physiol 20:938–947

Bevegård S, Holmgren A, Jonsson B (1960) The effect of body position on the circulation at rest and during exercise, with special reference to the influence on the stroke volume. Acta Physiol Scand 49:279–298

Bevegård S, Holmgren A, Jonsson B (1963) Circulatory studies in well trained athletes at rest and during heavy exercise, with special reference to stroke volume and the influence of body position. Acta Physiol Scand 57:26–50

Bourne GH (1961) Structural aspects of aging. Pitman Medical Publishing Co Ltd, London

Brandfonbrener M, Landowne M, Shock NW (1955) Changes in cardiac output with age. Circulation 12:557–566

Carlson LA, Pernow B (1961) Studies on the peripheral circulation and metabolism in man. Acta Physiol Scand 52:328–342

Cobb LA, Johnsson WP (1963) Hemodynamic relationships of anaerobic metabolism and plasma free fully acids during prolonged strenuous exercise in trained and untrained subjects. J Clin Invest 42:800–808

Conway J, Wheeler R, Sannerstedt R (1971) Sympathetic nervous activity during exercise in relation to age. Cardiovasc Res 5:577–581

Cournand A, Riley RL, Breed ES, Baldwin E deF, Richards DW (1945) Measurement of cardiac output in man using the technique of catheterization of the right auricle or ventricle. J Clin Invest 24:106–116

Davies DF, Shock NW (1950) Age changes in glomerular filtration rate, effective renal plasma flow and tubular excretory capacity in adult males. J Clin Invest 29:496–505

Dill DB, Consolazio CF (1962) Responses to exercise as related to age and environmental temperature. J Appl Physiol 17:645–753

Dill DB, Robinson S, Ross JC (1967) A longitudinal study of 16 champion runners. J Sports Med Phys Fitness 7:4–32

Emirgil E, Sobol BJ, Campodonico S, Herbert WH, Mechkati R (1967) Pulmonary circulation in the aged. J Appl Physiol 23:631–640

Fazekas JF, Alman RW, Bessman AN (1952) Cerebral physiology of the aged. Am J Med Sci 223:245–257

Foster GL, Reeves TJ, Meade JF (1964) Hemodynamic responses to exercise in clinically normal middle-aged men and in those with angina pectoris. J Clin Invest 43:1758–1768

Gloger von K (1972) Die Altersabhängigkeit des Pulmonalarteriendruckes während stufenweise gesteigerter Ergometerarbeit. Z Kreisl Forsch 61:728–737

Granath A, Strandell T (1964) Relationship between cardiac output, stroke volume and intracardiac pressures at rest and during exercise in supine position and some anthropometric data in healthy old men. Acta Med Scand 176:447–467

Granath A, Jonsson B, Strandell T (1961) Studies on the central circulation at rest and during exercise in the supine and sitting body position in old men. Acta Med Scand 169:125–126

Granath A, Jonsson B, Strandell T (1964) Circulation in healthy old men studied by right heart catheterization at rest and during exercise in supine and sitting position. Acta Med Scand 176:425–446

Grant RP (1956) Left axis deviation. An electrocardiographic – pathologic correlation study. Circulation 14:233–241

Grimby G, Nilsson NJ, Saltin B (1966) Cardiac output during submaximal and maximal exercise in active middle-aged athletes. J Appl Physiol 21:1150–1156

Grimby G, Häggendal E, Saltin B (1967) Local xenon 133 clearance from the quadriceps muscle during exercise in man. J Appl Physiol 22:305–310

Hansson JS, Tabakin BS, Levy AM (1968) Comparative exercise-cardiorespiratory performance of normal men in the third, fourth, and fifth decades of life. Circulation 37:345–360

Harris P, Heath D, Apostolopoulos A (1965) Extensibility of the human pulmonary trunk. Br Heart J 27:651–658

Hartley LH, Grimby G, Kilbom Å, Nilsson NJ, Åstrand I, Bjurö J, Ekblom B, Saltin B (1969) Physical training in sedentary middleaged older men. Scand J Clin Lab Invest 24:335–344

Hollman W (1963) Höchst- und Dauerleistungsfähigkeit des Sportlers. Johann Ambrosius Barth, München

Hollman W (1965) Körperliches Training als Prävention von Herz-Kreislauf-Krankheiten. Hippokrates Verlag, Stuttgart

Holmberg S, Serzysko W, Varnauskas E (1971) Coronary circulation during heavy exercise in control subjects and patients with coronary heart disease. Acta Med Scand 190:465–480

Holmgren A, Jonsson B, Sjöstrand T (1960) Circulatory data in normal subjects at rest and during exercise in recumbent position, with special reference to the stroke volume at different work intensities. Acta Physiol Scand 49:343–363

Jorfeldt L, Wahren J (1971) Leg blood flow during exercise in man. Clin Sci 41:459–466

Julius S, Amery A, Whitlock LS, Conway J (1967) Influence of age on the hemodynamic response to exercise. Circulation 36:222–230

Kjellberg SR, Rudhe U, Sjöstrand T (1949) The relation of the cardiac volume to the weight and surface area of the body, the blood volume and the physical capacity for work. Acta Radiol 31:113–122

König K, Reindell H, Mosshoff K, Roskamm H, Kessler M (1961) Das Herzvolumen und die körperliche Leistungsfähigkeit bei 20- bis 60 jährigen gesunden Männern. Arch Kreisl Forsch 35:37–45

König K, Reindell H, Roskamm H (1962) Das Herzvolumen und die Leistungsfähigkeit bei 60- bis 75 jährigen gesunden Männern. Arch Kreisl Forsch 39:143–150

Kohn RR, Rollerson E (1959) Studies on the mechanism of the age-related changes in swelling ability of human myocardium. Circ Res 7:740–747

Landowne M, Brandfonbrener M, Shock NW (1955) The relation of age to certain measures of performance of the heart and the circulation. Circulation 12:567–577

Lober H (1953) Pathogenesis of coronary sclerosis. Arch Pathol 55:357–365

Malmborg RO (1965) A clinical and hemodynamic analysis of factors limiting the cardiac performance in patients with coronary disease. Acta Med Scand Suppl 426:1–94

Master AM, Dublin LI, Marks HH (1950) The normal blood pressure range and its implications. JAMA 143:1464–1473

Morgan TE, Short FA, Cobb LA (1969) Effect of long-term exercise on skeletal muscle lipid composition. Am J Physiol 216:82–90

Norris AH, Shock NW, Yiengst MJ (1953) Age changes in heart rate and blood pressure responses to tilting and standarized exercise. Circulation 8:521–526

Renck H (1969) The elderly patient after anaesthesia and surgery. Acta Anaesthesiol Scand Suppl 34:1–136

Robinson S (1938) Experimental studies of physical fitness in relation to age. Arbeitsphysiologie 10:251–323

Shock NW, Yiengst MJ, Watkin DM (1953) Age change in body water and its relationship to basal oxygen consumption in males. J Gerontol 8:388–396

Sjöstrand T (1960) Functional capacity and exercise tolerance in patients with impaired cardiovascular function. In: Gordon BL (ed) Clinical cardiopulmonary physiology. Grune and Stratton Inc, New York, p 201

Strandell T (1963) Electrocardiographic findings at rest, during, and after exercise in healthy old men compared with young men. Acta Med Scand 174:479–499

Strandell T (1964a) Heart rate, arterial lactate concentration and oxygen uptake during exercise in old men compared with young men. Acta Physiol Scand 60:197–216

Strandell T (1964b) Heart rate and work load at maximal working intensity in old men. Acta Med Scand 176:310–318

Strandell T (1964c) Circulatory studies on healthy old men. Acta Med Scand Suppl 4:1–44

Strandell T (1970) Are there signs of incipient cardiac insufficiency in healthy elderly men? In: Symposium on incipient cardiac insufficiency. Sandoz Ltd, Basel, pp 203–208

Strandell T (1976) Cardiac output in old age. In: Caird FI, Dall JLC, Kennedy RD (eds) Cardiology in old age. Plenum Press, New York, p 81

Varnauskas E (1955) Studies in hypertensive cardiovascular disease with special reference to cardiac function. Scand J Clin Lab Invest Suppl 17

Wade OL, Bishop JM (1962) Cardiac output and regional blood flow. Blackwell Scientific Publications, Oxford

Wahren J, Saltin B, Jorfeldt L, Pernow B (1974) Influence of age on the local circulatory adaptation to leg exercise. Scand J Clin Lab Invest 33:79–86

Myocardium and Valves

A. POMERANCE

A. Introduction

If our standard for the normal in geriatric patients is accepted as the least degree of abnormality seen in this age group, then normal ageing itself causes relatively few changes in the heart. Even the almost universal coronary atherosclerosis is a disease and not an expression of normal ageing. Pathologists familiar with geriatric autopsies are well aware that the heart of a centenarian may be indistinguishable from that of a patient 50 years younger. However, in common with other organs the heart is increasingly likely to develop abnormalities with increasing age and any of the forms of cardiac pathology which occur in younger patients may also be seen in geriatric patients as well as several conditions which, for all practical purposes, are only found in patients over 70 years old (Fig. 1).

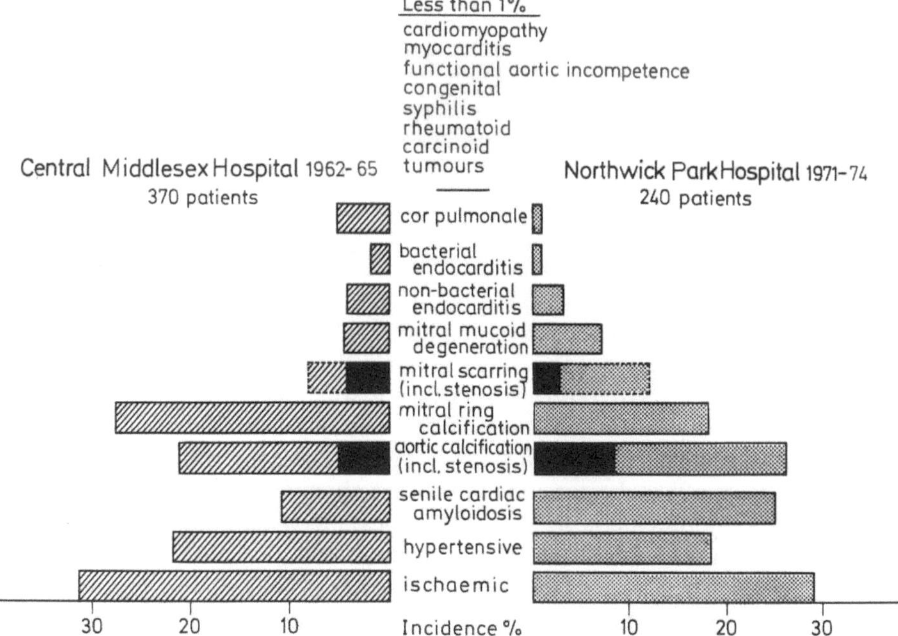

Fig. 1. Cardiac abnormalities found in two series of autopsies on geriatric patients dying in general hospitals. The studies were approximately 10 years apart. Both hospitals are within in Greater London area

B. Normal Ageing Changes

Changes in heart size with age can usually be attributed either to cardiovascular disease or to generalised body wasting. In individuals without cardiovascular disease, heart weight is related to body weight (REINER et al. 1959; REINER 1960). The age-related increase in relative heart weight noted by LINZBACH and AKUAMOA-BOATENG (1973a) was associated with an age-related increase in systolic blood pressure and the main condition contributing to increase in heart weight with increasing age in HODKINSON et al.'s series (1979) was ischaemic heart disease.

The quantity of collagen and elastic in the atria increases and the proportion of muscle decreases (DAVIES and POMERANCE 1972; MCMILLAN and LEV 1962). The amount of fat increases, particularly in the interatrial septum and occasionally tumour-like masses of adipose tissue may form in the interatrial septum and be associated with arrhythmias (PAGE 1970; REYES and JABLOKOW 1979). A slight increase in the amount of collagen in the interventricular septum with age has also been reported (LENKIEWICZ et al. 1972).

The quantity of *lipofuscin* in the myofibres increases steadily with age (MCMILLAN and LEV 1962; STREHLER et al. 1959). In routinely stained (haematoxylin and eosin sections, lipofuscin appears as yellow-brown intracytoplasmic granules located at the poles of the myofibre nuclei. It is better demonstrated (Fig. 2) by special staining methods such as Sudan dyes and is autofluorescent under ultraviolet light. It is generally accepted as being derived from lysosomes and recent ultrastructure observations have shown what appear to be mitochondrial remnants in the characteristic membrane-bound lipofuscin granules (KOOBS et al. 1978; STREHLER and MILDVAN 1962).

Although lipofuscin accumulation is clearly age related, being absent in childhood and invariably present in the elderly, there are considerable quantitative variations between individuals in the same age group (STEPIEN and BUCZYNSKI 1972). STREHLER and his colleagues (STREHLER 1967; STREHLER et al. 1959; STREHLER and MILDVAN 1962) found no correlation with sex or race although the highest rate of accumulation was in Japanese subjects. There was also no relation with heart size, other cardiac pathology or cardiac failure. Vitamin E deficiency and starvation, however, appear to accelerate the rate of lipofuscin deposition (KOOBS et al. 1978).

Lipofuscin accumulation seems to be a true manifestation of biological ageing and has generally been regarded as of no functional significance but recently KOOBS et al. (1978) have suggested that it may be related to the decline in cardiac efficiency of advanced age. Their hypothesis was that it was an indicator of peroxidative mitochondrial damage, which could result in impaired intracellular protein synthesis and therefore in reduced replacement of myofibre contractile proteins.

Basophilic myofibre degeneration is another change which is normally present to some degree in all elderly hearts. This appears as solid amorphous basophilic masses within the myofibres and is best demonstrated by PAS staining (Fig. 3). Histochemistry identifies the basophilic substance as an insoluble product of glycogen metabolism and the ultrastructure resembles that of nervous system corpora amylacea (KOSEK and ANGELL 1970; ROSAI and LASCANO 1970). As with lipofuscin the presence of basophilic myofibre degeneration is strongly age associated and has no known functional connotations although unusually well-marked basophilic de-

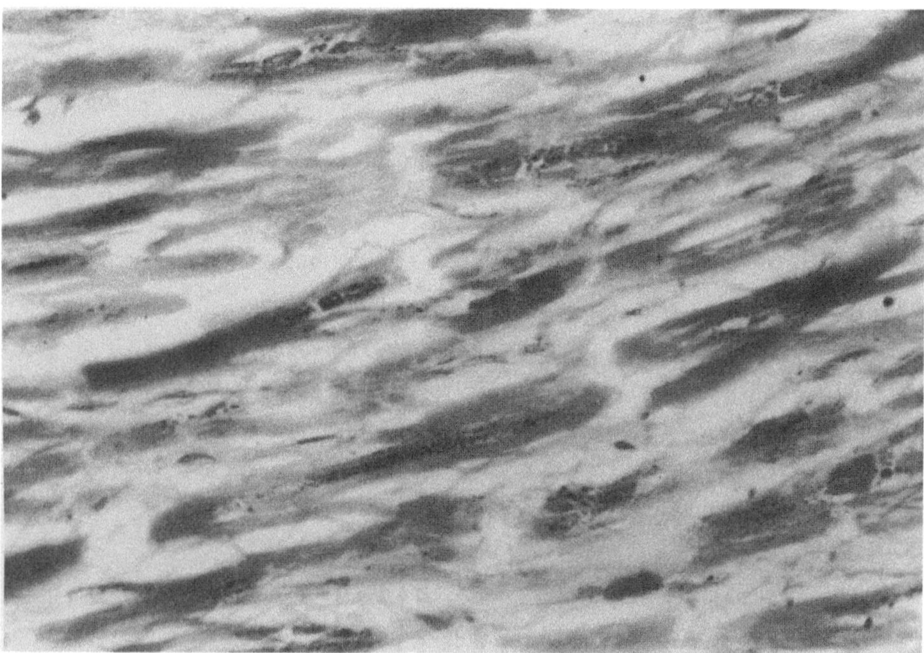

Fig. 2. Lipofuscin accumulation in myofibres. The pigment granules are most numerous adjacent to the myofibre nuclei and in the central part of the fibres. Schmorl's stain, × 360, reduced to 70%

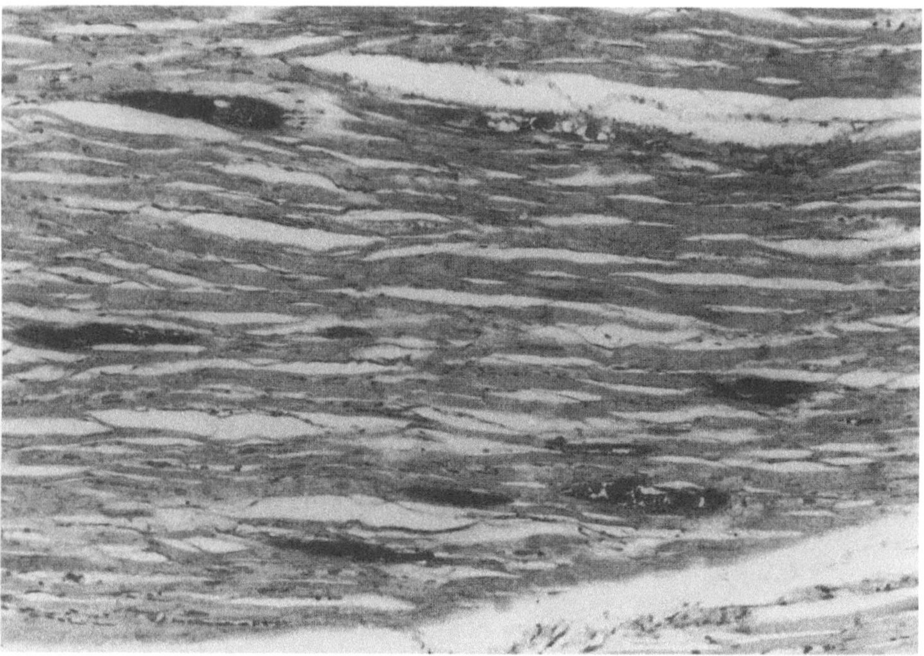

Fig. 3. Basophilic myofibre degeneration. Many of the myofibres contain darkly staining solid masses of amorphous material. PAS, × 180, reduced to 70%

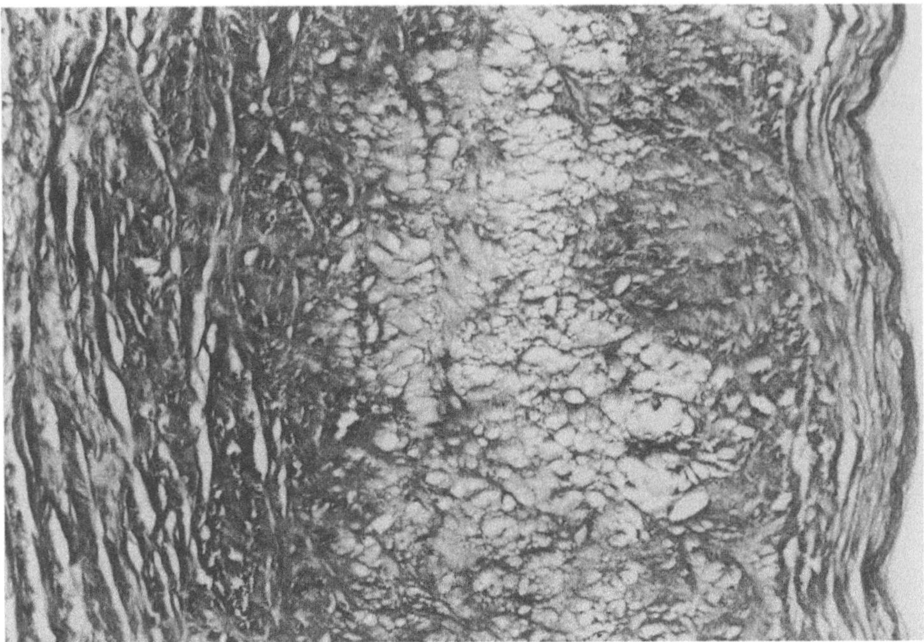

Fig. 4. Section of an anterior mitral cusp showing a band of lipid in the fibrosa just deep to the endocardium. Elastic van Gieson, × 100, reduced to 70%

generation is often associated with myxodema or cardiomyopathy (HAUST et al. 1962).

Endocardial ageing changes consist of thickening and increasing opacity of the endocardium of the atria and atrial surfaces of the atrioventricular valves with localised endocardial thickenings developing on the closure lines of the valves. Histologically the thickened endocardium shows proliferation of elastic and collagen progressing to fragmentation, disorganisation, and irregular staining of the elastic (McMILLAN and LEV 1959). The thickenings of the valve closure lines consist of localised fibroelastic proliferation sometimes with obvious fragmentation of the underlying elastic lamina.

These endocardial changes are clearly the result of mechanical factors, the diffuse endocardial thickening being a response to blood flow and those on the valve closure lines being caused by repeated impact.

Yellow areas of lipid appear on the ventricular surface of the anterior mitral cusp (see Fig. 15) in the 3rd or 4th decade and increase with advancing age (McMANUS and LUPTON 1963; POMERANCE 1967). These are also the result of normal haemodynamic factors, produced by pulsatile blood flow against the ventricular surface of the closed cusp. Histology (Fig. 4) shows a fine foamy sudanophilic appearance in the cusp fibrosa. The lipids appear identical to those found in uncomplicated vascular atheroma but, unlike the latter, thrombosis and secondary haemorrhage do not occur and calcification is unusual and always insignificant.

The collagen of the left side of the cardiac skeleton alters microscopically with age. It becomes denser with fewer nuclei and variable staining, the amount of mucopolysaccharide decreases and metachromasia is lost (SELL and SCULLY 1965; TORII et al. 1965). Lipid begins to appear in the 3 rd decade increasing progressively with age and fine powderly calcification usually develops in the aortic cusp bases around the 5 th decade and in the mitral ring around the 6 th decade (KIM et al. 1976; SELL and SCULLY 1965). Electron microscopic studies have shown an age-associated accumulation of residual bodies in the cytoplasm of the fibrocytes, and calcium deposition was closely associated with these cellular degradation products rather than with collagen or elastic (KIM et al. 1976).

With the possible exception of lipofuscin accumulation none of the changes which seem to be an invariable part of the ageing process appear to have any direct functional importance. Changes in myofibre enzymes with ageing have also been described in experimental animals (LIMAS 1971) but no similar findings have yet been reported in man and at present there seems to be no pathological basis for decline in cardiac efficiency which occurs in the elderly.

C. Myocardial Pathology

I. Ischaemic Heart Disease

Although coronary atherosclerosis is undoubtedly the most important and frequent cause of heart disease in middle and old age in the Western world, it is by no means synonymous with geriatric heart disease. In personally studied hospital autopsy material (Fig. 1) ischaemic myocardial pathology has been present in less than one-third of all elderly patients and even in those with cardiac failure the incidence was just under 50%. The type of ischaemic lesion present in the cardiac failure cases was usually either a recent localised transmural infarct or the more diffuse, mainly concentric and subendocardial type of fibrosis associated with three vessel coronary disease (Table 1).

Small microscopic foci of fibrosis are common in elderly hearts and appear to be of no clinical significance. They correlate poorly with coronary artery stenosis but increase in frequency with age (SCHWARTZ and MITCHELL 1962) and probably result from small foci of myocardial inflammation such as those not uncommonly observed in a variety of causes of death (DAVIS 1975).

The incidence of ischaemic heart disease is higher in non-hospital sudden deaths. In a personally reviewed series of 380 cases aged over 65 years, 62% had died of ischaemic heart disease. In contrast to the hearts of patients dying of ischaemic disease in hospital many of the hearts from the sudden death series had no infarcts or ischaemic fibrosis although severe coronary artery stenosis was always present in these cases.

Although the pathology of ischaemic heart disease differs little in patients over and under 65 years there are some aspects which are particularly associated with older patients and which reflect the atypical clinical features often seen in the elderly.

A high incidence of clinically unsuspected ischaemic pathology is likely to be found in geriatric autopsies unless ECGs have been routinely performed. In most reported series the figure has been about 20% (GJOL 1972) and many patients will

Table 1. Ischaemic pathology in patients over 65 years dying in hospital

	Cardiac failure 118 cases	No failure 139 cases
Recent infarction	13%	4%
Fibrosed infarct	9%	11%
Recent and fibrotic	11%	2%
Diffuse fibrosis	12%	5%
Total ischaemic pathology	45%	22%
Non-ischaemic fibrosis	6%	10%

have died of causes other than cardiac failure (Table 1). Large fibrous infarcts with no history suggestive of past infarction are rarely seen except in the elderly. These lesions have clearly followed extensive transmural necrosis, the aneurysm walls consisting mainly or wholly of fibrous tissue. Calcification is common as is endocardial thrombus deposition but embolisation from this source is surprisingly uncommon.

External cardiac rupture is a complication of myocardial infarction which is uncommon except in the elderly. It has been calculated (SIEVERS 1966) that the frequency increases by 3.6% per decade. In most recent reviews the incidence has been between 5% and 12% of fatal infarcts and most cases have been over 65 years with an increased prevalence in women.

There is no satisfactory explanation for the association between external cardiac rupture and advancing age. Ageing alone does not apparently produce any morphological changes which could weaken the left ventricle. It has been suggested (LONDON and LONDON 1965) that age-related alterations in myofibre cement lines and intercalated discs might predispose to myofibre fragmentation but there is at present no firm evidence for this hypothesis. An increase in cardiac ruptures has been reported following the introduction of external cardiac massage but recent studies (CHRISTENSEN and PEDERSEN 1976; RASMUSSEN et al. 1979) agree that these resuscitative measures are not responsible for the ruptures.

At autopsy or, occasionally, surgery the pericardial sac is tense, purple and distended by blood clot (Fig. 5). The rupture site is seen as a ragged tear on the epicardial surface, most often on the anterior wall of the left ventricle. On cutting through the rupture site an irregular transmural haemorrhagic track can usually be identified (Fig. 6) indicating that the rupture is a process of gradual dissection and not a "blowout." The rupture always occurs through an area of transmural recent infarction, often at its junction with uninfarcted myocardium, but the infarcted area may be surprisingly small. Complete occlusion of the relevant coronary artery is almost invariably present, often without marked underlying stenosis (PENTHER et al. 1977). There are rarely any fibrotic ischaemic lesions and it seems that fibrosis protects against rupture.

In most reported series precipitating factors have been postinfarction hypertension or continuing physical activity. These factors suggest that raised intraventricular pressures may be an important factor. However, immobilisation of patients

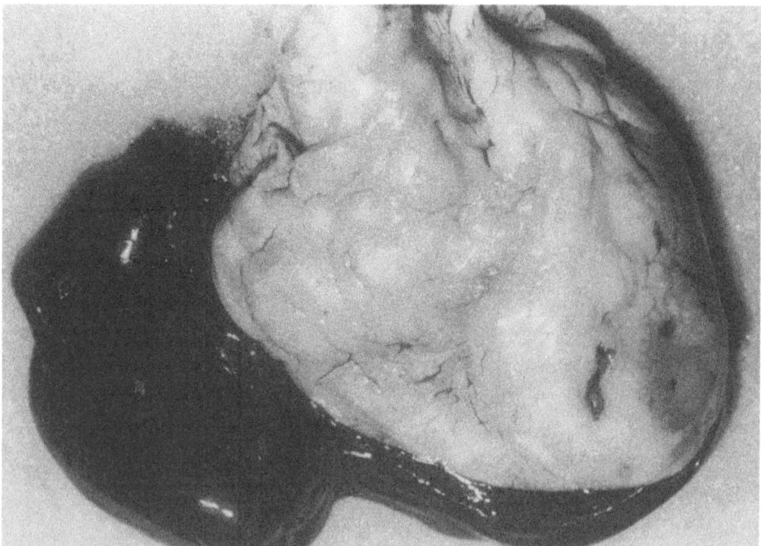

Fig. 5. External cardiac rupture. A ragged tear is visible on the anterior surface of the left ventricle near the interventricular groove. The heart is lying on a mass of blood clot which had been distending the pericardial cavity. From a previously fit and well 82-year-old woman who did suddenly

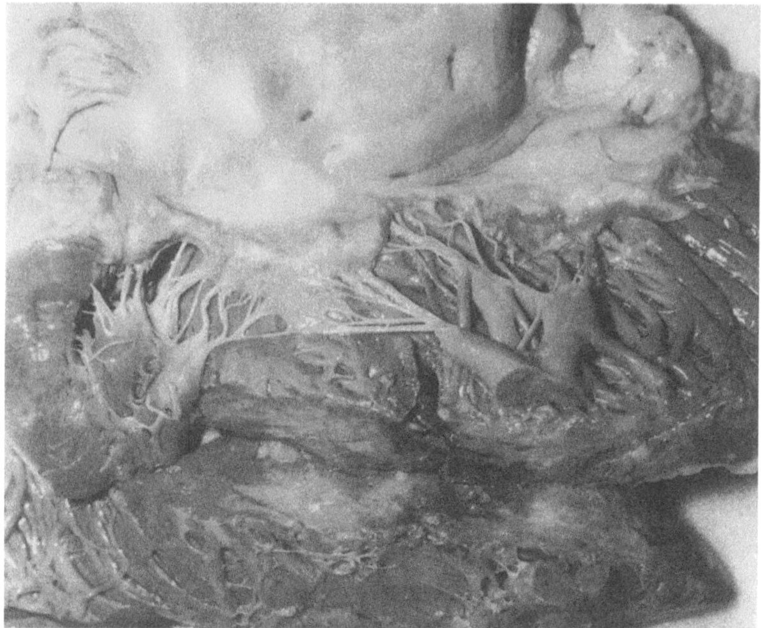

Fig. 6. Opened left side of heart with the ventricle cut transversely through an area of infarction. A haemorrhagic tract can be seen running through the infarct at the junction of posterior septum with free wall. Note also the nodular thickening of the apposing edges of the mitral valve cusps

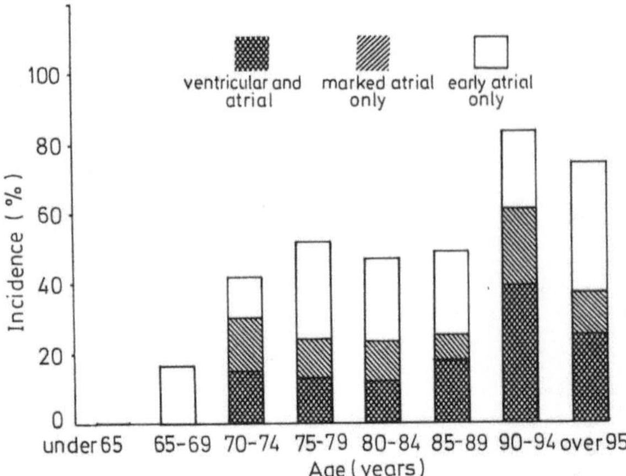

Fig. 7. The incidence of senile cardiac amyloidosis in relation to age

with known acute infarction failed to lower the incidence of cardiac rupture (Ras-mussen et al. 1979) and in Spiel et al.'s series (1979) raised blood pressure either before or after myocardial infarction could not be implicated as a risk factor for external cardiac rupture.

Transseptal and papillary muscle ruptures also complicate myocardial infarction in the elderly but unlike external cardiac rupture the incidence is no higher than in younger groups.

II. Senile Cardiac Amyloidosis

Senile cardiac amyloidosis is a form of primary amyloid which can justifiably be considered as a separate subgroup because of its distinctive age and pathological distribution and because it is immunologically distinct from other forms (Dorn-well et al. 1978; Westermark et al. 1977).

It is rare under 70 years but its prevalence increases sharply with age beyond this and almost 60% of patients aged over 90 show at least well-defined atrial deposits of amyloid (Fig. 7). In our most recent study (Hodkinson and Pomerance 1977) amyloid was demonstrable in the hearts of over 50% of 244 patients over 65 years. This was, however, limited to very fine atrial deposits in over half these cases and ventricular involvment was present in only 16.5%.

Senile cardiac amyloid appears to have been recognized first in 1876 (Soyka) but until the second half of the present century relatively few cases had been re-corded. Over the past 30 years many studies have appeared from several countries with reported incidences varying from under 2% to over 80% (Table 2). This wide range is clearly due to differences in sampling and staining techniques. Since senile cardiac amyloid is often limited to the atria and the deposits are relatively fine, retrospective studies based on samples from ventricles would clearly show a rela-tively low incidence as would those in which the initial suspicion of amyloid was based on routine haematoxylin and eosin-stained sections only.

Table 2. Reported series of senile cardiac amyloidosis 1950–1980

Country of origin	Authors	Stain used	Incidence	Sex ratio ♂:♀
United States	Josselson et al. (1952)	Methyl violet	2.5% over 70 years (10 cases)	4:1
Germany	Husselman (1955)	Methyl violet	12.5% over 70 years (69 cases)	3:2
United States	Mulligan (1958)	Methyl violet	1.5% over 70 years (17 cases)	6.4:1
United States	Buerger and Braunstein (1960)	Haematoxylin and eosin	3.6% over 70 years (42 cases)	0.85:1
England	Pomerance (1966)	Methyl violet	12.5% over 70 years (45 cases)	2:1
United States	Schwartz (1969)	Thioflavine S	83% over 70 years (151 cases)	–
Japan	Ikee (1970)	Congo red, Gentian violet Thioflavine T	37% over 70 years (46 cases)	0.7:1
Germany	Katenkamp and Stiller (1971)	Thioflavine S	91% over 70 years (70 cases)	1:1
Uganda	Drury (1973)	Congo red	10% over 70 years (10 cases)	–
Japan	Hinohara (1973)	Congo red	26.8% over 70 years (11 cases)	–
Italy	Serentha et al. (1973)	Congo red, Methyl violet, Thioflavine T	10% over 70 years (18 cases)	1:1.2
United States	Wright and Calkins (1975)	Congo red	55% over 60 years (55 cases)	–
England	Hodkinson and Pomerance (1978)	SAB, Congo red	53% over 65 years (118 cases)	0.87:1
Canada	Pomerance and Silver (1981)	SAB	53.6% over 65 years (59 cases)	–

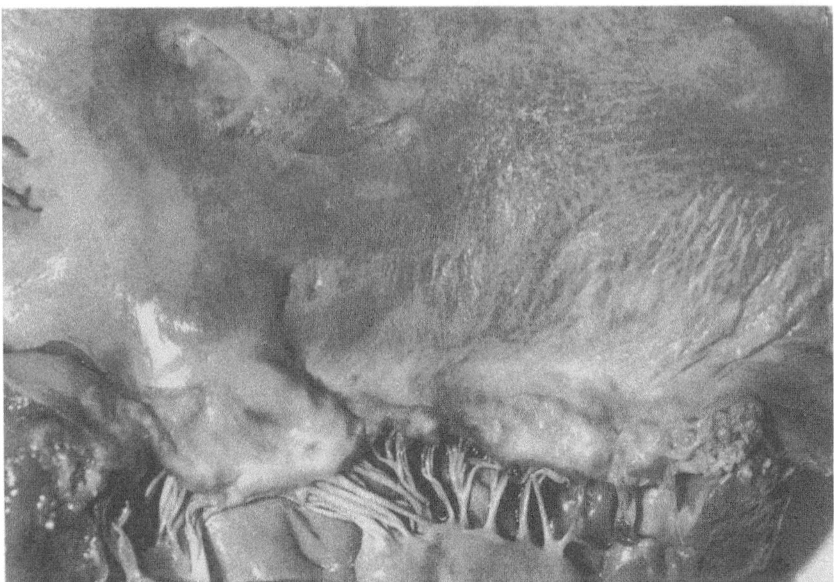

Fig. 8. Opened left atrium and upper ventricle showing numerous small closely set greyish nodules of amyloid in the atrial endocardium. Mitral ring calcification is also present. The calcified bar can be seen at the incision line at both sides of the left ventricle and causing mild distortion of the posterior mitral cusp. From a 72-year-old woman who died in congestive heart failure

Macroscopically there is frequently nothing to suggest cardiac involvment by amyloid. The large firm waxy heart of primary amyloid as seen in younger patients does not occur in the senile form. In our material there was no correlation whatsoever between heart weight and the presence or absence or cardiac amyloid. Careful inspection of the atrial endocardium may show tiny semitranslucent nodules which are easily overlooked in the fresh heart particularly if not numerous. These nodules become more conspicuous after fixation (Fig. 8) but are best demonstrated by application of an iodine solution.

Microscopically (Fig. 9) the earliest deposits are seen in the atrial capillaries and as fine insterstitial strands between the subendocardial myofibres. Electron microscopy has confirmed the close relationship between the amyloid deposits and capillaries (Tseng and Lim 1977). With increasing severity the size and number of foci of amyloid deposition increase as does the thickness of the interstitial strands, and broad bands of amyloid surround individual myofibres, eventually causing compression atrophy. This loss of muscle as the quantity of amyloid increases explains the absence of significant cardiac enlargement in even severely affected hearts. Nodular deposits of amyloid appear in the atrial endocardium forming the characteristic raised nodules which, when present, allow a confident diagnosis of cardiac amyloid macroscopically.

In severe cases small deposits of amyloid may be visible in valves but this finding is uncommon compared with the frequency of valve involvment in other types

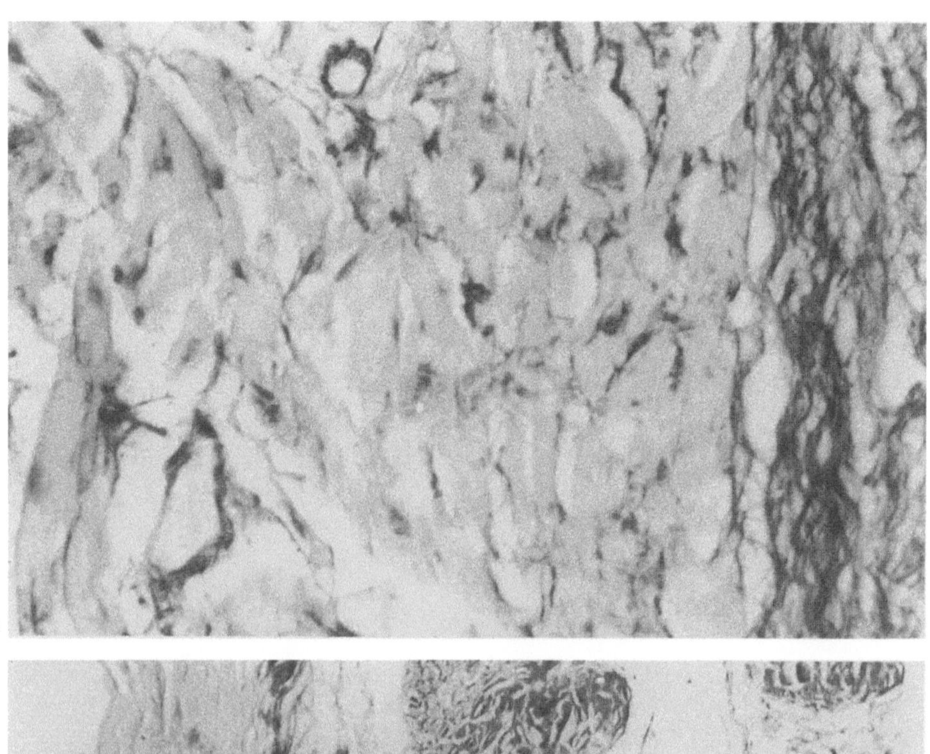

a

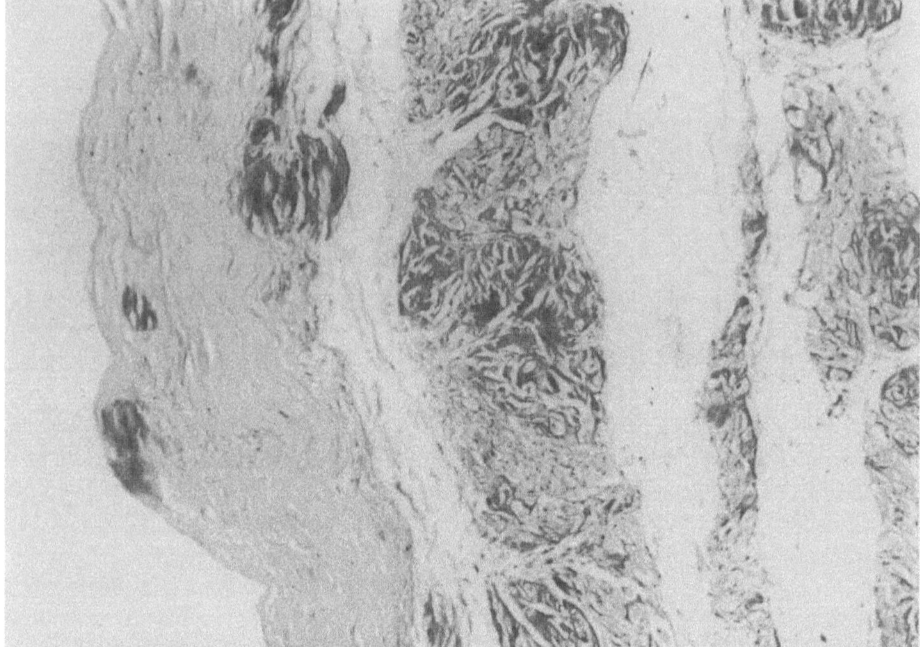

b

Fig. 9 a–c. Histology of senile cardiac amyloid. **a** Very early deposites in the atrium. Amyloid is seen as small dark foci in the capillary walls and thin dark strands of tissue between the myofibres. Sulphonated alcian blue, × 400, reduced to 70% **b** Section of atrium with well-marked amyloid. Nodular deposits of amyloid are present in the atrial endocardium and are surrounding, compressing, and in places completely replacing the myofibres. Crystal violet, × 100, reduced to 70% **c** Section through upper interventricular septum. The contractile myocardium on the right shows several large foci of amyloid. The bundle of His *(H)* on the left is free from amyloid. Sulphonated alcian blue, × 100, reduced to 75%

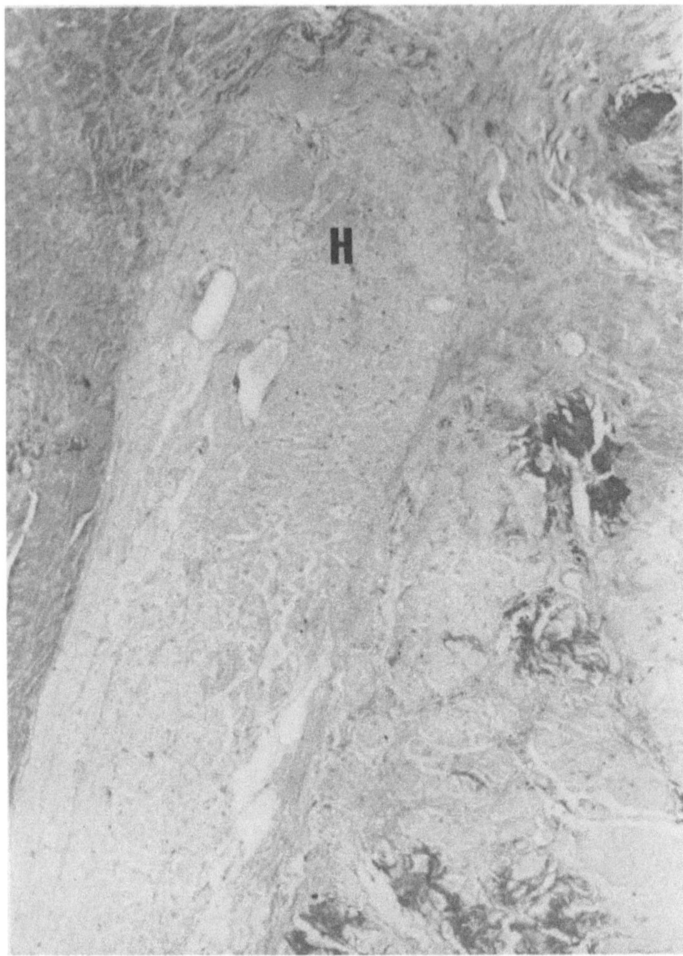

Fig. 9c
(legend see p. 53)

of cardiac amyloid (Buja et al. 1970). Conducting tissue is affected late, if at all (Ridolfi et al. 1977) and most cases of severe senile cardiac amyloid observed personally have not shown deposits in the conducting system (Fig. 9c).

Extra-cardiac deposits are often present in patients with severe cardiac involvement but have not been seen where amyloid was confined to the atria (Hodkinson and Pomerance 1977; Smith et al. 1979). The lungs are most frequently and most extensively involved, with small nodules of amyloid being present in vessels and alveolar septa. In other organs the deposits are limited to small foci in small vessel walls. Vessels in the usual biopsy sites may be affected but this occurs too rarely for rectal or tongue biopsies to be of any practical valve in the clinical diagnosis of this type of amyloid.

Until comparatively recently none of the generally used staining methods for identification of amyloid was entirely satisfactory in cardiovascular studies since they all showed an inverse relationship between specificity and sensitivity (Cooper

1969; Wright et al. 1969; Pomerance et al. 1976). Personal preference is for the sulphonated alcian blue (SAB) method (Lendrum et al. 1972) which, in the cardiovascular system, combines high sensitivity high specificity and good visual contrast. The staining reactions of senile cardiac amyloid are those generally accepted as characteristic of amyloid i.e. green/orange dichroism with alkaline Congo red and polarised light, fluorescence with Thioflavine T or S in ultraviolet light, metachromasia with methyl and crystal violet, jade green staining with SAB and a positive reaction for tryptophan. Resistance to potassium permanganate digestion identifies it as a primary amyloid (Romhanyi 1972; Smith et al. 1979; Wright and Calkins 1975). Its electron microscopic appearance is also characteristic of amyloid (Tseng and Lim 1977).

Recently Westermark and his colleagues (Cornwell et al. 1978; Westermark et al. 1977) succeeded in extracting a major amyloid fibroprotein from hearts which were severely affected by senile cardiac amyloid. This protein, which they have designated protein Asca, appeared to be unique for this type of amyloidosis, differing from other primary and secondary amyloid fibroproteins including the senile pancreatic and cerebral forms. It appeared to be immunologically identical in different individuals and could be demonstrated in the amyloid deposits but not in the normal heart tissues.

1. Age and Sex

All studies have agreed that the prevalence of senile cardiac amyloidosis increases sharply with age. In our most recent study, which used the very sensitive SAB stain, no amyloid was found in patients under 65 years but 84% of those over 90 years had at least minor atrial deposits and about one-half of these cases also had ventricular involvment. Curiously the condition seems to be less common in centenarians. Ischii and Sternby (1978) found only eight cases in their 23 centenarians and only one of three centenarians included in our study had cardiac amyloid. The reported sex incidence has varied (Table 2). In our material there was a significantly higher incidence in women in the series as a whole but when only cases with moderate or marked ventricular involvment were considered the ratio reversed to 12% of men compared with 8% of women. This suggests that although women are more prone to develop senile cardiac amyloid than men, they are less likely to be severely affected.

2. Clinical Features

As might be expected the clinical significance of cardiac amyloidosis is related to its severity. Small deposits, limited to the atria, appear insignificant, but larger amounts are likely to be associated with both atrial fibrillation and cardiac failure. In our study (Hodkinson and Pomerance 1977) both these clinical findings showed independent, statistically significant correlations with the degree of senile cardiac amyloidosis.

The high incidence of digitalis sensitivity in the elderly and the reported association between digitalis sensitivity and cardiac amyloid in younger patients (Buja et al. 1970) raises the possibility that senile amyloid may be responsible for digitalis sensitivity but we were unable to demonstrate any association between these two findings.

At present there is no satisfactory way of confirming a clinical suspicion of senile cardiac amyloid in vivo. Conduction abnormalities and ECG changes suggestive of ischaemia may be seen in patients with severe cardiac amyloidosis but such findings are inconstant. The sites usually biopsied are rarely involved in the senile form of amyloidosis and although the condition is one of those which may be associated with a raised alkaline phosphatase (HODKINSON and POMERANCE 1974), there are many other causes of raised alkaline phosphatase in the geriatric age group.

3. Pathogenesis

The immunological origin of amyloid is now well established but the exact reason for development of the senile cardiac form remains as unclear as that for other types of amyloid. Furthermore WESTERMARK'S recent immunochemical studies (1979) suggest that there may be two different forms of senile cardiac amyloid since the Asca protein could not be demonstrated where amyloid was confined to the atria.

Age-related amyloid is common in many animals (SCHWARTZ 1970; THUNG 1957) and in some is undoubtedly genetically determined. Genetically determined forms of amyloidosis are also well recognized in man but there is nothing so far to indicate that the senile form is one of this group. As can be seen from Table 2 it has been reported in many ethnic groups including Japanese, American Blacks, and Ugandan Africans as well as in Europeans and white North American populations. An age-related (SAA) serum protein substance has recently been described (ROSENTHAL and FRANKLIN 1975), which suggests that senile amyloid may be a direct expression of the immunological changes of senescence, but the subunit fibril protein of senile cardiac amyloid is different from the age-related SAA substance (WESTERMARK et al. 1977) and in our material there was no difference in serum immunoglobulins in patients with and without cardiac amyloid (MAUGHAN et al., to be published).

Associations with carcinomatosis, malnutrition, and chronic tuberculosis have been suggested in some of the earlier studies and we therefore examined these possibilities in our cases, together with possible associations with chronic infections and hypertension. No correlations were found with any of these factors and indeed the incidence of carcinomatosis was higher in the patients without amyloid.

4. Isolated Valvular Amyloid

Rarely the valves alone are distorted and thickened by nodules of material with the staining reactions of amyloid. Myocardial involvment is minimal or absent. This finding is of no clinical significance other than perhaps producing a systolic murmur. All three cases personally observed and the cases reported by JACOBOWITZ and DUSTIN (1974) were over 60 years.

III. Cardiomyopathies

1. Hypertrophic Cardiomyopathy

With the introduction of non-invasive diagnostic procedures such as echocardiography, it has become apparent that hypertrophic cardiomyopathy (idiopathic subaortic stenosis, asymetrical septal hypertrophy) is not the rarity it was previously thought to be and furthermore that it is not uncommon in the elderly (BERGER et al. 1979; PENTHER et al. 1970; WHITING et al. 1971). In recent studies from general community hospitals, up to 65% of cases diagnosed were over 60 years, as were almost one-third of the series of 47 autopsy cases studied by DAVIES et al. (1974). Patients have mainly been women and it has been suggested that they may have a less severe form of the disease and thus be more likely to survive into old age (KRASNOW and STEIN 1978). A high incidence of preceding hypertension was noted in PETRIN and TAVEL'S (1979) cases and these authors suggest that long-standing hypertension might induce development of hypertrophy in genetically predisposed subjects.

The diagnosis is not often made clinically in the elderly. Any signs or symptoms present are usually attributed to ischaemic or hypertensive heart disease (KRASNOW and STEIN 1978). BERGER et al. (1979) stress that failure to recognise hypertrophic cardiomyopathy in older patients is more likely to be due to failure to consider this diagnosis than to any differences in clinical features in comparison with younger patients. Many of the patients with hypertrophic cardiomyopathy diagnosed by echocardiography had no relevant symptoms and in our autopsy series almost half the elderly cases died of unrelated causes. Correct diagnosis is important since drugs used in other cardiac conditions may have an adverse effect while propanolol produces symptomatic improvement in a high proportion of cases (BERGER et al. 1979).

The *pathology* of hypertrophic cardiomyopathy in the elderly differs slightly from that in younger patients (POMERANCE and DAVIES 1975). The hearts tend to be heavier and the septal hypertrophy, although always present, is less conspicious because hypertrophy of the left ventricular free wall is usually also present. A characteristic subaortic fibrous band (Fig. 10) is visible in a high proportion of cases (PENTHER et al. 1970; POMERANCE and DAVIES 1975). This band is a mirror image of the aortic face of the anterior mitral cusp and is a form of friction lesion, caused by the systolic contact of cusp and septum. The band is diagnostic of hypertrophic cardiomyopathy and once formed does not regress even if the heart dilates and obstruction is no longer present. For pathologists it is, therefore, a valuable indicator of the correct diagnosis in an age group where hypertrophic cardiomyopathy might well otherwise not be considered.

Microscopically the foci of hypertrophied abnormally branched and orientated myofibres characteristic of hypertrophic cardiomyopathy are present but are usually less easy to find than in the hypertrophied septa of younger patients.

2. Congestive Cardiomyopathy

Since diagnosis of congestive cardiomyopathy demands exclusion of all possible causative pathology including coronary atherosclerosis, it is rarely made in the ge-

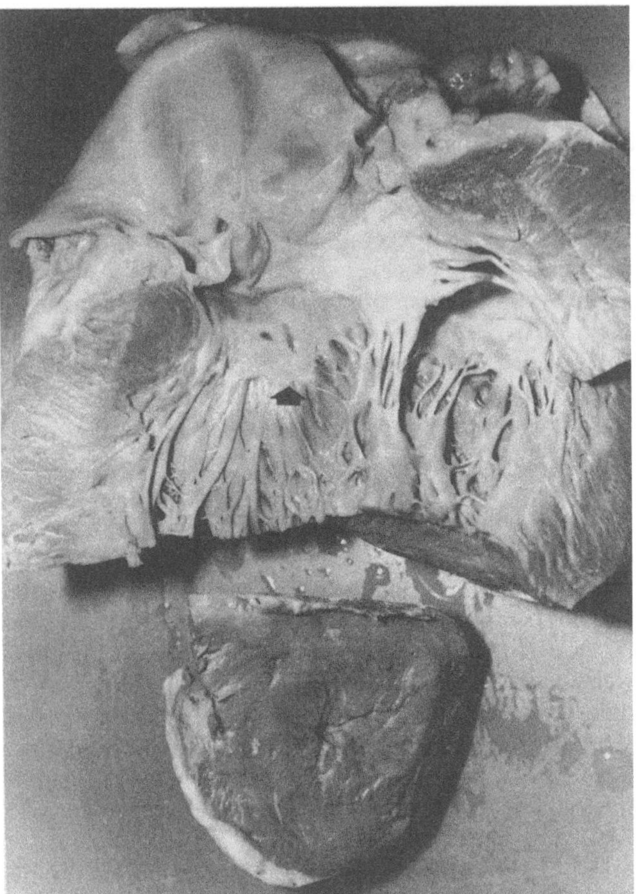

Fig. 10. Hypertrophic cardiomyopathy (idiopathic hypertropic subaortic stenosis). Opened left side of heart showing the typical small conical left ventricular cavity. The free wall is hypertrophied as well as the upper septum and a subaortic fibrous band characteristic of hypertrophic cardiomyopathy is present *(arrow)*. The aortic face of the anterior mitral cusp shows a corresponding flat fibrous thickening. From an elderly woman who died of congestive heart failure. She was known to have had arrhythmias for 2 years and an apical pansystolic murmur had been present

riatric age group. However, cases are occasionally seen and an example has been reported in a 96-year-old patient (Roberts and Ferrans 1975).

Macroscopically the heart of congestive cardiomyopathy is globular with a large dilated left ventricular cavity (Fig. 11) in contrast to the small conical cavity typical of hypertrophic cardiomyopathy. Thrombi are often seen in the interstices of the trabeculae of the ventricles together with small patches of white endocardial fibrous thickening. By definition, valves and coronary arteries must be normal and indeed the coronary arteries are usually strikingly free from atheroma. Histology is non-specific, usually consisting of myofibre hypertrophy and dilatation changes and mild interstitial fibrosis only.

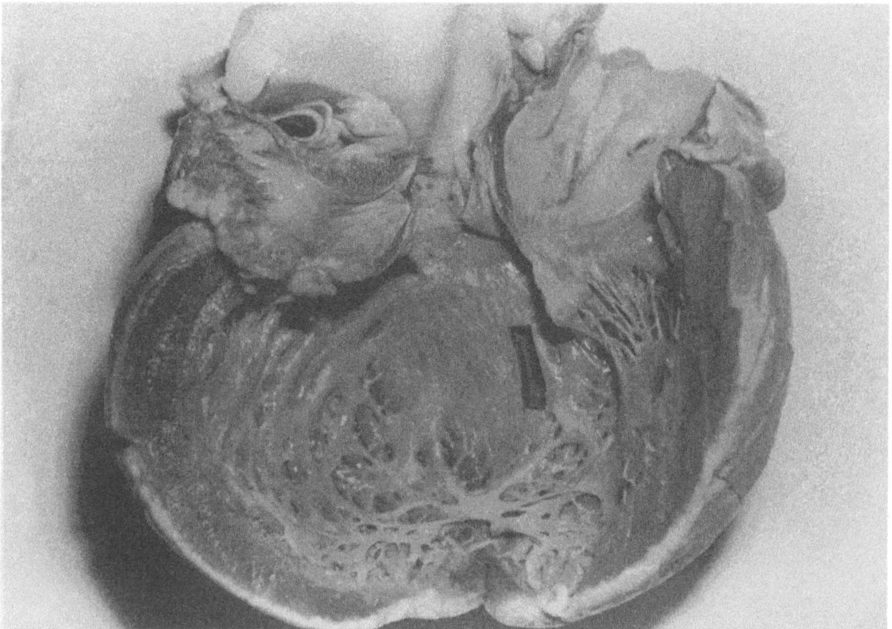

Fig. 11. Congestive cardiomyopathy. Opened left side of heart showing the typical globular dilated ventricular cavity with small patches of endocardial fibrous thickening and thrombi in the interstices near the apex. The ventricular wall is hypertrophied. The coronary arteries were widely patent with slight atheroma only. From an 82-year-old woman with a history of angina who died in congestive heart failure

Secondary cardiomyopathies are uncommon in all age groups, but with the exception of genetically determined metabolic and neuromuscular conditions all are at least as likely to be found in elderly patients as in middle age.

IV. Myocarditis

Myocarditis may occur in many virus and rickettsial infections of which Coxsackie is probably the most frequent in Europe and the North American continent (ABEL-MANN 1973; DAVIES 1975; KLINE et al. 1978; LANCET 1974). The inflammatory reaction is non-specific, consisting of varying proportions of polymorphs, eosinophils, chronic inflammatory cells, and histiocytes.

Occasional small aggregates of inflammatory cells are often found in the myocardium of patients dying of a wide range of conditions but they appear too insignificant to be of clinical importance and the diagnosis of myocarditis should not be applied to these lesions.

Myocarditis with conspicuous giant cells is seen in miliary tuberculosis and sarcoidosis as well as in an idiopathic form. Unsuspected miliary tuberculosis is still a comparatively common finding in the elderly. The myocardium may be involved in severe rheumatoid disease with development of granulomas similar to those seen

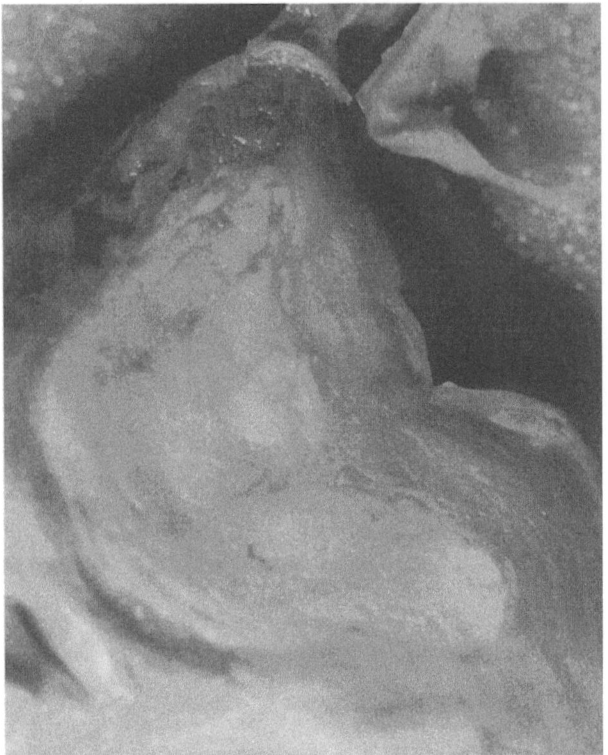

Fig. 12. Gumma. Section through the upper interventricular septum of a 77-year-old man showing a large caseous lesion just below the aortic valve ring. Courtesy of Dr. K. Misch

in subcutaneous tissues. These lesions often develop in the interventricular septum and may cause heart block (IVESON and POMERANCE 1977; ROBERTS et al. 1968). Gummas (Fig. 12) are now rare, at least in Britain, but the few cases found are usually in elderly patients. Myocardial necrosis with or without an inflammatory response has also been associated with a wide range of drugs (DAVIES 1975).

V. Metabolic Diseases

Apart from diabetes mellitus, which is a well-recognised predisposing factor in atherosclerosis (ROBERTSON and STRONG 1968), metabolic abnormalities are uncommon in all age groups but no less so in geriatric patients. Primary hemochromatosis is an occassional cause of cardiac failure (DI GIORGIO 1973) and a pathologically identical condition may develop after multiple blood transfusions. Grossly the heart is strikingly brown in colour and histology shows large amounts of brown pigment in myofibres, interstitial tissues and conducting system. This pigment gives a positive Prussian blue reaction. Chronic renal failure may also occasionally produce a sufficiently severe degree of oxalosis to affect the heart (SALYER and HUTCHINS 1974).

VI. Non-specific Myocardial Changes

Small foci of myofibre degeneration may be seen in many diseases associated with cardiac failure including severe anaemia, thyrotoxicosis, myxodema, and chronic alcoholism. Interstitial fibrosis is often also present in alcoholic heart disease (SCHENK and COHEN 1970), fatty degeneration of myofibres is common in anaemia and myxodematous hearts may have unusually well-marked degrees of basophilic myofibre change (see Sect. B).

VII. Tumours

Careful examination of the hearts of patients dying of malignant disease has shown cardiac metastases in 10%–15% of cases (DAVIES 1975) and metastatic tumours are therefore not uncommon in the elderly. Pancreas, breast, lung, and kidney are the most frequent primary sites.

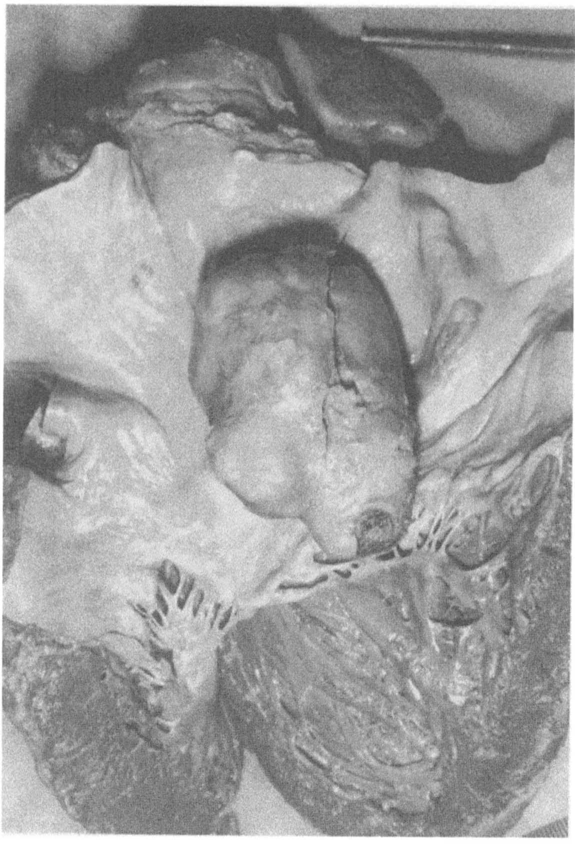

Fig. 13. Atrial myxoma. A large lobulated tumour is attached to the fossa ovale. Its apex is ulcerated and the mitral valve thickened. From a 73-year-old woman with a history of "heart trouble" for about 30 years

Primary cardiac tumours are rare, as at all ages. Most are myxomas, undiagnosed antemortem although patients often have had a long history of heart disease. HUDSON (1962) illustrates a case in a 95-year-old woman. Myxomas usually form smooth rounded tumours attached to the margins of the septum secundum (Fig. 13). They are distinguished from atrial thrombi by their firm attachment to the atrial septum, often by a definite pedicle and by the absence of mitral or tricuspid stenosis although some degree of mechanically produced valvular thickening is usual with tumours that are large enough to impinge on the valve cusps. Histologically they consist of characteristic lepidic cells in a myxomatous stroma.

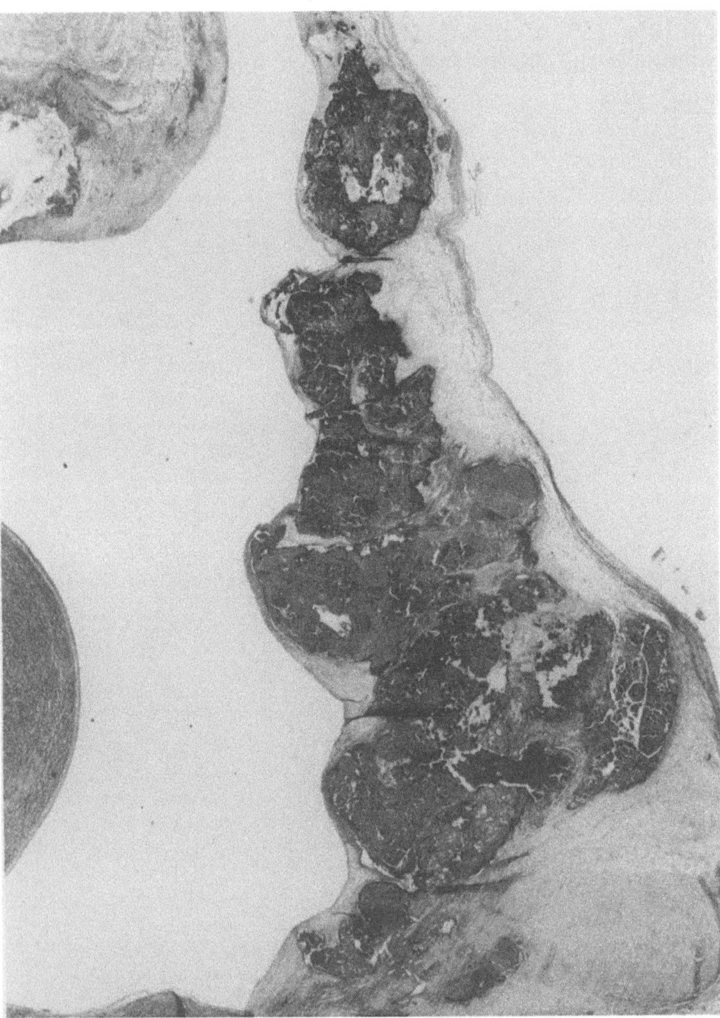

Fig. 14. Section of aortic valve cusp showing severe degenerative calcification. Solid darkly staining masses of calcium are distending the fibrosa. The changes are most extensive at the base of the cusp and do not extend to the free edge. No evidence of previous valvulitis is present. Haematoxylin and eosin, × 16, reduced to 80%

D. Valve Pathology

Valve disease in the elderly is predominantly the result of degenerative changes affecting the fibrosa. In most cases the degenerative process is an exaggeration of the normal ageing changes already described and results in aortic sclerosis and stenosis and mitral ring calcification. In a substantial minority it consists of mucoid degeneration with consequent expansion of the valve cusps and mitral systolic prolapse.

I. Aortic Sclerosis and Stenosis

In the aortic valve, degenerative calcification affects the fibrosa of the valve cusps. Solid masses of calcium develop, usually starting at the bases of the cusps where traumatic damage is greatest due to repeated flexion. With increasing severity the calcific masses expand along the fibrosa but rarely extend beyond the linea alba (Fig. 14). The valvular endocardium and free edges of the cusps are rarely involved if at all, a feature which makes for easy distinction from calcification following rheumatic or other inflammatory valve disease. Other features which distinguish degenerative from postinflammatory calcification are the absence of commissural adhesions and distortion of the free edges of the cusps in degenerative valve disease

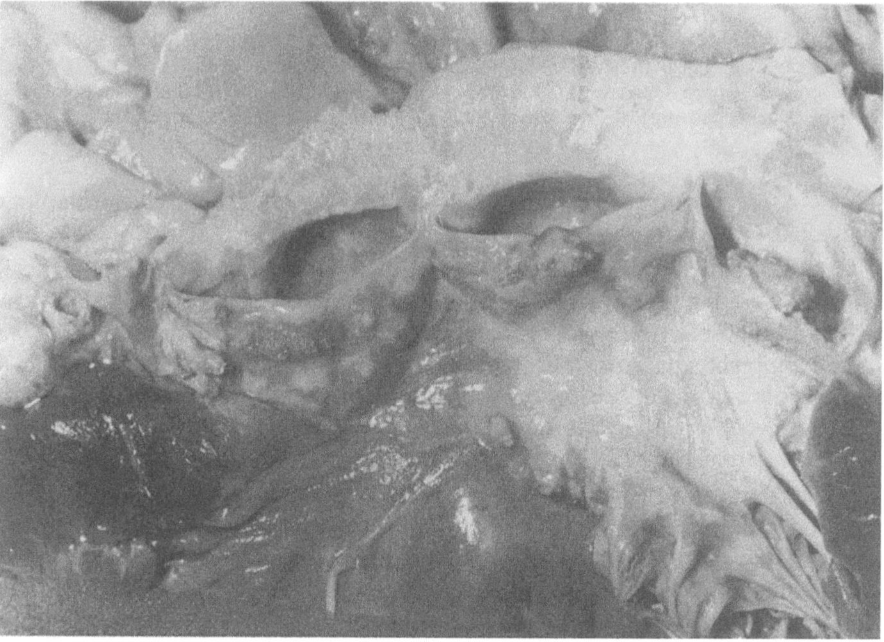

Fig. 15. Severe degenerative aortic valve calcification with superimposed thrombotic endocarditis. Nodular masses of calcium are distorting all three aortic valve cusps and vegetations can be seen on the nodulae Arantii and at the edge of the bisected left coronary cusp. Early mitral ring calcification is visible at the junction of membranous and musculature septum with the anterior mitral cusp, and a large plaque of lipid and several smaller plaques are also visible on the aortic face of the anterior mitral cusp

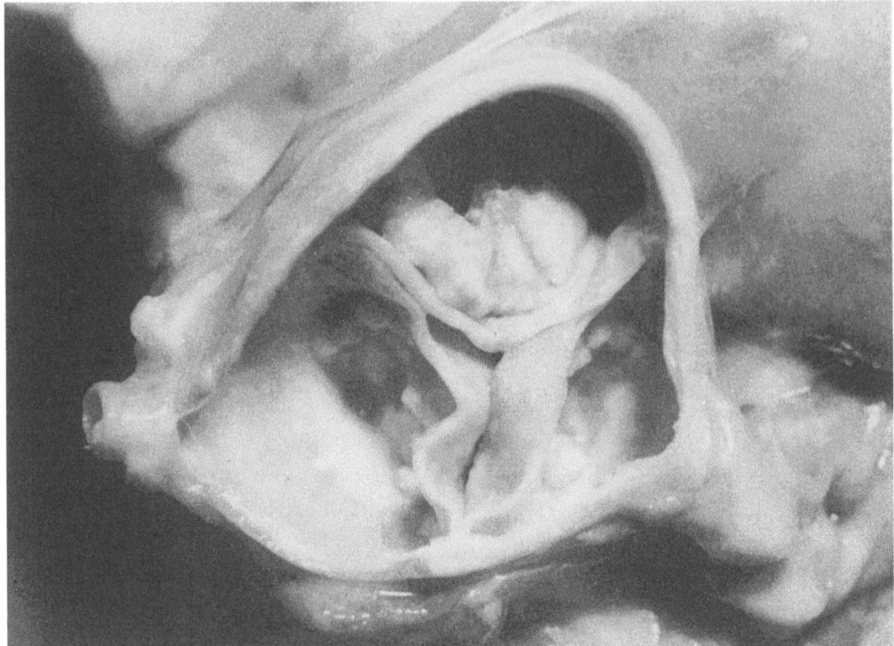

Fig. 16. Aortic stenosis due to degenerative calcification. The unopened aortic valve is seen from above. A large mass of calcium almost fills the non-coronary sinus and multiple smaller nodules are distorting the coronary cusps. The cusps show no significant thickening of free edges, contraction or commissural adhesions. The orifice is triradiate

and microscopically the small thick-walled vessels typical of postinflammatory valve pathology are absent.

In most patients the degree of valvular distortion is mild and the clinical effects consist of production of the systolic murmur of aortic sclerosis only. However, as with all valve deformities, there is an increased risk of endocarditis (Fig. 15). Aortic sclerosis appears unimportant in the genesis of cardiac failure. In personally studied cases it was one of the few conditions which was more common in patients who had not been in cardiac failure. The incidence of aortic sclerosis in these cases was 24% compared with 18% in failure cases.

Degenerative calcification is, however, the cause of most true *aortic stenosis* in geriatric patients. Previously normal three cusped valves may develop sufficiently severe calcification to immobilise the cusps (Fig. 16). This is responsible for most isolated aortic stenosis in patients over 75 years (POMERANCE 1972). Calcification in a congenitally bicuspid valve is the single most common cause of isolated aortic stenosis in adults (BACON and MATTHEWS 1959; POMERANCE 1972; ROBERTS 1970). The calcium is of the same degenerative type as in the older patients, primarily involving the cusp fibrosa and particularly the raphe of the conjoined cusp (Fig. 17). It appears about a decade before that in the normal three cusped valves, being accelerated by the mechanical stresses resulting from the abnormal anatomy and inability to open fully (EDWARDS 1961, 1962).

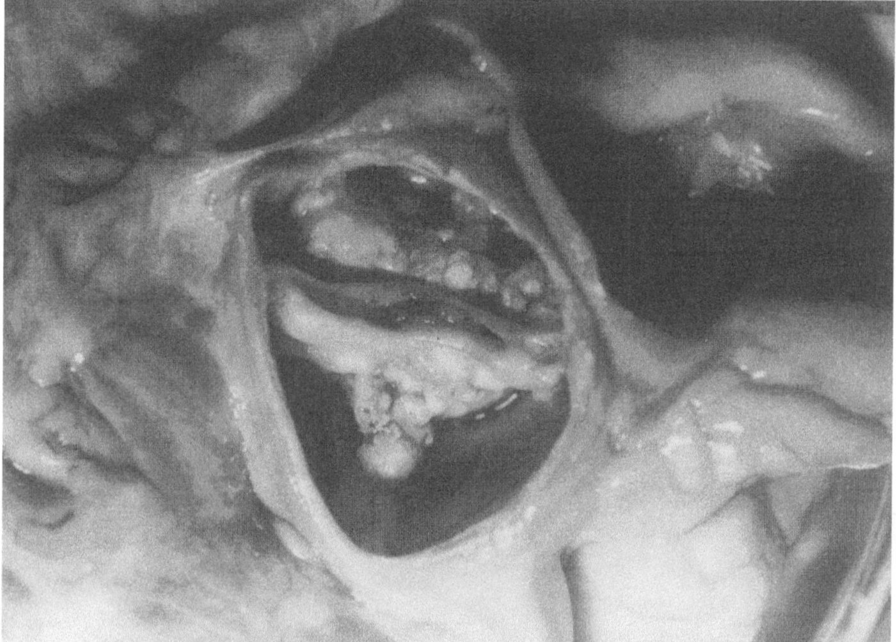

Fig. 17. Aortic stenosis due to degenerative calcification in a congenitally bicuspid aortic valve. The valve is viewed from above. The raphe between the congenitally fused cusps *(below)* is heavily calcified and large nodular masses of calcium are also distorting both the fused and the single cusp. Thrombotic endocarditis is further occluding the stenotic slit-like orifice

Although degenerative valve calcification is clearly an age-related condition it is not clear why it develops to a greater degree in some individuals than in others. Although men seem affected more than women the difference is not statistically significant (POMERANCE et al. 1978). As deposition of calcium appears related to mechanical factors an association with hypertension or cardiac hypertrophy is suggested but none has been found. Relevant metabolic factors also need to be considered but no correlation with serum calcium, phosphate or alkaline phosphatase has been found and histological comparison of bone density in patients with and without degenerative calcification has also shown no correlation (POMERANCE et al. 1978).

II. Mitral Ring Calcification

In the mitral apparatus degenerative calcification affects the valve ring, and cusp involvment is usually relatively minor and secondary. The sequence of pathological changes is the same as in the aortic cusp fibrosa with focal calcification usually appearing first in the part of the ring where the medial mitral commissure and muscular and membranous septum meet (Figs. 15, 18, 34) and in the centre of the posterior cusp attachment.

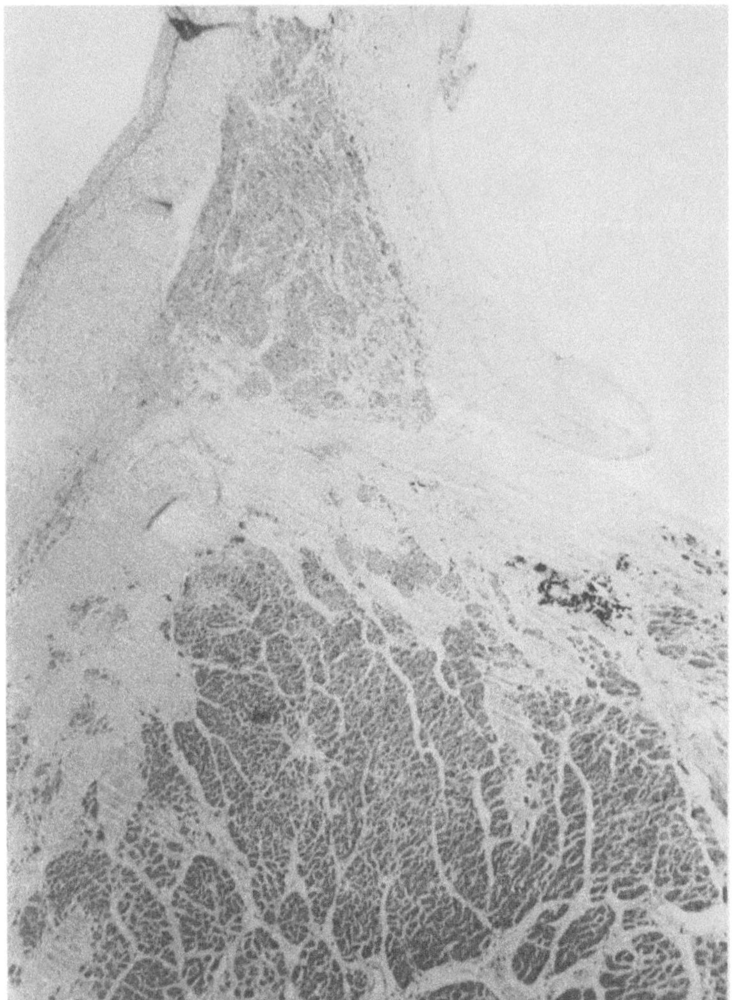

Fig. 18. Very early mitral ring calcification. Section through the interventricular septum showing the bundle of His *(upper centre)*. Early calcification is present at the junction of the ring fibrosa and ventricular muscle. Haematoxylin and eosin, × 40, reduced to 80%

Macroscopically the early lesions appear as small nodules and spicules which are clearly of no clinical significance. Larger calcified masses, even if localized, often produce sufficient cusp distortion to cause incompetence (Fig. 19). Extension in length and thickness eventually transforms the entire intramyocardial ring into a rigid C- or J-shaped bar, which may reach 2 cm diameter (Figs. 20 and 21). When calcification involves the entire ring the normal systolic contraction of the atrioventricular orifice is prevented with resulting mitral incompetence. Extension of calcium into the subvalve angle is common and may form a prominent ridge over which the posterior mitral cusp becomes stretched and to which the chordae tendinae become adherent. Occasionally the calcified bar undergoes central necro-

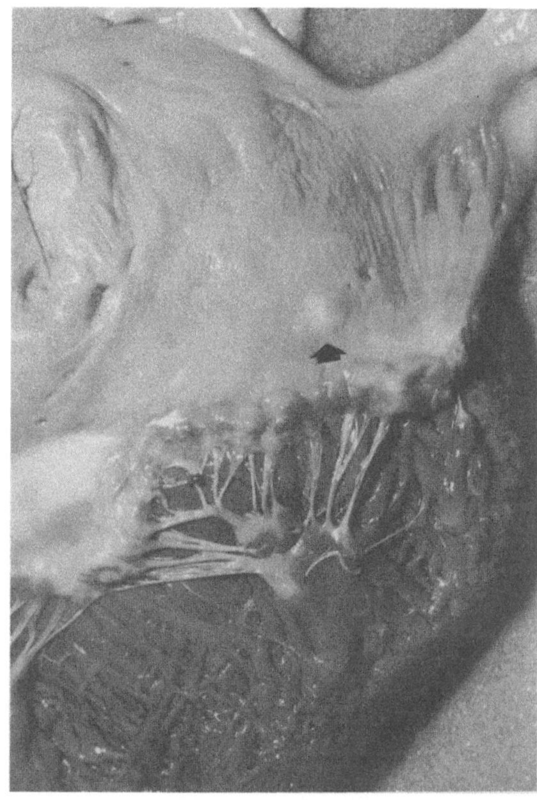

Fig. 19. Mild mitral ring calcification with mitral incompetence. There is a spur of calcium distorting the posterior mitral cusp adjacent to the cut edge. A patch of endocardial fibrous thickening in the atrial wall just above and medial to the spur *(arrow)* is caused by the incompetent jet

sis resulting in a caseous looking "abscess", which may reach a considerable size (Fig. 22). Such lesions can easily be mistaken for a tuberculoma or gumma.

Masses of calcium may erode through the atrial surface of the valve cusps (Fig. 20) and the exposed calcium provides a site for thrombus deposition. These thrombi may reach considerable size and be a source of major emboli (FULKERSON et al. 1979; GUTHRIE and FAIRGRIEVE 1963; KORN et al. 1962; POMERANCE 1970). Emboli consisting of calcific debris only have also been recorded (FULKERSON et al. 1979; RIDOLFI and HUTCHINS 1976). Bacterial endocarditis may result from infection of these thrombi.

Thrombi and infected vegetations based on mitral ring calcification are characteristically found at the base of the valve cusps in contrast to the usual site on contact margins or jet lesions. A high incidence of ring abscesses has been noted in infective endocarditis based on mitral ring calcification (MAMBO et al. 1978).

Microscopically (Figs. 18 and 23) basophilic solid masses of calcium are seen, initially localised to the ring fibrosa but with increasing size encroaching on the fibrosa of the valve cusp and extending into the septal ventricular myocardium.

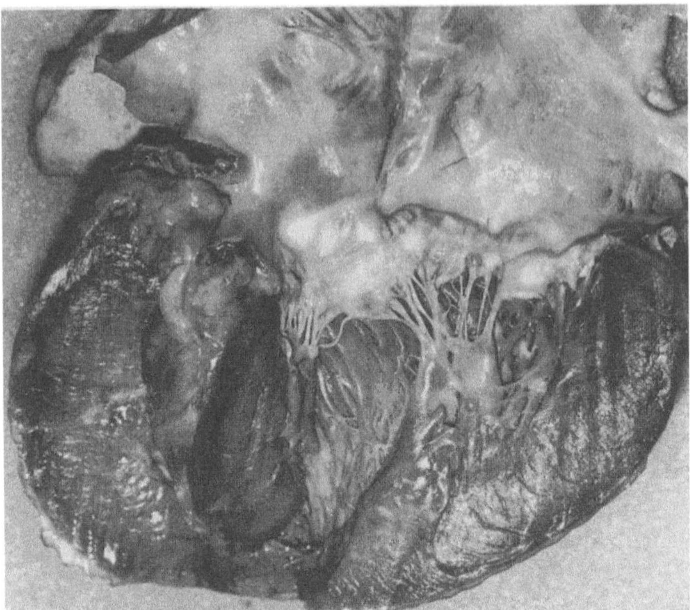

Fig. 20. Mitral ring calcification associated with hypertrophic cardiomyopathy. A spur of calcium has ulcerated through the atrial surface at the medial commissure. A marked degree of left ventricular hypertrophy is also seen and a subaortic fibrous band similar to that in Fig. 10 was also present

Rupture through into the subvalve angle is common and surrounding fibrosis is often present and may produce a marked degree of thickening in the subvalve angle. As in the aortic valve, thin-walled vessels, and mild chronic inflammatory cell infiltration are often present at the edge of the calcified areas but again the thick-walled small vessels of postinflammatory valve disease are absent. Cartilage and even, rarely, bone may be seen although this finding is much less frequent than in aortic valve calcification. Acute inflammation and necrosis may be present in the overlying cusp or in the adjacent myocardium, as may old or recent hemorrhage. Calcification may provoke a foreign body type giant cell reaction and occasionally a pallissaded fibroblastic reaction with necrosis, similar to a rheumatoid nodule, may be seen (Pomerance 1970).

Age and Sex. Mitral ring calcification is rare below 70 years and shows a marked and statistically significant correlation with advancing age beyond this (Pomerance et al. 1978) although, like senile cardiac amyloidosis, there is a fall in extreme old age. Ischii and Sternby (1978) observed only four cases amongst their 23 centenarians. The condition is significantly commoner in women, the reported ratios varying from 3:2 to over 4:1 (Pomerance et al. 1978; Simon and Liu 1954). Massive mitral ring calcification is almost entirely a disease of elderly women (Korn et al. 1962; Sugiura et al. 1977).

The *clinical significance* of mitral ring calcification is, predictably, related to severity. Minor degrees are usually of no clinical importance but patients with suf-

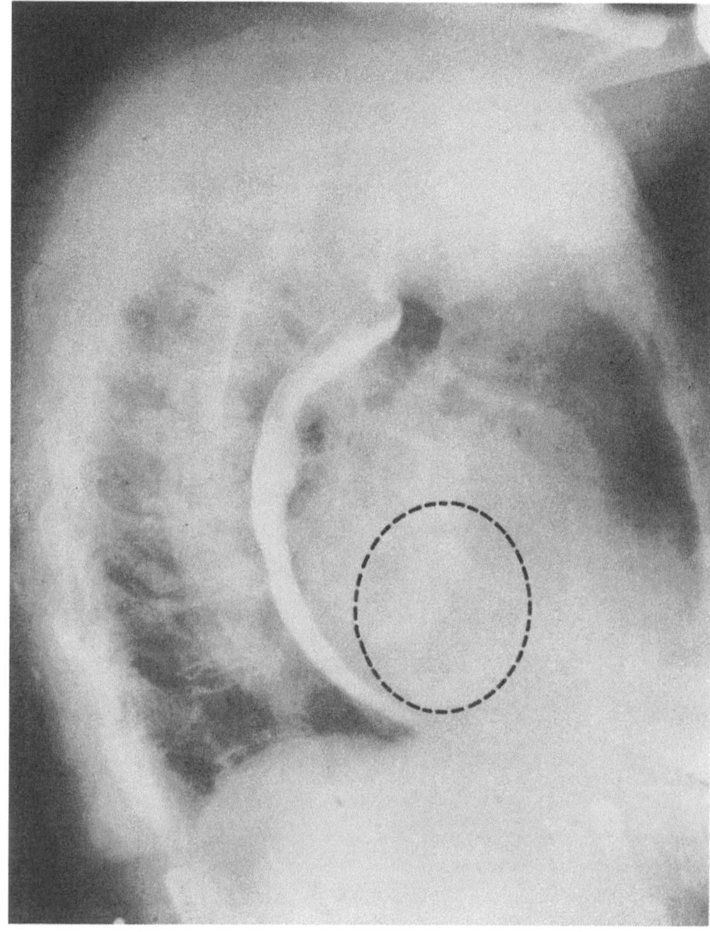

Fig. 21. Massive mitral ring calcification *(ringed)* seen in the lateral view of a barium swallow chest X-ray

ficient calcification to cause even localised distortion are likely to have systolic murmurs indicating mitral incompetence (DENHAM et al. 1977; FERTMAN and WOLFF 1946; GEILL 1951; POMERANCE 1970; SIMON and LIU 1954; SUGIURA et al. 1977). Mitral stenosis may be present in massive calcification if the calcium extends to the base of the valve cusps or forms a prominent subvalvar ring. Such marked degrees of ring calcification are easily seen on routine chest X-Rays (Fig. 21); less marked ring calcification requires echocardiography (Fig. 24) for clinical diagnosis.

Congestive cardiac failure due to massive mitral ring calcification is now well recognized (KORN et al. 1962; SUGIURA et al. 1977) but lesser degrees are rarely directly responsible for failure. However, the incidence of mitral ring calcification is considerably higher in patients with cardiac failure than without. In our recent study (HODKINSON and POMERANCE 1979) the comparative incidences were 26%

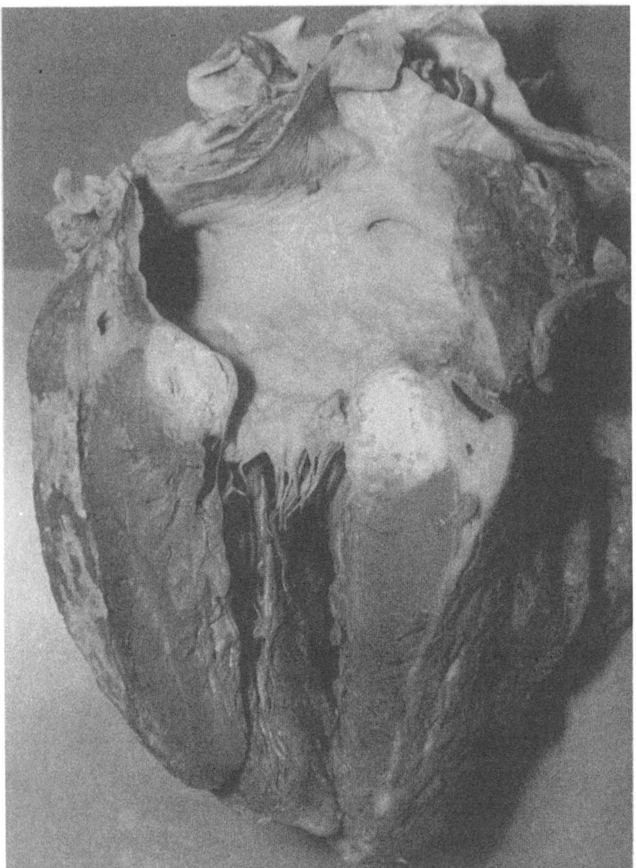

Fig. 22. Massive mitral ring calcification with caseous necrosis. From a 73-year-old woman who died of uraemia. Courtesy of Dr. C. Tribe

and 12% respectively. It seems likely that even the relatively minor functional impairment produced contributes to the polypathic cardiac failure which is so often encountered in the elderly.

Conduction disturbances are common, as might be anticipated from the anatomical relationships between the mitral ring and bundle of His (Fig. 18). They range from minor degrees of bundle branch block to complete heart block (KORN et al. 1962; LEV 1964; POMERANCE 1970; RYTAND and LIPSITCH 1946; SIMON and LIU 1954) and FULKERSON et al. (1979) also found evidence of diffuse conducting system disease in over half their series of 80 patients with roentgenographically proven mitral ring calcification. This series also showed a relatively high incidence of embolic complications.

Infective endocarditis is less frequent than would be expected from the degree of valvular deformity often present in this common disease but once developed is resistant to treatment (MAMBO et al. 1978).

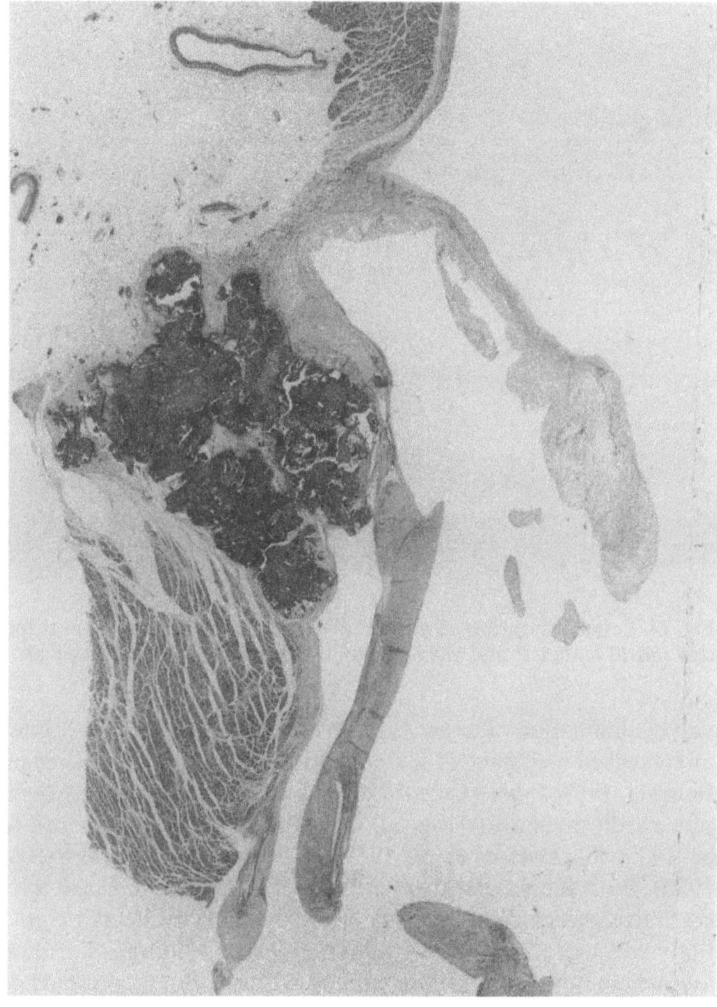

Fig. 23. Section through the posterior left ventricular wall showing a large nodular mass of calcium in the valve ring extending into the subvalve angle with a chorda tendina stretched over it. Haematoxylin and eosin, × 7, reduced to 80%

As with aortic valve calcification it is not entirely clear why only a minority of elderly patients should develop this exaggerated ageing change although the association with mechanical factors is stronger for mitral ring calcification. There is no correlation with rheumatic, rheumatoid or other inflammatory heart disease. Associations with diabetes mellitus (KIRK and RUSSELL 1969) and osteitis deformans (HARRISON and LENNOX 1948) have been reported although not present in our material. Metastatic calcification frequently affects the mitral ring and an increased incidence of soft tissue, tracheal, costal cartilage, and aortic calcification was noted by ISCHII and STERNBY (1978) in their patients with mitral ring calcification. However, no evidence of abnormal calcium metabolism has been found in degenerative

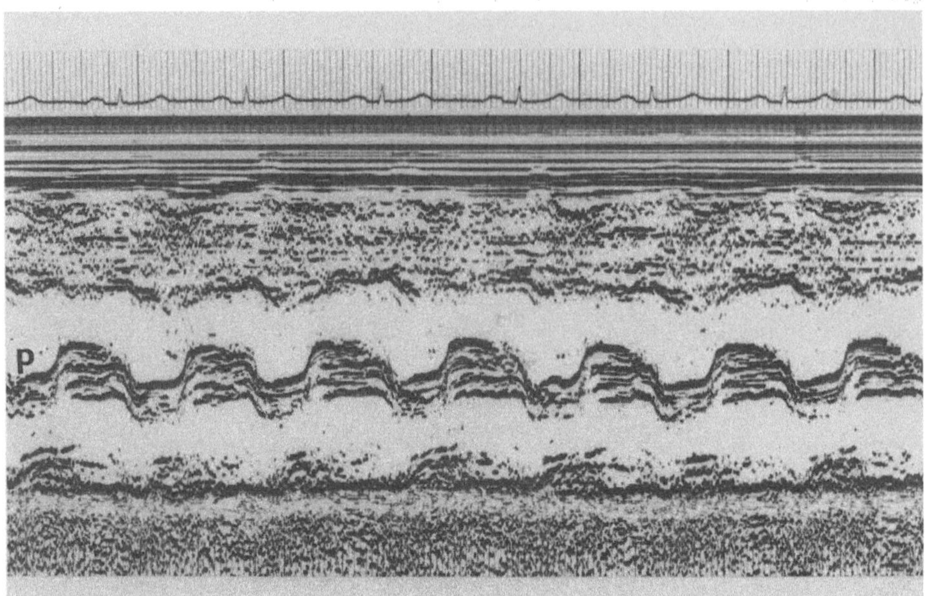

Fig. 24. Echocardiogram of mitral valve calcification showing multiple echoes in the posterior mitral leaflet *P* and slow diastolic closure rate. Courtesy of Dr. R. Pridie

valve calcification of either type (POMERANCE et al. 1978). Some studies have shown an increased incidence of systemic hypertension (FULKERSON et al. 1979; KIRK and RUSSELL 1969; POMERANCE 1970) and more recently an association with hypertrophic cardiomyopathy (Fig. 20) and aortic stenosis have been noted (DROBINSKI et al. 1979; FULKERSON et al. 1979; KRONZON and GLASSMAN 1978; SCHOTT et al. 1977). Both these conditions are associated with increased left ventricular systolic pressures. A significant correlation with increased heart weight after correction for body size was found in our material. These findings all indicate that mechanical factors are important in determining whether elderly patients do or do not develop significant mitral ring calcification.

The reason for the striking female predominance remains obscure. There is no correlation with parity (POMERANCE 1970). The prevalence of osteoporosis in elderly women has suggested the existence of a factor affecting the distribution of calcium between bone and soft tissue (BLANKENHORN 1964) but we have found no correlation between histologically measured osteoporosis and degenerative valve calcification. Possibly the mitral ring reacts differently to injury in women, a suggestion supported by the well-known female preponderance of rheumatic mitral stenosis although rheumatic carditis is equally common in both sexes.

III. Mucoid Degeneration – The Floppy Mitral Valve

This degenerative process also affects the fibrosa but involves mainly the central fibrous plate of the mitral valve cusps. In contrast to the rigidity and sclerosis of calcific degenerative disease, mucoid degeneration results in softening of the fi-

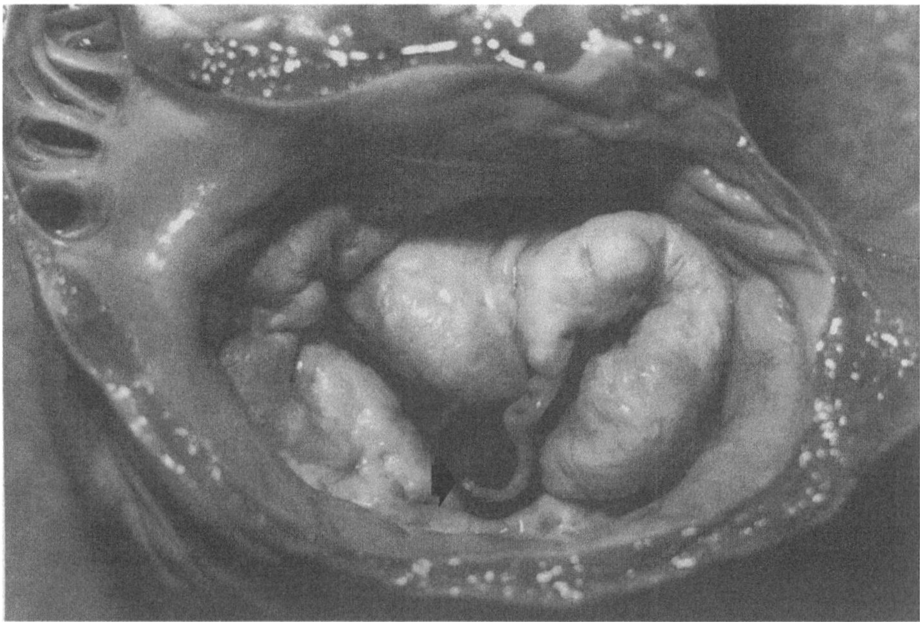

Fig. 25. Ruptured chorda tendina in mucoid degeneration. The mitral valve is seen from above and has been fixed in the systolic position showing prolapse into the left atrium. The *arrow* indicates a ruptured chorda tendina also prolapsing into the atrium

brosa, with consequent expansion of the cusps and stretching of the chordae tendinae and systolic mitral cusp prolapse. It seems probable that most cases of mitral valve prolapse and its numerous synonyms, (see JERESATY 1979) are due to primary mucoid degeneration, which is, therefore, a common condition. Its comparatively recent recognition is due more to the realisation that not all chronic valve disease is congenital or rheumatic rather than to any actual change in its prevalence. Mitral valve prolapse has been reported in between 6% and 10% of apparently healthy young subjects (DARSEE et al. 1979) and a similar figure of 5%–7% has been recorded for significant primary mucoid degeneration in autopsies on patients over 60 years (DAVIES et al. 1978; POMERANCE 1969). Most autopsy cases have been in elderly patients; the average age of a personally studied series was 73 years. DAVIES et al. (1978) found that the incidence tended to increase with age.

Macroscopically the primary change is usually confined to the mitral valve. Part or all of either or both cusps may be affected, the posterior being involved more often and usually more severely than the anterior. The most striking feature is expansion of the cusps, the posterior leaflet being up to twice the depth of the anterior instead of the normal half to two-thirds. Cusps are white, opaque, and voluminous resembling a partly collapsed parachute or balloon. Systolic prolapse can be easily demonstrable at post-mortem by gentle pressure on the fluid-filled left ventricle before opening or by fixation in the systolic position (Fig. 25). The mitral ring may also be dilated (BULKLEY and ROBERTS 1975; DAVIES et al. 1978). Similar changes may be present in the tricuspid valve although these are usually less severe. On sec-

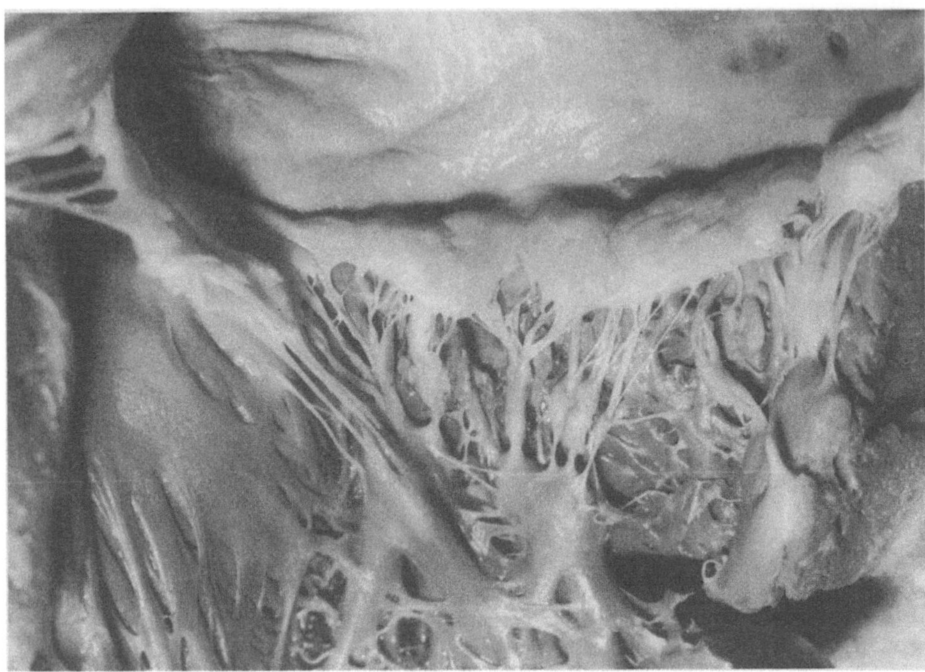

Fig. 26. Ballooning deformity (floppy valve) of the posterior mitral cusp. There is a large friction lesion on the ventricular endocardium below the junction of the two lateral scallops and chordae tendinae have become firmly incorporated into this fibrous plaque

Table 3. Pathology of primary mucoid degeneration compared with that of chronic rheumatic valve disease

Primary mucoid degeneration	Chronic rheumatic valve disease
Cusps expanded	Cusp contracts (fibrosis following inflammation)
No commissural adhesions	Commissural adhesions usually present
No calcification	Calcification common
Chordae thin and tapered	Chordae usually thickened fused and contracted
Ventricular mural friction changes often present	No mural friction changes
Only fibrosa affected	All valve layers involved
Cusp layers remain distinct	Disorganisation of cusp architecture and fibrosis
No vascularisation	Small thick-walled vessels usually present
Degenerative process	Inflammatory process

tioning, affected cusps often have a rather cartilaginous semi-translucent appearance. The chordae tendinae are long and thin, usually tapering from thickened leaflet insertions. Small areas of ulceration and thrombus are often seen on the atrial surfaces of the ectatic cusps, since these are easily traumatised in normal valve movement. Morphological evidence of mitral incompetence is often visible as marked atrial dilatation or jet lesions of the atrial endocardium. Left ventricular

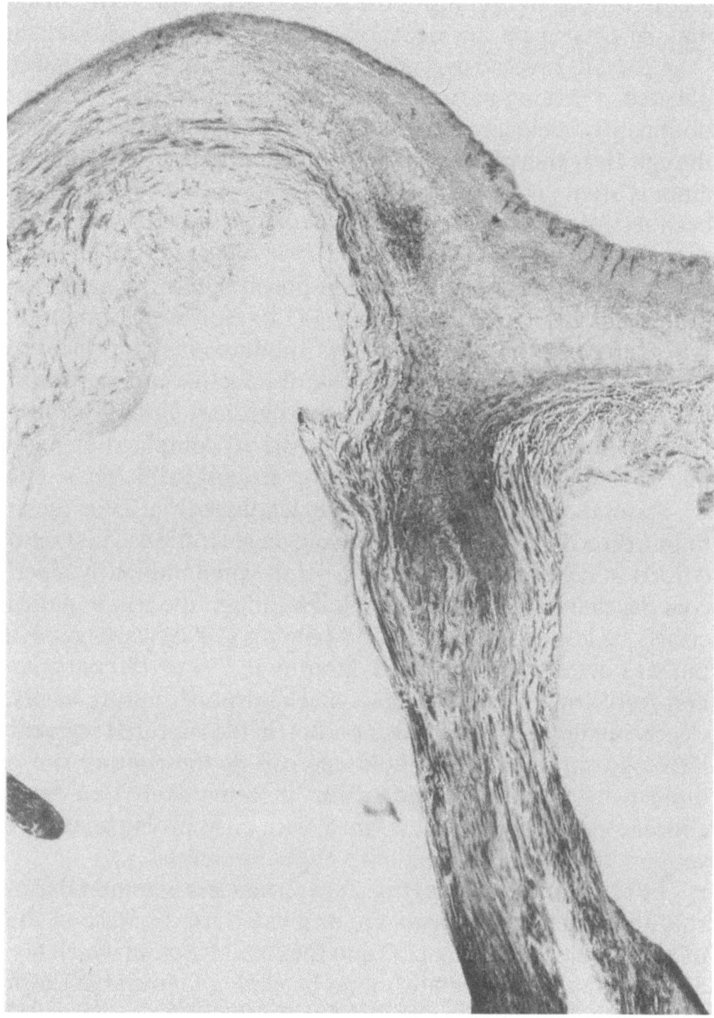

Fig. 27. Section through part of a mitral valve with mucoid degeneration. The normal dark staining dense collagen has been largely replaced by a loose connective tissue. Elastic van Gieson, × 20, reduced to 80%

friction lesions are common because the normal anatomical relationships between chordae tendinae and posterior ventricular wall are altered by the cusp prolapse (SALAZAR and EDWARDS 1970). When well marked these lesions may incorporate the chordae tendinae (Fig. 26) and the combination of valve deformity and chordal adhesion may mislead those unfamiliar with the pathology of mucoid degeneration into a diagnosis of chronic rheumatic valve disease. However, the pathologies of these two conditions have little in common (Table 3).

Microscopically (Fig. 27) a loose spongy myxoid tissue replaces the normally dense collagen of the cusp fibrosa. This has the staining characteristics of an acid mucopolysaccharide. The chordae tendinae may show similar changes. Some degree of fibrous thickening of the atrial endocardium is usual and small foci of fibrin may be present on, or incorporated near, the endocardial surface.

Clinically mucoid degeneration is almost always a benign condition unless complicated. The long natural history ensures that cases seen at autopsy will be predominantly in elderly subjects and the condition is often clinically unsuspected. Although clear morphological and clinical evidence of well-marked mitral incompetence is often present, this incompetence appears very well tolerated. Patients have been recorded known to have murmurs for over 20 years (ALLEN et al. 1974; BITTAR and SOSA 1968; DAVIES et al. 1978; JERESATY 1979; TRESCH et al. 1979) and about half the patients included in hospital autopsy series have died of unrelated causes (DAVIES 1978; POMERANCE 1975). However, primary mucoid degeneration is not infrequently complicated by "spontaneous" rupture of the chordae tendinae and it also carries an increased risk of infective endocarditis. It seems that elderly patients are probably at greater risk from these complications (TRESCH et al. 1979). Unexplained sudden death is an occasional complication and the condition is also one of those which often contributes to polypathic heart failure.

Spontaneous rupture of chordae tendinae (Fig. 25) is the usual cause of cardiac failure directly resulting from mucoid degeneration. This complication has been recorded in between 11% and 13% of the predominantly elderly patients with mucoid degeneration dying in hospital although the risk in patients as a whole would clearly be less. In JERESATY's 350 patients (1979) it was reported in only five cases but was detected by echocardiography in 7% of 190 patients by CHANDRARATNA and ARONOW (1979). The exact mechanism of rupture varies. In many cases it is clearly related to mucoid degeneration in the ruptured segment of chorda; in others histology shows only fibrinoid necrosis at the rupture site or rather corrugated bundles of collagen. In these cases it seems likely that excessive tension on the chordae alone is responsible since, with cusp prolapse, there is loss of the normal support from the coapting cusp edges in systole.

Infective endocarditis (Fig. 28) appears less common than spontaneous chordal rupture but elderly patients are at greater risk because of the increased liklihood of bacteraemia (see Sect. DV) and the small thrombi which are often present on the atrial surface of the ectatic cusps provide a favourable site for growth of microorganisms. Vegetations also develop on the jet lesions caused by the mitral incompetence. These are usually found on the interatrial septum or on the posterior atrial wall.

Sudden death is fortunately not a common complication of mucoid degeneration (DAVIES et al. 1978; JERESATY 1979). Its mechanism is still not understood. Although ischaemia-like chest pain and ECG changes are often present in otherwise asymptomatic mitral valve prolapse (GOOCH et al. 1972), there is usually no morphological evidence of coronary artery insufficiency. The possibility of an associated cardiomyopathy has been raised and abnormal histochemistry, increased interstitial fibrosis and mitochondrial degenerative changes have recently been reported (MALCOLM et al. 1979; MASON et al. 1978).

The aetiology of primary mucoid degeneration is still not determined. The association of similar valve pathology with connective tissue disorders such as Marfan's syndrome (McKUSICK 1972) with minor skeletal abnormalities (DEVEREUX et al. 1976; GOOCH et al. 1972; SALOMON et al. 1975; UDOSHI et al. 1979) and the oc-

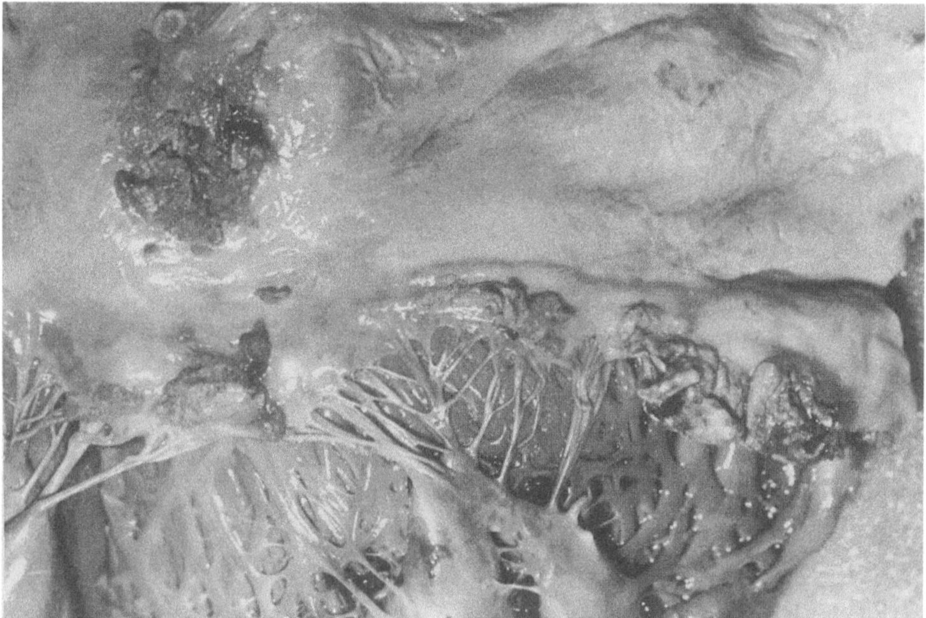

Fig. 28. Infective endocarditis on mucoid degeneration. The posterior mitral cusp is expanded and large vegetations are present on the apposing edges of both mitral cusps and also on the jet lesion on the atrial septum

casional familial cases suggest that genetic factors may be concerned. The predominance of elderly patients in autopsy series and the existence of a similar age-related valve degeneration in dogs (POMERANCE and WHITNEY 1970) suggest that ageing may be a factor. DAVIES et al. (1978) suggested that the development of mucoid degeneration may be analogous to the changes developing in skin with advancing age.

IV. Chronic Inflammatory Valve Disease

1. Rheumatic Valve Disease

With the virtual disappearance of rheumatic carditis in Great Britain, chronic rheumatic valve deformities are now seen mainly in the elderly. In our most recent study the incidence was 3% and earlier series have reported an incidence of about 5% (BEDFORD and CAIRD 1960; POMERANCE 1965).

Minor degrees of postinflammatory valvular scarring (Fig. 29) are rather more common and their incidence has not decreased significantly. These lesions are of no clinical significance other than as a cause of mitral murmurs (DENHAM et al. 1977) and possibly as predisposing to endocarditis (OKA and ANGRIST 1967; OKA et al. 1968).

The pathology of rheumatic valve disease does not differ significantly from that in younger patients. Mitral valve changes range from relatively minor degrees of

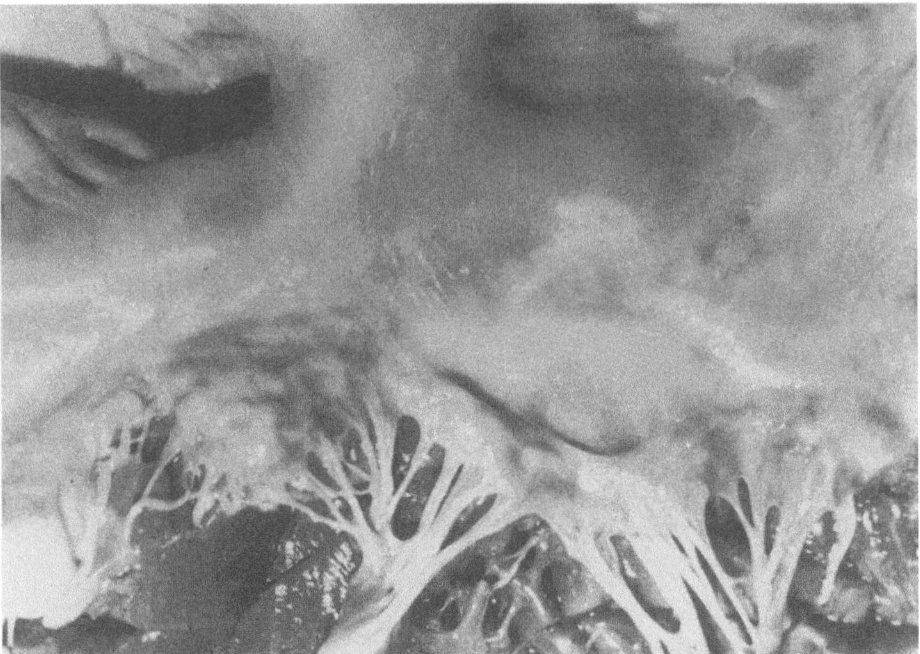

Fig. 29. Minor postinflammatory scarring of the anterior mitral cusp. Part of the posterior mitral cusp is also included and shows a mild degree of ballooning deformity due to mucoid degeneration

cusp scarring and commissural adhesions to grossly thickened and distorted cusps with adherent thick and contracted chordae tendinae (Fig. 30). Aortic cusps show thickening and contraction usually with fused commissures (see Fig. 32). Calcification is common in both valves and mainly affects the fused commissures. *Histologically* normal valve architecture is disorganised with irregular fibrosis involving all layers of the cusps and small thick-walled vessels are usually present. Fibrin deposits at varying stages of organisation are often seen, together with small filiform processes (Lambl's excrescences) with a characteristic laminar fibro-elastic structure which are derived from partially detached fibrin deposits. Progression of the valve deformity is the result of a continuing cycle of fibrin deposition, organisation to fibrous tissue, and increasing deformity which attracts further fibrin deposition. It is not due to continuing inflammatory activity (MAGAREY 1949).

Although the pathological features are still widely accepted as pathognomonic of rheumatic valve disease, they are actually non-specific sequelae of severe valvulitis with thrombus formation and their invariable relationship with rheumatic carditis is now being debated. Many elderly patients give no history of past rheumatic fever and while poor memory must account for some of these cases, there is increasing evidence for a non-rheumatic origin in others. The comparatively recent decline in chronic rheumatic heart disease has been in cases with rheumatic histories while those with no relevant histories have not declined (VENDSBORG et al. 1968). Many organisms are well known to affect the pericardium and myocardium and it is im-

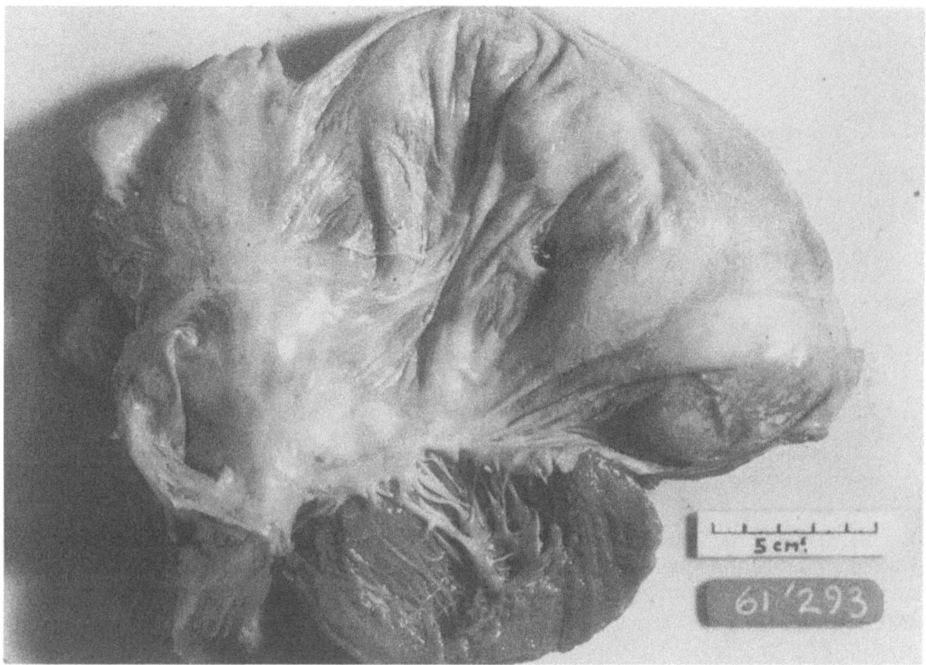

Fig. 30. Rheumatic mitral valve disease with marked left atrial dilatation. The mitral valve cusps are contracted and thickened and the chordae are thickened and fused

probable that the valves are spared. Indeed routine sections of mitral valves in unselected autopsies not infrequently show a mild valvulitis. In Britain and the United States Coxackie, ECHO, psittacosis, and mycoplasma are the most likely causative agents (BURCH et al. 1970; BURCH and GILES 1972; LANCET 1971, 1974; WARD 1975, 1978). Once valve damage has occurred the same cycle of fibrin deposition and organization operates as in rheumatic valvulitis, with eventual fibrous thickening and distortion.

2. Rheumatoid and Other Inflammatory Diseases

Rheumatoid disease occasionally affects the heart. Rheumatoid granulomas form in the fibrosa of the aortic and mitral cusps as well as in the myocardium (CARPENTER et al. 1967; ROBERTS et al. 1968). In the mitral valve they are usually of no practical importance (IVESON and POMERANCE 1977) but in the aortic valve the resultant fibrous thickening and contraction of the cusps produces aortic incompetence. Because the granulomas rarely reach the endocardial surface the active stage is not associated with thrombus deposition and therefore commissural adhesions do not form and there is no stenosis.

Ankylosing spondylitis (BULKLEY and ROBERTS 1973; GRAHAM and SMYTHE 1958) and Reiter's disease (PAULUS et al. 1972) are other systemic inflammatory diseases which may rarely cause aortic incompetence in the elderly.

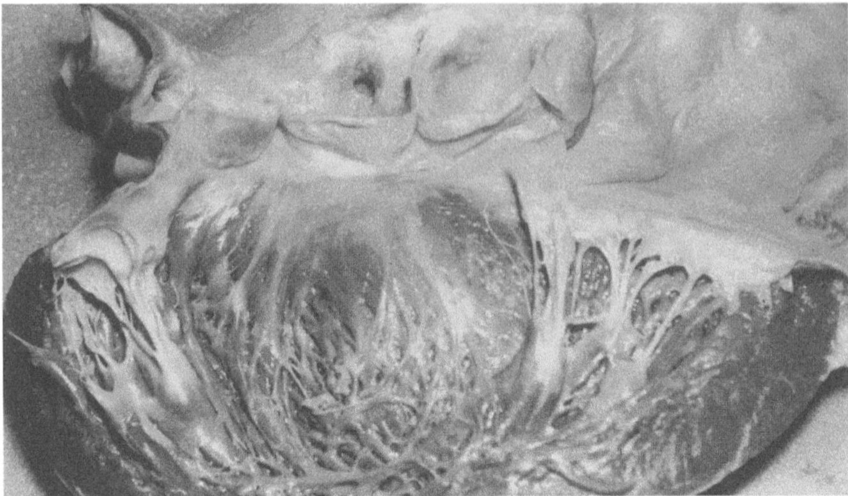

Fig. 31. Senile aortic incompetence. The aortic valve cusps have cord-like thickening of the free edges indicating incompetence due to aortic ring dilatation. The left ventricle is dilated and hypertrophied. From a 77-year-old woman with known aortic incompetence for 5 years before death

Syphilis is now rare in Britain although this is clearly not a universal finding. SUGIURA et al. (1975) found syphilitic aortic regurgitation in over 21% of their series of 1,000 elderly patients.

The aortic incompetence in all these three conditions is secondary to inflammatory dilatation of the aorta and there are no inflammatory changes in the valves themselves. The valve pathology is similar in all, with widened commissures due to the aortic dilatation and cord-like thickening of the free edges of the valve cusps due to exposure to the regurgitant blood stream. A similar appearance is seen in some cases of the idiopathic aortic incompetence of the elderly (Fig. 31). This condition was noted in 4.4% of BEDFORD and CAIRD'S (1960) cases although it has been very uncommon in more recent material. The underlying pathology in these cases is probably varied. Some show minor non-specific inflammatory aortic scarring but most appear to be due to hypertension and dilatation of the aortic ring with age (GOULEY and SICKEL 1943) and show only minor cystic degeneration and loss of elastica.

V. Infective Endocarditis

This condition has increasingly become a disease of elderly patients, often with no preceding valve disease (HUGHES and GAULD 1966; LANCET 1967; LERNER and WEINSTEIN 1966). In a recent study of 70 cases from this country one-third of the patients were over 60 years of age and the peak incidence was in the 7th decade (SCHNURR et al. 1977). The changing pattern has only been partly due to the introduction of antibiotics and decline in rheumatic fever. An important factor is increasing survival to ages where degenerative valve diseases become common as do conditions requiring diagnostic and surgical procedures likely to produce bacteremia.

In geriatric patients, as with many diseases in this age group, symptoms are often atypical and clinical diagnosis not made or delayed, the infective organism is likely to be a virulent one and many cases are not diagnosed ante mortem. Although *Streptococcus viridans* is still isolated in a high proportion of cases, *Staphylococcus pyogenes*, enterococci and pneumococci are now the commonest organisms. Fungal infections are becoming more frequent, usually associated with long-term antibiotics, steroids or treatment of malignancy. Blood cultures may be negative, possibly just because of previous antibiotics or poor bacteriological technique, but uraemia or prolonged infection alone may be responsible.

Macroscopically infective endocarditis is characterised by vegetations which are nodular, usually friable masses generally found on the atrial surfaces of the atrioventricular valves or the ventricular surfaces of the aortic valves. The pulmonary valve is rarely affected. They also form on the jet lesions produced by valvular incompetence (see Fig. 28). The vegetations vary from pinhead size to large masses which may almost block the valve orifices; the very large vegetations are usually due to fungal infections. Perforations of the cusps are common, particularly with pyogenic staphyloccal and pneumococcal infections. Abscesses of the aortic or mitral valve rings (Fig. 32) form if infection extends to these structures (MAMBO et al. 1978; SHELDON and GOLDEN 1951).

Microscopically the vegetations consist of fibrin, red cells, leucocytes, and micro-organisms. The underlying cusps show inflammation with necrosis. Small abscesses and focal inflammatory cellular infiltration are often present in the myocardium and occasionally the abscesses may be visible to the naked eye.

The underlying valve pathology may be rheumatic or congenital, as in younger patients, the congenital deformity usually being a bicuspid aortic valve. Infection on degenerative valve diseases has been discussed in the appropriate sections. Pacemaker wires and prosthetic valves, being foreign bodies, also predispose to infection. However, in geriatric patients the largest single group are those with no obvious underlying abnormality (Table 4) (APPLEFIELD and HORNICK 1974; SCHNURR et al. 1977; THELL et al. 1975). In many of these cases minor postinflammatory changes can often be found on careful inspection of the infected valves and such minor pathology is easily destroyed or overlooked. It is also likely that the high incidence in some reported series was due to failure to recognise mucoid degeneration since this condition has only come into prominence relatively recently. However, even allowing for such cases it is clear that many instances of infective endocarditis in the elderly do arise on previously normal valves and there is good evidence that the endocarditis then has developed as a result of stress. Valvular swelling and oedema can be induced experimentally by a variety of stress producing stimuli including surgery and infection (OKA et al. 1968) and similar lesions can often be seen in patients dying in hospital. They appear as minute translucent nodules along the closure lines of the cusps. The endocardium over these lesions is easily traumatised and small thrombi form and if bacteraemia then occurs these thrombi are colonised and develop into bacterial vegetations (OKA et al. 1968). The same stages in development of infected vegetations can be seen in human heart valves.

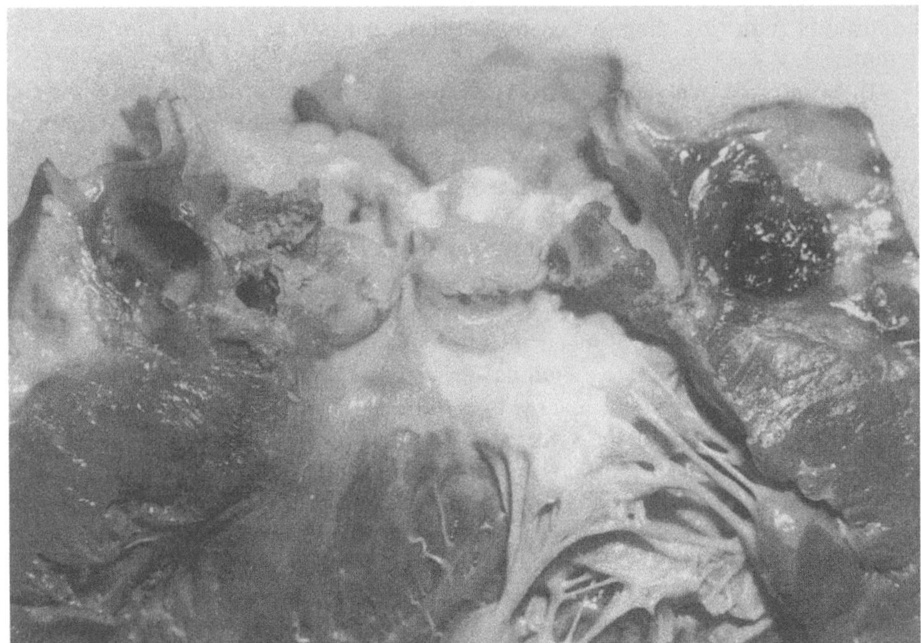

Fig. 32. Infective endocarditis (staphylococcal) of aortic valve with ring abscess. Both the aortic and the mitral cusps show thickening contraction and commissural adhesions due to previous rheumatic carditis. The left coronary cusp is perforated and the coronary sinus communicates with a cavity which is partly filled by blood clot. From a 72-year-old woman with rheumatic fever in childhood and typical clinical signs of infective endocarditis which failed to respond to treatment

Table 4. Underlying valve abnormalities in infective endocarditis (autopsy cases)

Underlying pathology	Under 65 years (29 cases)	Over 65 years (21 cases)
Inflammatory (including rheumatic)	20% ($^2/_5$ rheumatic)	19% (all rheumatic)
Congenital	14%	10%
Floppy valve	14%	14%
Degenerative calcific	0	14%
Iatrogenic (including pacemakers, prostheses)	30%	10%
Normal	20%	38%

VI. Non-Bacterial Thrombotic Endocarditis

This conditions is common in the elderly, simply because of its association with disseminated malignancy and other wasting diseases. It is seen most often with carcinoma of the pancreas, stomach or lung (POMERANCE 1975) but may also be found in well-nourished patients without malignant disease.

As in infective endocarditis NBTE is characterised by vegetations on the closure lines of the cusps (Fig. 33), almost always mitral or aortic. The vegetations vary in size and colour and are macroscopically indistinguishable from those of infective endocarditis. Histologically they differ in the absence of inflammatory reac-

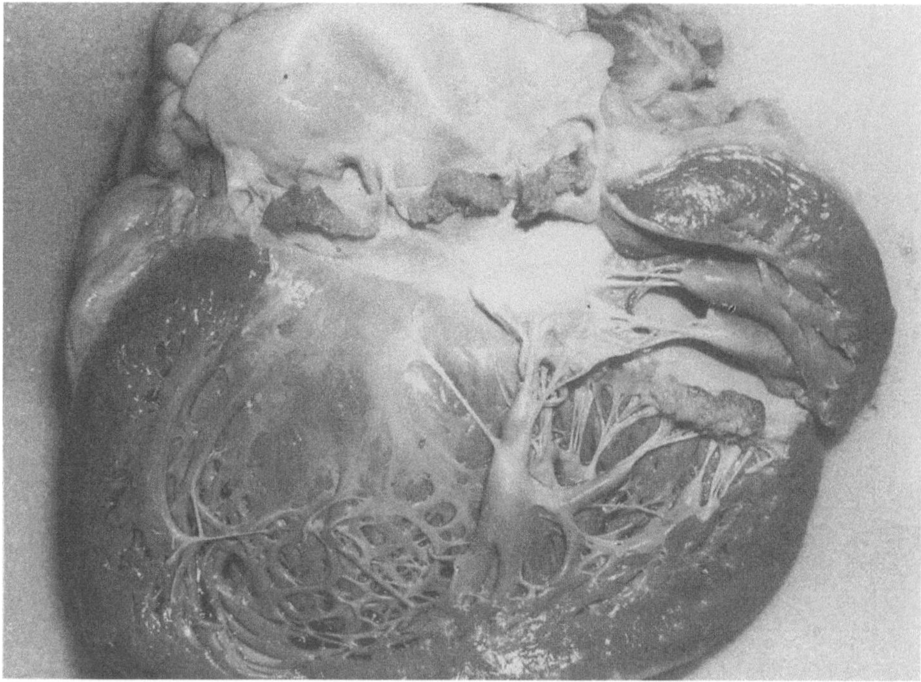

Fig. 33. Non-bacterial thrombotic endocarditis. There are large vegetations on the closure lines of all three aortic cusps and on the posterior mitral cusp. The patient died of cardinomatosis from a pancreatic primary

tion or micro-organisms and by the lack of significant pathology in the underlying valve cusps although minor postinflammatory changes are often present (ELIAKIM and PINCHAS 1966) and predispose to deposition of thrombus.

In most elderly patients NBTE is an incidental facet of terminal disease. However, systemic emboli are common and occasionally symptoms from cerebral emboli may be the first sign of a still treatable neoplasm (ASHENHURST and CHERTKOW 1962; BRYAN 1969; DEPPISCH and FAYEMI 1976; ROSEN and ARMSTRONG 1973; WOOLEY et al. 1970).

VII. Uncommon Valve Abnormalities

It should be remembered that even rare forms of acquired heart disease are at least as likely to be seen in elderly as in young patients.

Carcinoid heart disease affects the pulmonary and tricuspid valves which are incompetent and stenotic with thickened and contracted cusps. Fibrous plaques may also be present in the right atrial endocardium, extending from the thickened cusps on to the ventricular endocardium.

Papillary endocardial "tumours" (HEATH and THOMPSON 1967; NASSAR and PARKER 1971; POMERANCE 1975) are sea anemone like lesions (Fig. 34) usually found on the mitral or aortic cusps but which may arise on any cusp or cavity en-

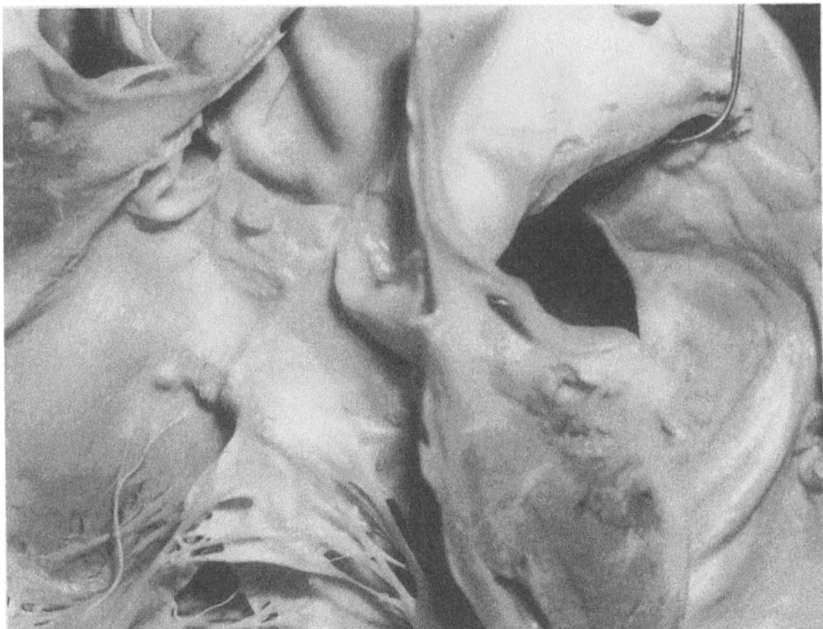

Fig. 34. Multiple cardiac pathology. The heart has been opened to show the mitral valve and left ventricular outflow and part of the left atrium, behind. The edge of a large atrial septal defect can be seen. A papillary tumour is attached to the linea alba of the non-coronary aortic cusp and mitral ring calcification is present and can be seen at the junction of mitral valve and membranous and muscular septum. (The papillary tumour was photographed after fixation and the characteristic frond-like structure could no longer be demonstrated macroscopically.) From a 74-year-old woman being treated for congestive cardiac failure for some months before her sudden death. Courtesy of Dr. K. Misch

docardium. Most reported cases and most of those seen personally have been in elderly patients. The "tumours" are not true neoplasms but are derived from the filiform Lambl's excrescences present in almost all elderly or damaged valves. They grow by accretion and organisation of fibrin (MAGAREY 1949). Most are of no clinical significance but occasionally they may form a ball-valve over a coronary ostium or be sources of emboli (HARRIS and ADELSON 1965).

VIII. Prosthetic Valve Pathology

Open heart surgery has now been established sufficiently long for its late sequelae to be appearing in geriatric patients and valve replacement in patients over 65 years is now also a common procedure. Late complications of valve replacement are thrombosis, infection, and mechanical dysfunction (ROBERTS et al. 1973; SILVER 1978). Thrombosis may impede ball or disc movement, may be sufficient to occlude the valve orifice and may be responsible for cerebral or coronary emboli (Fig. 35). Infected vegetations maybe grossly indistinguishable from non-infected thrombus. The causative organism is often a fungus. Mechanical dysfunction results from

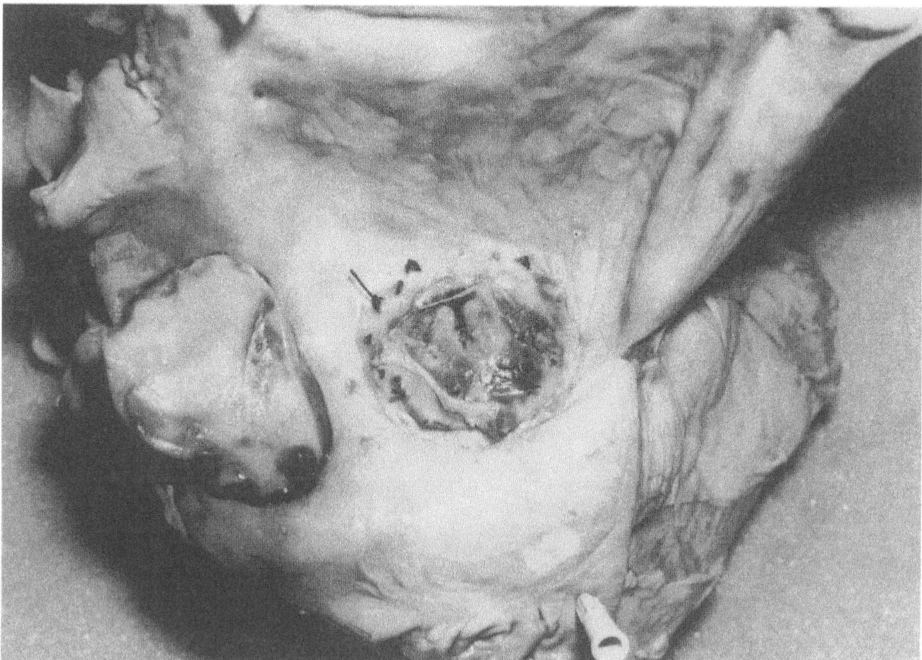

Fig. 35. Late thrombosis of prosthetic mitral valve. The opened left atrium is viewed from above and shows a large pannus of thrombus almost completely occluding the mitral orifice. Thrombus is also protruding from the atrial appendage *(left)*. From a 70-year-old woman who developed intractable congestive heart failure 6 years after mitral valve replacement

wear on the ball or disc which may then become fixed in either open or closed position or may shrink, escape or fragment, usually with catastrophic stenosis or incompetence.

IX. Cardiac Pathology and Congestive Cardiac Failure

A probable cause and effect relationship between congestive heart failure in the elderly and marked degrees of most of the pathological changes described in the present chapter is self evident, but the importance of the less severe changes is not so clear cut. While some functional effects appear inevitable with anything other than the mildest morphological changes, individually these seem insufficient to cause cardiac failure in most patients. Nevertheless, apart from aortic sclerosis and non-bacterial thrombotic endocarditis, most of the cardiac abnormalities found in elderly patients are found more commonly in those who had been in congestive cardiac failure than those who had not (HODKINSON and POMERANCE 1979; LINZBACH and AKUAMOA-BOATENG 1973 b; METIVIER 1971; POMERANCE 1965) and the probable explanation is that the effects of even minor functional abnormalities are cumulative. Multiple pathology is common in the hearts of elderly patients (Fig. 34) and patients in cardiac failure have a higher incidence of multiple pathology than those not in failure (HODKINSON and POMERANCE 1979; LINZBACH and AKUAMOA-

Boateng 1973 b; Metivier 1971; Pomerance 1965) and it is, therefore, reasonable
to suggest that the combined functional impairment of two or more relatively
minor abnormalities would be sufficient to precipitate cardiac failure even though
individually they would not do so.

Acknowledgments. Many of the illustrations in this chapter have appeared in earlier publications and I am grateful to the editors and/or publishers of Pomerance and Davis, Pathology of the Heart; Caird, Dall and Kennedy, Cardiology in old age; Silver, Cardiovascular
pathology; The Pathology Annual 1977; The British Heart Journal; and The Journal of
Clinical Pathology for permission to reproduce them. I should also like to thank Mr.
R. Blake for the photographic printing and Mrs. V. Pilbrow for secretarial assistance.

References

Abelmann WH (1973) Viral myocarditis and its sequelae. Ann Rev Med 24:145
Allen H, Harris A, Leatham A (1974) Significance and prognosis of an isolated late systolic
    murmur. Br Heart J 36:525
Applefield M, Hornick B (1974) Infective endocarditis in patients over age 60. Am Heart
    J 88:90
Ashenhurst EM, Chertkow G (1962) Cerebral embolism from nonbacterial thrombotic en-
    docarditis. Can Med Assoc J 86:313
Bacon APC, Matthews MB (1959) Congenital bicuspid aortic valves and the aetiology of
    isolated aortic valvular stenosis. Q J Med 28:545
Bedford PD, Caird FI (1960) Valvular disease of the heart in old age. Churchill Livingstone,
    Edinburgh London New York
Berger M, Rethy C, Goldberg E (1979) Unsuspected hypertrophic subaortic stenosis in the
    elderly diagnosed by echocardiography. J Am Geriat Soc 27:178
Bittar N, Sosa JA (1968) The billowing mitral valve leaflet. Report on fourteen patients. Cir-
    culation 38:763
Blankenhorn DH (1964) The relation of age and sex to diffuse aortic calcification in man.
    J Gerontol 19:72
Bryan CS (1969) Nonbacterial thrombotic endocarditis with malignant tumours. Am J Med
    46:787
Buerger L, Braunstein H (1960) Senile cardiac amyloidosis. Am J Med 28:357
Buja LM, Khoi NB, Roberts WC (1970) Clinically significant cardiac amyloidosis. Clinico-
    pathologic findings in fifteen patients. Am J Cardiol 26:394
Bulkley BH, Roberts WC (1973) Ankylosing spondylitis and aortic regurgitation. Circula-
    tion 48:1014
Bulkley BH, Roberts WC (1975) Dilatation of the mitral annulus. A rare cause of mitral
    regurgitation. Am J Med 59:457
Burch GE, Giles TD (1972) The role of viruses in the production of heart disease. Am J Car-
    diol 29:231
Burch GE, Giles TD, Colcolough HL (1970) Pathogenesis of „rheumatic" heart disease: cri-
    tique and theory. Am Heart J 80:556
Carpenter DF, Golden A, Roberts WC (1967) Quadrivalvular rheumatoid heart disease as-
    sociated with left bundle branch block. Am J Med 43:922
Chandraratna PAN, Aronow WS (1979) Incidence of ruptured chordae tendinae in the mi-
    tral valvular prolapse syndrome. Chest 75:3
Christensen JB, Pedersen OL (1976) Cardiac rupture after acute myocardial infarction. Dan
    Med Bull 23:235
Cooper JH (1969) An evaluation of current methods for the diagnostic histochemistry of
    amyloid. J Clin Pathol 23:410
Cornwell GG, Natvig JB, Westermark P, Husby G (1978) Senile Cardiac amyloid: Demon-
    stration of a unique fibril protein in tissue sections. J Immunol 120:1385

Darsee JR, Mikolich JR, Nicoloff NB, Lesser LE (1979) Prevalence of mitral valve prolapse in presumably healthy young men. Circulation 59:619

Davies MJ (1975) Myocarditis. Chap 6. In: Pomerance A, Davies MJ (eds) Pathology of the heart. Blackwells, London

Davies MJ, Pomerance A (1972) Quantitative study of ageing changes in the human sino-atrial node and internodal tracts. Br Heart J 34:150

Davies MJ, Pomerance A, Teare RD (1974) Pathological features of hypertrophic obstructive cardiomyopathy (HOCM). J Clin Path 27:529

Davies MJ, Moore BP, Braimbridge (1978) The floppy mitral valve. Study of incidence, pathology, and complications in surgical necropsy and forensic material. Br Heart J 40:468

Denham MJ, Pomerance A, Hodkinson HM (1977) Pathological validation of auscultation of the elderly heart. Postgrad Med J 53:66

Deppisch LM, Fayemi AO (1976) Nonbacterial thrombotic endocarditis. Am Heart J 92:723

Devereux RB, Perloff JK, Reichek N, Josephson ME (1976) Mitral valve prolapse. Circulation 54:3

Di Giorgio AJ (1973) Primary hemochromatosis; easily missed cause of cirrhosis, diabetes, and heart failure. Geriatrics 28:131

Drobinski G, Thery JM, Tereau Y, Tereau A, Bejean-Lebuisson, Evans JI, Kelessides C, Chomette G, Grosgogeat Y (1979) Echocardiographical, hemodynamic, and anatomical features of calcification of the mitral ring. Arch Mal Coeur 72:706

Drury RAB (1973) The cardiac pathology of elderly Ugandan Africans. East Afr Med J 50:566

Edwards JE (1961) The congenital bicuspid aortic valve. Circulation 23:485

Edwards JE (1962) On the etiology of calcific aortic stenosis. Circulation 26:817

Eliakim M, Pinchas S (1966) Degenerative verrucous endocardiosis. A clinical-pathological study of 45 cases with reference to a protracted form of the disease. Isr J Med Sci 2:42

Fertman MH, Wolff L (1946) Calcification of the mitral valve. Am Heart J 31:580

Fulkerson PK, Beaver BM, Auseon JC, Graber HL (1979) Calcification of the mitral annulus. Etiology, clinical associations, complications and therapy. Am J Med 66:967

Geill T (1951) Calcification of left annulus fibrosus. J Gerontol 6:327

Gjol N (1972) Cardiac rupture. Geriatrics 27:126

Gooch AS, Vicencio F, Maranhao V (1972) Arrhythmias and left ventricular asynergy in the prolapsing mitral leaflet syndrome. Am J Cardiol 29:611

Gouley BA, Sickel EM (1943) Aortic regurgitation caused by dilatation of aortic valve orifice and associated with characteristic valvular lesions. Am Heart J 26:24

Graham DC, Smythe HA (1958) The carditis and aortitis of ankylosing spondylitis. Bull Rheum Dis 9:171

Guthrie J, Fairgrieve J (1963) Aortic embolism due to myxoid tumour associated with myocardial calcification. Br Heart J 25:137

Harris LS, Adelson L (1965) Fatal coronary embolism from a myxomatous polyp of the aortic valve. An unusual cause of sudden death. Am J Clin Pathol 43:61

Harrison CV, Lennox B (1948) Heart block in osteitis deformans. Br Heart J 10:167

Haust MD, Rowlands DT, Garancis JC, Landing BH (1962) Histochemical studies on cardiac „colloid". Am J Path 40:185

Heath D, Thompson IM (1967) Papillary „tumours" of the left ventricle. Br Heart J 29:950

Hinohara S (1973) Cardiac amyloidosis. Jpn J Med 12:231

Hodkinson HM, Pomerance A (1978) Cardiac amyloidosis in the elderly associated elevation of serum alkaline phosphatase. Age Ageing 3:76

Hodkinson HM, Pomerance A (1977) The clinical significance of senile cardiac amyloidosis; a prospective clinico pathological study. Q J Med 46:381

Hodkinson HM, Pomerance A (1979) The clinical pathology of heart failure and atrial fibrillation in old age. Postgrad Med J 55:251

Hodkinson I, Pomerance A, Hodkinson HM (1979) Heart size in the elderly; a clinicopathological study. J R Soc Med 72:13

Hudson REB (1962) Cardiovascular pathology. Edward Arnold, London

Hughes P, Gauld WR (1966) Bacterial endocarditis, a changing disease. Q J Med 35:511

Husselmann H (1955) Beitrag zum Amyloid-Problem auf Grund von Untersuchungen an menschlichen Herzen. Virchows Arch [Pathol Anat] 27:607

Ikee Y (1970) Pathological studies on amyloidosis – histopathology of senile cardiac amyloidosis. Acta Pathol Jpn 20:423

Ischii T, Sternby NH (1978) The pathology of centenarians. I. The cardiovascular system and lungs. J Am Geriat Soc 26:108

Iveson JMI, Pomerance A (1977) Cardiac involvement in rheumatoid disease. Clin Rheumat Dis 3:467

Jacobovitz D, Dustin P (1974) Right heart valvular amyloidosis in a patient with duodenal carcinoid tumours. J Pathol 112:195

Jeresaty RM (1979) Mitral valve prolapse. Raven Press, New York

Josselson AJ, Pruitt RD, Edwards JE (1952) Amyloid localized to the heart. Analysis of 29 cases. Arch Pathol 54:359

Katenkamp D, Stiller D (1971) Histotopographic studies on senile cardiac amyloidosis. Pathol Eur 6:109

Kim KM, Valigorsky JM, Mergner WJ, Jones RT, Pendergrass RF, Trump BF (1976) Ageing changes in the human aortic valve in relation to dystrophic calcification. Hum Pathol 7:47

Kirk RS, Russell JGB (1969) Sub-valvular calcification of mitral valve. Br Heart J 31:684

Kline IK, Kline TS, Saphir O (1978) Myocarditis in senescence. Am Heart J 65:446

Koobs DH, Schultz RL, Jutzy RV (1978) The original of lipofuscin and possible consequences to the myocardium. Arch Pathol Lab Med 102:66

Korn D, DeSanctis RW, Sell S (1962) Massive calcification of the mitral annulus: a clinicopathological study of 14 cases. New Engl J Med 267:900

Kosek JC, Angell W (1970) Fine structure of basophilic myocardial degeneration. Arch Path 89:491

Krasnow N, Stein RA (1978) Hypertrophic cardiomyopathy in the aged. Am Heart J 96:326

Kronzon I, Glassman E (1978) Mitral ring calcification in idiopathic hypertrophic subaortic stenosis. Am J Cardiol 42:60

(Lancet, anonymous) (1967) Bacterial endocarditis: a changing pattern. Lancet 1:605

(Lancet, anonymous) Aetiology of acquired valvar heart disease. Lancet 1:897

(Lancet, anonymous) Viruses and heart disease. Lancet 2:991

Lendrum AC, Slidders W, Fraser DS (1972) Renal hyalin. A study of amyloidosis and diabetic fibrinous vasculosis with new staining methods. J Clin Pathol 25:373

Lenkiewicz JE, Davies MJ, Rosen D (1972) Collagen in human myocardium as a function of age. Cardiovasc Res 6:549

Lerner PI, Weinstein L (1966) Infective endocarditis in the antibiotic era. New Engl J Med 274:199, 259, 323, 388

Lev M (1964) Anatomic basis for atrio-ventricular block. Am J Med 37:742

Limas CJ (1971) Ageing of the myocardium. Acta Cardiol 26:249

Linzbach AJ, Akuamoa-Boatenge E (1973a) The alterations of the ageing human heart. I. Heart weight with progressing age. Klin Wochenschr 51:156

Linzbach AJ, Akuamoa-Boateng E (1973b) The alterations of the ageing human heart: II. Polypathy of the heart with progressing age. Klin Wochenschr 51:164

London RE, London SB (1965) Rupture of the heart. A critical analysis of 47 consecutive autopsy cases. Circulation 31:202

Magarey FR (1949) On the mode of formation of Lambl's excrescences and their relation to chronic thickening of the mitral valve. J Pathol Bact 61:203

Malcolm AD, Chayen J, Cankovic-Darracott S, Jenkins BS, Webb-Peploe MM (1979) Biopsy evidence of left ventricular myocardial abnormality in patients with mitral-leaflet prolapse and chest pain. Lancet 1:1052

Mambo NC, Silver MD, Brunsdon DFV (1978) Bacterial endocarditis of the mitral valve associated with annular calcification. Can Med Assoc J 119:323

Mason JW, Koch FH, Billingham ME, Winkle RA (1978) Cardiac biopsy evidence for a cardiomyopathy associated with symptomatic mitral valve prolapse. Am J Cardiol 42:557

McKusick VA (1972) Heritable disorders of connective tissue, 4th ed. Mosby, St Louis

McManus JFA, Lupton CH (1963) Lipid deposits in the aortic cusp of the mitral valve. Arch Pathol 75:674

McMillan JB, Lev M (1959) The ageing heart. I. Endocardium. J Gerontol 14:268

McMillan JB, Lev M (1962a) The ageing heart. Myocardium and epicardium. In: Shock N (ed) Biological aspects of ageing. Columbia University Press, New York

McMillan JB, Lev M (1962b) The ageing heart. II. The valves. J Gerontol 19:1

Metivier J (1971) Clinical and anatomic study of cardiopathies in the elderly (subjects over age 70 years). Ann Med Interne (Paris) 122:367

Mulligan RM (1958) Amyloidosis of the heart. Arch Pathol 65:615

Nassar SGA, Parker JC (1971) Incidental papillary endocardial tumour; its potential significance. Arch Pathol 92:370

Oka M, Angrist A (1967) Mechanism of cardiac valvular fusion and stenosis. Am Heart J 74:37

Oka M, Belenky D, Brodie S, Angrist A (1968) Studies of bacterial susceptibility of heart valves. Lab Invest 19:113

Page DL (1970) Lipomatous hypertrophy of the cardiac interatrial septum: its development and probable clinical significance. Hum Pathol 1:151

Paulus HE, Pearson CM, Pitts W (1972) Aortic insufficiency in five patients with Reiter's syndrome. A detailed clinical and pathological study. Am J Med 53:464

Penther P, Cousteau JP, Gay J (1970) Some peculiar aspects of obstructive cardiomyopathy of subjects over 55 years of age (with reference to 14 cases). Arch Mal Coeur 63:1230

Penther Ph, Gerbaux A, Blanc JJ, Morin JF, Julienne JL (1977) Myocardial infarction and rupture of the heart; a macroscopic pathologic study. Am Heart J 93:302

Petrin TJ, Tavel M (1979) Idiopathic hypertrophic subaortic stenosis as observed in a large community hospital: Relation to age and history of hypertension. J Am Geriatr Soc 27:43

Pomerance A (1965) Pathology of the heart with and without cardiac failure in the aged. Br Heart J 27:697

Pomerance A (1966) The pathology of senile cardiac amyloidosis. J Path Bact 91:357

Pomerance A (1967) Ageing changes in human heart valves. Br Heart J 29:222

Pomerance A (1969) Ballooning deformity (mucoid degeneration) of atrio-ventricular valves. Br Heart J 31:343

Pomerance A (1970) Pathological and clinical study of calcification of the mitral valve ring. J Clin Pathol 23:354

Pomerance A (1972) The pathogenesis of aortic stenosis and its relation to age. Br Heart J 34:569

Pomerance A (1975) Endocarditis, chap 13. In: Pomerance A, Davies MJ Pathology of the heart. Blackwell, London

Pomerance A, Davies MD (1975) Pathological features of HOCM in the elderly. Br Heart J 37:305

Pomerance A, Silver M (1981) Age related cardiovascular changes and mechanically induced endocardial pathology. In: Silver M (ed) Cardiovascular pathology. Churchill Livingstone, Edinburgh London New York

Pomerance A, Whitney JC (1970) Heart valve changes common to man and dog. A comparative study. Cardiovasc Res 4:61

Pomerance A, Slavin G, McWatt J (1976) Experiences with the SAB stain in cardiac pathology. J Clin Pathol 29:22

Pomerance A, Darby AJ, Hodkinson HM (1978) Valvular calcification in the elderly: Possible pathogenic factors. J Gerontol 33:672

Rasmussen S, Leth A, Kjoller E, Pedersen A (1979) Cardiac rupture in acute myocardial infarction. A review of 72 consecutive cases. Acta Med Scand 205:11

Reiner L, Mazzoleni A, Rodriguez FL, Freudenthal RR (1959) The weight of the human heart. I. „Normal" cases. Arch Pathol 68:58

Reyes CV, Jablokow VR (1979) Lipomatous hypertrophy of the interatrial septum. Am J Clin Pathol 72:785

Ridolfi RL, Hutchins GM (1976) Spontaneous calcific emboli from calcific mitral annulus fibrosus. Arch Pathol 100:117

Ridolfi RL, Bulkley BH, Hutchins GM (1977) The conduction system in cardiac amyloidosis. Am J Med 62:677

Roberts WC (1970) The structure of the aortic valve in clinically isolated aortic stenosis. An autopsy study of 162 patients over 15 years of age. Circulation 42:91

Roberts WC, Ferrans VJ (1975) Pathologic anatomy of the cardiomyopathies. Idiopathic dilated and hypertrophic types, infiltrative types and endomyocardial disease with and without eosinophilia. Hum Pathol 6:287

Roberts WC, Kehoe JA, Carpenter DF, Golden A (1968) Cardiac valvular lesions in rheumatoid arthritis. Arch Intern Med 122:141

Roberts WC, Bulkley BH, Morrow AG (1973) Pathologic anatomy of cardiac valve replacement. A study of 224 necropsy patients. Prog Cardiovasc Dis 15:539

Robertson WB, Strong JP (1968) Atherosclerosis in persons with hypertension and diabetes mellitus. Lab Invest 18:538

Romhanyi G (1972) Differences in ultrastructural organization of amyloid as revealed by sensitivity or resistance to induced proteolysis. Virchows Arch [Pathol Anat] 357:29

Rosai J, Lascano EF (1970) Basophilic (mucoid) degeneration of myocardium. Am J Pathol 61:99

Rosen P, Armstrong D (1973) Non-bacterial thrombotic endocarditis in patients with malignant neoplastic diseases. Am J Med 54:23

Rosenthal CJ, Franklin EC (1975) Variation with age and disease of amyloid. A protein related serum component. J Clin Invest 55:746

Rytand DA, Lipsitch LS (1946) Clinical aspects of calcification on the mitral annulus fibrosus. Arch Intern Med 78:544

Salazar AE, Edwards JE (1970) Friction lesions of ventricular endocardium; relating to chordae tendinae of mitral valve. Arch Pathol 90:364

Salomon J, Shah PM, Heinle RA (1975) Thoracic skeletal abnormalities in idiopathic mitral valve prolapse. Am J Cardiol 36:32

Salyer WR, Hutchins GM (1974) Cardiac lesions in secondary oxalosis. Arch Intern Med 134:250

Schenk EA, Cohen J (1970) The heart in chronic alcoholism. Clinical and pathologic findings. Pathol Microbiol 35:96

Schnurr LP, Ball AP, Geddes AM, Gray J, McChie D (1977) Bacterial endocarditis in England in the 1970's: A review of 70 patients. Q J Med 46:499

Schott CR, Kotler MN, Parry WR, Segal BL (1977) Mitral annular calcification. Clinical and echocardiographic correlations. Arch Intern Med 137:1143

Schwartz CJ, Mitchell JRA (1962) The relation between myocardial lesions and coronary artery disease. Brit Heart J 24:761

Schwartz P (1969) Cardiovascular amyloidosis in the aged. Geriatrics 24:S 1

Schwartz P (1970) Amyloidosis; causes and manifestation of senile deterioration. Charles C Thomas, Springfield, Illinois, USA

Sell S, Scully RE (1965) Ageing changes in the aortic and mitral valves; histologic and histochemical studies, with observations on the pathogenesis of calcific aortic stenosis and calcification of the mitral annulus. Am J Pathol 46:345

Serentha P, Baldonie, Bratina G, Galetti G (1973) Cardiac amyloidosis in old age. G Gerontol 21:496

Sheldon WH, Golden A (1951) Abscesses of valve rings of heart, frequent but not well recognised complication of acute bacterial endocarditis. Circulation 4:1

Sievers J (1966) Cardiac rupture in acute myocardial infarction. Geriatrics 21:125

Silver MD (1978) Late complications of prosthetic heart valves. Arch Pathol Lab Med 102:281

Simon MA, Liu F (1954) Calcification of mitral valve annulus and its relationship to functional valvular disturbance. Am Heart J 48:497

Smith RRL, Hutchins GM, Moore GW, Humphrey RL (1979) Type and distribution of pulmonary parenchymal and vascular amyloid. Correlation with cardiac amyloidosis. Am J Med 66:96

Soyka J (1876) Über amyloide Degeneration. Prag Med Wochenschr 1:165

Spiel R, Dittel M, Jobst Cb, Kiss H, Nobis H, Prachar H, Enenkel W (1979) Ventricular rupture during acute myocardial infarction. Z Kardiol 68:147

Stepien A, Buczynski E (1972) Comparative studies on content of lipofuscin in the heart. Pathol Pol 23:451

Stiller D, Katenkamp D (1971) Senile cardiac amyloidosis. Dtsch Gesundheitswes 26:2178

Strehler BL (1967) The nature of cellular age changes. Symp Soc Exp Biol 21:149

Strehler BL, Mildvan AS (1962) Studies on the chemical properties of lipofuscin age pigments. In: Shock N (ed) Biological aspects of ageing. Columbia University Press, New York

Strehler BL, Mark DD, Mildvan SA, Gee MV (1959) Rate and magnitude of age pigment accumulation in the human myocardium. J Gerontol 14:430

Sugiura M, Hiraoka K, Ohkowa S, Shimada H (1975) A clinicopathological study on the heart diseases in the aged. The morphological classification of the 1000 consecutive autopsy cases. Jpn Heart J 16:526

Sugiura M, Uchiyama S, Kuwako K, Ohkawa S, Hiraoka K, Ueda K (1977) A clinicopathological study on mitral ring calcification. Jpn Heart J 18:154

Thell R, Martin FH, Edwards JE (1975) Bacterial endocarditis in subjects 60 years of age and older. Circulation 51:174

Thung PJ (1957) The relation between amyloid and ageing in comparative pathology. Gerontology 1:234

Torii S, Bashey RJ, Nakao K (1965) Acid mucopolysaccharide composition of human heart valve. Biochim Biophys Acta 101:285

Tresch DD, Siegel R, Keelan MH, Gross CM, Brooks HL (1979) Mitral valve prolapse in the elderly. J Am Geriat Soc 27:421

Tseng HL, Lim BS (1977) Electron microscopic study of senile cardiac amyloidosis. Micron 8:33

Udoshi MB, Shah A, Fisher VJ, Dolgin M (1979) Incidence of mitral valve prolapse in subjects with thoracic skeletal abnormalities – A prospective study. Am Heart J 97:303

Vendsborg P, Hansen LF, Olesen KH (1968) Decreasing incidence of a history of acute rheumatic fever in chronic rheumatic heart disease. Cardiology 53:332

Ward C (1975) Virus valvular heart disease. Am Heart J 90:804

Ward C (1978) "Rheumatic" heart disease, psittacosis and the importance of epidemiology. Am Heart J 95:266

Westermark P (1979) Senile amyloidosis. G Gerontol 27:563

Westermark P, Natvig JB, Johansson B (1977) Characterization of an amyloid fibril protein from senile cardiac amyloid. J Exp Med 146:631

Whiting RB, Powell WJ, Dinsmore RE, Sanders CA (1971) Idiopathic hypertrophic subaortic stenosis in the elderly. New Engl J Med 285:196

Wooley CF, Baba N, Ryan JM (1970) Nonbacterial thrombotic endocarditis. Clinical recognition. Arch Intern Med 125:126

Wright JR, Calkins E (1975) Amyloid in the aged heart, frequency and clinical significance. J Am Geriatr Soc 23:97

Wright JR, Calkins E, Breen WJ, Stolte G, Schultz RT (1969) Relationship of amyloid to ageing. Medicine 48:39

Valvular Disease of the Heart

F.I. CAIRD

A. Epidemiology of Valvular Disease

Classical cardiological teaching is that valvular heart disease, except aortic stenosis, is rare in old age. That this is not so was clearly shown by pathological investigations (FRIEDBERG and TARTAKOWER 1931), and by clinical studies reviewed by BEDFORD and CAIRD (1960).

I. Rheumatic Heart Disease

The current prevalence of rheumatic heart disease in the general elderly population is of the order of 2%–3%, and about 4% among elderly hospital patients (DROLLER and PEMBERTON 1953; BEDFORD and CAIRD 1960; POMERANCE 1976; KENNEDY et al. 1977). The prevalence of rheumatic heart disease in old age is the resultant of the incidence of rheumatic fever during the childhood and adolescence of the present elderly population, and the natural history of established rheumatic heart disease in middle age. The incidence of rheumatic fever fell during the first half of this century (SIEVERS and HALL 1971), and the prevalence of rheumatic heart disease in old age will thus decline in future.

II. Non-rheumatic Mitral Disease

Clinically significant non-rheumatic mitral valve disease probably contributes a further 1%–2% to the hospital prevalence of mitral disease in old people (POMERANCE 1976).

III. Aortic Valve Disease

Aortic stenosis of various aetiologies is found in 4%–5% of old people (ACHESON and ACHESON 1958; BEDFORD and CAIRD 1960; POMERANCE 1976; KENNEDY et al. 1977). No secular change in the prevalence of aortic stenosis is likely, except in so far as cases of rheumatic aetiology may decline. Aortic incompetence without stenosis, due to a wide variety of causes (see Sect. C.III.1), is encountered in perhaps a further 1%–2% of old people (POMERANCE 1976; KENNEDY et al. 1977). The prevalence of 4% given by BEDFORD and CAIRD (1960) is undoubtedly too high.

The total prevalence of valvular disease of all kinds in the elderly population is thus considerable, and the resulting clinical and diagnostic problems are common.

B. Mitral Valve Disease

I. Age Changes in the Mitral Valve

Changes in the mitral valve and its valve ring which are attributable to the ageing process are well described (MCMILLAN and LEV 1959; SELL and SCULLY 1965; POMERANCE 1976). Nodular thickening of the atrial surfaces of the cusps occurs at their points of apposition during systole, which are presumably the sites of maximum mechanical stress. There is a decrease in the number and size of nuclei in the fibrous stroma of the valve ring, accumulation of lipid, degeneration of collagen, and calcific change. Simple age changes in the mitral valve are unlikely either to be of haemodynamic significance or to produce physical signs.

II. Rheumatic Mitral Disease

1. Pathology

The pathology of rheumatic mitral disease in old people is essentially identical to that in younger patients. The principal features are fibrotic disorganisation of the valve architecture and scarring of the cusps, thickening and contracture of the chordae, and commissural adhesion, fusion, and calcification. Whether all such valvular abnormalities are truly rheumatic in origin is uncertain; some cases may have other inflammatory aetiologies (POMERANCE 1976).

2. Clinical Features

40% of elderly patients with rheumatic mitral valve disease give a history of rheumatic fever or chorea in early life. The age at the occurrence of the first rheumatic manifestation is identical to that found in large series of cases of acute rheumatic fever (BEDFORD and CAIRD 1960), but elderly patients may possibly have suffered fewer overt recurrences of rheumatic activity (HEBBERT and RANKIN 1954). Mitral disease may only become clinically apparent for the first time 60 years after the initial episode of rheumatic fever (CURRENS 1967).

Mitral incompetence is the predominant lesion in most elderly patients with rheumatic heart disease, only about one-third having predominant mitral stenosis (BEDFORD and CAIRD 1960). One-half also have aortic valve disease; two-thirds of these have aortic incompetence, and one-third aortic stenosis with or without incompetence. 40% of elderly patients with rheumatic mitral disease seen in hospital show evidence of cardiac failure. One-third, particularly of those with mitral stenosis, are in atrial fibrillation, while systemic embolism is a major feature in perhaps 6%, again especially in those with mitral stenosis.

The physical signs of mitral valve disease in the elderly parallel those in younger patients. Left ventricular hypertrophy predominates in those with mitral incompetence, and a right ventricular impulse may be evident in those with predominant mitral stenosis. The auscultatory signs are also essentially the same. When a loud first heart sound is heard in an elderly patient with tachycardia or cardiac failure, a careful auscultatory search should be made for other signs of mitral disease. This should be repeated once resolution of cardiac failure or reduction in heart rate has been accompanied by an increase in cardiac output, and thus in the reappearance of the flow-dependent diastolic murmur. An opening snap is not infrequent (CAIRD et al. 1973), and when the cardiac output is low may be the only auscultatory sign of mitral stenosis.

P mitrale and right ventricular hypertrophy may be found in mitral stenosis, and left ventricular hypertrophy is to be expected in predominant mitral incompetence. The chest radiograph is of great value since left atrial enlargement may well be evident, but both Kerley's lines and definite evidence of pulmonary hypertension (other than increase in size of the upper lobe veins) are relatively unusual.

In mitral stenosis, the rapid filling wave in early diastole may be absent on the apex cardiogram, and in patients in sinus rhythm, outward movement of the left ventricle during atrial systole may be slow (CAIRD 1976). Echocardiography has been little reported in the diagnosis of rheumatic mitral valve disease in the elderly, but the patterns seen would be expected to resemble those in younger patients.

3. Haemodynamics

Radionuclide studies of the circulation in elderly patients with mitral disease are compared in Table 1 with findings in normal elderly subjects and patients with other forms of heart disease (CAIRD 1980). In atrial fibrillation, cardiac output is considerably reduced, pulmonary mean transit time prolonged, and pulmonary blood volume increased. In cardiac failure these changes are greater, and except in respect of pulmonary blood volume, exceed those found in cardiac failure without valvular disease.

4. Complications

The important complications of rheumatic mitral disease in old age are atrial fibrillation, arterial embolism and cardiac failure. There are clear interrelations between these three occurrences. 60% of elderly hospital patients with rheumatic mitral disease and atrial fibrillation are in cardiac failure, as against 25% of those with sinus rhythm (BEDFORD and CAIRD 1960). Systemic embolism is also associated with atrial fibrillation in patients with mitral stenosis, though in mitral incompetence, coincident myocardial infarction with left ventricular endocardial thrombosis is the usual cause.

5. Prognosis

The principal determinents of prognosis in rheumatic mitral valve disease in old age are cardiac rhythm and cardiac failure. The survival of patients in sinus rhythm without cardiac failure probably differs little from that of other old people of the same age, but if atrial fibrillation or cardiac failure is present, only 10%–15% survive 3 years or more (BEDFORD and CAIRD 1960). The type of valve lesion is of lesser importance, though survival appears slightly better in mitral incompetence than in mitral stenosis.

Table 1. Radionuclide circulatory studies in valvular disease in old age (For methods, see CAIRD, 1980)

Patient group	Rhythm[a]	Heart failure	No.	Cardiac index[b] (litres/min/m^2)	Blood volume[b] (litres/m^2)	Mean circulation time[b] (s)	Pulmonary mean transit time[b] (s)	Pulmonary blood volume[b] (ml/m^2)
Normal[a]	SR	No	12	3.62 ± 1.19	3.30 ± 0.72	58 ± 11	4.8 ± 1.2	276 ± 63
Left ventricular hypertrophy[d]	SR	No	17	3.55 ± 1.19	4.07 ± 0.66	78 ± 22	6.4 ± 1.7	357 ± 10
Cardiac failure[d]	SR	Yes	13	2.96 ± 1.23	4.43 ± 1.31	102 ± 40	10.0 ± 4.1	456 ± 158
Atrial fibrillation[d]	AF	No	14	2.82 ± 0.67	4.53 ± 0.96	88 ± 21	9.6 ± 3.1	441 ± 160
Mitral disease	SR	No	2	2.92	3.23	67	4.2	203
Mitral disease	AF	No	4	2.28 ± 0.37	3.82 ± 0.86	102 ± 30	10.2 ± 2.7	382 ± 90
Mitral disease	SR	Yes	7	1.78 ± 0.31	4.10 ± 0.83	136 ± 29	15.7 ± 7.1	457 ± 202
Mitral disease	AF	Yes	7[c]	2.31 ± 0.82	4.33 ± 1.01	126 ± 55	12.8 ± 7.0	461 ± 236
Aortic valve disease	SR	No	7	3.67 ± 1.36	3.95 ± 1.34	68 ± 16	7.7 ± 1.4	476 ± 179
Aortic valve disease	SR[e]	Yes	8	2.65 ± 1.58	4.80 ± 1.69	126 ± 57	11.8 ± 5.7	466 ± 214

[a] SR, sinus rhythm; AF, atrial fibrillation
[b] Mean$\pm$SD
[c] Two observations on two patients
[d] From CAIRD (1980)
[e] One with AF

6. Treatment

The treatment of rheumatic mitral disease in the elderly is usually medical. However, symptomatic mitral valve disease with moderate or severe disability should be considered an indication for operation in elderly as well as in younger patients (OH et al. 1973; STARR and LAWSON 1976; DE BONO et al. 1978). STARR and LAWSON (1976) described 89 patients over the age of 60 treated by mitral valve replacement. The hospital mortality was 16%, but 60% survived 5 years, and 40% 10 years after the operation. Early deaths are mostly due to myocardial infarction and low output states, and late deaths to cardiac failure and endocarditis. Technical improvements in prosthetic valves have in particular been associated with a reduction in the rate of postoperative thrombo-embolic complications. Functional improvement after operation is often very gratifying and patients incapacitated for many years may well be restored to activities normal for their age.

III. Calcification of the Mitral Ring

1. Pathology

The frequency at autopsy of calcification of the mitral ring increases from 6% in men aged 70–79 to 19% in men aged over 90, and from 12% to 40% respectively in women (POMERANCE 1976); at all ages it is about twice as common in women as in men. Lesser degrees of calcification take the form of small localised nodules, usually at the middle of the junction of the medial commissure of the posterior cusp and ventricular wall. This is close to the bundle of His, and the condition may thus be associated with atrioventricular block. More extensive deposits extend into the angle under the valve, forming a ridge over which the cusp is stretched, and to which the chordae may adhere. Distortion and upward displacement of the cusp result in mitral incompetence, and very gross lesions may give rise to minor degrees of obstruction (KIRK and RUSSELL 1969). The most massive lesions transform the whole mitral ring into a rigid calcified bar, which may undergo softening and be mistaken for an inflammatory lesion. Microscopically the calcified lesion consists of an amorphous eosinophilic material, which may be surrounded by inflammatory tissue, or on occasions transformed into cartilage and bone.

The pathogenesis of mitral ring calcification is unknown, and it has been regarded as an exaggerated age change (POMERANCE 1976). If this is so, it is difficult to see why it is so much more frequent in women than in men.

2. Clinical Features

Calcification of the mitral ring is usually asymptomatic, the only evidence being the radiological appearance of an obliquely set horseshoe of calcium seen on radiographs of the chest. Severe calcific changes may produce clinically apparent mitral incompetence (less often stenosis), and on occasions complete heart block (RYTAND and LIPSITCH 1946; SIMON and LIU 1954; KORN et al. 1962; KIRK and RUSSELL 1969). The physical signs resemble those of rheumatic mitral disease, and the electrocardiogram may show atrial fibrillation and atrioventricular conduction defects. The diagnosis is made from the chest X-ray, and should give rise to no difficulty.

IV. Mucoid Deformity of the Mitral Valve

1. Pathology

Mucoid deformity of the mitral valve is a common pathological finding with many names (Pomerance 1976), and is found in 5% of elderly hearts. In its gross form part or all of the affected cusp, usually the posterior, stretches and increases in size and depth, coming to resemble an opaque white parachute or deflated balloon. The chordae are also lengthened, but are not fused or contracted, though they may become adherent to the mural endocardium. Areas of ulceration and thrombus deposition are common on the abnormal cusp, and infective endocarditis may develop. The principal haemodynamic consequence is mitral incompetence, which results from overshoot of the cusp into the left atrium during systole.

Microscopically the orderly arrangement of the collagen of the fibrous layer of the cusp is replaced by areas of loose spongy mucoprotein or mucopolysaccharide material, but in contrast to the disorganisation seen in rheumatic mitral disease, the normal anatomical layers are preserved, and there is neither abnormal vascularisation nor other evidence of inflammation. Similar changes may occur in the chordae and may lead to their rupture. Uninvolved chordae may also rupture as a result of the gross mechanical disturbance produced by the cusp abnormality.

The pathogenesis of this interesting condition is unknown, but as with calcification of the mitral valve ring, an exaggerated age change is certainly a possibility.

2. Clinical Features

Clinical evidence of mitral valve prolapse is not unduly rare in old age. The characteristic physical sign is a late systolic murmur, sometimes initiated by a systolic click, without evidence of mitral obstruction (Epstein and Coulshed 1973). Atrial fibrillation, ventricular ectopic beats and cardiac failure are not unusual. The electrocardiogram shows no signs of cardiac infarction, as is usually the case with ischaemic papillary muscle dysfunction (see Sect. B.V), and there is no X-ray evidence of calcification of the mitral ring. The echocardiogram shows the abnormal movement of the valve (Dillon et al. 1971; Popp et al. 1974). In asymptomatic cases the prognosis appears good, but once cardiac failure has developed, survival usually seems short.

V. Papillary Muscle Dysfunction

Papillary muscle dysfunction has been clearly recognised as a cause of mitral incompetence following acute cardiac infarction (Heikillä 1967), the mechanism being disorganisation of papillary muscle contraction, allowing systolic prolapse of part of the mitral valve into the left atrium. Persistent functional abnormality following papillary muscle infarction is probably not rare (de Pasquale and Burch 1966). The diagnosis should be suspected when there is an apical pansystolic murmur, sometimes with a third heart sound, but without evidence of mitral obstruction, in a patient whose electrocardiogram shows evidence of past, usually inferior, myocardial infarction. The prognosis seems in general to be good.

Rupture of papillary muscle or of its attached chorda is a rare but dramatic complication characteristically occurring a few days after cardiac infarction. Chordal rupture may also complicate mucoid degeneration of the mitral valve. Successful surgical treatment has been reported in old age (STARR and LAWSON 1976; DE BONO et al. 1978).

VI. Left Atrial Myxoma

Left atrial myxoma is a condition which is uncommon at any age but may be rarely encountered in the elderly (GOODWIN 1963; HARVEY 1968). Rapidly advancing symptoms of mitral obstruction, usually of less than 2 years duration, contrast with the much longer duration of symptoms in rheumatic mitral disease. Systemic emboli are common, but episodes of syncope due to intermittent complete obstruction of the mitral valve are relatively infrequent. The combination of emboli, variable mitral murmurs, a raised ESR and abnormality of the plasma proteins may suggest bacterial endocarditis, but blood cultures are negative. These features should suggest the possibility of the diagnosis, and echocardiography (NASSER et al. 1972) or angiocardiography should be carried out as a matter of urgency, since any surgical treatment must be undertaken before there is irreversible cardiac deterioration.

C. Aortic Valve Disease

I. Age Changes in the Aortic Valve

Age changes in the aortic valve resemble those in the mitral valve (McMILLAN and LEV 1959; SELL and SCULLY 1965; POMERANCE 1976). Valvular thickening ranges in severity from a palpable ridge along the attachment of the cusps, which is almost universal by middle age, to extensive calcific changes in the cusp fibrosa, involving the basal parts but not usually the free edges of the cusps. These changes are best termed "aortic valvular sclerosis," to distinguish them from changes in the aorta itself; they seem likely to be due to the repeated mechanical stresses of normal valve action over many years.

II. Aortic Stenosis

1. Pathology

Three different forms of aortic stenosis are encountered in old age (POMERANCE 1972). These are postinflammatory stenosis, degenerative calcification, and degenerative changes in bicuspid valves.

In postinflammatory stenosis the commissures are fused and the cusps contracted, so that the valve orifice becomes a central triangle or circle. If commissural fusion is asymmetrical, the orifice is eccentric or angled, but its apex remains approximately central. The original inflammatory process is probably usually rheumatic, but it is certainly possible that non-rheumatic infections may be the cause of isolated cases (POMERANCE 1976).

Degenerative calcification of tricuspid valves is macroscopically different, in that the commissures are not fused, and the cusps are not contracted. The orifice is thus triradiate, and the cusps are immobilised by extensive calcification extending out from their bases. This condition can be regarded as an extension of the changes of aortic valvular sclerosis. It is the commonest cause of aortic stenosis over the age of 75 (POMERANCE 1972).

In calcification of a congenital bicuspid valve, there are only two cusps, and the larger has a fibrous ridge on its aortic aspect, indicating the line of failure of cusp development. The orifice is transverse or slightly crescentic. The calcific changes resemble those seen in tricuspid valves, and are probably produced prematurely by abnormal mechanical stresses. However, congenital bicuspid valves without stenosis are also encountered in old age (POMERANCE 1976).

2. Clinical Features and Diagnosis

The majority of cases of aortic stenosis in old age have no cardiac symptoms. Approximately one-third are dyspnoeic, commonly because of cardiac failure (BEDFORD and CAIRD 1960). A varying proportion have angina pectoris, mostly in association with ischaemic heart disease. Syncopal attacks, often exertional, occur in up to 30%. In terminal cardiac failure, there may be episodes of "chronic syncope," with impairment of consciousness, sweating, restlessness, confusion, irregular bradycardia, and hypotension (KUMPE and BEAN 1948).

Most of the classical physical signs of aortic stenosis can be demonstrated in severe cases in the elderly: a slowly rising pulse, reduced pulse pressure, left ventricular hypertrophy, a cardiac impulse with a clear atrial component, a long, loud, and harsh basal ejection murmur with a thrill and depression, and reversed splitting of the second heart sound. Expiratory accentuation of the ejection murmur may sometimes be obvious (CAIRD and DALL 1979). Two-thirds of cases show evidence of aortic incompetence, and when this is severe the bisferiens pulse may be apparent.

In less severe cases the diagnosis is more difficult. The slowly rising pulse is absent and the pulse pressure normal, but the ejection murmur, maximum in the right second space but often widely audible over the praecordium and at the apex, can still be heard and the second heart sound is reduced in intensity.

The electrocardiogram usually shows clear evidence of left ventricular hypertrophy, but the difficulties of diagnosis of minor degrees of left ventricular hypertrophy (ROMHILT et al. 1969) are such that it may not be apparent (FORKER et al. 1970). Some 5%–10% of cases show left bundle branch block. Sinus rhythm is usual, even in the presence of congestive heart failure. The chest X-ray will show left ventricular enlargement, particularly if there is cardiac failure or aortic incompetence. Lateral chest X-rays, chest screening, and body-section radiography may show calcification of the aortic valve, which when present, is evidence of severe stenosis (GLANCY et al. 1969). The echocardiographic demonstration of aortic stenosis is difficult.

The principal problems of diagnosis are those of distinguishing between aortic stenosis and aortic valvular sclerosis without obstruction, between aortic stenosis and incompetence and other causes of aortic incompetence (see Sect. C.III.2) and between aortic stenosis and hypertrophic obstructive cardiomyopathy (see Sect. D.III).

The clinical distinction between aortic stenosis and aortic valvular sclerosis is based on the presence in the former of left ventricular hypertrophy and of changes in the second heart sound, and on the loudness and length of the ejection murmur. In aortic stenosis the systolic murmur is loud, and longer than in aortic valvular sclerosis; phonocardiography may be of help in making the distinction (ARAVANIS and LUISADA 1957). Reduced intensity and reversed splitting of the second heart sound can usually be demonstrated in aortic stenosis. For a confident diagnosis of aortic stenosis, clinical, electrocardiographic, or radiological evidence of left ventricular hypertrophy must be present, but left ventricular hypertrophy due to other causes may coexist with aortic valvular sclerosis.

The diagnosis of aortic stenosis is more often missed than made in error (ANDERSEN et al. 1975), though a certain diagnosis may at times be impossible (RODSTEIN and ZEMAN 1967).

3. Haemodynamics

Systolic gradients across the aortic valve can be as great in the elderly as in younger patients (FINEGAN et al. 1969; AUSTEN et al. 1970; ROBERTS et al. 1971; STARR and LAWSON 1976), and calculated valve areas as small. In elderly patients with aortic stenosis without cardiac failure, cardiac output is well maintained, but falls substantially if failure develops (Table 1). In the absence of cardiac failure, the increase in pulmonary mean transit time and pulmonary blood volume is slight and comparable to that in elderly patients with left ventricular hypertrophy due to hypertension or ischaemic heart disease, but both measurements are considerably increased in those with heart failure.

4. Prognosis

The prognosis of asymptomatic aortic stenosis in old age is good (BEDFORD and CAIRD 1960), and there appear to be no symptoms (e.g. angina) which are associated with a worse outlook. But once cardiac failure has developed, few patients survive more than 3 years.

5. Treatment

Medical treatment of cardiac failure may result in short-lived improvement, but surgical treatment has much to offer severely disabled patients (AUSTEN et al. 1970; OH et al. 1973; STARR and LAWSON 1976; DE BONO et al. 1978). In STARR and LAWSON's series of 221 aortic valve replacements over the age of 60, the hospital mortality was 16%, but the survival rate at 5 years was 68% and at 10 years 41%. Symptomatic improvement is usually striking. It is clear that operation should be offered to many more elderly patients than at present.

III. Aortic Incompetence

1. Pathology

The numerous causes of aortic incompetence in the elderly may be divided into those in which the primary abnormality is in the aortic valve, and those in which it is in the aortic root. Any of the types of aortic stenosis, but particularly the postinflammatory variety with contraction of the cusps, may produce aortic incompetence, which is present in some two-thirds of elderly patients with aortic stenosis (BEDFORD and CAIRD 1960). A second much rarer condition in which the valve is primarily affected is the aortic incompetence of rheumatoid disease (CLARK et al. 1957). Granulomata in the fibrous part of the valve result in fibrous thickening and contracture of the cusps, without commissural adhesions (POMERANCE 1976). Other valvular causes include cusp rupture and infective endocarditis.

There are in addition several forms of aortic incompetence in which the aortic root is primarily involved. Syphilitic aortic incompetence is now a relative rarity, though in recent years one-third of all cases have been encountered in old age (HEGGTVEIT 1964; PREWITT 1970). Dilatation of the valve ring stretches the cusps and widens the commissures; damage to the free edges of the cusps by the regurgitation leads to their becoming sclerotic and rolled. Other conditions producing essentially similar results are the aortic incompetence of ankylosing spondylitis (BULKLEY and ROBERTS 1973), giant cell arteritis, cystic medionecrosis, and chronic dissecting aneurysm (LEVINE et al. 1951).

There remains a group of cases in which none of these pathologies is apparent. The aorta shows no distinctive macroscopic features, but the incompetence is due to dilatation of the aortic ring. Microscopic changes in the aorta are similarly slight, though there may be destruction and fibrous scarring of the medial elastic tissue (POMERANCE 1976). Exaggeration of the dilatation of the aorta that occurs with normal ageing (SUTER 1897) would seem the most likely cause, and high blood pressure may perhaps accelerate the process in some cases.

2. Clinical Features and Diagnosis

40% of cases of rheumatic heart disease in old age show aortic incompetence in addition to signs of mitral disease (BEDFORD and CAIRD 1960), but only very rarely without such signs. The combined lesion is commoner in men than women, as in middle age. The early diastolic murmur is almost always soft and short. Severe aortic incompetence is unusual, but there is often left ventricular hypertrophy.

When aortic incompetence complicates aortic stenosis, the features of the latter will be present, in particular depression of the aortic component of the second heart sound, and the diastolic murmur is again usually short and soft.

Syphilitic aortic incompetence is often accompanied by evidence of tabes dorsalis or taboparesis (BEDFORD and CAIRD 1960). The aortic incompetence is usually severe, with a collapsing pulse, high pulse pressure, and left ventricular hypertrophy and dilatation. There is almost always an aortic ejection murmur, the second heart sound is loud and ringing, and the diastolic murmur is long and widely heard over the praecordium. The chest X-ray characteristically shows irregular dilatation of the aorta, and calcification in its ascending part. The serological tests for syphilis are usually positive, or are known to have been so in the recent past. The prognosis is usually poor (BEDFORD and CAIRD 1960).

The rarer causes of aortic incompetence may be diagnosed from the clinical features of the associated conditions, such as rheumatoid arthritis, ankylosing spondylitis or giant cell arteritis. The diagnosis of incomplete aortic rupture may only be possible in retrospect, as when death finally occurs from complete aortic dissection.

"Isolated aortic incompetence" is best regarded as a clinical syndrome, with a number of causes, which share the common feature of the presence of aortic incompetence without evidence of other valve disease or of syphilis (BEDFORD and CAIRD 1960). The condition is almost always asymptomatic and its haemodynamic impact clinically slight. The pulse and pulse pressure are commonly normal and there is only rarely evidence of left ventricular hypertrophy. There is often an aortic ejection murmur, but the second heart sound is normal or loud, and the early diastolic murmur short. There may be electrocardiographic evidence of left ventricular hypertrophy, but the chest X-ray is usually unhelpful, since aortic dilatation is rarely severe enough to be clearly recognised. The prognosis is good.

3. Treatment

Surgical treatment is only rarely required for aortic incompetence in the elderly, but STARR and LAWSON (1976) report 17 patients and DE BONO et al. (1978) nine in whom the valve lesion had varying causes. STARR and LAWSON (1976) suggest that all patients with symptoms should be offered operation, unless there is evidence of serious disease of other organs.

D. Other Valve Disease

I. Tricuspid Valve Disease

1. Pathology

Age changes in the tricuspid valve resemble those in the mitral, but are commonly less severe.

Rheumatic tricuspid stenosis is extremely rare in the elderly (BEDFORD and CAIRD 1960) because it is usually a manifestation of severe rheumatic heart disease, the prognosis of which is such that the great majority of the cases are likely to die in middle age (COOKE and WHITE 1941). Tricuspid stenosis in carcinoid heart disease is also very rare, but its pathological appearances are characteristic (POMERANCE 1976).

2. Tricuspid Stenosis

Tricuspid stenosis is manifest by gross elevation of the venous pressure during all phases of the cardiac cycle, with hepatic enlargement and often ascites, but without evidence of frank cardiac failure. Dyspnoea is often disproportionately slight. The electrocardiogram usually shows atrial fibrillation, but when sinus rhythm is maintained, a tall pointed P wave without right axis shift is often combined with first degree heart block (GOODWIN et al. 1957; KITCHIN and TURNER 1964). The chest X-ray shows enlargement of the right atrium.

3. Tricuspid Incompetence

Tricuspid incompetence is common in old age because it almost always accompanies substantial elevation of the right ventricular diastolic pressure (KORNER and SHILLINGFORD 1957), and thus complicates right heart failure of any cause. The venous pulse shows a large positive systolic wave, and there is usually a pansystolic murmur maximal at the left lower sternal edge, with obvious accentuation on inspiration.

The electrocardiogram is that of the causative heart disease, and on the chest X-ray there is usually dilatation of the superior vena cava.

Tricuspid incompetence is often transient and variable, disappearing over a period of days as right heart pressures fall towards normal, and recurring if they rise again. Persistent "organic" tricuspid incompetence due to destructive changes in the valve is usually associated with tricuspid stenosis, and is thus decidedly rare in old age.

II. Pulmonary Valve Disease

A very occasional case of pulmonary incompetence complicating severe chronic pulmonary hypertension in chronic lung disease is encountered in old age. The early diastolic murmur is heard only at the left sternal edge, and there is clear evidence of right but not left ventricular hypertrophy and dilatation. There are no peripheral signs of aortic incompetence.

III. Multiple Valve Disease

Multiple valve disease is not rare in old age. Combined mitral and aortic incompetence was found in 29% of cases of rheumatic heart disease and mitral disease, and aortic stenosis in a further 14% (BEDFORD and CAIRD 1960). Surgical treatment carries a considerable operative mortality (OH et al. 1973), but the 5-year survival approaches 50% (STARR and LAWSON 1976).

One potentially important differential diagnosis is hypertrophic obstructive cardiomyopathy (WHITING et al. 1971; POMERANCE and DAVIES 1975; KRASNOW and STEIN 1978). Obstruction to left ventricular ejection results in an ejection murmur, but this is relatively poorly conducted to the neck, and the aortic component of the second heart sound is normal. There is usually evidence of mitral incompetence. The physical signs thus resemble those of multiple valve disease, but the chest X-ray only rarely shows evidence of calcification of the aortic valve, and the echocardiogram has many characteristic features (KRASNOW and STEIN 1978). The diagnosis is important because treatment with beta-adrenergic blocking drugs may be useful (KRASNOW and STEIN 1978), and surgical treatment may benefit more severe cases (SWAN et al. 1971).

E. Endocarditis

I. Infective Endocarditis

1. Pathology

Infective endocarditis may involve both normal and abnormal valves in the elderly (POMERANCE 1976). The nodular masses of fibrin and red blood cells, with inflammatory cells and micro-organisms, are usually found on the atrial surfaces of the mitral valve and the ventricular surfaces of the aortic valves along the lines of closure. Vegetations may also form at the sites of jet lesions on the endocardium. There are usually necrotic changes in the underlying valve, frequently with perforation of cusps and rupture of chordae. Extension of the infection into the valve rings may result in heart block, and the myocardium often contains embolic abscesses.

2. Clinical Features

WEDGWOOD (1976) has reviewed the clinical features of the disease as it is encountered in old age. An obvious source of infection is relatively uncommon, and fewer than half the cases now seen are due to *Streptococcus viridans*. Negative blood cultures are not uncommon, and have many causes, including the prior use of antibiotics and the presence of unusual organisms or fungi; some may in fact be due to non-bacterial thrombotic endocarditis (see Sect. E.II).

The principal symptoms are those of "toxaemia", with weight loss, anorexia, and weakness. Symptoms of fever are less frequent, but psychiatric disturbances are common (GLECKLER 1958). The toxaemic symptoms are likely to be attributed to malignant disease, and the psychiatric to cerebral arteriosclerosis.

The principal physical signs are fever and a heart murmur, but neither may be present initially. Fever may be slight or intermittent, and its detection may require repeated recording of the temperature. The murmur may be soft, or regarded as of no significance. Congestive heart failure may be present and atrial fibrillation is not rare (EISINGER 1971).

The crucial investigation is blood culture, which may need to be repeated several times. In patients with teeth, *Streptococcus viridans* is the usual infecting organism, and in those in whom infection follows genito-urinary operations or procedures, *Streptococcus faecalis* or other organisms.

Acute bacterial endocarditis is perhaps not clearly separable from the subacute variety, and more cases with symptoms of short duration are being recognised in the elderly. A clinically short illness can be caused by *Streptococcus viridans*, but the common organism is *Staphylococcus aureus*. There are severe toxaemic and febrile symptoms, and often intracutaneous haemorrhages; cerebral manifestations may be due to staphylococcal meningitis. Diagnosis and treatment are a matter of great urgency, but the prognosis is extremely poor.

3. Treatment

Penicillin remains the mainstay of treatment in cases due to *Streptococcus viridans*, and should be given by intravenous infusion when gross muscle wasting makes repeated injections distressing (WEDGWOOD 1976). Cases due to other organisms should be treated with single or combined antibiotics, as appropriate to the bacterial sensitivities, with careful monitoring of blood levels. Treatment should be continued until there are clear clinical signs of improvement, with reduction in heart rate, fall in erythrocyte sedimentation rate, and disappearance of red cells from the urine.

The poor prognosis of bacterial endocarditis in the elderly is mainly due to delay in diagnosis and initiation of treatment, as well as to the frequent occurrence of damage to the aortic valve, with serious haemodynamic consequences. A mortality rate of 30% is acceptable (WEDGWOOD 1976). Prevention is therefore the more important, and antibiotic cover should be given for 24–48 h to all old people with known valvular disease who have a dental extraction, or undergo any genito-urinary procedure.

II. Non-bacterial Thrombotic Endocarditis

Non-bacterial thrombotic endocarditis (NBTE) is a common pathological finding at autopsy in the elderly (POMERANCE 1976). The vegetations occur at the same sites as those of bacterial endocarditis, and are indeed macroscopically indistinguishable from them. Microscopically, however, they contain neither micro-organisms nor inflammatory cells, and there is no inflammatory change in the valve itself. Thrombotic endocarditis is usually only diagnosed at autopsy, but it may be suspected in cases of "bacterial endocarditis with persistently negative blood cultures", and in preterminal embolic arterial occlusion.

References

Acheson RM, Acheson ED (1958) Coronary and other heart disease in a group of Irish males aged 65–85. Br J Prev Soc Med 12:147–153
Andersen JA, Hansen BF, Lyngborg K (1975) Isolated valvular aortic stenosis. Acta Med Scand 197:61–64
Aravanis C, Luisada AA (1957) Obstructive and relative aortic stenosis: differential diagnosis by phonocardiography. Am Heart J 54:32–41
Austen WG, De Sanctis RW, Buckley MJ, Mundth ED, Scannell JG (1970) Surgical management of aortic valve disease in the elderly. J Am Med Assoc 211:624–626
Bedford PD, Caird FI (1960) Valvular disease of the heart in old age. Churchill London
Bulkley BH, Roberts WC (1973) Ankylosing spondylitis and aortic regurgitation. Circulation 48:1014–1027
Caird FI (1976) Valvular heart disease. In: Caird FI, Dall JLC, Kennedy RD (eds) Cardiology in old age. Plenum Press, New York London, pp 231–247
Caird FI (1980) Radionuclide studies of the circulation in the elderly. J Clin Exp Gerontol 2:23–40
Caird FI, Dall JLC (1979) Cardiovascular system. In: Brocklehurst JC (ed) Textbook of geriatric medicine and gerontology, 2nd edn. Churchill Livingstone, Edinburgh London, pp 125–127
Caird FI, Kennedy RD, Kelly JCC (1973) Combined apexcardiography and phonocardiography in investigation of heart disease in old age. Gerontol Clin 15:366–377
Clark WS, Kulka JP, Bauer W (1957) Rheumatoid aortitis with aortic regurgitation. Am J Med 22:580–592
Cooke WT, White PD (1941) Tricuspid stenosis. Br Heart J 3:147–165

Currens JH (1967) Rheumatic heart disease from ages 71 to 98. JAMA 199:849–851
de Bono AHB, English TAH, Milstein BB (1978) Heart valve replacement in the elderly. Br Med J 2:917–919
de Pasquale NP, Burch GE (1966) The necropsy incidence of gross scars or acute infarction of the papillary muscles of the left ventricle. Am J Cardiol 17:169
Dillon JC, Haine CL, Chang S, Feigenbaum H (1971) Use of echocardiography in patients with prolapsed mitral valve. Circulation 43:503–507
Droller H, Pemberton J (1953) Cardiovascular disease in a random sample of elderly people. Br Heart J 15:199–204
Eisinger AJ (1971) Atrial fibrillation in bacterial endocarditis. Br Heart J 33:739–741
Epstein EJ, Coulshed N (1973) Phonocardiogram and apex cardiogram in systolic click-late systolic murmur syndrome. Br Heart J 35:260–275
Finegan RE, Gianelli RE, Harrison DC (1969) Aortic stenosis in the elderly. New Engl J Med 281:1261–1264
Forker AD, McCallister BD, Giuliani ER, Osmundson PJ (1970) Atypical presentations of patients with calcific aortic stenosis. JAMA 212:774–779
Friedberg CK, Tartakower T (1931) Über den günstigen Verlauf des endokarditischen Herzklappenfehlers. Z Klin Med 116:759–803
Glancy DL, Freed TA, O'Brien KP, Epstein SE (1969) Calcium in the aortic valve. Ann Intern Med 71:245–250
Gleckler WJ (1958) Diagnostic aspects of subacute bacterial endocarditis in the elderly. Arch Int Med 102:761–765
Goodwin JF (1963) Diagnosis of left atrial myxoma. Lancet 1:464–468
Goodwin JF, Rab SM, Sinha MH, Zoob M (1957) Rheumatic tricuspid stenosis. Br Med J 2:1383–1389
Harvey WP (1968) Clinical aspects of cardiac tumors. Am J Cardiol 21:328–343
Hebbert FJ, Rankin J (1954) Mitral valve disease over the age of fifty. Acta Med Scand 150:101–118
Heggtveit HA (1964) Syphilitic aortitis: a clinicopathological autopsy study of 100 cases 1950 to 1960. Circulation 29:346–355
Heikillä J (1967) Mitral incompetence complicating acute myocardial infarction. Br Heart J 29:162–169
Kennedy RD, Andrews GR, Caird FI (1977) Ischaemic heart disease in the elderly. Br Heart J 39:1121–1127
Kirk RS, Russell JGB (1969) Subvalvular calcification of the mitral valve. Br Heart J 31:684–692
Kitchin A, Turner R (1964) Diagnosis and treatment of tricuspid stenosis. Br Heart J 26:354–379
Korn D, de Sanctis RW, Sell S (1962) Massive calcification of the mitral annulus. New Engl J Med 267:900–909
Korner P, Shillingford JP (1957) Tricuspid incompetence and right ventricular output in congestive heart failure. Br Heart J 19:1–7
Krasnow N, Stein RA (1978) Hypertrophic cardiomyopathy in the aged. Am Heart J 96:326–336
Kumpe CW, Bean WB (1948) Aortic stenosis. Medicine (Baltimore) 27:139–185
Levine E, Stein M, Gordon G, Mitchell N (1951) Chronic dissecting aneurysm of the aorta resembling chronic rheumatic heart disease. New Engl J Med 244:902–906
McMillan JB, Lev M (1959) The aging heart. J Gerontol 14:268–283
Nasser WK, Davis RH, Dillon JC, Tavel ME, Helman CH, Feigenbaum H, Fisch C (1972) Atrial myxoma. Am Heart J 83:810–824
Oh W, Hickman R, Emanuel R, McDonald L, Somerville J, Ross D, Ross K, Gonzalez-Lavin L (1973) Heart valve surgery in 114 patients over the age of 60. Br Heart J 35:174–180
Pomerance A (1972) Pathogenesis of aortic stenosis and its relation to age. Br Heart J 34:569–574
Pomerance A (1976) Pathology of the myocardium and valves. In: Caird FI, Dall JCL, Kennedy RD (eds) Cardiology in old age. Plenum Press, New York London, pp 11–55

Pomerance A, Davies MJ (1975) Pathological features of hypertrophic obstructive cardio-
    myopathy in the aged. Brit Heart J 37:305–312
Popp RL, Brown OW, Silverman JF, Harrison DC (1974) Echocardiographic abnormalities
    in the mitral valve prolapse syndrome. Circulation 49:428–433
Prewitt TA (1970) Syphilitic aortic insufficiency. J Amer Med Ass 211:637–639
Roberts WC, Perloff JK, Constantino T (1971) Severe aortic valvular stenosis in patients
    aged over 65. Amer J Cardiol 27:497–506
Rodstein M, Zeman FD (1967) Aortic stenosis in the aged. Clinical pathological correla-
    tions. Amer J Med Sci 254:577–584
Romhilt DW, Bove KE, Norris RJ, Conyers E, Conradi S, Rowlands DT, Scott RC (1969)
    A critical appraisal of the electrocardiographic criteria for the diagnosis of left ventric-
    ular hypertrophy. Circulation 40:185–195
Rytand DA, Lipsitch LS (1946) Clinical aspects of calcification of the mitral annulus fi-
    brosus. Arch Intern Med 78:544–564
Sell S, Scully RE (1965) Aging changes in the aortic and mitral valves. Am J Path 46:345–365
Sievers J, Hall P (1971) Incidence of acute rheumatic fever. Br Heart J 33:833–836
Simon MA, Liu SF (1954) Calcification of the mitral valve annulus and its relation to func-
    tional valve disturbances. Am Heart J 48:497–505
Starr A, Lawson R (1976) Cardiac surgery in the elderly. In: Caird FI, Dall JLC, Kennedy
    RD (eds) Cardiology in old age. Plenum Press, New York London, pp 369–396
Suter F (1897) Über das Verhalten des Aortenumfanges unter physiologischen und patho-
    logischen Bedingungen. Arch Exp Path Pharmakol 39:289–332
Swan DA, Bell B, Oakley CM, Goodwin JF (1971) Analysis of symptomatic course and
    prognosis and treatment of hypertrophic obstructive cardiomyopathy. Br Heart J
    33:671–685
Wedgwood J (1976) Remediable heart disease. In: Caird FI, Dall JLC, Kennedy RD (eds)
    Cardiology in old age. Plenum Press, New York London, pp 249–265
Whiting RB, Powell WJ, Dinsmore RE, Sanders CA (1971) Idiopathic hypertrophic subaor-
    tic stenosis in the elderly. New Engl J Med 285:196–200

Cardiac Arrhythmias

R. Harris

A. Introduction

The aging human heart shows an increased incidence of age-associated cardiac arrhythmias (Harris 1970, 1976) which appear related to alterations in the electrical activity of the heart with age and the ionic movements across the excitable membranes in the old myocardium. Long-term recordings of electrocardiograms in a normal population confirm that the incidence of ectopic activity increases with age and that important arrhythmias and frequent ectopic beats in old age are indications of underlying cardiac disease rather than a benign part of the aging process (Raftery and Cashman 1976).

Cardiac arrhythmias are considerably more serious in old age because they further compromise the blood supply of vital body organs already impaired by aging changes and disease. Atrial and ventricular tachycardias in excess of 140 beats per minute significantly reduce peripheral blood perfusion. Elderly patients with cerebral or carotid artery narrowing often manifest diffuse or focal cerebral insufficiency during cardiac arrhythmias. Transient cardiac arrhythmias are more likely to produce symptoms of diffuse cerebrovascular insufficiency rather than focal, neurologic signs. Cardiac dysrhythmias may be important causes of otherwise unexplained giddiness, falls, blackouts, and confusional states in the elderly.

Cardiac arrhythmias also contribute to heart failure. When the heart rate is rapid, the prolonged contraction duration of the old heart compromises ventricular filling and causes incomplete relaxation between beats leading to a higher left ventricular end-diastolic pressure, a higher pulmonary venous pressure, and a greater tendency toward congestive heart failure. The prolonged contraction duration, as studied in the old rat myocardium, is attributed to the slow removal of calcium from the contractile proteins which is independent of the catecholamine content of the myocardium. This sequestration of calcium from the contractile proteins is primarily a function of the sarcoplasmic reticulum (Lakatta et al. 1975).

The management of cardiac arrhythmias requires (1) appreciation of the etiology, nature, background, and clinical circumstances at the onset of the arrhythmia (see Sect. B.I), (2) correct diagnosis of the arrhythmia (see Sect. B.II), and (3) selection of the appropriate drugs and therapy that will correct cellular abnormalities, electrophysiologic dysfunction, and the disease factors responsible for them (see Sect. C).

This chapter presents the information needed to improve the medical skills of physicians in managing their aging patients with cardiac arrhythmias. It is intended to supplement the standard texts on this subject and is best used in conjunction with them.

B. Diagnostic Considerations

I. Etiology

1. Physiologic Causes

Cardiac arrhythmias are characterized by disturbances in the order, rate, depolarization, regularity, and/or origin of the heart beat. Until recently, clinical cardiac arrhythmias were attributed to abnormalities of conduction, automaticity, or a combination of both. Now, most cardiac arrhythmias are attributed to reentry as a result of unidirectional block and a critical delay in conduction. Under certain circumstances hyperkalemia, hypercalcemia, and various drugs affecting the transmembrane differential may also convert fast response Purkinje fibers to functionally slow response fibers. Additional mechanisms include early and delayed afterdepolarizations, which can induce "triggered" arrhythmias, phase 4 depolarizations, and abnormal automaticity in partially depolarized fibers (ROSEN et al. 1980).

Cardiac arrhythmias may also result from abnormalities of impulse formation arising from physiologic factors and enhanced automaticity. For example, the rate of firing of the cardiac pacemaker cells is controlled by the activity of the autonomic nervous system and the local chemical environment of the pacemaker cells. The autonomic nervous system, and especially the balance between the sympathetic and vagal drives, is fundamental in the genesis of cardiac arrhythmias. Increased vagal activity may depress the automaticity of the sinoatrial (SA) node and shift the site of the origin of the impulse to another pacemaker proximal to the atrioventricular (AV) node (low atrial rhythm) or to cells in the His–Purkinje system which are less strongly influenced by vagal activity. At the atrium and ventricular levels, it is not always clear whether autonomic nervous system activity preferentially induces a reentrant or automatic phenomenon (COUMEL et al. 1979). Conditions that reduce the level of extracellular potassium or increase exposure to catecholamines enhance automaticity in the Purkinje fibers or myocardial cells and may precipitate arrhythmias. Carbon dioxide retention (not uncommon in the elderly patient with pulmonary disease) may increase the excitability of the heart muscle. Hypoxia and exposure to mechanical or thermal injury may also produce cardiac arrhythmias.

2. Aging Changes

Anatomic, biochemical, and electrophysiologic changes of aging in the old heart may alter its normal physiologic properties and produce greater excitability, irritability, and slowed conduction. New techniques using bundle of His recordings have demonstrated that the ability of the old heart to conduct rapidly occurring impulses from the atria through the atrioventricular junction to the ventricle diminishes. Microelectrode recordings of atrial action potentials also demonstrate age-related changes in cardiac membranes. For example, the rat myocardium shows three major electrophysiologic changes with advancing age: (1) the maximum rate of rise of phase 0 decreases, (2) the plateau phase of repolarization becomes more prominent, and (3) the time necessary to achieve 95% repolarization increases. Conduction velocity decreases with age (ROBERTS and GOLDBERG 1975). The decrease in the maximum rate rise of the action potential explains some changes in the conduction velocity and contractility of the heart in older animals and people (CAVOTO et al. 1974).

Age-related changes in the intracellular sodium and potassium contents of the aging rat heart may also be major determinants in its increased resting action potential. Trend analysis of the Na influx rates in atrial muscle of rats shows a significant increase with age except for a decrease at 24 months. Intracellular sodium concentration significantly increases from 1 to 3 months and a significant decrease at 6 months is followed by leveling off. Potassium influx rates remain relatively constant at all ages (GOLDBERG et al. 1975). Intracellular potassium concentration exhibits an initial significant decrease from 1 to 3 months followed by a significant increase at 6 months, which remains unchanged through 28 months. Right atrial tissue removed at heart surgery from older people shows a higher stimulation threshold, which precludes endocardial pacing on tissue (BUSH et al. 1971).

Some atrial arrhythmias in the aged arise from the anatomic heart changes attributed to the aging process, such as focal thickening of the elastic and reticular nets and infiltration of fat in and about the region of the SA node and the internodal tracts. These changes represent a slow and continuous process that begins at about 60 years of age. They are unrelated to coronary artery disease, and partially account for the ease with which atrial arrhythmias are induced in elderly hearts (DAVIES and POMERANCE 1972).

3. Disease

Atrial pathology may be caused by disease such as nonspecific inflammation, degenerative and fibrotic processes, and ischemic states secondary to disease of the sinus node artery or its parent artery. Such atrial pathology may produce atrial arrhythmias (TITUS 1973).

Arteriosclerosis, acute coronary thrombosis, or shock, which decreases the blood supply to the sinus node, may also induce serious ventricular arrhythmias. Some of these may be due to myocardial infarction or cardiac chamber dilatation, which alter the action potential and produce excessive stretch, hypoxia, electrolyte disturbances, and greater potassium accumulation. Chronic or recurrent ventricular tachycardia with or without associated myocardial ischemia may also arise from reentry as a result of a basic inhomogeneity between normal working myocardium and abnormal, impaired ventricular muscle.

4. Iatrogenic (Drug-Induced) Factors

Some drugs used in treatment may produce cardiac arrhythmias by abolishing the normal physiologic overdrive suppression mechanism that ordinarily enables the sinus node to initiate the heart beat. As a result, catecholamines and digitalis may reverse the response of the automaticity cells to overdrive so that overdrive, instead of depressing, actually enhances automaticity and the possibility of escape rhythms (CRANEFIELD et al. 1973).

The clinical effects of cardioactive drugs depend also upon the mechanism and the magnitude of abnormalities of sinoatrial dysfunction. A pharmacologic agent with negligible effects on the normal sinus node may exert profound adverse effects on the sinus node and sinoatrial junction in the elderly patient with sick sinus syndrome. Thus, a specific cardioactive drug like digitalis may act differently in the presence of abnormal intrinsic sinoatrial function than in its absence (Jordan et al. 1979).

Digitalis toxicity is an especially common iatrogenic cause of multifocal ventricular extrasystoles, paroxysmal supraventricular tachycardia, atrial fibrillation with block, or other arrhythmias in elderly patients.

Diuretics producing electrolyte imbalance and tricyclic antidepressant drugs producing myocardial toxicity may also precipitate iatrogenic arrhythmias of the aged. Caffeine and alcohol too may precipitate arrhythmias in some sensitive individuals with or without organic heart disease.

II. Types of Common Arrhythmias and Management

1. World Health Organization Classification

Although the World Health Organization's comprehensive classification of cardiac arrhythmias (1979) provides a useful scheme for classifying the disturbances of cardiac rhythms (Tables 1–5), this chapter is limited to the identification of the more common cardiac arrhythmias and their management in the elderly. (Heart block is discussed elsewhere in this volume.)

2. Normal Supraventricular Rhythms

These rhythms originate in the sinus node, atrium, or atrioventricular junction. They are characterized by QRS complexes of normal duration up to 0.10 s (greater when aberrant ventricular conduction is present).

a) Sinus Rhythm

Normal sinus rhythm is characterized by regular impulse formation in the sinoatrial node and a normal resting heart rate in old age between 44 and 100 beats per minute. The intrinsic pacemaker rate in isolated heart preparations decreases with age because of basic changes in the pacemaker cells. In the intact animal, the effects of sympathetic influences on the heart rate vary with age, animal species, and the environment. Reflex control of the heart rate is altered in old age because of diminished reactivity of chemoreceptor and baroreceptor reflexes and increased vagal tone. As a result, hypoxia and hypercarbia increase the heart rate less in older than in younger people.

b) Sinus Arrhythmia

This benign arrhythmia is common in the elderly where the degree of variation with respiration increases. In phasic sinus arrhythmia, the sinus rate accelerates with inspiration and decreases with expiration. Nonphasic sinus arrhythmia, due to shifting of the pacemaker stimulus within the sinus node, is unrelated to inspiration or expiration. No treatment is required.

Table 1. World Health Organization (1979) classification of cardiac arrhythmias according to impulse origin

1. Supraventricular
   I. Sinoatrial (SA) node
   II. Atrium [excluding SA node and
      atrioventricular (AV) junction]
     A. Right
     B. Left
     C. Multifocal
     D. Unspecified
   III. AV junction
   IV. Unspecified supraventricular
 	
2. Ventricular
   I. Right
   II. Left
   III. Septal
   IV. Multifocal
   V. Unspecified
 	
3. Impulse origin undetermined
   (supraventricular or ventricular)
	4. Artificial pacemaker
	   I. Atrial pacing
	     A. No sensing function
	       (asynchronous, fixed rate)
	     B. Atrial sensing, inhibited mode
	     C. Atrial sensing, triggered mode
	   II. Ventricular pacing
	     A. No sensing function
	       (asynchronous, fixed rate)
	     B. Atrial sensing, triggered mode
	     C. Ventricular sensing,
	       inhibited mode
	     D. Ventricular sensing,
	       triggered mode
	   III. Atrioventricular pacing
	     A. No sensing function
	       (asynchronous, fixed rate)
	     B. Ventricular sensing,
	       inhibited mode

Table 2. World Health Organization (1979) classification of cardiac arrhythmias according to discharge (impulse) sequence

1. Single or up to two consecutive discharges
   I. Premature impulses (excluding
      manifest parasystolic impulses)
     A. Extrasystoles
       a) Doublet (couplet)
       b) Bigeminy
       c) Trigeminy, quadrigeminy, etc.
       d) R on T phenomenon
       e) Other patterns
     B. Captures
     C. Unspecified
   II. Escapes
 	
2. Regular rhythms
   I. At inherent rate
     (including escape rhythm)
   II. Bradycardia
   III. Accelerated rhythm
   IV. Tachycardia
   V. Flutter
     A. Typical
     B. Atypical
	3. Irregular rhythms
	   I. At inherent rate
	     (including escape rhythm)
	     A. Respiratory
	     B. Nonrespiratory
	       a) Ventriculophasic
	       b) Arrest
	       c) Other
	   II. Bradycardia
	     A. Respiratory
	     B. Nonrespiratory
	       a) Ventriculophasic
	       b) Arrest
	       c) Other
	   III. Accelerated rhythm
	     A. Respiratory
	     B. Nonrespiratory
	       a) Ventriculophasic
	       b) Arrest
	       c) Other
	   IV. Tachycardia
	     A. Respiratory
	     B. Nonrespiratory
	       a) Ventriculophasic
	       b) Arrest
	       c) Other
	   V. Fibrillation

Table 3. World Health
Organization   (1979)
classification of cardiac
arrhythmias according
to rate of discharge

1. 20 or less/min
2. 21–30/min
3. 31–40/min
4. 41–50/min
5. 51–100/min
6. 101–150/min
7. 151–200/min
8. 201–250/min
9. More than 250/min

c) Wandering Pacemaker

In this benign disorder, the pacemaker impulse wanders to different parts of the
sinus node, atria, and AV node. The pacemaker impulse is in the head, body, or
tail of the sinus node when the electrocardiogram shows an upright P wave preceding the QRS complex in limb leads and a P-R interval of 0.12 s or longer (Fig. 1).

d) Extrasystoles

Extrasystoles originate in the sinus node, atria, atrioventricular junction, or ventricles as a result of increasing myocardial irritability and other changes of aging and
disease. The normal upper limits are a frequency of 5% for supraventricular and
10% for premature ventricular beats in persons over 60 years of age (SIMONSON
1972). People over the age of 65 have a 10% incidence of atrial premature contractions and a 6% incidence of ventricular premature contractions (MIHALICK
and FISCH 1974).

Supraventricular extrasystoles have a narrow QRS complex of 0.10 s or less.
An extrasystole with a QRS complex wider than 0.10 s may represent a supraventricular beat with aberrant conduction or a ventricular extrasystole. Such impulses
are generally supraventricular when they have a preceding P wave and no fully
compensatory interval.

An AV junctional extrasystole is identified by a QRS interval of normal width,
a short P-R interval less than 0.12 s and retrograde P waves in leads II and III preceding the QRS complex (Fig. 1). An absent P wave or a retrograde P following
the QRS interval (ROSEN 1973) may also characterize these beats. Such extrasystoles do not require treatment.

3. Abnormal Supraventricular Arrhythmias

The frequency of atrial arrhythmias increases between the 7th and 10th decades.
Fast supraventricular arrhythmias include sinus tachycardia, ectopic atrial
rhythms, atrial flutter, and atrial fibrillation which may be paroxysmal or nonparoxysmal. Different etiologic factors and mechanisms may be responsible (see
Sect. B.I).

Table 4. World Health Organization (1979) classification of cardiac arrhythmias according to impulse conduction

1. Conduction from a pacemaker
   (exit of an impulse)
   I. Normal or presumably normal
   II. First degree block
   III. Second degree block
      A. Type I (Wenckebach)
      B. Type II (Mobitz II)
      C. Advanced
   IV. Unspecified block
      (concealed discharge)
   V. Impaired conduction presumably due
      to physiologic refractoriness
      A. Delayed conduction
      B. Intermittent failure

2. Atrioventricular conduction
   I. General classification
      A. Normal
      B. First degree block
      C. Second degree block
         a) Type I (Wenckebach)
         b) Type II (Mobitz II)
         c) Advanced
      D. Third degree block
      E. Unspecified block
      F. Impaired conduction presumably
         due to physiologic refractoriness
         a) Delayed conduction
         b) Intermittent failure
         c) Persistent failure
            (duration unspecified)
      G. Short P-R interval
      H. Alternation of conduction
   II. Bundle branch and fascicular
      conduction
      A. Normal
      B. Right bundle branch block
         (RBBB)
         a) Incomplete
            (1) Intermittent (transient,
               nonpermanent)

         (2) Persistent (duration
            unspecified)
         b) Complete
            (1) Intermittent (transient,
               nonpermanent)
            (2) Persistent
      C. Left bundle branch block (LBBB)
         a) Incomplete
            (1) Intermittent
            (2) Persistent
         b) Complete
            (1) Intermittent
            (2) Persistent
      D. (Left) Anterior fascicular block
         (LAFB)
         a) Intermittent
         b) Persistent
      E. (Left) Posterior fascicular block
         (LPFB)
         a) Intermittent
         b) Persistent
      · F. Combinations of bundle branch
         and fascicular block (specify)
      G. Impaired conduction presumably
         due to physiological refractoriness
         aberrant conduction)
         a) Right
         b) Left
         c) Right and left
         d) Unspecified

3. Intramyocardial conduction
   I. Intra-atrial conduction delay
      (including aberrant atrial conduction)
   II. Intra-atrial block
   III. Unspecified (nonspecific) intra-
      ventricular conduction delay or block
4. Ventriculoatrial conduction

a) Sinus Tachycardia

Sinus tachycardia is present when the heart beat originates in the sinoatrial node and the heart rate is over 100 beats per minute. When the heart rate is faster than 150, other supraventricular tachycardias should be suspected. Temporary sinus tachycardia is a normal response to ordinary physical activity, eating, anxiety, pain, caffeine, nicotine, epinephrine, atropine, amyl nitrate, and quinidine. Unexplained persistent sinus tachycardia is abnormal. Treatment is directed at eliminat-

Table 5. World Health Organization (1979) classification of cardiac arrhythmias according to special aspects related to impulse formation and/or conduction

1. Artificial pacemaker function
   I. Normal
   II. Defective
     A. Pacing
     B. Sensing
     C. Pacing and sensing
2. Concealed conduction
   I. In a pacemaker
   II. In the AV junction
   III. In the subjunctional region
   Effect of concealment (applicable to all
     sites mentioned above)
     A. Impairment of conduction
     B. Facilitation of conduction
     C. Resetting of subsequent
       discharge
     D. Combinations
3. Coupling interval
   I. Constant (80 ms or less)
   II. Variable
4. Entrance block (protection)
   I. Parasystole
     A. Intermittent
     B. Persistent
   II. Other
5. Enhancing mechanisms
   I. Supernormality
     A. Of conduction
     B. Of excitability
   II. Other
6. Gap phenomena
   I. In the AV conduction system
     A. During anterograde conduction
     B. During retrograde conduction
	II. In other parts of the heart
	7. Isorhythmic dissociation
	8. Multiform configuration of wave forms
	   I. Bidirectional (alternating)
	   II. Fusions
	     A. Atrial
	     B. Ventricular
	   III. Torsade de pointes
	   IV. Unspecified
	9. Preexcitation
	   I. Atrial
	     A. Intermittent
	     B. Persistent
	   II. Ventricular
	     A. WPW pattern
	       a) Intermittent
	       b) Persistent
	     B. Short PR syndrome
	       a) Intermittent
	       b) Persistent
	10. Reentry
	   I. Atrial
	   II. AV junctional
	   III. Ventricular
	   IV. Combined atrial and ventricular
	   Further specifications, applicable to
	     above:
	     A. Concealed
	       a) Single
	       b) Repetitive
	     B. Manifest
	       a) Single
	       b) Repetitive

ing the underlying cause, such as chronic anxiety, heart failure, hemorrhage, occult infection, fever, shock, hyperthyroidism, or anemia. When no etiology can be found and the patient is disturbed by the tachycardia, oral propranolol or reserpine may be tried.

b) Ectopic Atrial Rhythms

Paroxysmal supraventricular tachycardia usually results from reentry within the AV junction and frequently utilizes an accessory atrioventricular node bypass tract. In humans it may also be initiated by a properly timed atrial premature beat, junctional ectopic beats with an atrial echo, or a ventricular ectopic beat with an atrial echo and ventricular reciprocal beat (TICZON and WHALEN 1973).

The electrocardiogram of paroxysmal atrial tachycardia shows abnormal P waves at a rate of 140–240 beats per minute that consistently precede normal ap-

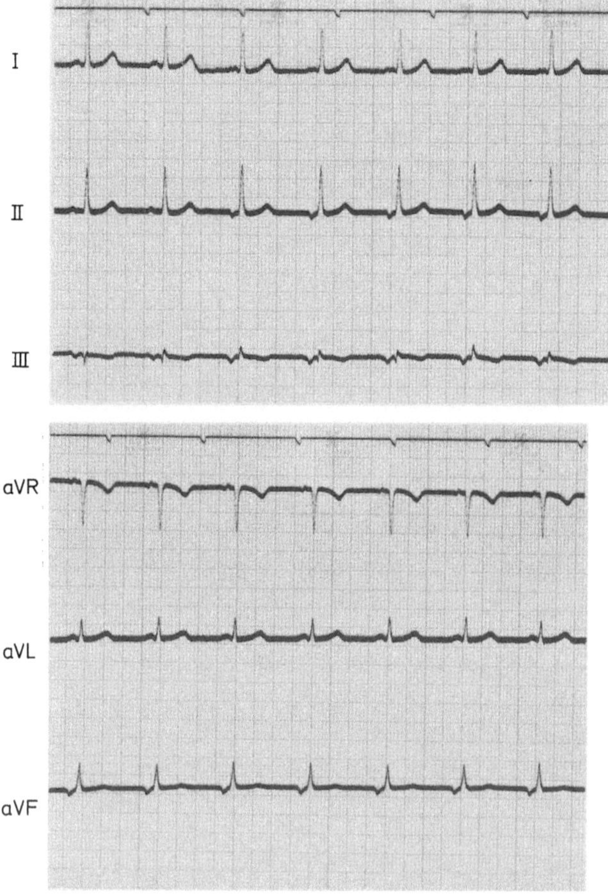

Fig. 1. Wandering pacemaker. First two sinus beats are followed by a shift to AV junction rhythm characterized by a shorter P-R interval (0.10 s), lower, notched P waves in lead 1, and inverted P waves in leads 2 and 3

pearing QRS complexes. The electrocardiogram of atrioventricular junctional tachycardia is similar except for the presence of retrograde P waves in leads II, III, and aVF, a P-R interval less than 0.12 s; an absent P wave preceding QRS complexes; or a retrograde P wave after the QRS complex. For both, the QRS complex is normal in width unless bundle branch block is present. At faster heart rates, atrioventricular heart block is common in the aged because of an impaired atrioventricular conduction system. Since the surface electrocardiogram does not always permit an accurate diagnosis of atrial activity, paroxysmal supraventricular tachycardia is a good term to use when the exact origin of the supraventricular rhythm is uncertain.

Management requires identification and correction of the predisposing and precipitating factors within the context of the clinical situation. Underlying complications, including drug intoxication, heart failure, hypokalemia, thyrotoxicosis,

Table 6. Availability status of different classes of antiarrhythmic agents

	Therapeutically available in the United States	Investigational in the United States	Experimental only
Class I	Quinidine Procainamide Lidocaine Phenytoin Disopyramide	Tocainide Mexiletine Aprindine N-acetyl Procainamide (NAPA)	Ajmaline Ethmozin Encainide
Class II	Propranolol Timolol	Alprenolol Oxprenolol Metoprolol Atenolol Nadolol Acebutolol	
Class III	Bretylium		Amiodarone Sotalol
Class IV	Verapamil (I.V.)	Nifedipine	Diltiazem Dimeditiapramine (R011-1781)

hypoxia, pericarditis, and myocardial infarction should be treated. In the absence of serious complications, simple reassurance, oxygen, sedation, and rest should be prescribed. These measures permit the arrhythmia to return spontaneously to sinus rhythm in a few hours. Vagotonic maneuvers, including the Valsalva maneuver, coughing, gagging, and self-induced vomiting may be tried. Carotid sinus pressure is sometimes helpful, but should be performed carefully under cardiographic monitoring in the aged who may have a sensitive carotid sinus reflex and widespread atherosclerosis in the carotid or basilar arteries. Carotid sinus pressure slows sinus tachycardia, terminates paroxysmal supraventricular tachycardia, or produces atrioventricular block with slowing of the ventricular rate (see also Sect. B.III).

In the usual variety of paroxysmal supraventricular tachycardia, the antegrade "slow" pathway may slow further and/or block when propranolol, digoxin, or verapamil is given. The retrograde fast pathway may be suppressed by the same agents, but it is specifically sensitive to the class I antiarrhythmics drugs: quinidine, procainamide, and disopyramide (Table 6). When quinidine is used in refractory atrial arrhythmias, it is best to monitor the patient for several hours after the quinidine has been stopped to make sure paroxysmal ventricular tachycardia or fibrillation do not complicate quinidine therapy.

If the arrhythmia does not respond to pharmacologic therapy, synchronized DC cardioversion may be tried. It is best performed when the patient has had no digitalis or after digitalis has been discontinued for several days. Temporary pervenous right atrial or right ventricular pacing has also been used to terminate paroxysmal supraventricular tachycardias refractory to drugs.

Edrophonium bromide (Tensilon), other cholinergic drugs, and pressor agents used to treat paroxysmal supraventricular tachycardia can be dangerous in old people but may be helpful in an emergency (Fig. 2). When edrophonium is used,

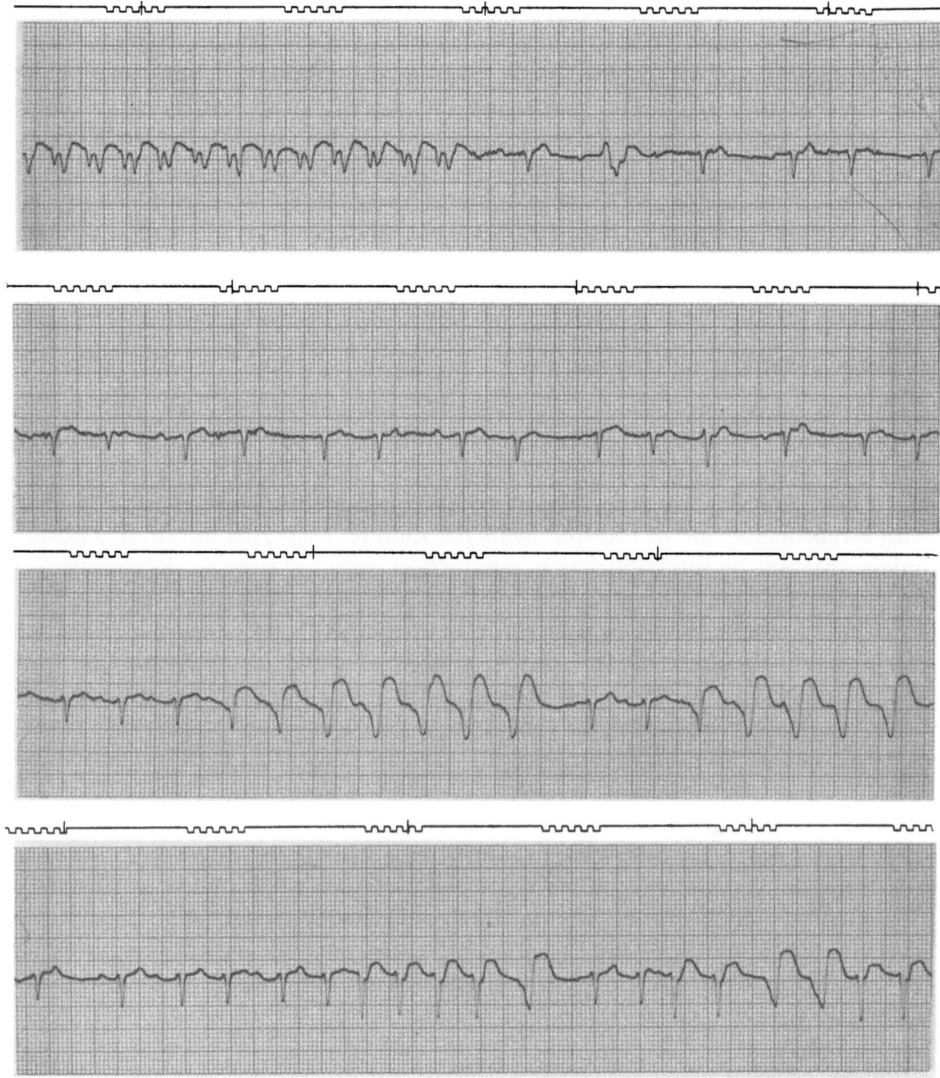

Fig. 2. Continous electrocardiographic recording in a 79-year-old man suffering from severe pulmonary insufficiency, acute hypoxia, and paroxysmal supraventricular tachycardia with a heart rate of 200 beats per minute and intraventricular conduction defect. Midway along the *top strip*, intravenous administration of endrophonium bromide (Tensilon) temporarily restored sinus rhythm. When tachycardia recurred *(third strip)*, another injection temporarily restored sinus rhythm. Subsequent injections failed to affect this arrhythmia

a syringe containing 1 mg atropine sulfate should be available to counteract any severe cholinergic reaction.

Patients with recurrent paroxysmal supraventricular tachycardia should be advised not to smoke or to drink coffee and other beverages with high caffeine content. Maintenance digitalis therapy and/or a combination of one or more antiarrhythmic agents (quinidine, propranolol, procainamide, and diphenylhydantoin) may be tried prophylactically in long-term management of these tachycardias.

Nonparoxysmal atrial arrhythmias occur most commonly in patients with digitalis intoxication or chronic lung disease as a result of an enhanced automatic pacemaker. They are characterized by an atrial rate between 70–180 beats per minute and a ventricular rate determined by the presence or absence of AV block. Multifocal atrial tachycardia is characterized by multiform P waves which precede QRS, an atrial rate greater than 100 beats per minute, varying P-R intervals, and irregular R-R intervals. Treatment with antiarrhythmic agents and electrocardioversion often fails and the mortality rate is high (Donoso 1973).

c) Atrial Flutter

This arrhythmia almost always occurs in older subjects with organic heart disease or pulmonary embolism. The electrocardiogram shows saw-toothed or undulating atrial "F" waves, at a rate of 300–320 beats per minute. These are clearest in leads II, III, aVF, and V1. Impaired atrioventricular conduction often causes 2:1 block with a ventricular rate of 150–160 beats per minute. The QRS duration is normal unless aberrant or intraventricular conduction defect is present. Recommended treatments include pharmacologic conversion with digoxin, digoxin, and quinidine, a combination of digoxin and propranolol, procainamide, electrical conversion with direct current cardioversion, or rapid atrial pacing. In some situations, it is advisable to resort initially to cardioversion if the patient is in heart failure or shock as a result of the arrhythmia. This arrhythmia responds so readily to cardioversion that many cardiologists consider it the treatment of choice at all ages.

Digitalis is useful to slow the ventricular rate and to convert atrial flutter to atrial fibrillation or sinus rhythm in elderly patients not already on digitalis. Pharmacologic conversion with quinidine or procainamide works in about 50%–60% of patients with atrial flutter. The patient should first be digitalized to prevent rapid ventricular rates during the 1:1 AV conduction since the anticholinergic effects of these drugs accelerate the atrioventricular node conduction as the atrial rate slows.

d) Atrial Fibrillation

The incidence of atrial fibrillation is 8% in people over 65 years of age (Mihalick and Fisch 1974). Paroxysmal atrial fibrillation occurs in routine electrocardiograms of asymptomatic elderly people and more commonly in patients with pulmonary embolism, myocardial infarction, acute pericarditis, decompensated lung disease, hypoxemia, thyrotoxicosis, coronary heart disease, sick sinus syndrome, atrial septal defect, and after thoracotomy.

Treatment of the underlying cause often restores sinus rhythm spontaneously. If not, digitalis alone or in conjunction with quinidine converts atrial fibrillation to sinus rhythm in about 80% of patients with arteriosclerotic heart disease and in about 40% with rheumatic heart disease. Other class I antiarrhythmic agents may work when these drugs fail (Figs. 3–6). Propranolol may also be tried as a drug of second choice.

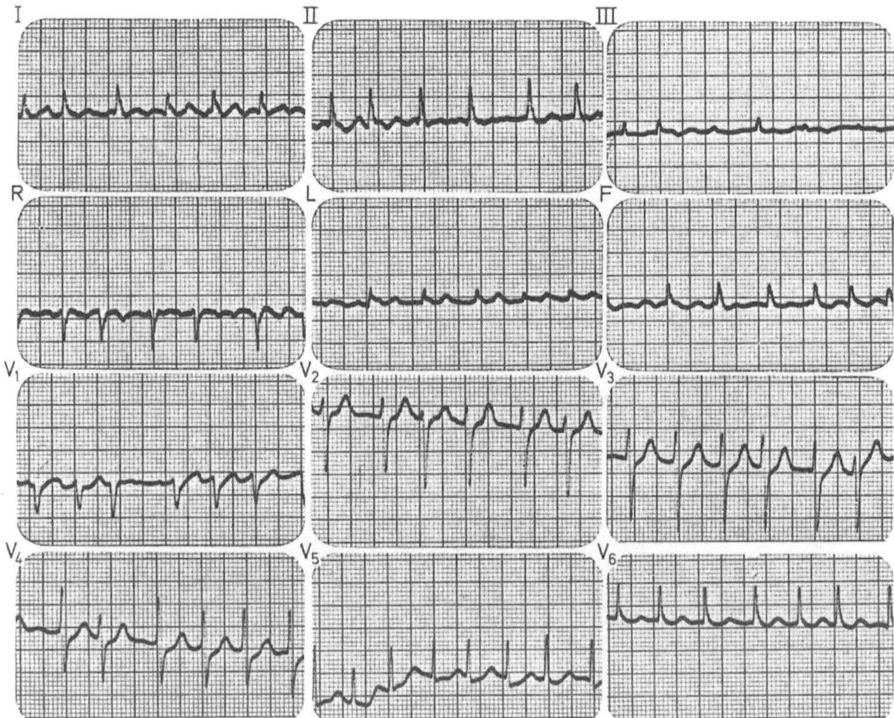

Fig. 3. Electrocardiogram shows paroxysmal atrial flutter fibrillation of recent onset in previously healthy 70-year-old woman

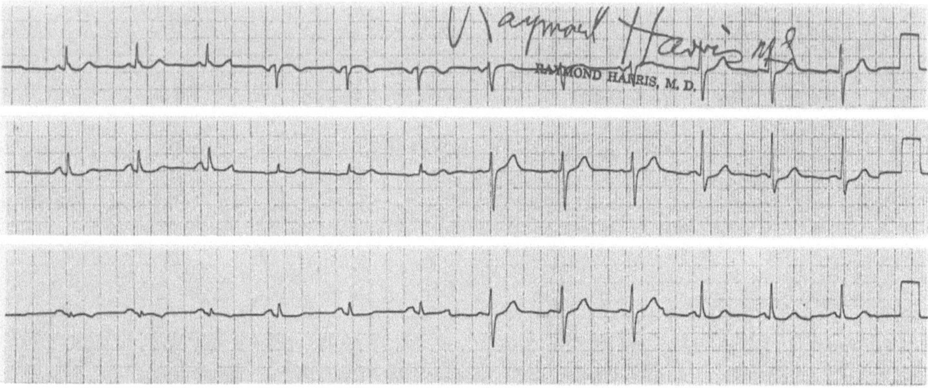

Fig. 4. Electrocardiogram 1 day later in the same patient as in Fig. 3. It was taken 24 h after the patient received 1 mg digoxin followed by 200 mg quinidine sulfate every 2 h for five doses and shows sinus rhythm

Direct current cardioversion of atrial fibrillation in elderly patients has been recommended to improve their cardiovascular circulation and to reduce the danger of emboli (STERN 1979). Synchronized DC cardioversion restores sinus rhythm in about 92% of patients unresponsive to drug therapy and in whom hyperthyroidism and electrolyte imbalance have been excluded. The decision to use cardioversion

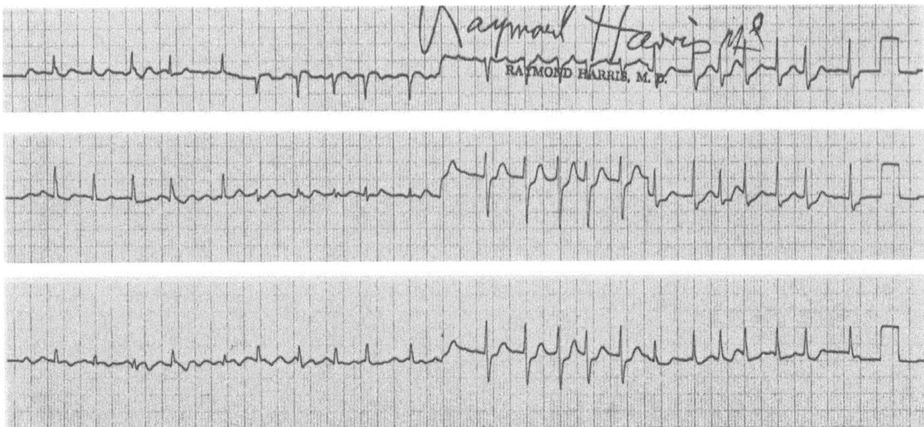

Fig. 5. Electrocardiogram taken 1 day later than that in Fig. 4 in the same patient shows return of paroxysmal atrial fibrillation after quinidine was discontinued because of severe diarrhea and nausea

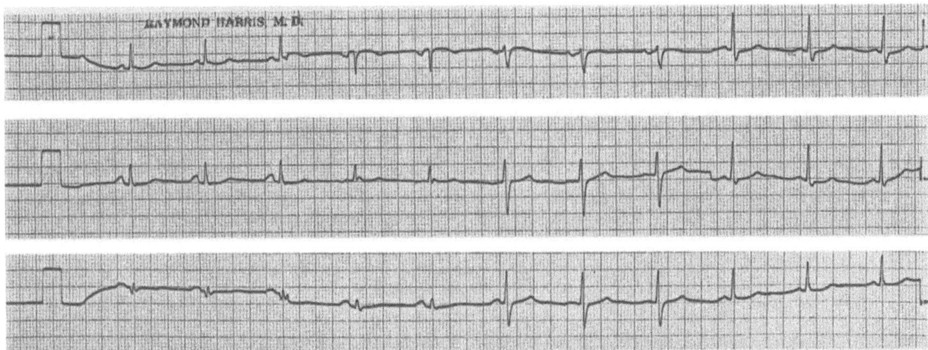

Fig. 6. Taken 1 day later than in Fig. 5 in the same patient, this electrocardiogram shows the return of sinus rhythm after the oral administration of 200 mg disopyramide and two additional doses of 100 mg each given 4 h apart. The patient was on a daily maintenance dose of digoxin (0.25 mg). She experienced no side effects from this combination of drugs

must consider that the elderly patient tolerates slow atrial fibrillation without difficulty and sinus rhythm after cardioversion may last from a few seconds to a few years. Furthermore, sinus node pathology makes cardioversion more hazardous. After conversion, the sick sinus node may fail to take over and atrial fibrillation or a more dangerous fatal arrhythmia may follow. For this reason, the insertion of a temporary transvenous ventricular pacemaking catheter should be considered before cardioversion to reduce the dangers of asystole or other arrhythmias in patients with sick sinus syndrome. Anticoagulation therapy for 7–10 days prior to elective conversion is preferable in patients with systemic embolism, mitral stenosis, cardiomyopathy, or chronic atrial fibrillation.

Many elderly patients tolerate well chronic atrial fibrillation with a ventricular heart rate of 60–80 beats per minute. Digoxin should be given to maintain this heart rate. Propanolol may be added when rapid atrial fibrillation fails to respond to the digoxin, but not to those with incipient or actual heart failure.

e) Sinus Bradycardia

Asymptomatic sinus bradycardia with a resting rate of less than 60 beats per minute is found in physically fit individuals and in the elderly where it may be an expression of vagotonia, malfunctioning sinus node, or increased carotid sinus sensitivity. Digitalis, beta-adrenergic blocking agents, glaucoma, increased intracranial pressure, and obstructive jaundice also cause sinus bradycardia. Sinoatrial block should be suspected in patients with sinus bradycardia in the range of 40–50 beats per minute. This diagnosis is made more easily when the electrocardiogram shows at times a heart rate double that of the bradycardia.

Treatment of asymptomatic sinus bradycardia is unnecessary, but a permanent artificial pacemaker may be needed in patients with cerebral symptoms or syncope resulting from the reduced cardiac output when the sinus bradycardia is 40 beats or less per minute. Before a pacemaker is prescribed, other causes for these symptoms should be excluded. A permanent pacemaker should be inserted only if the patient becomes symptomatic during continuous electrocardiographic monitoring which shows a slow heart rate or an arrhythmia. Symptoms in the absence of severe bradycardia or arrhythmias usually exclude a disorder of the sinus node as the primary cause. In these patients, continuous Holter electrocardiographic monitoring, the determination of corrected sinus recovery time, and the estimated sinonodal conduction are useful to detect sinonodal dysfunction. Normal Holter ambulatory electrocardiography and functional testing of the sinus node constitute strong evidence against significant sinus node dysfunction. Bundle of His recordings may be clinically helpful in selecting appropriate atrial or ventricular sites for permanent pacemaker implantation. Disease of the AV conducting system rules out the use of atrial pacemakers (see also Sect. B.III).

4. Ventricular Arrhythmias

a) Extrasystoles

Ventricular extrasystoles are frequent in older people as a result of their greater myocardial irritability and more severe organic heart disease. A frequency of 10% is not unusual in persons over 60. Many elderly patients with ventricular premature beats are asymptomatic and rarely require treatment.

The appearance of frequent multifocal, complex ventricular premature contractions is an ominous sign of pending ventricular tachycardia or fibrillation. They increase the risk of sudden death, especially in patients with myocardial infarction or severe coronary artery disease and/or cardiomyopathy, and require prompt evaluation with ambulatory Holter monitoring and treadmill exercise testing. Indications for drug treatment include ventricular extrasystoles that occur more frequently than five beats per minute, appear close to the preceding T wave, or are multifocal. Digitalis toxicity should be excluded as a cause of multifocal ventricular extrasystoles in patients on digitalis. Ventricular arrhythmias associated with hemodynamic and symptomatic consequences in patients with coronary ar-

Table 7. Clinical pharmacology of antiarrhythmic agents

Drug	Daily oral dose	Initial IV dose	Maintenance IV dose	GI absorption
Quinidine	1.2– 2.4 g	–	–	>95%
Procainamide	1 – 6 g	100 mg IV every 5 min to 1 g	20–80 µg/kg	75%–95%
Propranolol	40 –500 mg	0.1 mg/kg		20%–50%
Phenytoin	300 –500 mg	50–100 mg/IV every 5 min to 1 g		Slowly
Lidocaine		1 mg/kg bolus × 3	20–50 µg/kg/min	<35%
Disopyramide	400 –800 mg (150 mg every 6 h)	2 mg/kg	0.4 mg/kg/h	>95%

tery disease or myocardial infarction should be treated although there is insufficient evidence that long-term drug prophylaxis actually decreases the incidence of sudden death.

Quinidine sulfate, procainamide, disopyramide, and other class I antiarrhythmic agents are useful in treating patients with frequent ventricular extrasystoles (Table 7). In those without impending or actual heart failure, propranolol alone or combined with procainamide often controls the more ominous ventricular extrasystoles.

b) Ventricular Tachycardia

Intermittent paroxysmal ventricular tachycardia may be found in routine electrocardiograms of asymptomatic elderly patients or in those who complain of dizziness, "blackout spells," or falling. Fifty percent of paroxysmal ventricular tachycardias occur during a myocardial infarction and often constitute the first evidence of infarction. Sustained ventricular tachycardia unrelated to myocardial infarction occurs more frequently after the 5th decade and may be precipitated by straining at stool or digital stimulation of the rectum in some patients.

The electrocardiogram usually shows wide QRS complexes (0.12 s or more), a heart rate of 100 beats or greater per minute, and inverted retrograde P waves after QRS complexes. When it is difficult to distinguish supraventricular tachycardia with aberrant conduction from paroxysmal ventricular tachycardia, a useful rule of thumb is that supraventricular tachycardia is a more likely diagnosis in the presence of right bundle branch block pattern and regular ventricular rhythm; and ventricular tachycardia, in the presence of left bundle branch block pattern and slight irregularity of the ventricular rhythm.

Recurrent paroxysmal ventricular tachycardia is best managed pharmacologically with quinidine sulfate (400 mg every 6 h), disopyramide (150–200 mg every 6 h), or a combination of these drugs and propranolol (20–100 mg every 6 h). Disopyramide is contraindicated in elderly men with prostatic disease, who have a higher risk of urinary retention, and in people with glaucoma. If these drugs are

Table 7. (continued)

Peak levels after oral dose	Plateau on chronic oral dose	$t_{\frac{1}{2}}$ (PO unless otherwise specified)	Therapeutic range plasma level	Protein binding	Metabolism	Excreted unchanged in urine
1.5–2 h	2–3 days	6–7 h	2–6 µg/ml	80%	Liver	20%–50%
1 –1.5 h	2 days	3–4 h	3–10 µg/ml	15%–25%	Liver	50%–60%
1 –4 h	2.5 days	2–3 h	40–200 ng/ml	90%	Liver	< 2%
6 h	6–7 days	24 h	10–18 µg/ml	85%	Liver	< 5%
		30 min (IV)	2–5 µg/ml	10%–50%	Liver	<10%
0.5–3 h		6 h	2–4 µg/ml	50%	Liver	40%–60%

poorly tolerated or ineffective, procainamide (500–1,500 mg every 4 h) or the newer antiarrhythmic agents (tocainide, mexiletine, aprindine, or acebutolol, where available) may be useful. Programmed electric stimulation at arrhythmia centers may be imperative to establish more precise dosages and combinations of these drugs when ventricular arrhythmias resist ordinary drug therapy.

Synchronized DC electric cardioversion effectively terminates 98% of episodes of acute, uncomplicated tachycardia. When it cannot be given or fails, a lidocaine drip infusion or oral procainamide may be tried. In critically ill patients, a drip infusion of procainamide may be given intravenously at a rate of 100 mg/min under continuous electrocardiographic monitoring. This drug should be stopped with the appearance of a widening QRS interval, additional arrhythmias, shock, or other toxic signs. Bretylium has proven useful in serious situations when other drugs fall to control this arrhythmia.

After the paroxysmal ventricular tachycardia has reverted to sinus rhythm, the standard or new antiarrhythmic agents may be used to maintain a therapeutic blood level (Table 7). When drug therapy or cardioversion fail to control paroxysmal ventricular tachycardia, electric pacemaking to override the arrhythmia, surgical ventricular aneurysmectomy, or both may be necessary. Permanent cardiac pacing helps to control recurrent ventricular tachycardias in patients with sinus bradycardia and/or atrioventricular block.

c) Ventricular Fibrillation

This lethal arrhythmia requires immediate defibrillation by electric countershock and appropriate antiarrhythmic drugs, such as lidocaine, procainamide, and propranolol, to prevent recurrence. The use of bretylium has again found favor in this complication despite its hypotensive and other toxic effects. Intravenously injected diphenylhydantoin or potassium chloride may control refractory digitalis-induced ventricular tachycardia or fibrillation that fails to respond to other agents. The underlying cause of the ventricular fibrillation should always be corrected.

5. Special Arrhythmia Syndromes

a) Sick Sinus Syndrome

This syndrome is caused by the impaired function of the sinoatrial node and an abnormally unresponsive atrioventricular junctional pacemaker which arise from the degenerative changes of aging and disease. In this condition, the sinus node and its approaches may be replaced partially or completely by fibrous or sclerotic tissue. Although some vascular changes may be noted (about 25% of patients with this syndrome have clinical coronary artery disease), the sinus arteries are often intact.

Presenting symptoms and signs include fatigue, light-headedness, palpitations, angina, dizziness, sudden falls, recurrent syncope, transitory cerebral ischemic attacks (see Sect. B.II.5.b), and congestive heart failure. The sick sinus syndrome should be diagnosed or suspected in elderly patients with widespread abnormalities of impulse formation and conduction, such as sinus bradycardia, sinoatrial block, paroxysmal or chronic atrial tachycardia, tachybradycardia, chronic atrial fibrillation with slow ventricular responses due to concealed conduction, and concomitant disease of the AV junction and distal conduction pathways (FERRER 1973).

In the absence of clear-cut symptoms and electrocardiographic documentation of the sinus node syndrome, sinus node recovery time and other electrophysiologic testing may be necessary to make the correct diagnosis. Their principal value is to determine if the disorder is functional or organic. Prolonged sinus node recovery time and failure of atropine to accelerate the sinus node occur in 50%–80% of patients with sick sinus syndrome.

Slow atrial rhythm is part of the sick sinus syndrome. It originates as an escape rhythm that arises when sinus rhythm fails. It is characterized by a regular and relatively slow rate of 50–80 beats per minute; a P wave which shows abnormal notching and precedes every QRS complex; and a difference in size, occasionally in width, from the sinus P wave. The P-R interval may be normal or slightly longer than 0.20 s, but different from the P-R interval of the normal sinus rhythm arising in the sinoatrial node (FERRER 1980).

In the absence of serious symptoms, conservative therapy of the sick sinus syndrome is best. Procainamide or small doses of digoxin may be worthwhile in some patients with atrial tachycardia. Digitalis should be used with caution, if at all, because even small amounts may be toxic (MARGOLIS et al. 1975). In the absence of heart failure, beta-adrenergic blocking agents which decrease conduction in the AV node may be tried alone or with small amounts of digoxin to control the heart rate in patients with tachyarrhythmia syndromes. Digitalis toxicity should be suspected when atrial fibrillation becomes atrial flutter after digitalis is given.

Artificial cardiac pacemakers may be necessary in patients with disturbances of consciousness, syncope, recurrent arrhythmias, and tachybradycardia syndromes. They permit the use of digitalis and other antiarrhythmic agents to control the tachyarrhythmia and/or heart failure without fear of aggravating the bradycardia (HARRIS 1976). A ventricular pacemaker is best in patients with sick sinus syndrome and atrioventricular conduction disturbances. When a normal contraction sequence is desirable, atrial or AV sequential demand units may be used to improve cardiac function by making use of the atrial contraction in patients with normal atrioventricular conduction.

b) Cardiogenic Neurology

Episodic sick sinus syndrome reflects an atriopathy which is responsible for cardiogenic embolization in at least 25% of patients with strokes. Many transient cerebral insufficiency attacks (TIAs) in patients with sick sinus syndrome are caused by emboli from the left atrial appendage. ABDON (1979 a, b, 1981) found the overall incidence of cerebral embolization exceeded 7%/year in patients with episodic sick sinus syndrome. At postmortem examination, three out of four patients with sick sinus syndrome had thrombi in their left atrial appendages. In the general population, 9% of elderly patients were found to have episodic sick sinus syndrome. The sick sinus syndrome, even if only periodically present, carries a high unpredictable risk for systematic embolization and may be responsible for some of the other vague mental and neurologic conditions found in old age. The prophylactic use of dipyridamole (Persantine), aspirin, or anticoagulation therapy to prevent cerebral embolization from the left atrial appendage should be considered in patients with sick sinus syndrome.

Nonembolic cerebrovascular insults to the aging brain may occur in patients with cardiac arrhythmias when their arterial blood pressure drops below the critical level for brain circulation. Patients with cardiac arrhythmias (other than atrial fibrillation) are more likely to develop symptoms and signs of diffuse cerebral ischemia (syncope, confusion, or dizziness) than the focal neurologic deficit found in most cerebral transitory ischemic attacks (HARRIS 1981).

c) Acute Stokes-Adams Syndrome

This syndrome is the most serious and dramatic cerebrovascular insult induced by cardiac arrhythmias. It is associated with transient episodes of syncope which arise from the poor cardiac output as a result of excessively slow heart rates due to sinoatrial block, marked sinus bradycardia, complete AV heart block or fast rates due to supraventricular or ventricular tachycardia and fibrillation. When a thorough history and physical examination do not document an arrhythmia as the cause of syncope, a 24-h Holter monitor electrocardiographic recording often permits detection of the arrhythmia and its correlation with the attack. A provocative treadmill exercise test also helps identify the underlying heart disease and arrhythmia (see Sect. B.III).

Emergency treatment of the acute attack includes cardiopulmonary resuscitation to maintain ventilation and circulation and cardioversion to restore sinus rhythm if ventricular tachycardia or fibrillation is present. Supportive measures to maintain adequate oxygenation, vital signs, and blood pressure should be instituted. Temporary cardiac pacing may be necessary in patients with cardiac arrest.

Pharmacologic treatment and artificial pacemaking are also indicated in patients with recurrent Stokes-Adams attacks due to arrhythmias to prevent their recurrence (see Sect. C). In patients with ventricular standstill or symptomatic slow heart rates, a permanent artificial demand pacemaker is essential. For clinically significant ventricular tachycardias associated with bradycardia, a permanent de-

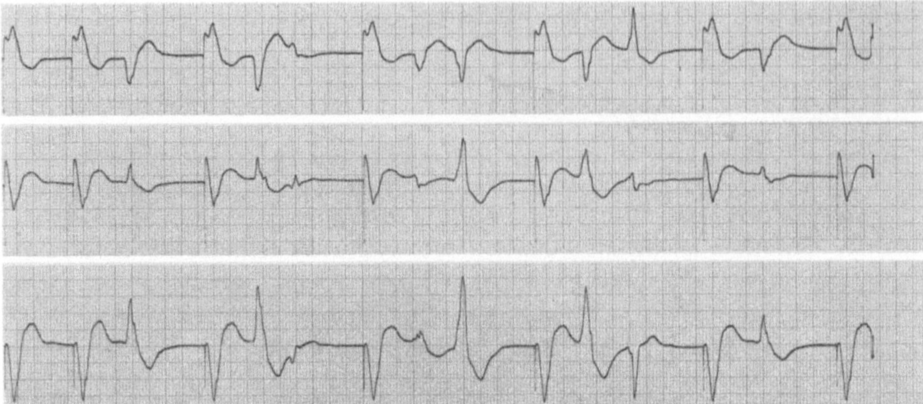

Fig. 7. Rhythm strip showing pacemaker-induced arrhythmia. Pacemaker beat *(identified by spike)* is coupled with ventricular extrasystoles producing bigeminy and trigeminy

mand ventricular pacemaker is recommended. In selected patients with sinus node disease, ventricular failure and intact AV conduction, atrial pacing may be more beneficial than ventricular pacing. Atrial pacing often improves cardiac hemodynamics while ventricular pacing may cause further deterioration of ventricular function, especially in patients with retrograde ventriculoatrial conduction. Atrioventricular sequential demand pacing represents the most advanced type of therapy currently available for patients with sick sinus syndrome and should be inserted if the aim of the pacemaker treatment is to improve their cardiac hemodynamics.

d) Pacemaker Arrhythmias

The introduction of cardiac pacemakers into medical practice has spawned a variety of iatrogenic pacemaker arrhythmias. These range from simple disorders of the cardiac rhythm produced by battery failure to more complex arrhythmias originating from runaway pacemakers, intermittent wire breaks and reentry arrhythmias caused by pacemaker stimulation (Fig. 7).

The advent of more sophisticated demand pacemakers has led to unusual but normal rhythms due to the interplay between the artificial pacemaker beats and the patient's own beats. It is therefore important that the physician be familiar with the type and characteristics of the pacemaker. Newly developed pacemakers offer a greater and more flexible variety of programmable modes that ensure better atrial input, ventricular-inhibited demand pacemaking and AV sequential fixed rates. These pacemakers permit alterations in heart rate, pulse width, and sensitivity levels by externally controlled programmers.

The principal arrhythmia arising from asynchronous (fixed rate) pacemaker is competition from the patient's own conducted or ectopic beats (Fig. 7). Pacemaker parasystole may also develop in patients with fixed-rate ventricular pacemakers in which the artificial stimulus competes with the intrinsic conducted beat for control of the ventricular rhythm. When runaway pacemaker arrhythmias occur, the pacemaker can be deactivated immediately by cutting the lead wire.

Competition from pacemaker-induced ventricular arrhythmias may increase mortality. When competition from ventricular premature beats develops in a patient with a pacemaker, increasing the pacing rate or administering antiarrhythmic agents may suppress it. The newer, R-wave sensitive, noncompetitive demand pacemakers now available prevent such competition and should be installed when the older asynchronous types are replaced.

III. Special Diagnostic Procedures

1. Carotid Sinus Massage

Carotid sinus massage enhances the ability of the routine surface electrocardiogram to determine whether an arrhythmia is supraventricular or ventricular in patients with atrial flutter, in 2:1 atrioventricular conduction when atrial flutter waves are unclear, or in paroxysmal ventricular tachycardia where the P wave is concealed in the QRS complex or the T wave. Carotid sinus massage prolongs the atrioventricular conduction time and either terminates the arrhythmia or moves the P wave out of the QRS complex, so that it becomes more visible.

Carotid sinus massage for therapeutic or diagnostic purposes in aged patients with syncope should not be routinely performed because it may obliterate the carotid artery flow to the brain, cause cerebrovascular thrombosis, or produce noxious inhibitory or excitatory cardiac effects. Inhibitory vagal stimulation can slow or stop the discharge of sinoatrial impulses (producing sinus bradycardia or sinoatrial arrest), depress the conduction of impulses from the sinus node to the atria (producing sinoatrial block), or depress the atrioventricular node (prolonging the P-R interval and causing AV block). Excitatory cardiac effects may initiate atrial flutter or atrial fibrillation, increase the rate of atrial flutter, transform atrial flutter to atrial fibrillation, increase ectopic ventricular impulse formation, or paradoxically facilitate or reverse atrioventricular conduction from the ventricles to the atria.

A hypersensitive carotid sinus must be differentiated from other more common causes of dizziness or syncope, such as cardiac arrhythmias, vasovagal response, postural hypotension, or cerebrovascular insufficiency. This diagnosis is established when gentle compression over the bifurcation of the carotid artery sinus during electrocardiographic monitoring reproduces these complaints. Carotid sinus denervation is a simple, effective treatment for this complication.

In elderly patients with hypersensitive carotid reflex, cholinergic drugs such as neostigmine, morphine, and related medications which potentiate the vagal form of this reflex should be avoided. Digitalis also sensitizes this vagal type of reflex and increases the risk of cerebral complications. During anesthesia and operation, vigorous manipulation of the head and neck should be avoided in order not to provoke the hyperactive carotid sinus reflex.

2. Continuous Ambulatory Electrocardiographic Monitoring

Ambulatory electrocardiographic monitoring with a Holter-type recorder is invaluable to document and establish the definitive diagnosis of a cardiac arrhythmia, determine its mechanism, assist in the evaluation of the treatment of recurrent arrhythmias and identify potential rhythm and conduction disturbances as the basis for recurrent paroxysmal symptoms arising from a disturbance of the heart rhythm. This method is superior to the conventional 12-lead electrocardiographic determination for evaluating patients with syncopal or presyncopal episodes whose resting electrocardiogram may be normal and for correlating symptomatology with the presence or absence of an arrhythmia, especially during exercise, sleep, psychological stress, and eating. It helps to establish a cardiac diagnosis in the elderly patient whose electrocardiogram shows occasional ventricular premature contractions and whose light-headedness or dizziness is not reproduced by carotid sinus massage, turning the head from side to side, or arising quickly from a supine position. Continuous electrocardiographic monitoring in patients with heart rates under 40, or occasional sinus pauses to a maximum of 2 s during sleep may confirm an apparent sick sinus syndrome or exclude it in favor of vertebrobasilar insufficiency when the patient's complaints appear unrelated to a heart rhythm disturbance.

Elderly patients with intermittent symptoms of cerebrovascular insufficiency should be studied by ambulatory electrocardiographic monitoring to rule out intermittent cardiac arrhythmias or conduction abnormalities. Patients with bifascicular block on the resting electrocardiogram may also benefit from a Holter recording, even in the absence of symptoms of cerebrovascular insufficiency. The majority of these patients may exhibit periods of complete heart block (months or years prior to the development of complete AV heart block) which are too brief to produce clinical symptoms. Detection of these episodes by Holter monitoring permits the institution of appropriate therapy in advance of symptoms. Ambulatory Holter monitoring is also useful in patients with the tachybradycardia arrhythmia syndrome to study the effect of therapy. Another use is to assess elderly patients with chest pain, transient neurologic symptoms, and nocturnal complaints and to detect coronary-prone patients, who are at greater risk of sudden death from cardiac arrhythmias.

When the cause of the syncopal episodes is a slow ventricular rate, a permanent demand ventricular pacemaker may correct the problem. When the syncopal episode is due to impaired cardiac output resulting from a decreased cerebral blood flow associated with bursts of ventricular tachycardia, it is helpful to insert a permanent demand ventricular pacemaker to maintain a suitable cardiac rate and use antiarrhythmic drugs to control the ventricular tachycardia.

3. Other Specialized Diagnostic Recordings

a) Esophageal Leads

This lead, obtained by inserting an esophageal electrode catheter into the esophagus, records the electric potential from the back of the heart. It is useful to clarify the relationship between the atrial and ventricular complexes when the P waves are obscured or absent on the surface electrocardiogram.

b) Intracardiac Recordings

Intracardiac leads can be used to identify an arrhythmia when an esophageal lead fails to do so, and to measure the sinus node recovery time, the main unidirectional sinoatrial conduction time, and the physiologic responses to premature atrial stimulation. Additional tests to measure sinus node function include the administration of atropine, sinus node recovery time after atropine, conduction of the first ten beats after cessation of pacing, and measurement of intrinsic heart rate after the administration of atropine and propranolol (GANN et al. 1979).

Bundle of His studies record the presence and site of atrioventricular delay and block within or below the AV node. The combination of atrial stimulation and Bundle of His recording improves the diagnosis of sinoatrial disease and other conduction system disturbances.

Intraventricular electric recordings can determine if an arrhythmia is ventricular or supraventricular and evaluate the therapeutic efficiency of acutely administered drugs in patients with arrhythmias. Programmed electric stimulation of the ventricle has proven useful to determine if the patient is "arrhythmia-prone" and the best drugs to use in the treatment of otherwise refractory ventricular arrhythmias. These techniques are also used in the mapping of electric conduction in the heart to determine the mechanisms of the arrhythmia and the value of surgical intervention to prevent recurrent, refractory arrhythmias.

4. Treadmill Exercise Stress Testing

Under proper conditions which limit exercise to a tolerable level, treadmill exercise testing is safe and useful to determine the exercise tolerance of elderly patients with angina pectoris and to detect transient changes in cardiac rhythm and conduction which may develop during exercise or immediately thereafter.

C. Therapeutic Considerations

I. Drug Therapy

1. Clinical Pharmacokinetics

Clinical pharmacokinetics is the application of pharmacokinetics (study of drug disposition) to the treatment of patients. An understanding of the general principles of pharmacokinetics enables the clinician to use more effectively the available antiarrhythmic agents and to anticipate the individual drug requirements for elderly patients with age-related changes, and altered drug dispositions due to disease (RICHEY and BENDER 1977). Attention to clinical pharmacokinetic principles requires that dosage of antiarrhythmic agents be individualized according to the patient's weight, age, and other factors which affect the disposition of a particular drug in the body. The choice of a particular dosage interval also depends upon the half-life of the drug, its therapeutic index, and the consideration of the patient's convenience. Subsequent adjustment in dosage may be required because of toxicity or the lack of therapeutic response. Measurements of the blood or plasma levels of the drugs are helpful in making appropriate adjustments to drug therapy, particularly during long-term administration (Table 7) (HARRISON et al. 1977). The correct dose for every elderly patient must be empirically determined and individualized.

2. Age-Related Considerations

Factors influencing drug activity with advancing age include: alterations in the gastrointestinal absorption of drugs, distribution of drugs, regional blood flow, tissue and plasma protein binding, drug metabolism, hepatic blood flow, excretion of drugs, end-organ sensitivity, drug interaction, and other aging changes discussed elsewhere in this volume. Elderly patients are generally more sensitive to cardiovascular drugs because of these factors and therefore usually require smaller doses and more careful supervision than younger people. Although some changes in sensitivity to cardiovascular drugs with increasing age occur at the effector organ level, more important are the age-related changes in renal and hepatic clearances which are impaired with age, the decrease in lean body mass, which results in much of the metabolically active tissue being replaced by fat, and the altered distribution of drugs in the elderly, resulting from changes in body composition, plasma protein binding, and regional blood perfusion. Plasma albumen decreases with age. Peripheral blood flow is redistributed in favor of the cerebral and coronary circulations, thereby reducing blood flow to the kidneys, liver, mesentery, and skin. These factors vary individually in aged persons, but influence the rate and extent to which a drug is made available to receptors for interaction and the duration of its effects. Unless drug dosages are appropriately age adjusted and individually and empirically prescribed, drug toxicity arising from these age-related changes may increase mortality in the elderly.

Quinidine and digitalis illustrate the value of paying attention to these age-related considerations. The hepatic biotransformation and renal excretion of quinidine decrease with age so that the half-life of quinidine (7.3 h) in healthy individuals aged 34 years or less becomes significantly prolonged and the rate of total clearance reduced in healthy volunteers 60 years of age or older (Ochs et al. 1978). The decreased rate of quinidine clearance in the elderly predisposes to excessive drug accumulation and toxicity unless the dosage is appropriately adjusted.

The increased incidence of digitalis toxicity in the elderly is mainly attributable to their contracted space of distribution for digoxin as a result of decreased lean body mass and to their reduced renal excretion. Consequently, the same dose of digoxin (metabolized and excreted mainly by the impaired kidney) produces an increased half-life and a serum digoxin level nearly twice as high in the elderly as in the young. Although most forms of digitalis can be used in the aged, digoxin with its shorter half-life (36 h when renal function is normal) is generally preferred because of its greater margin of safety in elderly patients. To avoid toxicity, digoxin is best given without a loading dose and in lesser amounts than those given to younger people. If there is no acute emergency, a daily oral maintenance dose of 0.25 mg may be given until a steady digitalized state is achieved in 7–10 days (Doherty 1979). In emergencies, a larger dose given intravenously may be necessary.

3. Clinical Pharmacology of Antiarrhythmic Agents

Each antiarrhythmic agent is characterized by individual unique electrophysiologic properties and specific patterns of absorption, distribution, and elimination which are described in regular pharmacologic texts. Age factors, associated disease, concomitant therapy, drug interactions, and individual patient differences and predispositions alter the usual dosage requirement (Table 7).

Drug interactions are an important aspect of the treatment of cardiac arrhythmias in the aged. For example, drugs, such as phenobarbital or phenytoin, that induce drug-metabolizing enzymes in the liver may significantly shorten the duration of quinidine action by increasing its rate of elimination. Occasionally, the prothrombin time will increase after quinidine therapy is begun in patients on warfarin therapy.

Pharmacodynamic interactions may also occur. Quinidine, an α-adrenergic blocking agent, is likely to interact with drugs that cause vasodilatation or decreased blood volume. Powerful loop diuretics, such as furosemide, may cause marked hypotension in patients on quinidine.

Similarly, the concomitant use of quinidine and digoxin may significantly elevate serum digoxin levels as a result of the displacement of the digoxin by quinidine molecules from binding sites in skeletal muscle and other tissues, or the reduction by quinidine of the renal clearance of digoxin (DOHERTY et al. 1980). Such interactions increase the potential for toxic effects for digoxin with its 2:1 toxic:therapeutic ratio. For this reason, frequent dose adjustments and serum digoxin assays must be performed when quinidine is concomitantly administered with digoxin.

Drug interactions may also occur between tricyclic antidepressants and guanethidine, clonidine, alpha-methyldopa (Aldomet), lidocaine, and L-dopa. Treatment is complex and must be individualized (JEFFERSON 1975). The tricyclic antidepressants exert a direct myocardial depressant activity and effect on the adrenergic neurons through their anticholinergic activity, which can lead to arrhythmias, blood pressure abnormalities, and congestive heart failure (JEFFERSON 1975). In man, toxic doses of the tricyclic drugs are capable of causing a wide variety of rate and rhythm disturbances, heart block, and even sudden death. The direct arrhythmogenic effects of the tricyclic antidepressants may depend upon interference with sodium–potassium transport across cell membranes and other factors, including dose, presence of other drugs, and the premorbid condition of the patient.

Digitalis glycosides exert their antiarrhythmic effects indirectly on the autonomic nervous system. Other antiarrhythmic drugs act mainly on the cardiac cell membrane to produce specific ionic currents and also affect the autonomic nervous system. All β-adrenergic-blocking drugs affect cardiac rhythm through their actions on β-adrenergic receptors, but their other important electrophysiologic effects may vary (BIGGER 1980).

Antiarrhythmic drugs may be grouped into four classes according to their most significant electrophysiologic actions on cardiac muscle (Table 8). This classification facilitates the rational choice of a regimen of antiarrhythmic agents and helps predict adverse reactions when different agents are combined (SINGH 1979). Table 6 lists the conventional and new investigative drugs according to their electrophysiologic class and availability.

a) Class I Antiarrhythmic Drugs

Quinidine is effective for the acute or long-term treatment of supraventricular and ventricular arrhythmias. It is the most dependable drug for converting atrial fibril-

Table 8. Comparative mechanisms of action of antiarrhythmic agents

| Class I | 1) Essentially local anesthetics on nerve
2) Depress phase 4 depolarization
3) Variable effect on action potential duration
4) Depress upstroke velocity of phase 0 (i.e., reduce "membrane responsiveness")
   a) Increase threshold of excitability
   b) Reduce conduction velocity
   c) Prolong effective refractory period | Class III | Dominant property: Uniform prolongation of the action potential duration
   a) Depress phase 4 depolarization
   b) Prolong absolute refractory period
   c) Depress excitability |
| Class II | 1) Common property: Sympathetic antagonism
2) Depress phase 4 depolarization
3) Other electrophysiologic properties uncertain | Class IV | Dominant property: Inhibit slow channel activity
   a) Depress phase 4 depolarization
   b) Depress conduction in fibers with slow-channel dependent action potentials |

lation to normal sinus rhythm and maintaining it. Drug-induced premature ventricular beats, atrioventricular block, QRS widening, ventricular tachycardia, and even ventricular fibrillation may occur when the plasma quinidine level exceeds the therapeutic plasma concentration level of 2.0–6.0 µg/ml.

Procainamide hydrochloride (Pronestyl) is indicated in the treatment of premature ventricular contractions, ventricular tachycardia, atrial fibrillation, and paroxysmal atrial tachycardia. Oral or intramuscular therapy is preferable. The intravenous route should be reserved for life-threatening arrhythmias that do not respond to oral or intramuscular therapy. Since a lupus erythematosus-like syndrome may develop in patients on long-term procainamide therapy, the serum antinuclear antibody titer should be determined regularly in patients receiving procainamide for a long time or showing symptoms of a lupus-like reaction. A significant rise in this titer is an indication for stopping this drug.

Lidocaine is effective against ventricular arrhythmias of many etiologies. It is usually the agent of first choice in a ventricular arrhythmia unless the patient is overly sensitive and becomes confused or toxic on normal or less than normal therapeutic serum levels (Table 7). It is effective in about 87% of ventricular arrhythmias and in only 20% of supraventricular arrhythmias. Ninety percent is metabolized in the liver and 10% is excreted unchanged through the kidney. In rats, the depressant effect of lidocaine on atrial pacemakers increases with age but decreases with age on ventricular pacemakers (Goldberg and Roberts 1978).

Diphenylhydantoin sodium (Dilantin) may be given intravenously to control digitalis-induced arrhythmias. It is contraindicated in patients with a high degree of heart block or marked bradycardia and should be used cautiously in patients with hypotension and severe myocardial insufficiency. The liver is the site of biotransformation of this drug. Consequently, the patient's age can affect the disposition of this drug since elderly patients often have impaired liver function. For this reason, plasma dilantin levels should be taken frequently in elderly patients on this drug to prevent toxic responses, including ataxia, confusion, and other neurologic complaints.

Disopyramide (Norpace) is a new antiarrhythmic agent with actions and versatility resembling those of quinidine. Its most frequent side effects are constipation and urinary hesitancy due to its anticholinergic effects. Blurred vision and urinary retention may necessitate stopping the administration of this drug in older people. See Table 6 for other class I antiarrhythmic agents.

b) Class II Antiarrhythmic Drugs

β-adrenergic-receptor-blocking agents are useful in treating cardiac arrhythmias due to excessive catecholamine release, increased levels of circulating catecholamines, and increased sensitivity of the heart to catecholamines related to pheochromocytoma, thyrotoxicosis, exercise, or digitalis excess. These agents are effective in the treatment of acute and chronic supraventricular arrhythmias and ventricular arrhythmias unresponsive to first-line agents. Propranolol hydrochloride (Inderal) with a biologic half-life of 2–3 h, is an important member of this group. It is particularly useful in the management of paroxysmal supraventricular tachycardias, persistent symptomatic sinus tachycardia, and arrhythmias due to thyrotoxicosis, particularly when digitalis is contraindicated or does not adequately control ventricular rate. Propranolol is better tolerated but less effective than quinidine or procainamide in treating chronic ventricular arrhythmias. It is contraindicated in patients with bronchial asthma, markedly impaired myocardial contractility and in those who have actual heart failure or who are borderline compensated and may go into heart failure. It is not a drug of first choice in the elderly whose myocardium is already compromised by age and disease and in whom this drug may further depress myocardial contractility and precipitate cardiac failure. Other β-adrenergic-blocking agents belonging to this group of drugs now being investigated do not have the drawbacks of propranolol. Practolol is promising for the treatment of cardiac arrhythmias, but is not available for clinical use in all countries. See Table 6 for additional, newly developed class II antiarrhythmic drugs.

c) Class III Antiarrhythmic Drugs

Bretylium, an older drug now achieving greater recognition in the treatment of ventricular fibrillation refractory to conventional therapy, is recommended for the treatment of life-threatening ventricular arrhythmias that fail to respond to adequate doses of a first-line antiarrhythmic drug. Ventricular fibrillation that fails to respond to repeated DC countershocks may respond to the combination of bretylium tosylate and countershock. It acts directly on the myocardium and on adrenergic nerve transmission. Severe hypotension may result from its blocking effects on the sympathetic nervous system. See Table 6 for other class III antiarrhythmic drugs.

d) Class IV Antiarrhythmic Drugs

Verapamil is useful in the treatment of supraventricular arrhythmias. Consult Table 6 for other class IV antiarrhythmic drugs.

II. Electric Methods

1. Direct Current Cardioversion

Direct current cardioversion is most effective against arrhythmias caused by continuous reentry, such as atrial flutter, atrial fibrillation, paroxysmal supraventricular tachycardia, ventricular tachycardia, or ventricular fibrillation. It must be individualized to meet the needs of each patient. It is especially indicated for rapid tachyarrhythmias that cause shock, cardiac pain, hypotension, failure, or other hemodynamic embarrassment. It is effective for treating atrial fibrillation of recent onset that does not convert following medical treatment and control of the underlying cause. Many cardiac arrhythmias will respond to an initial shock of 25 J/s. If not, a repeat shock with higher dosage may succeed. Cardioversion is ordinarily not indicated in digitalis-induced arrhythmias, but at times may be necessary to convert life-threatening paroxysmal atrial tachycardia with blocked sinus rhythm when potassium, procainamide, or other medications have failed. The response of ventricular fibrillation to immediate unsynchronized electric conversion with a full dose of 400 J is surprisingly good in most patients except for those in heart failure or cardiogenic shock.

2. Pacing

a) Temporary

When medical measures fail to convert an acute arrhythmia, temporary cardiac pacing may be necessary to override supraventricular and ventricular arrhythmias or arrhythmias associated with the Wolff-Parkinson-White syndrome. Temporary transvenous catheter pacing may be necessary in patients with acute myocardial infarction complicated with atrioventricular block, bundle branch block, symptomatic sinus bradycardia, or excessive ventricular irritability. Careful electrocardiographic monitoring and a trial of temporary pacing may also be necessary in patients with symptomatic sinus node malfunction before permanent pacemakers are installed. Many forms of recurrent sustained ventricular tachycardias can now be terminated by programmed ventricular simulation.

b) Permanent

Permanent cardiac pacing may be indicated in elderly patients with intermittent, acquired, or complete atrioventricular heart block, symptomatic bradycardia due to sick sinus syndrome, or atrial fibrillation with slow ventricular rate.

Transvenous endocardial pacing is the method of choice whenever permanent pacing is necessary. This method avoids thoracotomy, general anesthesia and carries only a small operative mortality. Noncompetitive demand pacemakers are preferable to the older fixed rate units. These avoid competitive rhythms and the potential hazards of ventricular fibrillation. A wide variety of noncompetitive demand pacemakers are now available which will ordinarily not be polarized when the intrinsic beats occur at normal rates. Competition from ventricular premature contractions in patients with pacemakers that have externally adjustable cardiac rates can be suppressed either by increasing the pacing rates noninvasively or by administering antiarrhythmic drugs. More recently, permanent pacing-activated radiofrequency ventricular pacemakers have become available for the self-termination of recurrent ventricular tachycardias refractory to medical management (RUSKIN et al. 1980).

References

Abdon N-J (1979a) The sick sinus syndrome: A common diagnostic and therapeutic challenge in the elderly. In: Harris R (ed) Geriatric medicine, Lesson 12. Physicians Programs, New York

Abdon N-J, Jönsson BM (1979b) High risk of systemic embolization in episodic sick sinus syndrome (abstract). Pace 2:(Sept–Oct) A-50

Abdon N-J (1981) Cardiogenic neurology. Doctoral Dissertation, University of Lund, Malmö, Sweden

Bigger JT Jr (1980) Management of arrhythmias. In: Braunwald E (ed) Heart disease – A textbook of cardiovascular medicine. W.H. Saunders Co., Philadelphia London Toronto, Chap 20, pp 691–743

Bush HL, Gelband H, Hoffman BF, Malm JR (1971) Electrophysiological basis for supraventricular arrhythmias following surgical procedures for aortic stenosis. Arch Surg 103:620–625

Cavoto FV, Kelliher GJ, Roberts J (1974) Electrophysiological changes in the rat atrium with age. Am J Physiol 226:1293–1297

Coumel P, Leclercq N-F, Attuel P, LeVallée J-P, Flammang D (1979) Autonomic influences: Sympathetic drive and its genesis of ventricular arrhythmias. In: Narula OS (ed) Cardiac arrhythmias: Electrophysiology, diagnosis, and management. Williams and Wilkins, Baltimore, Chap 24, pp 457–473

Cranefield PF, Wit AL, Hoffman BF (1973) Genesis of cardiac arrhythmias. In: Donoso E (ed) Symposium cardiac arrhythmias. American Heart Association Monograph No 40. American Heart Association, New York, p 24

Davies MJ, Pomerance A (1972) Quantitative study of aging changes in the human sinoatrial node and internodal tracts. Br Heart J 34:150–152

Doherty JE (1979) Diagnosis and management of congestive heart failure in the elderly patient. In: Harris R (ed) Geriatric medicine, Lesson 10, Physicians Programs, New York

Doherty JE, Straub KD, Murphy ML, de Soyza N, Bissett JK, Kane JJ (1980) Digoxin-quinidine interaction: Changes in canine tissue concentration from steady state with quinidine. Am J Cardiol 45:1196–1200

Donoso E (1973) Introduction. In: Donoso E (ed) Symposium cardiac arrhythmias. American Heart Association Monograph No 40. American Heart Association, New York, p 1–2

Ferrer MI (1973) The sick sinus syndrome. In: Donoso E (ed) Symposium cardiac arrhythmias. American Heart Association Monograph No 40. American Heart Association, New York, pp 67–73

Ferrer MI (1980) Significance of slow atrial rhythm. Am J Cardiol 45:176–177

Gann D, Tolentino A, Samet P (1979) Electrophysiologic evaluation of elderly patients with sinus bradycardia. An Intern Med 90:24–29

Goldberg PB, Roberts J (1978) Physiological and pharmacological changes of rat cardiac pacemakers with increasing age. In: Roberts J, Adelman RC, Cristobalo VJ (eds) Pharmacological intervention in the aging process. Plenum Press, New York, pp 315–318

Goldberg PB, Baskin SI, Roberts J (1975) Effects of aging on ionic movements of atrial muscle. Fed Proc 34:188–190

Harris R (1970) The management of geriatric cardiovascular disease. J.B. Lippincott, Philadelphia Toronto

Harris R (1976) Cardiac arrhythmias in the aged. In: Caird FI, Dall JLC, Kennedy RD (eds) Cardiology in old age. Plenum Press, New York, Chap 17, pp 315–346

Harris R (1981) Cerebrovascular insults during senescence. In: von Hahn HP, Andrews J (eds) Geriatrics for everyday practice. S Karger AG, Basel, Chap 1, pp 1–14

Harrison DC, Meffin PJ, Winkle RA (1977) Clinical pharmacokinetics of antiarrhythmic drugs. Prog Cardiovasc Dis 20:217–242

Jefferson JW (1975) A review of the cardiovascular effects and toxicity of tricyclic antidepressants. Psychosom Med 37:160–179

Jordan J, Yamaguchi I, Mandel WJ (1979) The effects of drugs on normal and abnormal sinus node function. In: Narula OS (ed) Cardiac arrhythmias: Electrophysiology, diagnosis, and management. Williams and Wilkins, Baltimore, Chap 12, pp 207–239

Lakatta EG, Gerstenblith G, Angell CS, Shock NW, Weisfeldt ML (1975) Prolonged contraction duration in aged myocardium. J Clin Invest 55:61–68

Margolis JR, Strauss HC, Miller HC, Gilbert M, Wallace AG (1975) Digitalis and the sick sinus syndrome. Clinical and electrophysiologic documentation of severe toxic effect on sinus node function. Circulation 52:162–169

Mihalick MJ, Fisch C (1974) Electrocardiographic findings in the aged. Am Heart J 87:117–128

Ochs HR, Greenblatt DJ, Woo E, Smith TW (1978) Reduced quinidine clearance in elderly persons. Am J Cardiol 42:481–485

Raftery EB, Cashman PMM (1976) Long-term recording of the electrocardiogram in a normal population. Postgrad Med J 52 (Suppl 7):32–37

Richey DP, Bender AD (1977) Pharmacokinetic consequences of aging. Ann Rev Pharmacol Toxicol 17:49–65

Roberts J, Goldberg PB (1975) Changes in cardiac membranes as a function of age with particular emphasis on reactivity to drugs. In: Cristofalo VJ, Roberts J, Adelman RC (eds) Explorations in aging. Plenum Press, New York, pp 119–148

Rosen KM (1973) Junctional tachycardia: Mechanisms, diagnosis, differential diagnosis and management. In: Donoso E (ed) Symposium cardiac arrhythmias. American Heart Association Monograph No 40. American Heart Association, New York, pp 86–96

Rosen MR, Fisch C, Hoffman, BF, Danilo P, Lovelace DE, Knobel SB (1980) Can accelerated atrioventricular junctional escape rhythms be explained by delayed afterpolarizations? Am J Cardiol 45:1272–1284

Ruskin JN, Garan, H, Poulin F, Harthorne JW (1980) permanent radiofrequency ventricular pacing for management of drug-resistant ventricular tachycardia. Am J Cardiol 46:317–321

Shapiro AJ, Rosen MR (1979) Pharmacology of antiarrhythmic drugs. In: Cardiac arrhythmias – a clinician's guide to diagnosis and management. Biomed Inform Corp, New York, pp 17–23

Simonson E (1972) The effect of age on the electrocardiogram. Am J Cardiol 29:64–73

Singh BN (1979) Drug lag in therapy of arrhythmia and angina. Part I. Primary Cardiol 5 (No 12):45–53

Stern S (1979) Discussion. In: Busse EW (ed) Cerebral manifestations of episodic cardiac dysrhythmias. Excerpta Medica, Princeton, New Jersey, p 80

Ticzon AR, Whalen RW (1973) Refractory supraventricular tachycardias. In: Donoso E (ed) Symposium cardiac arrhythmias. American Heart Association Monograph No 40. American Heart Association, New York, pp 74–85

Titus JL (1973) Anatomy of the conduction system. In: Donoso E (ed) Symposium cardiac arrhythmias. American Heart Association Monograph No 40. American Heart Association, New York, pp 4–11

WHO/ISFC Task Force (1979) Classification of cardiac arrhythmias and conduction disturbances. Am Heart J 98:263–267

Heart Block

A. E. TÀMMARO

A. Introduction

This chapter deals with the problems of main geriatric interest which arise from the presence of sinoatrial, atrioventricular, and intraventricular blocks. The heart block develops mainly in elderly subjects and its incidence increases progressively with increasing age. However, this is not the only reason the heart block deserves particular attention from a geriatric point of view. As age advances, conduction disorders vary etiologically, pathologically, and clinically. They have therefore been indicated by MICHEL (1975) as ranking among the most topical problems of geriatric cardiology together with unstable angina.

B. Prevalence

The prevalence of conduction disorders in young and adult subjects as well as among elderly in- and outpatients is reported in Tables 1–3.

With regard to young and adult people (Table 1) it should be pointed out that the minimum admission age was 40 and 45 years respectively in the reports of SIEG-MAN-IGRA et al. (1978) and YANO et al. (1975). This may account for the relatively high incidence of conduction disturbances in comparison with the other studies.

With ageing a distinct and progressive increase in conduction disturbances takes place. Incidence, in fact, has been shown to be appreciably higher in the aged

Table 1. Prevalence of conduction disturbances in young and adult people

Report	JOHNSON et al. (1960)	SIEGMAN-IGRA et al. (1978)	YANO et al. (1975)	ROTMAN and TRIEBWASSER (1975)
N	67,375	4,706	6,217	237,000
AVB 1				
AVB 2				
AVB 3				
RBBB	0.16			0.16
LBBB	0.02			0.05
LAH		2.16	1.30	
RBBB+LAH				

All values are expressed as percentages. AVB 1, AVB 2, and AVB 3: first, second, and third degree atrioventricular block; RBBB: right bundle branch block; LBBB: left bundle branch block; LAH: left anterior hemiblock

Table 2. Prevalence of conduction disturbances in old people at home

Report	OST-RANDER et al. (1965)	EDMANDS (1966)	KENNEDY and CAIRD (1972)	KITCHIN et al. (1973)	CAMPBELL et al. (1974)	SIEGMAN-IGRA et al. (1978)
N	603	1,560	400	482	2,254	408
Age	Over 60	Over 52	Over 65	Over 62	Over 65	Over 60
AVB 1					0.9	
AVB 2					1 [a]	
AVB 3						
RBBB	2.0	2.0	3.5	2.3	1.9	
LBBB	1.7	1.4	2.5	0.6	1.4	
LAH					1.6	4.22
RBBB+LAH					0.7	

Values are expressed as percentages. AVB 1, AVB 2, and AVB 3: first, second, and third degree atrioventricular block; RBBB: right bundle branch block; LBBB: left bundle branch block; LAH: left anterior hemiblock.
[a] One case in 2,254

Table 3. Prevalence of conduction disturbances in old institutionalized people

Report	MIHALICK and FISCH (1977)	LUISADA (1977)	TAMMARO (1977)	LOEB and MORIN (1978)	BEGGIATO and PRATIS (1978)	SULLO et al. (1979)
N	671	455	1,792	429	1,660	516
Age	Over 70	Over 65	Over 60	Over 60	Over 60	Over 70
AVB 1	10.0	25.0		2.33		8.5
AVB 2				2.55		1.16
AVB 3		0.9		0.23		0.38
RBBB	7.1	10.5			4.4	13.5
LBBB	4.9	7.7			4.7	4.66
LAH	11.0	27.5	8.48		6.6	21.7
RBBB+LAH	0.5	9.0	2.29		2.1	7.55
LPH		0.6			0.8	0.58
RBBB+LPH					0.2	
SAB				0.47		0.58

All values are expressed as percentages. AVB 1, AVB 2, and AVB 3: first, second, and third degree atrioventricular block; RBBB: right bundle branch block; LBBB: left bundle branch block; LAH: left anterior hemiblock; LPH: left posterior hemiblock; SAB: sinoatrial block

at home (Table 2) and even higher in hospitalized elderly patients (Table 3). The lower prevalence found in the former group of subjects may be explained, at least in part, by the fact that these undoubtedly constitute the healthier part of the aged population, even though there is no binding relationship between conduction disorders and presence of heart disease. Furthermore, in the case of geriatric patiens the subjects' age may affect the results of such surveys and account for the differences. It has been observed that by classifying elderly people according to age the prevalence of conduction disturbances increases considerably as age advances (CAMPBELL et al. 1974; MIHALICK and FISCH 1974; TAMMARO 1977; BEGGIATO and

PRATIS 1978; SULLO et al. 1979). This trend has proved to be statistically significant (BEGGIATO and PRATIS 1978).

These data demonstrate that left anterior hemiblock is the most frequent conduction disorder in elderly subjects, while the difference in incidence between right and left bundle branch block tends to decrease and even completely disappear. The prevalence of sinoatrial block proves to be low and also in agreement with the percentage (0.33%) reported by PUECH et al. (1970). However these authors, who carried out a study on 1185 hospitalized subjects aged 70 years and over, found a considerably higher percentage of advanced second degree and third degree atrioventricular blocks (9.45%). This incidence is also clearly higher than that reported by SHAW and ERAUT (1970), who observed an incidence of 1‰ in patients aged over 75 years and less than 0.5‰ in subjects aged between 65 and 75. In most studies higher incidence in the male sex was observed.

C. Pathology and Common Causes

I. Sinoatrial Block

The pathological aspecs of this conduction disorder have been poorly investigated. The available reports agree in indicating that sinoatrial block may very seldom be the consequence of an occlusion of the sinus node artery. It has also been reported that in very few cases the sinus node artery might present a form of fibromuscular dysplasia associated with a marked reduction in the arterial lumen and followed by death due to cardiac arrest (JAMES and MARSHALL 1976). The most frequent finding is represented by a considerable reduction in the muscular and P cells associated with fibrosis and fibroelastosis, and also occasionally with interruption of internodal tracts. More rarely either amyloid or fatty infiltration has been found (BALSAVER et al. 1967; WAREMBOURG et al. 1974; DAVIES 1976; BALDI et al. 1977; DEMOULIN and KULBERTUS 1978). Changes in the atrioventricular node, in the His–Purkinje system, and in the common myocardium are also observable quite frequently. The occurrence of sinoatrial block may also be associated with an increase in the vagal tone. This is not uncommon in the elderly because of carotid sinus hypersensitivity (DIGHTON 1975; PFISTERER et al. 1977).

II. Atrioventricular Block

The lesions resulting in chronic atrioventricular block are only occasionally found either in the atrioventricular node or in the proximal parts of His's bundle. This localization was observed in 13% of subjects by DAVIES (1976) and in 2 out of 59 subjects by SUGIURA et al. (1975), while in most cases the lesions are found in either the branching portion of the bundle or in the bundle branches: 17.5% and 49.1% (DAVIES 1976). The latter two localizations were found in about 90% of the patients studied by HARRIS et al. (1969).

The lesion found most frequently is a bilateral idiopathic fibrosis of the conduction tissue with loss of specific fibers and without marked myocardial or vascular involvement. Two hypotheses have been put forward to explain how this damage may occur. According to LEV (1964), it is caused by an enhanced fibrocalcific infiltration usually developing in advanced age in the central fibrous body, in the valvular rings, and in the membranous and upper muscular portion of the interventricular septum. LEV named this process "sclerosis of the left side of the cardiac skeleton". Conduction tissue fibrosis is believed to set in as a result of its compression against the hardened structures of the left side of the cardiac skeleton. Lev's disease may be responsible for complete atrioventricular block with narrow QRS complexes on the ECG, as expression of the proximal localization of the pathological lesions.

However, this hypothesis accounts for only a small number of the blocks occurring in the elderly. Conduction system fibrosis is more often to be ascribed to a primitive degenerative process which affects especially the middle and distal region of the branches and is called Lenegre's disease from the name of the reporting author (1964). The localization differences are not always evident and a clear distinction between these forms is therefore not always possible.

Ischemia was responsible for heart block in 16.8% of the cases reported by DAVIES (1976). Conduction disturbances usually occur as a consequence of anteroseptal infarction, but more seldomly as a consequence of inferior necroses. The role played by coronary arteriosclerosis in the genesis of chronic atrioventricular blocks is generally considered as unimportant (PUECH et al. 1970; DAVIES 1976; KENNEL et al. 1973; DEEG and SCHNEIDER 1977). By contrast, OKADA and FUKUDA (1978) regarded coronary arteriosclerosis and primitive fibrosis of the conduction tissue as the principal causes of heart block in the elderly, while in young and adult subjects collagenosis, myocarditis, and ischemia are believed by these authors to be involved more frequently.

The heart blocks developing in the acute phase of the myocardial infarction are not characterized by any peculiar geriatric aspect. Among infarcted patients the average age has been found to be higher in those exhibiting conduction disturbances (DE PASQUALE and BRUNO 1976). Recently in a group of patients aged over 70 years and admitted to a coronary care unit, it was observed that all conduction disorders, except complete atrioventricular block, were more frequent among those with myocardial infarction (BERMAN 1979).

In patients aged over 80 the number of pacemaker implantations and the sum of atrioventricular blocks resulted significantly higher in the subgroup with the lower values of HDL-cholesterol, which is generally regarded as negative risk indicator for atherosclerosis but in this group failed to show relationships with history or ECG signs of ischemic heart disease, premature beats, right and left bundle branch block (SCHNEIDER et al. 1980).

The transient occurrence of complete heart block and other conduction disorders, primarily left anterior hemiblock, was also observed in the course of Prinzmetal's angina (BOTTI 1966; PELLEGRINO and PRENCIPE 1974; LÉVI et al. 1979). These transient conduction disorders deserve particular attention since in the elderly, Prinzmetal's angina is not at all rare and its clinical picture is even more difficult to evaluate than in the adult.

The common His's bundle may also be damaged by calcific infiltration usually originating from the mitral valvular ring. Calcification of this structure is a quite frequent finding (about 10% of cases) in elderly subjects. Unlike calcification of the aortic ring, it appears to be significantly associated with ageing (SUGIURA et al.

1976; Pomerance et al. 1978; Kronzon and Glassman 1978). Calcification of the mitralic ring is particularly frequent in the presence of obstructive hypertrophic cardiomyopathy in elderly patients (66% of cases) while it is rather rare in the young and in the adult (14%, Kronzon and Glassman 1978). On the other hand, conduction disturbances are rather frequent in hypertrophic and congestive cardiomyopathy, particularly in subjects of very advanced age (Waisser et al. 1975; Hess et al. 1977; Kuhn et al. 1978; Probst et al. 1979; Camerini et al. 1980). In this connection it should be stressed that in the last few years it has been repeatedly reported that these forms in elderly people are more frequent than is generally believed (Himbert et al. 1972; Waisser et al. 1975; Hamby and Aintablian 1976; Krasnow and Stein 1978; Tarquinii et al. 1978; Berger et al. 1979).

Amyloidosis is thought to cause conduction disturbances by some investigators (Bridgen 1964; Buja et al. 1970; Missmahl 1971). However, this relationship was not confirmed in a successive clinicopathological study (Hodkinson and Pomerance 1977).

Conduction disorders are frequently encountered among subjects with alcoholic cardiomyopathy; the most frequent forms are represented by first degree atrioventricular block and bundle branch blocks (Burstin and Piza 1967; Mösslacher et al. 1969; Parker 1974; Bashour et al. 1976). The "pure" form of alcoholic cardiomyopathy is rare in the elderly owing to frequent coexistence of arteriosclerotic damage. However, in old patients it may be possible that alcoholism represents a contributory cause of conduction disorders.

The atrial septum defect, which is not uncommonly found in advanced age, is often associated with heart block (Rodstein 1977; Thormann et al. 1979).

Among general diseases with clinical pictures which quite frequently include conduction disturbances, diabetes mellitus, and some collagen disease such as scleroderma and giant cell arteritis are most often encountered in old age. Dromotropic disturbances, and in particular those localized at the intraventricular level, are also found in a high percentage of old patients with chronic obstructive pulmonary disease (Levine and Klein 1976).

Familial forms of heart block have not been considered to be of geriatric interest, but recent investigation has pointed out that these forms not uncommonly become clinically evident in late adult or even in advanced age and progress further in following years (Schneider et al. 1978; Kiriyama et al. 1979; Stephan 1979).

Transient conduction disorders, up to complete heart block, were also observed in the presence of hyperkalemia (Punja et al. 1973; Fazzini et al. 1974; Monsallier et al. 1976; Shapiro 1979). Hyperkalemia may appear more readily in elderly subjects as a consequence of either renal insufficiency or abuse of potassium sparing drugs, the pharmacological effects of which elderly people are more responsive to.

Elderly subjects, and in particular those suffering from conduction disturbances, are more prone to develop even severe forms of heart block of iatrogenic origin. Among the drugs which may be dangerous in this respect, in addition to digitalis and antiarrhythmic agents characterized by a marked negative dromotropic effect, an important role is played by phenothiazines and tricyclic antidepressant agents, which are widely used in the geriatric field (Rodstein 1977; Kantor et al. 1978; Rodstein and Oei 1979).

III. Intraventricular Block

The pathological and etiological considerations contained in the previous paragraph are also appropriate for the intraventricular blocks. Rather disappointing results have been obtained from anatomoelectrocardiographic correlations. Electrocardiographic patterns of localized conduction disorders, such as bundle branch blocks and fascicular blocks, are almost always associated with a widespread involvement of the conduction system (DEMOULIN and KULBERTUS 1972; ROSSI 1976). It has been observed, however, that damage of His's bundle may result in electrocardiographic patterns of localized block (FABREGAS et al. 1976). On the other hand, severe histopathological alterations of the left bundle branch have been found in subjects showing no electrocardiographic abnormalities (ROSSI 1964). The electrocardiographic pattern of right bundle branch block associated with left anterior hemiblock in an elderly subject without evidence of heart disease usually suggests the presence of Lev's disease. These forms are generally characterized by a favorable prognosis and only seldomly progress to complete heart block. On the other hand, occurrence of monofascicular block accompanied by a rather rapid progression to a bifascicular block in subjects of late adult or senile age without signs of heart disease suggests the presence of Lenegre's disease and should be regarded as a forewarning sign of complete heart block (ROSENBAUM et al. 1970).

Ischemic heart disease was present in 41% of patients with left anterior hemiblock (ROSENBAUM et al. 1970) and in 23% of patients with bifascicular blocks (KULBERTUS et al. 1978). Therefore it plays an important role in the genesis of these conduction disorders. However, the significance of such a causal relationship should not be overemphasized, as ischemic heart disease per se is present in a high percentage of elderly subjects.

Transient left anterior hemiblock may appear either in the presence of acute myocardial ischemia or even during an exercise test (KULBERTUS and HUMBLET 1972; HEGGE et al. 1973). In these cases the conduction disorder may be due either to a reduction in the blood supply to the left anterior fasciculus or to diffuse ischemia of the left anterior wall with consequent delay in the activation of this region (CASTELLANOS and MYERBURG 1976).

Left anterior hemiblock and bifascicular blocks are often associated with the presence of arterial hypertension: 53.9% and 52.0% respectively in the case reports of ROSENBAUM et al. (1970) and KULBERTUS et al. (1978). There is therefore no doubt that an etiological relationship exists between hypertension and intraventricular blocks, even though its underlying mechanisms are not completely clear (ROSENBAUM et al. 1970).

D. General Clinical Aspects

I. Sinoatrial Block

With regard to the electrocardiographic patterns of sinoatrial block, there are no significant differences between adults and the elderly. In the latter the block is often transient and secondary to carotid sinus hypersensitivity. Particularly in the presence of sinus bradycardia, the occurrence of a sinoatrial block is suggestive of marked sinus node dysfunction, which, from a functional point of view, results in an increase in the sinus node recovery time and in the sinoatrial conduction time. In one- to two-thirds of cases (BENSAID et al. 1973), sinoatrial block is associated with tachycardia, atrial flutter, or atrial fibrillation, thus giving rise to the so-called sick sinus syndrome.

In recent investigations it has been observed that in a high percentage of subjects with sinoatrial block, atrioventricular and intraventricular conduction disturbances are also present (POP et al. 1977; BALDI et al. 1977; SANTINI et al. 1976; MORET et al. 1979).

II. Atrioventricular Block

Isolated first degree atrioventricular block becomes progressively more frequent with advancing age and is usually well tolerated by old subjects because it does not affect hemodynamics. Furthermore no significant correlations were demonstrated with the presence of heart disease (MIHALICK and FISCH 1977).

Second degree atrioventricular blocks are of importance in the elderly mainly in view of their hemodynamic consequences and also because they may progress to complete heart block. Mobitz type I block (Wenckebach) is generally suggestive of conduction impairment at proximal level (NARULA et al. 1971; BAROLD and FRIEDBERG 1974), even though a distal lesion cannot be ruled out (WAXMAN and CASTELLANOS 1979). However, these authors share the opinion that Mobitz type II block is indicative of damage localized in the distal part of the conduction system and is therefore more prone to progress to complete heart block. With the exception of those accompanied by marked bradycardia, second degree atrioventricular blocks are generally well tolerated by old patients (FRANKE et al. 1976).

Old people are much more sensitive to the hemodynamic consequences of complete heart block than the young and adults. Subsidiary pacemakers show difficulties in initiating the heartbeat and low frequency discharge rate so that asystole and marked bradycardia occur more easily. Moreover, as localized or generalized blood flow deficits frequently coexist, even a short-lasting bradycardia can give rise to the low output syndrome and above all to cerebral symptoms.

The occurrence of such symptoms in an old subject with atrial fibrillation should always lead to the suspicion of complete heart block. The presence of R–R intervals of longer than 1,300 ms on the surface electrocardiogram, especially if they occur fairly constantly, is strongly suggestive of partial heart block, which may easily become complete (SÖDERSTRÖM 1958). Furthermore, the association of complete heart block and atrial flutter or fibrillation is accompanied by a significant increase in the incidence of systemic embolism (FAIRFAX et al. 1976), which is usually rare in subjects with heart block alone (REED et al. 1973).

III. Intraventricular Block

The fundamental investigations carried out by ROSENBAUM et al. (1970) significantly contributed to the establishment of the diagnostic criteria and to the clarification of some clinical aspects of the intraventricular conduction disturbances in relation

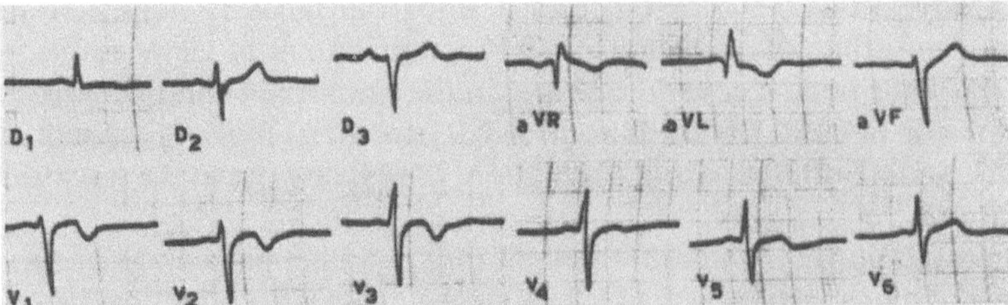

Fig. 1. Electrocardiographic tracing of left anterior hemiblock. Note the following patterns: (1) QRS axis over $-45°$ (in this case, $-60°$), (2) Q1–S3 pattern, and (3) appearance time of the intrinsicoid deflection in aVL is more than 45 ms and is more delayed than in V5 and V6. Moreover, a thickened terminal positivity in aVR and deep S waves in V5 and V6 are present. (TAMMARO and FORIN 1977)

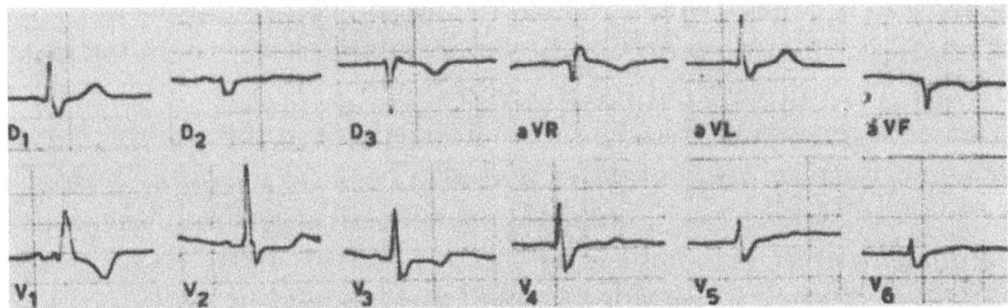

Fig. 2. Electrocardiographic tracing of left anterior hemiblock and right bundle branch block. Note the presence of the typical ECG pattern of left anterior hemiblock associated with evidence of right bundle branch block. (TAMMARO and FORIN 1977)

to the trifascicular nature of the His–Purkinje system (see Chap. 2). As a result, the concept of monofascicular (right bundle branch block, isolated left anterior, or posterior hemiblock), bifascicular (left bundle branch block, right bundle branch block associated with either left anterior or left posterior hemiblock), and trifascicular block (right bundle branch block associated with both left anterior and left posterior hemiblock) was introduced.

The electrocardiographic criteria for the diagnosis of these blocks in the elderly do not differ from the conventional ones established by ROSENBAUM et al. (1970). Figures 1 and 2 show the tracings of left anterior hemiblock isolated and associated with right bundle branch block, which are often found in elderly patients. The diagnosis of left posterior hemiblock is based on the presence of an electrical QRS axis of about $+120°$, with S1–Q3 pattern and QRS complexes of normal duration in the absence of right ventricular hypertrophy, vertical heart, or a large lateral infarction. It appears clear from this that the diagnosis of left posterior hemiblock is not based on purely electrocardiographic criteria but is the result of clinicoelectrocardiographic considerations.

It has been shown that left anterior hemiblock may mask either signs of myocardial ischemia (VOLPE 1978), inferior and anteroseptal myocardial infarction (CRISTAL et al. 1975; ALTIERI and SCHAAL 1973; HORWITZ and MEDRANO 1976), or simulate the presence of anteroseptal infarction (FARNHAM and SHAH 1976). In doubtful cases a careful evaluation of signs and symptoms as well as more thorough instrumental investigations are needed.

The presence of a left bundle branch block and, according to some investigators, left anterior hemiblock may lead to an increase in the preejection period and in the preejection/ejection period ratio, which could be wrongly attributed to reduced myocardial contractility and considered as a polycardiographic index of reduced cardiac performance (BRODER and POLANSKY 1971; MORAGREGA et al. 1976; BORRONI et al. 1977; LUISADA 1977). Such possible interference should be kept in mind since the systolic time intervals are receiving increasing attention as reliable noninvasive indices of myocardial functionality.

Recent studies carried out on patient materials consisting either exclusively (INOHUE et al. 1979) or prevalently (WYSE et al. 1979) of elderly subjects have confirmed that intraventricular conduction disturbances are often associated with sinoatrial node dysfunction. In patients with intraventricular blocks the incidence of ventricular extrasystoles has also been found to be significantly higher than in subjects with normal conduction. The highest incidence of ventricular extrasystoles has been observed in subjects with bifascicular blocks (WATANABE et al. 1973).

E. Symptomatology

The clinical manifestations of heart block are due either to marked bradycardia with consequent reduction of cardiac output or to ventricular asystole resulting in syncopal attacks of the kind of the Morgagni-Adams-Stokes syndrome (MAS attacks). In both cases the symptoms of cerebral origin are predominant. In the former case transient and partial alterations in the level of consciousness, as well as dizziness, general weakness, visual impairment, unsteadiness of gait, and paresthesias may develop. MAS attacks represented the most frequent cause of hospitalization for old patients with advanced heart block (86.6%) as described by PUECH et al. (1970).

These attacks are characterized by sudden and transient loss of consciousness (syncope) without warning signs, with diffuse pallor and quick return to consciousness (within 30 s), occasionally accompanied by flushing due to the dilatation of peripheral skin vessels on resumption of cardiac activity. These clinical signs are of diagnostic value (SIDDONS 1976). The pulse is extremely slow or even imperceivable, the blood pressure falls, the heart sounds are absent, and mydriasis may be present. In the elderly the clinical picture of MAS attack is characterized by a marked polymorphism and is often atypical (BERNARDI et al. 1977).

In elderly patients this syndrome usually develops in the presence of sinoatrial block, second degree type Mobitz II atrioventricular block with high atrioventricular ratio, complete heart block, and more seldomly as a consequence of supraventricular or ventricular tachyarrhythmias leading to cerebral ischemia. Ventricular tachycardia gives rise to MAS syndrome in 10%–25% of patients with heart block (HARRIS 1976).

These clinical manifestations are of particular interest in geriatrics for two reasons: firstly because the underlying conditions are particularly frequent in old people, and secondly because the extracardiac conditions capable of producing consciousness disorders and other symptoms which may be wrongly attributed to heart block frequently occur in old age.

F. Diagnosis

I. General Diagnostic Aspects

In the presence of such symptomatology a careful clinical evaluation is needed. A careful clinical history should first of all elucidate the circumstances in which the attack has appeared and ascertain whether there may have been any precipitating factors, such as posture changes, head or neck movements, carotis sinus pressure, or forewarning manifestations such as dizziness, visual disturbances, nausea, pallor and hyperventilation.

The general physical examination is usually not of great help in diagnosing this syndrome and further investigations are needed. Identification of a cardiac cause is essential at all ages, but the evaluation of the possible existence of a conduction disorder, whether manifest or latent, is imperative in the elderly. Conduction disorders and precocious or complex ventricular ectopias may be revealed by the baseline electrocardiogram. If the tracing is not diagnostic, continuous heart monitoring is indicated. This technique has been reported to be of great help in old subjects with symptoms attributable to reduction or arrest of cerebral blood flow (LEVIN 1976; GORDON 1978). Electrocardiography of His's bundle has also been of considerable diagnostic help in old subjects with syncopal attacks and no evidence of severe conduction disturbances (JEDYNAK and LANFRANCHI 1979).

As stated by SIDDONS (1976) about a third of patients with complete heart block present no syncope, while an extreme bradycardia (below 40 beats/min) may lead to the so-called low-output syndrome with signs of cerebral ischemia, physical weakness, and cardiac and/or renal failure; these were observed in 21.4% of the patients studied by PUECH et al. (1970).

Besides acute and transient manifestations, the consequences of chronic heart block with stable reduction in heart output should also be taken into consideration. Even in this case the most important clinical manifestations are represented by the signs and symptoms of cerebral ischemia. Symptoms of chronic encephalopathy, such as inanition, irritability, mental confusion, drowsiness, loss of recent memory, and weight loss were observed in some patients with chronic heart block (DALESSIO et al. 1965). All of these patients were aged more than 70 years and had been suffering from heart block for over 3 months. Isoproterenol administration was followed by an increase in heart rate with no modification in the cerebral symptoms, which markedly improved only after an artificial pacemaker was implanted. PUECH et al. (1970) found signs of ischemic encephalopathy in 13.4% of their patients, aged more than 70 years, with chronic heart block. The symptomatology subsided either partially or completely following acceleration of cardiac rate, which in the majority of the cases was obtained by heart pacing. As the treatment of chronic encephalopathy in the elderly is nearly always disappointing, the identification of a causative factor as heart block to which a more effective therapy could be applied is of great importance.

II. Differential Diagnosis of Syncope

The forms of syncope occurring more frequently in advanced age and thus requiring differentiation from the MAS attack are sinocarotid, cough, and micturition syncopes.

Sinocarotid syncope is typical for elderly subjects, especially if heart disease coexists (HERON et al. 1965). Its higher incidence in old age is to be attributed to the increased reactivity of the carotid sinus and is elicited by mechanic stimulation of the sinocarotid area, which may be followed by marked bradycardia, asystole, and peripheral vasodilation. Loss of consciousness occurs only in about a third of the cases. Other symptoms are vertigo, mental confusion, and focal neurological signs (MANKIKAR and CLARK 1975; JOHNSON 1976; WOLLNER and SPALDING 1978). The nature of the syncope is confirmed by a marked bradycardic response to the sinocarotid area massage. In elderly subjects this maneuver should be performed very cautiously and only on one side of the neck (SMIDDY et al. 1972). With this caution the maneuver has proved not to be dangerous even on very old subjects (MANKIKAR and CLARK 1975). The treatment consists of administration of atropine and, in refractory cases, of carotid sinus denervation.

Cough syncope results in a transient loss of consciousness after prolonged or violent coughing attacks. In less severe cases the symptomatology is limited to vertigo and mental cloudiness. This kind of syndrome is attributed to two mechanisms: (1) to a reduction in the venous return to the heart secondary to the increased intrathoracic pressure and (2) to a baroceptor reflex caused by pressor stimulation originating in the thoracic aorta and transmitted to sinocarotid reflexogenic areas with resultant blood pressure fall (JOHNSON 1976; WOLLNER and SPALDING 1978).

With regards to micturition syndrome, its geriatric significance is controversial. According to JOHNSON (1976) this form of syncope is more frequent in young and adult people, while SOLINAS and NOTARISTEFANO (1977) are of the opposite opinion. If it occurs at the beginning of the micturition and particularly when this is forced because of prostatic enlargement, it may be attributed to a mechanism such as that of the Valsalva maneuver, based on an increase in the intrathoracic pressure. Another mechanism consists of a sudden cessation of the peripheral vasoconstriction reflex starting from the distended bladder (DONKER et al. 1972; DEBARGE et al. 1974; WOLLNER and SPALDING 1978). Upright posture after prolonged bed rest, a high room temperature, and alcohol ingestion are precipitating factors for the occurrence of syncope.

When investigating the causes of syncope it should not be overlooked that a wide variety of drugs used in geriatric practice may be involved in its development, such as vasodilators, antihypertensives, quinidine, and quinidine-like agents, prenylamine, phenothiazines, and tricyclic antidepressants.

G. Prognosis

Prognostic evaluation of the various forms of heart block in the aged is made difficult by the frequent coexistence of organic heart disease. The latter often affects the natural history of these patients regardless of the conduction disorder, thus being of decisive importance for the subsequent course of the situation.

In complete heart block, prognosis depends on whether the disorder is tolerated from a hemodynamic point of view and on the presence, if any, and the severity of symptoms. The best prognosis is observed in symptom-free patients with a heart rate exceeding 40 beats/min, which increases by at least 5 beats/min on exercise and in the presence of narrow QRS complexes on the surface electrocardiogram (SIDDONS 1976). According to the data reported by AMIKAM et al. (1976), patients with complete heart block and MAS attacks present a 1-year mortality of 50% and a 5-year mortality of 75%.

The sinoatrial block, if transient and not associated with marked bradycardia may be well tolerated by elderly patients. On establishing a prognosis for these patients, the frequent coexistence of atrioventricular and intraventricular conduction disturbances, which may impair the effectiveness of a subsidiary pacemaker, should be taken into consideration.

First degree atrioventricular blocks are well tolerated by the elderly and their presence is not associated with an increase in morbidity or mortality.

With regards to second degree atrioventricular blocks, Mobitz type II block shows the worst prognosis because of frequent progression to complete heart block as a consequence of the distal localization of the underlying conduction tissue damage (EL SHERIF et al. 1976).

Attempts aiming at the prognostic evaluation of patients with intraventricular blocks led to controversial results because of lack of uniformity of the case materials and methods. The left axial deviation and the left anterior hemiblock per se have not proved to be associated with a higher mortality, morbidity, or progression to complete heart block (BLACKBURN et al. 1967; CAIRD et al. 1974; YANO et al. 1975; MIHALICK and FISCH 1977; TAMMARO and FORIN 1977). The right and left bundle branch blocks have been shown to be associated with higher mortality (CAIRD et al. 1974). As far as right bundle branch block is concerned, other studies have demonstrated no significant association with increased incidence of heart disease (EDMANDS 1966; MIHALICK and FISCH 1977), although a significant association has been shown among subjects with left bundle branch block.

Bifascicular blocks, and in particular right bundle branch block associated with left anterior hemiblock, have been investigated from a prognostic point of view for their possible role as forerunner of complete heart block and hence as a possible indication for the preventive implantation of an artificial pacemaker. The evolution of a bifascicular block toward complete heart block was demonstrated in a number of retrospective investigations and determined quantitatively in 9%, 13.6%, and 21% of the subjects followed up for 6.3, 19, and 58 months respectively (WATT and PRUITT 1969; SCANLON et al. 1970; KULBERTUS 1973). More recent studies based on the prospective follow-up of patients with bifascicular blocks indicate that this kind of progression was overestimated since lower percentages of evolution toward complete heart block have been found: 2% during 34 months (KULBERTUS et al. 1978) and 11% during 5 years (DHINGRA et al. 1979a).

These studies showed no significant progression differences among the various forms of bifascicular blocks. Among the subjects with bifascicular block a higher incidence of sudden death was observed (CHIANG et al. 1970; DHINGRA et al.

1979 a). The prognostic value of either intermittent or incomplete intraventricular blocks depends mainly on their frequent appearance as forerunners of either stable or complete conduction disturbances.

The presence of a bifascicular block should therefore not be regarded as an unfavorable prognostic sign, also in order not to arouse unjustified alarm in patients. The clinical and prognostic significance of such conduction disorders should be assessed by a careful examination of the general and cardiological condition of the patient. In this connection the occurrence of even slight and transient symptoms revealing bradycardia and asystole episodes, if any, is of great importance. The presence of organic heart disease has a definite prognostic importance since subjects with bifascicular block and organic heart disease showed a significantly higher incidence of spontaneous atrioventricular block as well as sudden and cardiovascular mortality if compared with primary conduction disease patients (DHINGRA et al. 1979 b). According to the results of a study carried out by the same group (DHINGRA et al. 1980) age per se cannot be regarded as determinant of risk of atrioventricular block or sudden death in patients with bifascicular block, with and without organic heart disease. Continuous heart monitoring and intracavitary electrocardiography may be of great help in clearing up either suspect or uncertain cases. Further improvement in the field of noninvasive recording techniques of the His potentials will be particularly useful for the elderly patient.

H. Treatment

I. Drug Treatment

In the presence of MAS attacks, if syncope does not subside spontaneously, heart resuscitation maneuvers, such as external cardiac massage, are needed. If feasible, external heart pacing may be helpful. Drug treatment is based on the intravenous administration of isoprenaline or orciprenaline. Steroids have also proved to be effective in some cases. If the attack is caused by sinoatrial block, which is often secondary to parasympathetic hypertone, atropine is better indicated. In any case, the patients should be carefully checked for the possible side effects of these drugs, which are particularly frequent and marked among elderly subjects.

In chronic heart block, acceleration of heart rate may be obtained in some cases with orciprenaline or sustained action isoprenaline. According to PUECH et al. (1970), medical treatment is justified only in the absence of syncope and with a fairly stable heart rate exceeding 35 beats/min. However, the effectiveness of long-term medication is unpredictable and the results obtained have proved rather disappointing.

II. Heart Pacing

The implantation of a permanent pacemaker represents the only effective treatment of chronic heart block. In the last decade.this therapeutic measure has been applied to a progressively increasing percentage of elderly subjects. At present, at least 80% of the subjects undergoing heart pacing are aged more than 60 years, and more than 90% in some reports. In the past 10 years a reduction in the percentage of pacemaker implantations for heart block has been observed, while among the paced persons the percentage of patients with heart failure and bradycardia as well as of those with sick sinus syndrome has shown an increase.

In patients with either complete or advanced heart block, even though intermittent, presenting with symptoms such as MAS attacks, vertigo, and low-output syndrome, the indication for pacing arises from the clinical criteria only. The presence of symptoms is an indication for pacing also in patients with sinoatrial block. When clinical signs of sinus node dysfunction are associated with changes in electrophysiological parameters of sinoatrial function and particularly in the case of prolonged sinus node recovery time symptoms are usually expected to appear within a short time and heart pacing is therefore indicated as a preventive measure.

The results of electrophysiological studies and of prospective follow-up of patients with bifascicular block have provided useful information regarding the indications for prophylactic heart pacing aiming at preventing symptoms and improving survival and life quality in these patients.

Heart pacing is indicated in symptomatic patients with prolonged H–V time on the His-bundle electrogram, even in the absence of documented heart block (SCHEINMANN et al. 1977; ALTSCHULER et al. 1979; NARULA and ALBONI 1979). This therapeutic measure is also indicated in asymptomatic patients with markedly prolonged H–V time if the duration of the bifascicular block is greater than 3 years and/or the block is associated with first degree atrioventricular block (VERA et al. 1976; HAFT 1977; DINI et al. 1978). Symptomatic patients without evidence of atrioventricular block and with normal electrophysiological parameters do not require prophylactic pacing (SCHEINMANN et al. 1977; NARULA and ALBONI 1979).

Until the late 1960s pacemakers were implanted under general anesthesia by inserting an epicardial electrode either by thoracotomy or through an epigastric transdiaphragmatic approach. Since then these techniques have been replaced by the transvenous implantation of an endocardial electrode. The implantation is done under local anesthesia and usually entails introducing the catheter electrode through the cephalic vein at the level of the deltoid-pectoral triangle. In advanced age the cephalic vein may be not available as a consequence of thrombosis or sclerosis. In this case the external jugular, subclavian, or axillary veins may be used. The transvenous technique was also successfully adopted for the emergency pacing of patients over 75 years (BARTECCHI 1979). The impulse generator is implanted subcutaneously in the anterior chest wall or in the axillary area.

This technique has proved particularly advantageous for elderly patients, enabling heart pacing to be applied even to patients of very advanced age because of reduced operative trauma, mortality, and complication rate (MATSUURA et al. 1978; MUGICA and BOUVRAIN 1979). Moreover, an early postoperative mobilization is possible. The implantation of a ventricular endocardial electrode is the measure of choice even in patients with sinoatrial block, because of the frequent coexistence of impaired atrioventricular conduction and the technical and economical problems connected with the implantation of a bifocal pacemaker.

Fixed-rate (asynchronous) pacemakers are at present used in very few cases. Fixed-rate pacing in a subject with only intermittent heart block may result in competition between conducted and artificial beats with a risk of dangerous arrhythmias. Use of demand (synchronous) pacemakers produces no risk of competition nor is spontaneous cardiac activity affected. Another advantage is that in this way the contribution of atrial systole to ventricular filling and cardiac output is maintained.

As reported in the past 10 years, complications occur in about a third of the patients. However, the complication rate has progressively and markedly decreased in the last few years as a result of technical improvements. Complications usually do not compromise the results of the intervention and their management is not particularly difficult in elderly subjects. Failure of the pacing system with recurrence of symptoms is the most frequent complication. In most cases this takes place following the displacement of the intracavitary electrode, which usually occurs within the first few days after implantation. Even though displacement of the electrode involves its penetration into the ventricular wall or the pericardium, it is not usually dangerous for the patient. A correct implantation technique and the proper use of improved electrodes enabled the incidence of displacements to be reduced (RETTIG et al. 1975; SIDDONS 1976).

Other complications may occur at the implantation site of the pacemaker: infection, hematoma, and skin necroses. They are more frequent in the elderly because of the thinness and lack of elasticity of the overlying tissue. However, in a fairly high percentage of cases these complications may be prevented by choosing carefully the implantation site and by a correct operative technique.

The results of heart pacing may be expressed as effects on survival and clinical picture. The study of survival of paced subjects has shown that after the introduction of heart pacing, life expectancy of these patients dramatically improves. The difference in survival between paced subjects and the general population matched for age and sex has shown a progressive reduction in the past few years. In a recent survey carried out on 427 patients who underwent heart pacing by transvenous endocardial electrode implantation (72.3% were over 65 years and only 8.9% under 55 years), it was shown that the survival differences with people of the same age and sex were negligible and not significant. Only women under 55 and men under 64 showed a statistically significant lower survival rate (FITZGERALD et al. 1979). This difference may result from the frequent association of heart block and coronary artery disease which is observed in middle age (GINKS et al. 1978). Average life expectation was over 10 years for the paced subjects in the age class 65–74 years and about 5 years for those aged more than 75 years.

A good rate of survival in elderly paced patients was also shown by surveys carried out in previous years (RETTIG et al. 1975; SIDDONS 1976; AMIKAM et al. 1976). In a group of patients aged more than 80 at the time of the pacemaker implantation, a 5-year survival of 45% was reported (STRAUSS and BERMAN 1978).

By comparing life expectancy of subjects over 70 with that of the whole group of paced patients, survival percentages of 90.0%, 82.1%, 74.1%, 67.2%, and 58.3%, and of 90.1%, 82.4%, 75.4%, 70.5%, and 66.7% after 1, 2, 3, 4, and 5 years respectively were found. Lower survival of older subjects after 4 years is linked to the natural lower life expectancy in this age group (AMIKAM et al. 1976).

Figure 3 shows the survival curve in a group of 139 patients over 80 years old paced for complete heart block as compared with the general population matched for age and sex. The life expectancy of the former corresponded to that of the latter

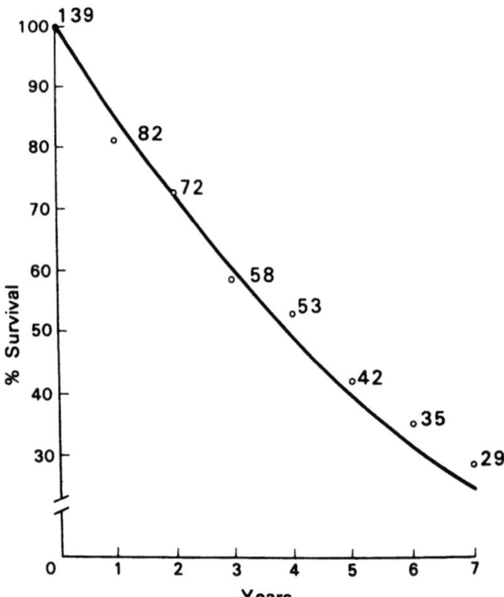

Fig. 3. Survival of 139 paced patients over 80 years old as compared with the general population matched for age and sex. *Solid line*, survival curve of the general population; *circles*, survival of the patients; *figures*, number at risk. (SIDDONS 1976)

without the greater mortality in the first year of pacing observed in other surveys (SIDDONS 1976).

Furthermore, the clinical picture is favorably affected by heart pacing. MAS attacks subside completely and the signs of low-output syndrome markedly improve in a high percentage of cases. In very old patients the grade of arteriosclerotic involvement of cerebral, coronary, and peripheral arteries is such as to limit the improvement which may be obtained by regulating heart rate. The psychological adaptation to the new situation following pacemaker implantation was more than satisfactory among old patients (RODSTEIN et al. 1977).

Methods for pacemaker control have considerably improved in the last few years, so that a correct and effective follow-up of these patients is now possible from this point of view as well. On the basis of all the above considerations it may therefore be stated that the implantation of an artificial pacemaker presents no particular difficulties in old age. The dramatic improvements in survival and in quality of life which follows this therapeutic measure is a very good reason for its widest application in the geriatric field.

References

Altieri P, Schall SF (1973) Inferior and anteroseptal myocardial infarction concealed by transient left anterior hemiblock. J Electrocardiol 6:257–258

Altschuler H, Fisher JD, Furman S (1979) Significance of isolated HV-interval prolongation in symptomatic patients without documented heart block. Am Heart J 97:19–26

Amikam S, Lemer J, Rogouin N, Peleg H, Riss E (1976) Longterm survival of elderly patients after pacemaker implantation. Am Heart J 91:445–449

Baldi N, Fonda F, Morgera T, Silvestri F, Camerini F (1977) La sindrome del seno malato. In: Furlanello F, Lanzetta T, Disertori M (eds) Le nuove frontiere delle aritmie. Picin, Padova, pp 304 ff

Balsaver AM, Morales AR, Whitehouse FW (1967) Fat infiltration of myocardium as a cause of cardiac conduction defect. Am J Cardiol 19:261–265

Barold SS, Friedberg HD (1974) Second degree AV-block: a matter of definition. Am J Cardiol 33:311–315

Bartecchi C (1979) Emergency transvenous (subclavian) cardiac pacing in elderly patients. J Am Geriat Soc 27:208–211

Bashour TT, Fahdul H, Cheng TO (1976) Multifascicular block in cardiomyopathy. Cardiology 61:89–97

Beggiato O, Pratis S (1978) I disturbi della conduzione intraventricolare dello stimolo negli anziani. Minerva Cardioangiol 26:325–329

Bensaid J, Guize L, Fernandez F, Schebat L, Lenegre J (1973) Bloc sinoauriculaire chronique et paralyse auriculaire permanente. Acta Cardiol 28:3–26

Berger M, Rethy C, Goldberg E (1979) Unsuspected hypertrophic subaortic stenosis in the elderly diagnosed by echocardiography. J Am Geriat Soc 27:178–182

Berman ND (1979) The elderly patient in the coronary care unit. II. Incidence and treatment of arrhythmias. J Am Geriat Soc 27:203–207

Bernardi A, Dalzocchio S, Montanari PV, Mansoldo G (1977) Problemi diagnostici differenziali della sindrome di M. A.S. nell'anziano. Acta Gerontol 27:272–284

Blackburn H, Vasquez CL, Keys A (1967) The aging electrocardiogram. A common aging process or latent coronary artery disease. Am J Cardiol 20:618–627

Borroni G, Bosisio P, Roncoroni G (1977) Blocco di branca sinistra intermittente: studio policardiografico di sette casi. Cardiol Prat 28:25–35

Botti RE (1966) A variant form of angina pectoris with recurrent transient complete heart block. Am J Cardiol 17:443–446

Bridgen W (1964) Cardiac amyloidosis. Prog Cardiovasc Dis 7:142–150

Broder G, Polansky BJ (1971) Prolonged pre-ejection period in left anterior hemiblock (abstr). Circulation 43–44 (suppl 2):145

Buja LM, Khoi NB, Roberts WC (1970) Clinically significant cardiac amyloidosis. Clinicopathological findings in 15 patients. Am J Cardiol 26:394–405

Burstin LS, Piza JE (1967) Cardiopatia alcoholica. Arch Inst Cardiol Mex 37:558–574

Caird FI, Campbell A, Jackson TFM (1974) Significance of abnormalities of electrocardiogram in old people. Br Heart J 36:1012–1018

Camerini F, Borgioni L, Fonda F, Klugman S, Mestroni L, Salvi A, Silvestri F (1980) La cardiomiopatia congestizia. In: DePonti C, Rovelli F (eds) Aggiornamenti in cardiologia 1980. Luigi Pozzi, Roma, p 126

Campbell A, Caird FI, Jackson TFM (1974) Prevalence of abnormalities of electrocardiogram in old people. Br Heart J 36:1005–1011

Castellanos A Jr, Myerburg RJ (1976) The hemiblocks in myocardial infarction. Appleton-Century-Crofts, New York, p 47

Chiang BN, Perlman LV, Fulton M, Ostrander LD, Epstein FH (1970) Predisposing factors in sudden death in Tecumseh, Michigan: a prospective study. Circulation 41:31–37

Cristal N, Ho W, Gueron M (1975) Left anterior hemiblock masking inferior myocardial infarction. Br Heart J 37:543–547

Dalessio DJ, Benchimol A, Dimond G (1965) Chronic encephalopathy related to heart block. Neurology 15:499–503

Davies MJ (1976) Pathology of the conduction system. In: Caird FI, Dall JLC, Kennedy RD (eds) Cardiology in old age. Plenum Press, London New York, pp 57–80

Debarge O, Christensen NJ, Corbett JL, Eidelman BH, Frankel HL, Mathias CJ (1974) Plasma catecholamines in tetraplegics. Paraplegia 12:44–49

Deeg P, Schneider KW (1977) Erregungsleitungsstörungen bei über 60jährigen. Z Kardiol Suppl 4 (abstr):19

Demoulin JC, Kulbertus HE (1972) Histopathological examination of left hemiblock. Br Heart J 34:807–814

Demoulin JC, Kulbertus HE (1978) Histopathological correlates of sinoatrial disease. Br Heart J 40:1384–1389

De Pasquale NP, Bruno MS (1976) Incidence and implications of abnormal intraventricular conduction in the coronary care unit. Cardiology 61:215–227

Dhingra RC, Wyndham C, Amat-y-Leon F, Denes P, Wu D, Sridhar S, Bustin AG, Rosen KM (1979 a) Incidence and site of atrioventricular block in patients with chronic bifascicular block. Circulation 59:238–246

Dhingra RC, Wyndham C, Bauernfeind R, Denes P, Wu D, Swiryn S, Rosen KM (1979 b) Significance of chronic bifascicular block without apparent organic heart disease. Circulation 60:33–39

Dhingra RC, Wyndham C, Deedwania PC, Bauernfeind R, Swiryn S, Best D, Rosen KM (1980) Effect of age on atrioventricular conduction in patients with chronic bifascicular block. Am J Cardiol 45:749–756

Dighton DH (1975) Sinoatrial block. Autonomic influences and clinical assessment. Br Heart J 37:321–325

Dini P, Santini M, Di Mascolo R, Boschetti C, Ialongo D, Rocchi M, Masini V (1978) Significato prognostico dell' intervallo HV in 66 pazienti con blocco di branca cronico. G Ital Cardiol 8:392–405

Donker DN, Robies de Medina EO, Kjeft S (1972) Micturition syncope. Electroencephalogr Clin Neurophysiol 33:328–331

Edmands RE (1966) An epidemiological assessment of bundle branch block. Circulation 34:1081–1087

El-Sherif N, Scherlag BJ, Lazzara R (1976) An appraisal of second degree and paroxysmal atrioventricular block. Eur J Cardiol 4:117–130

Fabregas RA, Tse WW, Han J (1976) Conduction disturbances of the bundle branches produced by lesions in the nonbranching portion of the His-bundle. Am Heart J 92:356–362

Fairfax AJ, Lambert CD, Leatham AL (1976) Systemic embolism in chronic sinoatrial disorders. N Engl J Med 295:190–192

Farnham DJ, Shah PM (1976) Left anterior hemiblock simulating anteroseptal myocardial infarction. Am Heart J 92:363–367

Fazzini PF, Marchi F, Sodi A (1974) Hyperkalemia in renal failure inducing AV-block. G Ital Cardiol 4:89–92

Fitzgerald WR, Graham IM, Cole T, Ewans DW (1979) Age, sex, and ischaemic heart disease as prognostic indicators in long-term cardiac pacing. Br Heart J 42:57–60

Franke H, Gall L, Chowanetz W (1976) Über das sogenannte Altersherz bei 50- bis 100jährigen. Z Kardiol 65:945–963

Ginks W, Siddons H, Leatham A (1978) Coronary artery disease as a cause of chronic disorders of impulse formation and propagation in middle age. In: 1st European Symposium on Cardiac Pacing. British Pacing Group, London, p 13

Gordon M (1978) Occult cardiac arrhythmia associated with falls and dizziness in the elderly: detection by Holter monitoring. J Am Geriatr Soc 26:418–423

Haft JI (1977) The HV interval and patients with bifascicular block. J Electrocardiol 10:1–3

Hamby RI, Aintablian A (1976) Hypertrophic subaortic stenosis is not rare in the eight decade. Geriatrics 31/7:71–74

Harris A, Davies M, Redwood D, Leatham A, Siddons H (1969) Aetiology of chronic heart block. Br Heart J 31:206–218

Harris R (1976) Cardiac arrhythmias in the aged. In: Caird FI, Dall JLC, Kennedy RD (eds) Cardiology in old age. Plenum Press, London New York, p 345

Hegge FN, Tuna N, Burchell HB (1976) Coronary arteriographic findings in patients with axis shifts or ST-segment elevation on exercise-stress testing. Am Heart J 86:603–615

Heron JR, Anderson EG, Noble IM (1965) Cardiac abnormalities associated with carotis sinus syndrome. Lancet 2:214–216

Hess OM, Turina J, Goebel NH, Grob P, Krayenbühl HP (1977) Zur Prognose der kongestiven Kardiomyopathie. Z Kardiol 66:351–360

Himbert J, Gay J, Paraiso N, Hanania G, Lenegre J (1972) Evolution des myocardiopathies primitives. Etude rétrospective de 218 observations anatomo-cliniques et de 254 traitements. Arch mal Coeur 65:35–50

Hodkinson HM, Pomerance A (1977) The clinical significance of senile cardiac amyloidosis: a prospective clinico-pathological study. Q J Med 46:381–387

Horwitz S, Medrano GA, Salator E (1976) Left fascicular block concealing anteroseptal infarction. Arch Inst Cardiol Mex 46:35–41

Inohue H, Ueda K, Ohkawa S, Kamata C, Mifune J, Sugiura M, Matsuo H (1979) Electro-physiologic study and prognosis of chronic bifascicular block. Jpn Heart J 20:141–151

James TN, Marshall TK (1976) De subitaneis mortibus. XVII. Multifocal stenoses due to fibromuscular dysplasia of the sinus node artery. Circulation 53:737–742

Jedynak C, Lanfranchi J (1979) Apport de l'électrocardiogramme hisien dans le diagnostic des syncopes du troisieme age. Rev Gériatr 4:151–160

Johnson RH (1976) Blood pressure and its regulation. In: Caird FI, Dall JLC, Kennedy RD (eds) Cardiology in old age. Plenum Press, London New York, p 112

Johnson RL, Averill KH, Lamb LE (1960) Electrocardiographic findings in 67,375 asymp-tomatic subjects. VI. Right bundle branch block. Am J Cardiol 6:143–151

Kantor SJ, Glassman AH, Bigger JT Jr (1978) The cardiac effects of therapeutic plasma con-centrations of imipramine. Am J Psychiat 135:534–538

Kennedy RD, Caird FI (1972) The application of the Minnesota code to population studies of the electrocardiogram in the elderly. Gerontol Clin 14:5–16

Kennel AJ, Titus JL, McCallister BD, Pruitt RD (1973) The vasculature of the atrioven-tricular conduction system in heart block. Am Heart J 85:593–600

Kiriyama T, Mizutani T, Kakusui K, Wada M, Isoda T, Inohue M, Okabe T, Taniguchi S, Kuribayasi T (1979) Familial heart block and sick sinus syndrome of adult onset. Jpn Heart J 20:441–459

Kitchin AH, Lowther CP, Milne JS (1973) Prevalence of clinical and electrocardiographic evidence of ischaemic heart disease in the older population. Br Heart J 35:946–953

Krasnow N, Stein RA (1978) Hypertrophic cardiomyopathy in the aged. Am Heart J 96:326–336

Kronzon I, Glassman E (1978) Mitral ring calcification in hydiopathic hypertrophic subaor-tic stenosis. Am J Cardiol 42:60–66

Kuhn H, Breithardt G, Knieriem H-J, Loogen F (1978) Endomyocardial catheter biopsy in heart disease of unknown etiology. In: Kaltenbach M, Loogen F, Olsen EGJ (eds) Cardiomyopathy and myocardial biopsy. Springer, Berlin Heidelberg New York, p 133

Kulbertus HE (1973) The magnitude of risk of developing complete heart block in patients with LAD-RBBB. Am Heart J 86:278–280

Kulbertus HE, Humblet L (1972) Transient hemiblock. An abnormal type of response to Masters two-step test. Am Heart J 83:574–576

Kulbertus HE, Rutten DL, Dubois M, Petit JM (1978) Prognostic significance of left ante-rior hemiblock with right bundle branch block in mass screening (abstr). Am J Cardiol 41:385

Lenegre J (1964) Etiology and pathology of bilateral bundle branch block in relation to complete heart block. Prog Cardiovasc Dis 6:409–444

Lev M (1964) Anatomic bases for atrioventricular block. Am J Med 37:742–748

Lévi S, Gerard R, Castellanos A, Gharhamani AR, Sommer LS (1979) Transient left ante-rior hemiblock during angina pectoris: coronarographic aspects and clinical signifi-cance. Europ J Cardiol 9:215–225

Levin EB (1976) Use of the Holter monitoring in the diagnosis of transient ischaemic at-tacks. J Am Geriatr Soc 24:516–521

Levine PA, Klein MD (1976) Mechanisms of arrhythmia in chronic obstructive lung disease. Geriatrics 31/11:47–56

Loeb G, Morin Y (1978) Troubles du rythme supraventriculaire et de la conduction auricu-lo-ventriculaire chez le sujet âgé. Sem Hop (Paris) 54:409–412

Luisada AA (1977) Using non invasive method to study the aging heart. Geriatrics 32/2:58–61

Mankikar GD, Clark ANG (1975) Cardiac effects of carotid sinus massage in old age. Age Ageing 4:86–94

Matsuura Y, Tamura M, Yamashina H (1978) Experiences of pace maker implantation in the patients more than 80 years of age (Japanese). J Jpn Assoc Thorac Surg 26:986–991

Michel D (1975) Aktuelle Probleme der geriatrischen Kardiologie. Aktuel Gerontol 5:255–263

Mihalick MJ, Fisch C (1974) Electrocardiographic findings in the aged. Am Heart J 87:117–128

Mihalick MJ, Fisch C (1977) Should ecg criteria be modified for geriatric patients? Geriatrics 32/2:65–72

Missmahl HP (1971) Myokardiopathie durch Amyloid. Verh Dtsch Ges Inn Med 77:359–365

Mösslacher H, Slany J, Hanak H, Stockinger L (1969) Alkoholmyokardiopathie. Z Kreisl 60:303–309

Monsallier JF, Carli A, Bleichner G, Grandadam P (1976) Troubles graves de la conduction révélant une hyperkaliémie ou une acidémie. Coeur Med Int 15:395–406

Moragrega AJL, Del Peral PJM (1976) Los intervalos sistolicos en los transtornos de conduccion intraventricular. Arch Inst Cardiol Mex 46:433–441

Moret R, Adamec R, François C (1979) Clinica e terapia della malattia del nodo del seno atriale o „SSS". In: De Ponti C, Rovelli F (eds) Progressi in cardiologia. Pozzi, Roma, p 23

Mugica J, Bouvrain Y (1979) Entrainement electrosystolique permanent chez 73 malades agés de plus de 90 ans. Bull Acad Nat Med (Paris) 163:433–436

Narula OS, Alboni P (1979) Prognostic value of HV interval in patients with chronic right bundle branch block and left axis deviation. G Ital Cardiol 9:111–116

Narula OS, Scherlag BJ, Samet P, Javier RP (1971) Atrioventricular block localization and classification by His-bundle recordings. Am J Med 50:146–165

Okada R, Fukuda K (1978) Morphological study of the conduction system in the aged cases with AV-block. Abstracts Sectional Sessions, XI. Int Congr Gerontology, Tokyo, p 91

Ostrander LD, Brandt RL, Kjelsberg MO, Epstein FH (1965) Ecg findings among the adult population of a total natural community, Tecumseh, Michigan. Circulation 31:888–898

Parker BM (1974) The effects of ethyl alcohol on the heart. JAMA 228:741–742

Pellegrino L, Prencipe D (1974) I disturbi della conduzione intraventricolare nell'angina pectoris „variant form" di Prinzmetal. Minerva Cardioang 22:32–37

Pfisterer M, Heierli B, Burkart F (1977) Hypersensitiver Carotissinus-Reflex bei älteren Patienten. Schweiz Med Wochenschr 107:1565–1567

Pomerance A, Darby AJ, Hodkinson HM (1978) Valvular calcification in the elderly: possible pathogenic factors. J Gerontol 33:672–675

Pop T, Effert S, Fleischmann D (1977) Die elektrophysiologische Konstellation des sogenannten Syndroms des kranken Sinusknotens. Z Kardiol 66:303–309

Probst P, Pachinger O, Murad AA, Leisch F, Kaindl F (1979) The HQ time in congestive cardiomyopathy. Am Heart J 97:436–441

Puech P, Grolleau R, Dufoix R (1970) Les troubles du rythme cardiaque chez le vieillard. Ann Cardiol Angéiol 19:251–256

Punja MM, Schneebaum R, Cohen J (1973) Bifascicular block induced by hyperkalemia. J Electrocardiol 6:71–76

Reed RL, Siekert RG, Merideth J (1973) Rarity of transient focal cerebral ischemia in cardiac disrhythmia. JAMA 223:893–895

Rettig G, Bette L, Doenecke P, Hoffmann W, Schieffer H, Sternitzke N (1975) Die Bedeutung der Schrittmachertherapie für die Geriatrie. Geriatrie 5:36–40

Rodstein M (1977) The ecg in old age: implications for diagnosis, therapy, and prognosis. Geriatrics 32/2:76–79

Rodstein M, Oei LS (1979) Cardiovascular side effects of long-term therapy with tricyclic antidepressants in the aged. J Am Geriatr Soc 27:231–234

Rodstein M, Zarit S, Savitsky E, Goldferer M (1977) Relation of long-term electronic cardiac pacing to mental status and adaptation in the institutional aged. J Am Geriatr Soc 25:534–540

Rosenbaum MB, Elizari MV, Lazzari JO (1970) The hemiblocks. Tampa Tracings, Oldsmar, p 123

Rossi L (1964) Discordant features in pathology of the bundle branches and related blocks. Acta Cardiol 19:286–304

Rossi L (1976) Histopathology of conducting system in left anterior hemiblock. Br Heart J 38:1304–1311

Rotman M, Triebwasser JH (1975) A clinical and follow-up study of right and left bundle branch block. Circulation 51:477–484

Santini M, Dini P, Di Mascolo R, Masini V (1976) Disturbi della conduzione associati a malattia del nodo del seno. G Ital Cardiol 6:876–791
Scanlon PJ, Pryor R, Blount SG Jr (1970) Right bundle branch block associated with left superior or inferior intraventricular block. Clinical setting, prognosis and relation to complete heart block. Circulation 42:1123–1133
Scheinman MM, Peters RW, Modin G, Brennan M, Mies C, O'Young J (1977) Prognostic value of infranodal conduction time in patients with chronic bundle branch block. Circulation 56:240–244
Schneider J, Boldt J, Leyhe A, Kaffarnik H (1980) HDL cholesterol, peripheral and coronary vascular disease in high age groups. Atherosclerosis 35:487–489
Schneider MD, Roller DH, Morganroth J, Josephson ME (1978) The syndromes of familial atrioventricular block with sinus bradycardia: prognostic indices, electrophysiologic and histopathologic correlates. Eur J Cardiol 7:337–351
Shapiro JB (1979) Bifascicular block produced by hyperkalemia. Cardiology 64:303–305
Shaw DB, Eraut D (1970) Prevalence and morbidity of heart block in Devon. Brit Med J 1:144–147
Siddons H (1976) Management of heart block. In: Caird FI, Dall JLC, Kennedy RD (eds) Cardiology in old age. Plenum Press, London New York, p 348
Siegman-Igra Y, Yahini JH, Goldbourt U, Neufeld HN (1978) Intraventricular conduction disturbances: a review of prevalence, etiology, and progression for ten years within a stable population of Israeli adult males. Am Heart J 96:669–679
Smiddy L, Lewis HD Jr, Dunn M (1972) The effect of carotid massage in older men. J Gerontol 27:209–211
Söderström N (1958) The diagnosis of partial AV-block and AS-syndrome in patients with atrial fibrillation. Cardiologia 33:397–406
Solinas P, Notaristefano A (1977) La sincope: inquadramento fisiopatologico e approccio diagnostico. In: Foresti A, Rovelli F (eds) Le emergenze in cardiologia. Pozzi, Roma, p 134
Stéphan M (1979) Défaut héréditaire de la conduction dans le systéme hisien. Arch Mal Coeur 72:62–71
Strauss HD, Berman ND (1978) Permanent pacing in the elderly. Pace 1:458–464
Sugiura M, Hirahoka K, Ohkawa S, Shimada H (1975) A clinico-pathological study of heart disease in the aged. Jpn Heart J 16:526–537
Sugiura M, Uchiyama S, Kuwako K (1976) A clinico-pathological study on the mitral ring calcification in the aged (Japanese). Jpn J Geriatr 13:189–192
Sullo B, Salvadorini F, Longi G (1979) I disturbi della conduzione dello stimolo negli anziani ricoverati. G Geront 27:135–147
Tàmmaro AE (1977) Diagnosi e significato prognostico delle turbe della conduzione intraventricolare nell'anziano. Acta Gerontol 27:249–253
Tàmmaro AE, Forin G (1977) Left fascicular hemiblocks in the elderly. J Am Geriatr Soc 25:439–442
Tarquinii M, Santoro A, Rossini G, Borgatti E (1978) Rilievi ecocardiografici di cardiomiopatia ipertrofica nell'anziano. G Gerontol 26:265–276
Thormann I, Paeprer H, Schmutzler H, Wegener W (1979) Vorhofseptumdefekt im Alter. Z Kardiol 67:488–502
Vera Z, Mason DT, Fletcher RD, Awan NA, Massumi RA (1976) Prolonged His-Q interval in chronic bifascicular block: relation to impending complete heart block. Circulation 53:46–55
Volpe U (1978) Left anterior hemiblock masking coronary insufficiency. Br Heart J 40:188–189
Waisser E, Gaasch WH, Quinones MA, Alexander JK (1975) His-bundle electrograms in patients with congestive cardiomyopathy. Eur J Cardiol 2:343–350
Warembourg H, Théry Cl, Lekieffre J, Delbecque H, Gosselin B (1974) Blocs sino-auriculaires et blocs auriculo-ventriculaires associés. Arch Mal Coeur 67:787–795
Watanabe Y, Pamintuan JC, Dreifus LS (1973) Role of intraventricular conduction disturbances in ventricular premature systoles. Am J Cardiol 32:188–195

Watt TB, Pruitt RD (1969) Character, cause and consequence of combined left axis deviation and RBBB in human electrocardiograms. Am Heart J 77:460–465
Waxman HL, Castellanos A (1979) Recent concepts in atrioventricular and fascicular block. Herz 4:12–20
Wollner L, Spalding JMK (1978) The autonomic nervous system. In: Brocklehurst JC (ed) Textbook of geriatrics and gerontology. Churchill Livingstone, Edinburgh London New York, pp 258–259
Wyse DG, McAnaulty JH, Rahimtoola SH, Murphy ES (1979) Electrophysiologic abnormalities of the sinus node and atrium in patients with bundle branch block. Circulation 60:413–420
Yano K, Peskoe SM, Rhoads GG, Moore JO, Kagan A (1975) Left axis deviation and left anterior hemiblock among 8,000 japanese-american men. Am J Cardiol 35:809–815

The Arterial and Venous System[*]

H. Haimovici

A. Introduction

I. Epidemiology

Epidemiology of vascular disorders in aging populations has focused almost exclusively on the arterial system. By contrast, the venous and lymphatic systems have received little or no attention as it is commonly assumed that they, especially the veins, undergo some nonspecific age-related changes consisting of increased tortuosity and phlebosclerosis.

The few epidemiologic comments to follow will therefore be confined to the arterial system, which is known to undergo complex age- and metabolic-related changes. Although epidemiologic investigations deal primarily with atherosclerosis of the coronary arteries, it is well documented that a relationship between arterial disease in any site is but one manifestation of a widespread disorder.

The geographic distribution of arterial processes, especially as related to *atherogenesis*, has shown great variations in patterns throughout the world (STRONG et al. 1971). As one could have anticipated, with increasing lifespan, especially in the Western world, the problem of vascular diseases with their multiple potential complications in the geriatric age group would be seen with greater frequency.

The degree of severity of the vascular lesions encountered in various geographic areas is variable. Many factors, as is known today, determine the nature and degree of arterial lesions. Most important among them is the dietary factor. Thus, the low incidence of atherosclerosis in certain populations, such as China or Japan, is attributed to the possible role of the unsaturated fatty acids in their diet. However, it should be pointed out that the nature of arterial lesions in the Orient, especially in Japan, is not related exclusively to atherosclerosis. A large percentage of these lesions are of an inflammatory nature, some of which is attributed to thromboangiitis obliterans (Buerger's disease) or Takayasu's disease. That diet may nevertheless play a role is exemplified by an increased incidence of atherosclerosis in the Japanese living in Hawaii and in the United States due to the high content of fat in the diet.

Many other similar examples of the roles of diet and geographic influence are well known through the findings of the International Atherosclerosis Project (STAMLER et al. 1971). Their data brought into focus the relative value of risk

---

[*] From the Vascular Surgical Service, Department of Surgery, Montefiore Hospital and Medical Center, and Albert Einstein College of Medicine, Bronx, NY

factors involved in the genesis of arterial diseases. The changing socioeconomic conditions prevailing throughout the world have shown an increasing frequency of dietary risk factors related to the development of atherosclerosis in some geographic regions where previously such disorders were infrequent or unknown.

Age-related vascular changes may be functional or organic (KOHN 1977). *Functional* changes are reflected in the loss of elastic properties of arteries leading to their rigidity. Increasing stiffness has been demonstrated in iliac arteries by increasing resistance to both longitudinal and circumferential stretch (ROACH and BURTON 1959). The age-related stiffness impairs pulsatile flow throughout the arterial system and thereby increases the load to the left ventricle. In spite of age-related changes in elastic properties, no correlation was found between the degree of atherosclerosis and loss of vessel compliance. Thus, these two processes may coexist but are not pathogenetically dependent.

Peripheral resistance increases with age, and inversely blood flow decreases. The latter change is, however, not present throughout the entire vascular tree. Thus, skeletal–muscle blood flow changes are only minimal in the absence of atherosclerosis. By contrast, perfusion, especially of digits or hand and foot, may be decreased significantly.

Organic changes consist of morphologic-age-related alterations, exclusive of atherosclerosis. The stiffness and dilatation of arteries are due to decreasing elastin and smooth muscle and progressive increase of collagen.

While atherosclerosis is more prevalent in older people, the pathogenesis of this process, is not always age related since it is not a universal phenomenon. As is well known today, many other factors underlie its development. Thus the basic morphologic–biochemical aging processes of the arteries do not necessarily lead to atherosclerosis. Their coexistence depends largely on different pathogenetic mechanisms.

II. Current Clinical Concepts

In the past 3 decades, great strides have been made in the diagnosis and management of vascular diseases in general. The awareness of such disorders being more common in the aging population has led to their earlier recognition and treatment. The newer noninvasive diagnostic modalities, along with the wider use of angiography, have led to a better understanding and treatment of these conditions.

This chapter will deal with the most common vascular disorders encountered in the geriatric patient. They will be confined to the following topics: occlusive arterial diseases, aneurysms, and acute venous thromboembolism.

B. Occlusive Arterial Diseases

I. Acute Arterial Disorders

1. Arterial Embolism

a) Cardiogenic Arterial Embolism

Arterial embolism is a complication of a preexisting cardiopathy and rarely of a proximal arterial lesion or the result of a cardiovascular procedure. The commonest origin of emboli is the left heart. While in the past, rheumatic heart disease (RHD) was the most frequent source of emboli (DALEY et al. 1951), followed by that of myocardial infarction (MI) and arteriosclerotic heart disease (ASHD) (HAI-MOVICI 1950), since about the 1950's the relative incidence of the nature of emboligenic cardiopathy has changed (DARLING et al. 1967).

Today, RHD is no longer as preponderant as before, in contrast to ASHD and MI. The latter two are seen more often as a result of increasing life span and the prevalence of atherosclerosis. Thus, the relative incidence for RHD before the 1950's was 40% and this has decreased to 22% in recent years. In contrast, the incidence of MI together with ASHD, previously 50.8%, has risen to 78% at present. Likewise, the ratio of ASHD to RHD, which was 1.5, has risen to 3.5. In addition, the coexisting peripheral atherosclerotic changes in those patients with ASHD is now found to be 84% compared to 50% previously. In brief, with an increasing life span and atherosclerosis, arterial embolism is today a problem preponderantly seen in the geriatric age group.

Mural thrombi associated with myocardial infarction may sometimes embolize long before clinical and electrocardiographic evidence of the origin becomes established. In a previous study, we found "silent" myocardial infarction to be present in over 11% of the patients. In such instances the differential diagnosis of embolism from arterial thrombosis may be difficult or even impossible.

Among rare etiologic factors of embolism are bacterial endocarditis, paradoxial thrombi, bullets, postoperative thrombi, atrial myxoma, and other tumors.

Clinical Manifestations. Peripheral emboli occur predominantly in the lower extremities. Their incidence, including the aortoiliac segment, ranges between 77% and 84%. In the upper extremities emboli lodge less frequently.

The common belief that arterial embolism is always characterized at onset by severe pain may be misleading. In a previous study based on the analysis of 330 cases of peripheral embolism, we found that *sudden onset* occurred only in 81%, of which 60% had pain and 21%, numbness and coldness. In the remainder, *progressive onset* was present in 12%, of which 7% had gradual pain, numbness, and coldness, and *silent arterial embolism* was diagnosed in 7%.

The initial site of pain appears to occur in the region of impaction of the embolus, while later pain is more peripheral and corresponds to muscle ischemia. Numbness, coldness, and tingling usually appear after pain. Absence of arterial pulsations, disappearance of the oscillometric index, absence of pulse waves (recorded by the Doppler ultrasonic velocity detector), or loss of muscular power and sensation with diminished reflexes are the main objective findings. Multiple emboli are not an infrequent occurence and are characteristic of the embolic nature of the arterial occlusion. Thus, in a series of 228 patients, 443 peripheral and visceral embolic events were diagnosed, of which 330 involved the extremities and 113, various visceral arteries.

Natural Course and Grading of Ischemia of Arterial Emboli. The natural course of arterial embolism of the lower extremity, based on location is shown in Table 1. In its simplest form, an embolism by itself occludes only a short segment of an artery. In the absence of spasm or secondary thrombosis, the restoration of the distal circulation may be effected by collateral channels. However, usually a peripheral

Table 1. Natural course of arterial embolism of the lower extremity, based on location of the occlusion

	Cases		Gangrene and early death		Gangrene and amputation		Recovery	
	N	%	*N*	%	*N*	%	*N*	%
Aorta	28	11.0	8	28.5	11	39.0	9	32.5
Iliac	53	20.8	4	7.5	32	60.4	17	32.1
Femoral	108	42.5	17	15.7	31	28.7	60	55.6
Popliteal	47	18.5	2	4.2	3	6.3	42	89.5
Tibial	18	7.2	0	0	1	5.5	17	94.5

arterial embolism occurs in a more complex clinicopathologic setting (HAIMOVICI 1950).

Although peripheral arterial emboli do not always lead to irreversible ischemic changes, it is significant that about half these patients may end up with gangrene of the extremity or die shortly after the onset of the acute arterial occlusion. Moderate ischemia with early pulse return occurred in 29.5% of cases and advanced ischemia in 22.2%, in a study previously reported. At onset of an arterial embolism, it is often difficult to forecast its outcome. Management of all cases should therefore be undertaken without delay.

The site of an embolic occlusion is generally easily identifiable. The clinical criteria, such as the level of the initial pain and that of disappearance of normal pulsations, the extent of the circulatory disturbances, and results of noninvasive diagnostic modalities are unquestionably useful. An additional criterion which may be helpful is that emboli usually lodge at arterial bifurcations. Unfortunately, in a certain number of patients with coexisting atherosclerotic disease, the exact localization of the embolus may be difficult to determine. Preoperative arteriography may be then essential.

Diagnosis of a peripheral arterial embolism is usually simple (Figs. 1 and 2). Conditions that may be confused with peripheral embolism are chiefly: phlegmasia cerulea dolens, acute arterial thrombosis, acute thrombosis of a popliteal aneurysm, acute thrombosis of a nonatherosclerotic artery, low flow syndrome due to circulatory failure, dissecting aortic aneurysm, and arterial spasm.

Upper extremity embolism incidence as found by CHAMPION and GILL (1973) based on 13 statistical studies with a total of 2,420 embolic episodes, occurred in 364 instances or 15% of cases. This average incidence corresponds to our own findings of 16% based on 330 embolic episodes. Being generally small, these emboli lodge in the majority of cases in the brachial (56.6%), followed by the axillary in 28.3%, and in the radial/ulnar in 15.2%. Differential diagnoses of upper limb emboli in the absence of a cardiopathy, are those originating from a thoracic outlet syndrome, acute thrombosis associated with trauma or atherosclerosis, from an infectious disease, or due to atheroemboli. The emboli resulting from these conditions are usually less dramatic than those from a cardiogenic source.

Visceral emboli occur less infrequently than generally recognized. If small, they are often clinically overlooked or remain unsuspected, whereas major embolic oc-

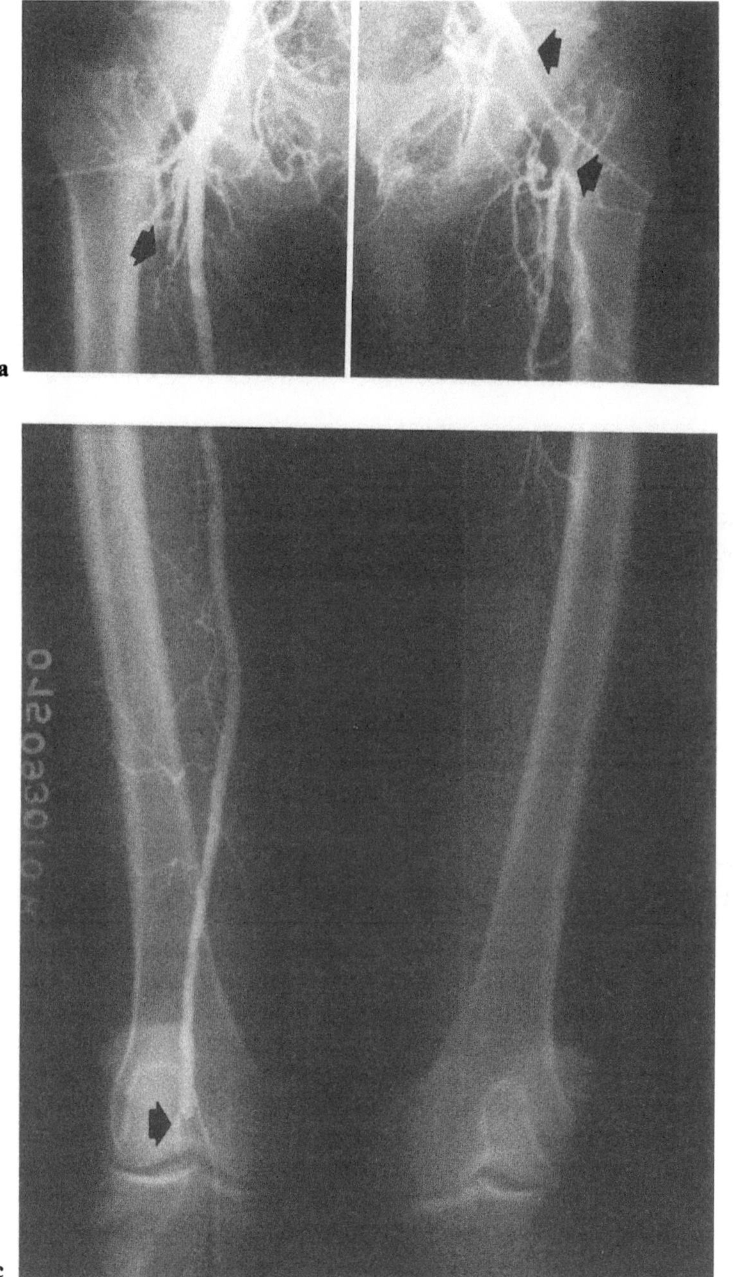

Fig. 1 a–c. Bilateral femoral arteriogram. **a** Embolism of left common femoral artery *(arrow)*, with complete occlusion including the entire superficial femoral and popliteal. **b** Embolism of right profunda femoris *(arrows)*. **c** Embolism of the right popliteal *(arrow)* HAIMOVICI 1982)

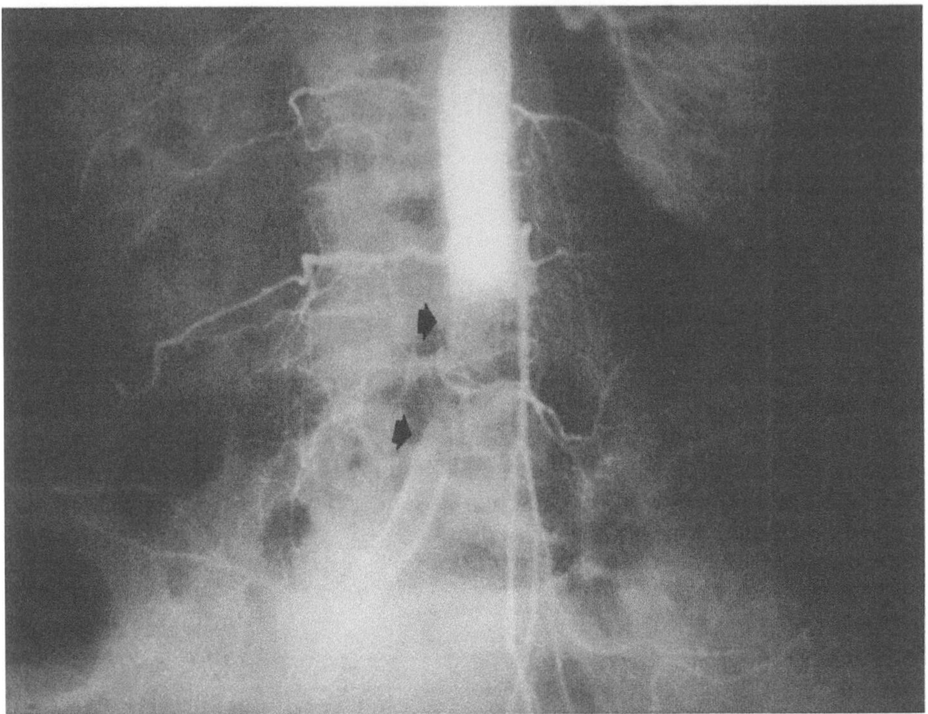

Fig. 2. Aortogram depicting a saddle embolus of the aortic bifurcation *(arrows)*, with complete occlusion of the left iliac and incomplete filling of the right iliac with a thrombus delineated by seeping radiopaque substance around it (HAIMOVICI 1982)

clusions display significant and often rapidly irreversible and lethal changes. Cerebral, mesenteric, and renal emboli are not uncommon, and they are often the cause of serious complications or death.

b) Noncardiogenic Arterial Embolism

α) *Atheroembolism.* Atheroembolism of atheromatous materials is being reported in recent years with increasing frequently (FLORY 1950; KAZMIER et al. 1966; KEMCZINSKI 1979; PANUM 1862). This may occur in two distinct forms: (1) as *microemboli* following release of cholesterol crystals or other debris of atheromatous components from an ulcerated plaque, and (2) as *macroemboli* resulting from major plaques usually mixed with thrombi and cholesterol crystals and lodging in major systemic arteries.

These emboli may occur spontaneously from an abdominal aneurysm or a nonaneurysmal lesion of the aorta; following surgical manipulation of the latter, or during aortic catheterization. The incidence ranges between 1.4% and 3%. The clinical spectrum of problems associated with microemboli are: (a) cyanotic or blue toes, (b) livedo reticularis, and (c) ulcerations or gangrene (especially of toes, but rarely of the fingers or hand). In a macroembolism of a major artery, the clinical picture is no different from that of an embolism of cardiac origin. Aortograms or peripheral arteriograms are often necessary to identify the source of the embolic nature of the vascular lesions. The treatment consists of nonsurgical or operative measures.

β) Acute Arterial Thromboembolism Complicating the Thoracic Outlet. Acute arterial thromboembolism of the upper extremity, associated with a thoracic outlet syndrome differs in many ways from a cardiogenic embolism, particularly in its pathophysiology and management. Indeed, the thromboembolic process originates in a damaged subclavian artery as a result of its prolonged compression by congenital or acquired anomalous anatomic structures at the thoracic outlet. Although these complications are seen mostly in the age group ranging between 20 and 50, occasionally such lesions may be encountered in older individuals. They are associated with cervical ribs, scalenus anticus, costoclavicular, and hyperabduction syndromes. These entitites, either alone or in combination, are responsible for the vascular complications described under this title. Recognition of the underlying thromboembolic process, the cause of the clinical manifestations, is the key to prevention and appropriate management (BERTELSEN et al. 1968; HALSTED 1916; JUDY and HEYMAN 1972; MARTIN et al. 1976).

c) Prognostic Factors

The major factors governing the results of treatment of an arterial embolism are related to duration of the occlusion, degree of ischemia, location and extent of the occlusion, and degree of skeletal muscle involvement (ERIKSSON and HOLMBERG 1977). With reference to the latter, in a number of cases of embolism, leg muscles may become edematous and preischemic. Because of the unyielding fascial compartments, the latter condition may turn into frank gangrene. To prevent such complications, it is imperative to perform fasciotomies without delay. Less frequently, but more threatening in the presence of severe muscle ischemia with necrosis and rhabdomyolysis is the occurrence of myoglobinuria and release of other metabolites from the necrotic muscle. The biochemical alterations may lead not only to loss of limb, but also loss of life.

Indeed the resulting metabolic complications and renal shutdown are associated with high morbidity and mortality rates. If recognized early, the revascularization syndrome can be forestalled by adequate alkalinization and hydration of the patient, along with fasciotomy, if necessary, of the involved limb (HAIMOVICI 1960, 1979).

Associated atherosclerosis with arterial embolism has become increasingly prevalent in the last few decades. Many of these patients have a past history of intermittent claudication, clearly suggesting the coexistence of peripheral arteriosclerotic occlusive disease. In these cases, results of embolectomy may be adversely affected by such lesions, especially in diabetic patients.

d) Treatment

An arterial embolism is generally a reflection of a life-threatening cardiopathy (BLAISDELL et al. 1978). Its management is that of the highest emergency and is directed toward: (1) the acute occlusion of the extremity and (2) the underlying heart disease. The latter condition will determine, to some extent, how aggressively one should proceed with the surgical treatment of the arterial embolism.

The patient's cardiac status must be assessed without delay, with attention directed toward its correction. Concurrently, with the management of the heart condition, one should initiate treatment of the acute ischemia of the limb.

As a first measure, the patient should be placed in the head-up position with the involved extremity on a pillow, to protect it from any pressure. Heparin should be administered intravenously as soon as possible. There is no contraindication to its administration, even if surgery is being contemplated within 2–3 h. Use of thrombolysins and low-molecular weight dextran are generally of limited value. Vasodilator drugs, preferably papaverine, when given intraarterially may be of some help. These medical, nonoperative measures are applicable during the period while the cardiac condition is being stabilized.

Embolectomy is the method of choice for managing arterial emboli. Few contraindications exist except in patients in whom conservative treatment appears adequate to prevent loss of limb. However, since the procedure can be carried out most of the time under local anesthesia, an embolectomy can be performed in almost every case. Use of the Fogarty catheter has simplified the operation, as it allows the operation to be carried out with ease, safety, and completeness. Its application to aortic and iliac emboli obviate the abdominal procedure and has considerably lowered operative morbidity and mortality (BYRNES and MACGOWAN 1975; FOGARTY and CRANLEY 1965; RAITHEL 1973a).

e) Late Arterial Embolectomy

Delayed arterial embolectomy may be indicated, provided the limb is still viable, even if only at a borderline level (HAIMOVICI 1959; JARRETT et al. 1979). While early embolectomy remains the overall undisputed principle, indications for late arterial embolectomy are based primarily on the physiologic state of the limb and less on the time elapsed before embolectomy. Limb salvage under these circumstances, as reported by a number of authors, ranged between 55% and 77%. In our own experience, 66.4% of limbs were saved.

Postembolic *gangrene* usually involves a wide segment of the limb, and is rarely limited to its distal areas. The gangrene affects not only the skin, but also the muscles, its extent depending usually on the level of the arterial occlusion. The more proximal (aortoiliac) the embolism, the more massive the ischemia. Amputation should be carried out at the level of tissue viability, rarely below but most often above the knee. Only in distal and segmental embolic occlusions (popliteal and tibial) does the gangrenous process remain confined to toes or distal foot.

2. Acute Arterial Thrombosis

Acute arterial thrombosis, as distinct from arterial embolism, may occur as a result of a great number of local arterial factors, or as a consequence of associated systemic diseases. Although these arterial occlusions are sudden, and cause serious tissue ischemia, their clinicopathologic features and their management are distinctive from those of an acute arterial embolism.

a) Acute Atherosclerotic Thrombosis

Atherosclerosis is the most common predisposing cause of acute thrombosis. It may occur in an asymptomatic ulcerated atherosclerotic plaque, or superimposed on a known, preexisting arteriosclerotic occlusive process, with a long-standing clinical history of arterial insufficiency (HAIMOVICI 1977).

The majority of cases of acute arterial thrombosis occur in the lower extremity, and only a small percentage in the upper. Thus RAITHEL (1973 b), in a series of 85 cases, reported its occurrence in 98% in the lower extremity, and only 2% in the upper. The relative incidence of acute arterial thrombosis distribution between the upper and lower extremities is in distinct contrast with that of arterial embolism in which involvement of the upper limb is somewhat greater.

The overall relative incidence of acute thrombosis and arterial embolism is not always easy to establish, especially in the elderly patients having a combined cardiopathy with peripheral arteriosclerosis. In a recent survey, I found that arterial embolism is more prevalent than acute thrombosis (56.6% embolism vs 43.4% thrombosis).

The type of clinical manifestations and their degree of ischemia are determined by two factors: (1) the location and extent of the thrombosis and (2) whether the thrombosis is primary or secondary to previous chronic arterial lesions.

Two clinicopathologic forms will be discussed here, since they are the most commonly encountered. *Acute aortoiliac thrombosis* is less frequent of the two types, and mimics that of a saddle embolism (DANTO et al. 1971). *Acute femoropopliteal thrombosis* is by far more frequent than aortoiliac involvement. The clinical background and appropriate arteriography will usually lead to the diagnosis.

Management as a rule is initiated by immediate intravenous heparin injection, using 1,000–2,000 units per hour, after having started with a loading dose of 4,000–5,000 units. Endarterectomy is rarely, if ever, useful in these acute arterial occlusions. A bypass graft may be necessary in the majority of cases, provided the run-off is adequately delineated.

b) Iatrogenic Acute Arterial Thrombosis

Peripheral arterial thrombosis secondary to injuries following their catheterization has been the subject of an increasing number of reports over the past 15 years (BRENER and COUCH 1973). With a widespread use of these procedures, thrombotic complications, while infrequent, may pose serious threat to limb or life. These complications occur either after angiography or blood-gas monitoring, or for therapeutic purposes. They may follow retrograde catheterization of the brachial and radial or transcutaneous catheterization of the femoral (ALPERT et al. 1976).

Recognition of these potential hazards and complications is essential for adequate and immediate treatment of the thrombotic lesion. Delay in their management may lead to irreversible changes with either partial loss of digits and gangrenous patchy skin, or rarely, loss of an entire extremity.

c) Acute Thrombosis of Small Arteries

Acute thrombosis of small arteries may occur in a wide and varied spectrum of entities. Their most common etiologic factors are: organic arterial diseases, posttraumatic occupational vasospastic syndromes, frostbite, collagen diseases, and hematologic disorders (HAIMOVICI 1977 b).

Of the *organic arterial diseases*, the most common are those associated with thromboangiitis obliterans, idiopathic acute thrombosis, and acute ischemia secondary to a low-flow syndrome (NcNamara et al. 1978). *Secondary Raynaud's* may be associated with acute thrombosis of small arteries, primarily of the hand. *Frostbite*, at the acute stage, is the result of vasoconstriction which, if unrelieved, may lead to severe ischemia as the result of superimposed acute thrombosis of the smaller arteries. Of the hematologic conditions, *polycythemia vera* is known to result in a certain percentage of cases with vascular complications, involving arteries as well as veins (Barabas et al. 1973). The nature of these complications is generally thrombotic and only occasionally embolic. The latter may occur as a result of arterioarterial embolism.

II. Chronic Arterial Conditions

1. Arteriosclerosis Obliterans

Arteriosclerosis is the most common cause of chronic arterial disease of the extremities. By contrast, thromboangiitis obliterans (TAO) is rarely seen today (Mckusick et al. 1962). The etiology and pathogenesis of arteriosclerosis, despite recent progress, have not been entirely elucidated. In its simplest definition, arteriosclerosis, a degenerative process, is characterized by lipid deposition in the intimal lining of the arteries, and by focal fibromuscular proliferation. At an advanced stage the endothelial lining is disrupted, leading to a thrombotic occlusion at the site of the atheromatous plaques. The atherosclerotic process usually involves somatic and visceral arteries to various degrees. The relative incidence of distribution of arterial lesions is largely lacking. Most studies have focused attention either on the peripheral arterial tree or individual visceral arteries. In general, it is recognized that the pathologic features of atherosclerosis are quite variable from individual to individual, and from one arterial segment to another. As a result, the patterns emerging from the innumerable combination of lesions are varied and complex (Wiest et al. 1980). However, in terms of location and extent of the atherosclerotic process in the lower extremity, it is possible to identify a certain number of regional patterns that lend themselves to an overall classification of three major groups: (1) aortoiliac, (2) femoropopliteal, and (3) tibioperoneal-pedal.

Although arteriosclerosis is a diffusely distributed process involving the intima, arteriography has disclosed that arteriosclerosis obliterans quite often may involve a single segment of the arterial tree. However, as the disease progresses, two or more segments may become occluded. Despite these lesions, a patent distal lumen (run-off or outflow tract) is often present, and is of great surgical significance.

Clinical manifestations and surgical management of arteriosclerosis obliterans may vary according to the location and extent of the occlusive process.

2. Aortoiliac Occlusion

Aortoiliac occlusion (Leriche Syndrome) is usually characterized by slow progression of occlusion of the terminal abdominal aorta and of the common iliac arteries. Although it occurs in younger persons, aortoiliac occlusion may also be seen in the elderly. This syndrome is well tolerated for quite a number of years before ischemic changes occur. Rest pain and gangrene may develop late in its evolution, and may be precipitated by some form of trauma or infection.

Evaluation of the aortoiliac lesions, in addition to the physical examination, may be achieved by noninvasive Doppler blood flow studies. If surgery is contemplated, a translumbar or transfemoral aortography is essential.

Arterial reconstruction is indicated in patients with nonhealing ulcers, or gangrenous changes of the toes. Although aortoiliac occlusive disease confined to this segment may go on for years before serious ischemic manifestations occur, in the combined pattern with distal occlusive disease, the process is progressive and usually requires reconstruction, mostly of the proximal arterial tree for adequate revascularization of the lower extremities (HAIMOVICI and STEINMAN 1969).

3. Femoropopliteal Arterial Occlusive Disease

The occlusive process of the femorpopliteal segment is the most common lesion in the lower extremity, especially in patients over 60. The relative incidence of the aortoiliac and femoropopliteal occlusion varies with the reported studies. However, the involvement of the superficial femoral (Fig. 3), either as an isolated lesion, or associated with the popliteal and tibial-peroneal arteries, is by far the most frequently encountered. The popliteal and leg arteries may be involved either independently or in association with the proximal arterial tree. The various occlusive arterial patterns have been reported elsewhere by the author (HAIMOVICI 1967 b, 1976 c).

Although the natural course of arteriosclerosis obliterans has not been entirely elucidated, various statistical studies show that of these patients slightly over 70% have only intermittent claudication. Ischemic rest pain, ischemic neuropathy, or both are seen in 16% of patients, while ischemic ulceration, gangrene, or both are seen in about 10%. Most published reports indicate that arteriosclerosis obliterans naturally tends to progress at rates that vary from patient to patient, and from location to location. Diabetes mellitus seems to accelerate the process and impart a more serious prognosis.

4. Peripheral Arterial Disease in Diabetes Mellitus

Vascular manifestations associated with diabetes represent today the gravest single factor underlying the morbidity and mortality of diabetic patients. The gravity of the vascular process stems from the wide involvement of virtually all arterial areas, peripheral as well as visceral (retina, kidney, heart, and brain).

It is noteworthy that the relative age-incidence in nondiabetic and diabetic patients varies inversely with the advance in decades. In our own studies of vascular lesions in these two groups of patients, there were slightly more than 50% under the age of 60, in the nondiabetic group, whereas only 33% were found in the diabetic. Conversely, after 60, the incidence in the diabetic group was 67% and 48.6% in the nondiabetic.

The *vascular lesions* encountered in diabetes vary with the size and location of the vessel. Basically, two major histologic types have been differentiated: arteriosclerotic (involving primarily the large and medium-sized arteries); and microangiopathic (involving arterioles and capillaries). Atherosclerosis is more diffuse

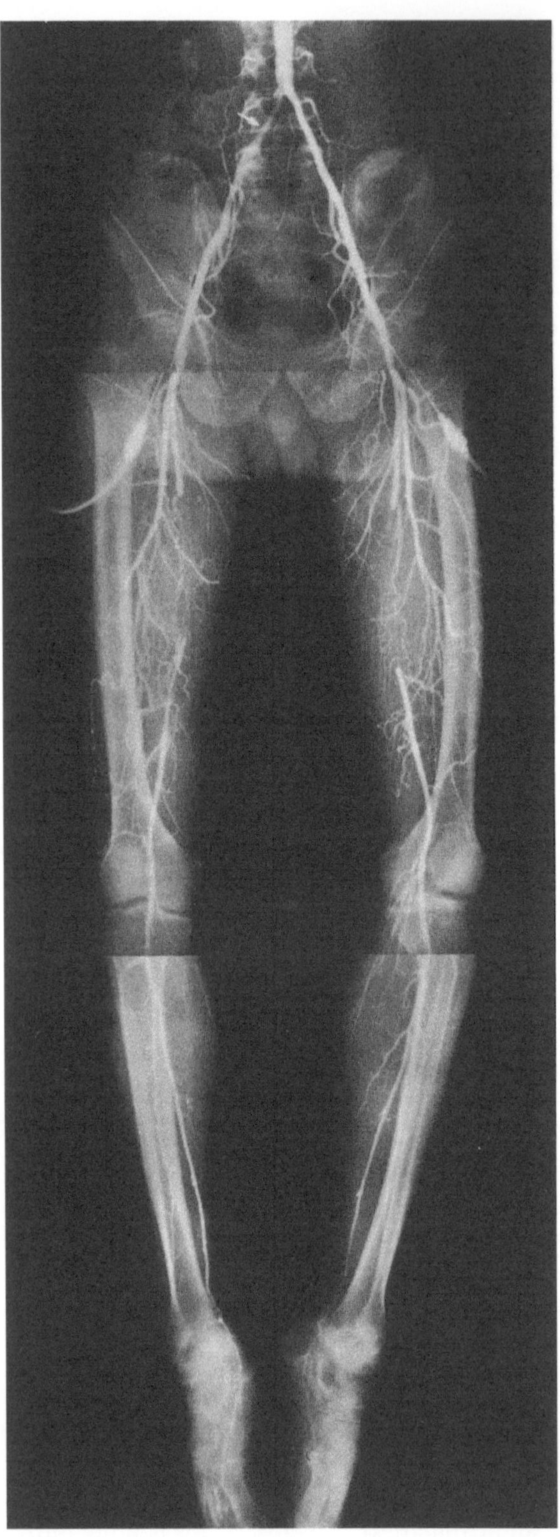

Fig. 3. Aortoarteriography of both lower extremities obtained through bilateral transfemoral arteriograms. Note complete occlusion of both superficial femoral arteries and inadequate opacification of right common iliac artery *(arrow)*. Patient had severe intermittent claudication bilaterally and underwent bypass grafts in each limb (Haimovici 1976)

in the diabetic. The site and extent of the initial atherosclerotic disease in larger arteries differs in diabetics from nondiabetic patients. In diabetes, the initial lesions involve the tibial and popliteal arteries, and less frequently the femoral artery or the aortoiliac segment (GENSLER et al. 1965).

Diabetic clinical lesions deserve a special mention. The clinical manifestations are frequently associated with, and sometimes dominated by, two other important clinical features: diabetic neuropathy and local infection. This association, in varying degrees, lends to the lesions a truly characteristic clinical picture, often referred to as the "diabetic foot." Because of the quasi specificity, these lesions justify a separate description. The clinical manifestations may be classified under the following four headings: (1) arteriosclerosis obliterans, (2) peripheral neuropathy, (3) infection, and (4) combined lesions. In managing a diabetic, one has to take into account the possibility of the three major factors, so as not to overlook any of them. The degree of participation of each of these three major etiologic factors is difficult to assess statistically. However, evaluation of each diabetic from this triple point of view is essential before deciding on the course to follow.

5. Evaluation of the Vascular Condition

Most patients present a history of intermittent claudication in the early stages of the process. In advanced cases, in addition to impaired walking ability, most patients complain of rest pain, ulcerations, or gangrene of toes associated with coldness and color changes of the skin.

Clinical examination provides the first criteria of the arterial condition: diminished, or absent, pulsations, color changes, decreased skin temperature, etc. The degree of patency of the major arteries, determined by palpation, are further checked by using an oscillometer at various levels of the limb, and by Doppler blood flow studies. Elevation-dependency may provide the velocity of color changes, consisting of rapid blanching of the toes and foot on elevation, and marked rubor on dependency. These color changes suggest poor collateral circulation. A sharp difference in skin temperature between the proximal and distal areas of the extremity would indicate a recent arterial occlusion. It is essential, both from history and from these preliminary findings, to determine whether the patient presents a chronic process of arterial insufficiency, or an acute occlusion, the latter offering a different clinical dimension and significance.

6. Instrumental Vascular Examination

Although the clinical history and the physical findings of peripheral arterial problems provide an overall estimation of the arterial insufficiency, a more quantitative estimate of the extent of arterial disease, and an objective means of assessing therapeutic results can be obtained both by noninvasive methods and arteriography (RAINES et al. 1976).

7. Noninvasive Methods

Although the oscillometer mentioned above may provide some information about the presence or absence of the major arterial pulsations, its accuracy remains, however, limited. The Doppler ultrasonic velocity detector (Darling et al. 1976), introduced in the last 5 years, is quite useful not only in vascular laboratories at the institutional level, but also in private offices. Essentially, it is designed to provide measurements of the arterial pressures as well as blood flow at various levels of the extremities. Such information may indicate the extent and approximate location of the arterial lesions. A great number of instruments are presently used for recording the limb systolic pressure and the pulse wave contour (Darling et al. 1976; Farrar et al. 1976). These evaluations obtained both before and after any therapeutic procedure offer at the same time a permanent record of the various findings (Verta et al. 1976). Other noninvasive techniques such as radioisotopes are more suitable in a vascular laboratory than in an office setting (Yao et al. 1973). It should be pointed out that while the noninvasive methods are quite useful in screening patients with complaints of arterial insufficiency, the information obtained fails to indicate the location and extent of the anatomic lesions of the arterial tree (McNamara et al. 1978).

8. Arteriography

Arteriography plays a decisive role in the evaluation and selection of patients for operation. The site, number, and extent of the arterial occlusions, the state of the proximal and distal arterial tree, and the degree of collateral circulation can only be determined by these means. A good arterial outline with a comprehensive visualization of the entire tree are prerequisites for a good angiographic study. Two methods of visualization are used: abdominal aortography, either by the translumbar technique or by the Seldinger method; and femoral arteriography. To achieve complete evaluation of the inflow and outflow arterial segments it is necessary to carry out a comprehensive arteriography from the abdominal aorta to the foot vessels. This method provides a complete view of the lesions and their integration into the rest of the vascular system.

9. Treatment

Selection of the type of treatment for arteriosclerosis obliterans of the lower extremity depends largely on the severity of the clinical manifestations. The latter are generally divided into three stages: Stage I, intermittent claudication; stage II, rest pain without lesions; and stage III, ulcers or gangrene.

a) Nonoperative Treatment

Intermittent claudication, stage I, rarely requires any specific active treatment. The oft prescribed vasodilator drugs are of little or no value. By contrast, walking a few miles a day may promote collateral circulation and may improve to some extent the intermittent claudication. The conservative treatment in such patients is all the more important in the elderly patients who sometimes also suffer from angina pectoris. The latter may be even more significant than the intermittent claudication. It may be brought on by prolonged walking. Under these circumstances, intermittent claudication might be considered a blessing in disguise. In the younger individuals, where intermittent claudication, especially if severe enough, interferes with gainful employment, one may consider surgical correction of the arterial lesions. Furthermore in the presence of severe ischemia of the extremities (stages II and III), the scope of medical management is necessarily limited. Relief of rest pain requires moderate to large amounts of analgesics or narcotics. Failure to achieve this is an indication for surgery.

b) Operative Treatment

In such patients, reconstructive arterial procedures (thromboendarterectomy, arterial grafts), lumbar sympatectomy, or a combination of these may yield gratifying results depending on the type of arterial lesions.

Thromboendarterectomy consists of the removal of the occluding block through a cleavage plane of the arterial wall. Indications for the procedure should usually be confined to short segmental occlusions. The greatest success obtained with this procedure is for lesions localized to the common iliac or common femoral arteries, whereas thromboendarterectomy in the superficial femoral or popliteal arteries is rarely as successful on long-term follow-up.

c) Intraluminal Angioplasty

In conjunction with the latter procedure an alternative nonsurgical method has been advocated in recent years. Introduced first by DOTTER and JUDKINS in 1964, it was received with a lot of skepticism by most vascular surgeons. Improvements in technique have recently revived this procedure, which is usually performed under local anesthesia, with fluroscopic monitoring. Most lesions are dilated by means of polyvinyl chloride balloon catheters, developed by Grunzig. This technique is mostly applicable in the dilatation of iliac-femoral-popliteal arterial stenosis, and occasionally for complete occlusions. The leg arteries are less suitable in most instances. Recent reports have indicated a substantial success in dilating or recanalizing the lesions in these arteries in approximately 80% of cases, with a follow-up of 1 year with a patency of 70%. It appears that a greater success is achieved in iliac stenosis than in the more distal vessels.

This procedure is now being tried in several centers in the United States and Europe, and although the accumulated experience so far is not substantial, the results are encouraging. The intraluminal angioplasty, as it is sometimes called, can be used either alone or in combination with vascular surgical procedures. Transluminal iliac dilatation may be associated with a femoropopliteal bypass, or a superficial femoral angioplasty may be associated with a femoropopliteal bypass graft. Further experience, and long-term evaluation is necessary before it is accepted on a wider scale both by surgeons and radiologists.

d) Bypass Grafts

Ever since introduction of the bypass principle in 1948, most occlusive arterial diseases have been treated by bridging the occluded areas with various types of grafts. Both autogenous vein grafts and fabric or synthetic tubes are used, the former being the material of choice, especially in the procedures for below the inguinal ligament. In the aortoiliac segment, Dacron grafts are almost universally used (EDWARDS 1978). Thromboendarterectomy is employed only for short segmental occlusions.

Recently introduced new grafts, the expanded polytetrafluoroethylene (PTFE) (VEITH et al. 1978), and glutaraldehyde-tanned umbilical cord vein are used as substitutes for vein grafts whenever the latter are not available. These are employed above and below the popliteal, in the anterior and posterior tibial and peroneal arteries. These grafts are of value in arterial reconstruction, especially in cases above the knee. The results of these grafts below the popliteal, however, are less encouraging.

e) Lumbar Sympathectomy

Lumbar sympathectomy, although used for over half a century is still a controversial procedure. Since the sympathectomy is designed only to promote development of collateral circulation, it is obviously a second best type of revascularization procedure. In spite of the fact that its objective is more limited than direct arterial reconstruction, lumbar sympathectomy is definitely indicated under certain conditions in advanced peripheral arterial disease, in which there is an obviously poor or absent run-off that precludes direct arterial surgery.

Combined procedures may often be necessary to overcome the multiplicity and great extent of arterial lesions. Thromboendarterectomy, or a bypass graft, may be combined with lumbar sympathectomy, especially in polysegmental occlusions or in diffuse obliterative disease of the distal arterial tree. These procedures are by no means competitive; rather, they supplement each other. The proximal procedures achieve their therapeutic effect by increasing the head pressure into the major collateral branches of the lower extremity, such as in the profunda femoris, while vasodilatation of the available collateral network is achieved by lumbar sympathectomy. This combined therapy, in our opinion, is always indicated when the popliteal-tibial system is diffusely or completely occluded. Relief of rest pain and healing of minor toe lesions may be obtained in a majority of cases.

f) Amputations

Six possible levels of amputation for ischemic gangrene are at: the toes, the transmetatarsal level, the ankle joint (Syme amputation), the supramalleolar level, the midleg (below-the-knee) and thigh (above-the-knee).

In recent years, better understanding of the peripheral vascular problems and the more extensive use of reconstructive arterial procedures have altered the outlook for patients with necrotic lesions of the toes or foot. As the result of these combined procedures, many patients with toe lesions may acquire sufficient collateral supply, sometimes preventing any loss of tissue, or permit only local minor amputations.

The choice of the level of amputation depends on the proper evaluation of both local factors and the patient's general condition. The local factors are the extent of gangrene or ulceration, the degree of infection, condition of adjacent areas, the degree of arterial impairment, and the severity of the pain.

The most common levels of amputations are the toes, either single or transmetatarsal, and the below-knee procedure. Conservation of the knee joint is an important consideration, especially in the elderly. Every effort should be made to avoid its loss. Above-knee amputation may be unavoidable if there is spreading gangrene and sepsis toward the knee joint.

A new concept in the management of lower extremity amputees by early or immediate fitting of prosthesis has been widely used for the past 15–20 years. The results obtained with this method promise to change the outlook for the geriatric amputee by expediting his or her rehabilitation.

g) Care of Ischemic Foot Lesions in Diabetic Patients

Management of ischemic foot lesions, especially in the elderly diabetic patient, has remained poorly defined, and the maneuvers designed to carry out this treatment are generally even more poorly understood. The major objectives for such treatment are generally even more poorly understood. The major objectives for such treatment are avoidance of any trauma to the ischemic foot, control of infection, control of pain, and preservation of muscle strength and joint motion.

Local care is essential. Adequate drainage from the necrotic lesions and presence of interdigital ulcers are often overlooked. The source of an abscess with minimal opening in these areas is not detected unless one examines methodically the various parts of the foot. The subungual infection, associated with an ingrown toenail is often the precipitating cause of gangrene. Black eschars should be elevated at the corners, allowing adequate drainage of the purulent material often trapped under them. The debridement of such scabs should be gentle, to avoid bleeding and further trauma of the ischemic tissues.

Control of pain is essential. This is particularly necessary in the preoperative period so as to have the patient in the horizontal position to reduce the edema and render the tissues more amenable to surgery.

Anesthesia of the foot due to diabetic neuropathy deprives the patient of the perception of pain accompanying infection and necrosis. Superficial lymphangitis and cellulitis, not responding promptly to systemic antibiotics, most often mask underlying abscesses, either in subcutaneous tissue or in the subfascial compartment. Debridement and wide drainage, followed by a continuous wet dressing, with an antibiotic solution for a week or 10 days may arrest the septic process.

These conservative measures cannot be overemphasized in the diabetic, and also in the nondiabetic. Careful, meticulous management of these local lesions may obviate loss of tissue and amputations.

C. Aneurysms

I. Abdominal Aortic Aneurysm

Aneurysms of the abdominal aorta have been encountered with greater frequency in the past 3 decades. Two factors seem to account for this incidence: (1) increased life span with a parallel increase in arteriosclerosis, and (2) greater awareness of the diagnosis of abdominal aortic aneurysms. As the longevity of the general population is increased, it seems reasonable to expect a further increase in the incidence of this condition.

1. Etiology

Aneurysms can be caused by a variety of agents that weaken the arterial wall. While in the past, mycotic, luetic, or traumatic lesions were important factors, today aneurysms of the abdominal aorta and of the major limb arteries are almost exclusively caused by arteriosclerosis. Most patients are elderly and exhibit varying degrees of cardiovascular disease. In our own experience, 75% of patients were in the 7th and 8th decade, and 87% of the entire group were males. Cardiovascular disease is often associated with abdominal aortic aneurysms, requiring proper evaluation before surgical correction of the lesion is undertaken. Old myocardial infarction, angina pectoris, and congestive heart failure are often found in these patients (BUSH et al. 1977). Other arteriosclerotic lesions, such as occlusive arterial disease of the lower extremities or aneurysms at other levels are frequently encountered (HAIMOVICI 1967a).

2. Natural Course of an Abdominal Aneurysm

The natural course of an untreated aortic aneurysm has been fairly well documented in recent years. Studies based on necropsy findings showed that a majority of patients died within 6–12 months after onset of symptoms, as a result of rupture of the aneurysm (DARLING et al. 1976). Studies based on clinical course have disclosed equally high mortality rates. Both these studies of untreated cases have shown that: (1) the survival rate of patients with abdominal aortic aneurysms is much lower than that of the normal population, especially after the age of 65, (2) there are no absolute criteria for predicting which case will rupture, since a substantial number of the so-called asymptomatic type eventually do rupture, and (3) rupture of the aneurysm is the greatest catastrophe in all cases, irrespective of whether they are symptomatic or asymptomatic.

3. Diagnostic Tests

In most instances, the diagnosis of an uncomplicated abdominal aneurysm can be made by clinical findings alone. However, since the advent of sonography or other noninvasive procedures the diagnosis is greatly facilitated (HERTLER and BEVEN 1978). Such tests may obviate the use of aortography and provide enough information, both for the diagnosis of the lesion and its extent. However, associated intraabdominal vascular lesions may require contrast visualization of the aorta, of its visceral arteries, as well as of the distal arterial tree in the lower extremities. Although the question of performing aortography in all cases of aortic aneurysm has been a controversial one, at the present time, due to low risk of complications, the procedure is being used more liberally than in the past.

4. Treatment

Since the untreated abdominal aortic aneurysm carries a high incidence of fatal or serious complications, such as rupture, embolism to the lower extremities, and infection, indication for its excision is widely accepted. With greater technical competence, operative mortality has decreased uniformly (STOKES and BUTCHER 1973).

Of the fatal complications following surgery, the most frequently encountered are myocardial infarction, cerebrovascular accidents, acute renal insufficiency, and hemorrhage from the operative site. Preoperative hypertension and cardiovascular-renal disease are the most significant factors adversely influencing survival after operation (BUSH et al. 1977).

Age, in itself, does not seem to contraindicate surgical resection of abdominal aneurysm. Indeed, recent studies have established that none of the known risk factors influence the operative mortality in patients 70 years and older. Elective surgery for asymptomatic or even expanding aneurysms in patients 80 years or older was reported to be associated with the mortality similar to the younger groups of patients. This is in contrast to the ruptured aneurysms in this old age group, in whom the operative mortality was 74%.

5. Ruptured Aneurysm

Rupture of an aneurysm is a catastrophic event, posing urgent problems in diagnosis and management. Successful outcome depends on prompt recognition and precise and rapid surgical management. The rupture of the abdominal aortic aneurysm occurs most commonly in the retroperitoneal space and more rarely, in the inferior vena cava or duodenum (DIGIOVANNI et al. 1975; ERNST et al. 1976).

The diagnosis of a ruptured abdominal aortic aneurysm is based on the presence of generalized excruciating abdominal pain or back pain, associated with the clinical picture of shock. Corroborating these two symptoms is the presence of the pulsatile and expansile abdominal mass. Before rupture, heralding symptoms occur rarely, and may account for only 15%–25% of the cases. In the majority of patients, examination discloses mild to severe shock associated with an enlarging or expanding pulsatile abdominal mass. Shortly after the onset, these patients may become oliguric or anuric (ABBOTT et al. 1975).

Based on the size of retroperitoneal hematoma, the degree of ruptured aneurysm may be classified as follows: group 1, intramural bleeding with a small hematoma confined to the immediate vicinity of the rupture; group 2, hematoma below the renal arteries, including the pelvis; group 3, hematoma extending above the renal arteries and to the pelvis; and group 4, free bleeding into the peritoneal cavity. There appears to be a correlation between the size and extent of the hematoma and the prognosis of survival (FITZGERALD et al. 1978).

The operative mortality in ruptured aneurysms is vastly different from the elective resection and ranges from 30%–76%. The factors influencing survival are duration and severity of the hypovolemic shock and acute renal shutdown. For the surgery to be successful, prompt recognition of these complications and immediate surgical intervention are essential.

6. Other Complications

Rupture into the inferior vena cava is uncommon but may be catastrophic if not recognized in time. The clinical picture of this complication is rather characteristic. The most important feature is a high output cardiac failure. The lower extremities may become enlarged, cold, and cyanotic. Oliguria and hepatomegaly with liver failure reflect the sudden hemodynamic changes in the visceral circulation. Prompt excision of the sac together with closure of the fistula between the aorta and the inferior vena cava, and implantation of a graft, are the essential steps for correction of this complication.

Aortoenteric fistula may occur either spontaneously or secondary to a suture line disrupture of an aortic graft. This uncommon complication is usually associated with a high mortality, even under favorable circumstances. The retroperitoneal sepsis associated with this complication leads to a high mortality rate both in the spontaneous and secondary cases.

Association of *horseshoe kidney* with an abdominal aortic aneurysm is rare. Their coexistence presents multiple challenges: preoperative diagnosis, difficulty in exposure and dissection of the aneurysm, preservation of renal vasculature (which is usually anomalous), and placement of the graft.

Mycotic aneurysms are fortunately rare, but are a most serious complication of abdominal aneurysms. The most common agents responsible for mycotic aneurysms are members of the *Salmonella* series. A variety of other organisms have also been isolated from aneurysmal tissue, including *Staphylococcus*, and *E. coli*. Prompt massive antibacterial therapy preceding surgical treatment often is the best chance for success in these once hopeless cases.

Ischemia of rectosigmoid colon is another complication. Ischemic changes of the sigmoid and the descending colon as a result of aortic resection are related to the operative management of the collateral circulation, especially of the inferior mesenteric and the other major branches of the abdominal aorta. The implantation of the stump of this latter artery into the prosthesis, in the event that ischemic changes are suspected, is mandatory at the time of the repair of the aneurysm.

Spinal cord ischemia may result from the permanent deprivation of blood supply to the spinal cord caused by interruption of the arteries placed in an anomalous position. Unfortunately such a complication cannot be foreseen, and little can be done after it happens.

II. Aneurysms of Visceral Branches of the Abdominal Aorta

Aneurysms of visceral branches of the abdominal aorta pose difficult diagnostic problems. Recent experience, using selective arteriography and other means have led to a reassessment of the incidence, clinical manifestations, and prognosis of these aneurysms. They may affect every branch of the abdominal aorta in varying degrees. There is increasing evidence that these aneurysms are less infrequent than the earlier literature would indicate. The presence of systemic arteriosclerotic lesions associated with vague abdominal discomfort should indicate the possibility of visceral artery involvement requiring aortography and selective arteriography. Noninvasive modalities are helpful in indicating the presence of anomalies. Once diagnosed, these aneurysms should be considered for surgical intervention in the majority of cases, in order to prevent the catastrophic outcome of sudden and fatal hemorrhage. Recent statistics of nonoperated cases fully justify a more aggressive attitude in the presence of a visceral aneurysm.

III. Peripheral Aneurysms

Aneurysms of the extremities occur mostly in the lower limb and rarely in the upper (HAIMOVICI 1976b). Those in the lower extremity originate infrequently in the iliac (Fig. 4), more often in the femoral, most commonly in the popliteal, and very rarely in the tibial arteries.

Irrespective of the involved arterial segment, the common denominator of all aneurysms is the underlying weakness of the arterial wall induced by arteriosclerotic lesions. Rarely are these due to mycotic, syphilitic, traumatic, or dissecting lesions. If untreated, these peripheral aneurysms result in a high incidence of arterial thrombosis and of gangrene, leading to amputation and sometimes even death. Although they may even rupture, this is a rare complication in contrast to that occurring in abdominal or thoracic aneurysms.

1. Femoral Aneurysms

Primary femoral aneurysms are generally of arteriosclerotic origin and of fusiform shape (ADISESHIAH and BAILEY 1977; HAIMOVICI 1976b). Their diagnosis can be made by palpation along the course of the femoral artery. Physical examination often permits accurate assessment of location and extent along with the patency of the vessel. If palpation indicates decreased pulsation and diminished arterial flow is suspected, arteriography should provide the information concerning the distal arterial tree and its degree of involvement with arteriosclerotic changes. In addition the aneurysmal sac is not always confined to the common femoral but involves the external iliac as well as the superficial femoral. Occasionally there is an associated profunda femoris aneurysmal dilatation and a coexisting popliteal le-

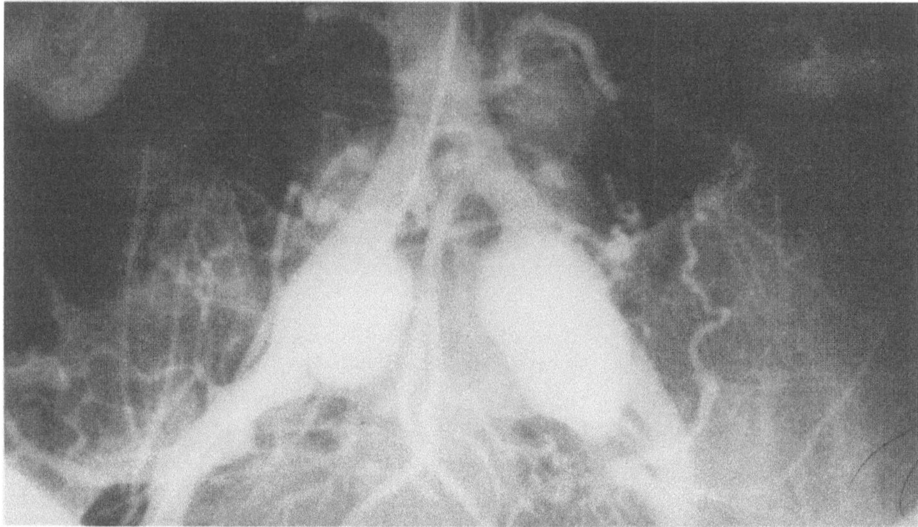

Fig. 4. Aortogram depicting bilateral iliac aneurysms (HAIMOVICI 1976)

sion. Femoral aneurysms are bilateral in about one-third of cases, and are associated with multiple aneurysms in other sites, in about 70% of cases.

B-Scan ultrasound has been used in recent years to evaluate the size of peripheral aneurysms. In the absence of an arteriogram the B-scan may provide valuable information, as reported in recent papers (Davis et al. 1977).

2. Popliteal Aneurysms

The popliteal is by far the most common site for aneurysmal dilatations (Chitwood et al. 1978). As in the case of the femoral in Scarpa's triangle, the popliteal has less protection by muscles and is subject to frequent bending. In the presence of arteriosclerotic changes, frequent flexion of the knee is recognized as a factor for predisposing to the dilatation of the vessel. Perhaps more than the bending of the knee, the poststenotic dilatation plays a role in the development of a popliteal aneurysm as a result of the compression of the artery by the tendon of the adductor magnus in the lower thigh, and also possibly of the arcuate popliteal ligament behind the knee. The popliteal aneurysmal sac is almost always elongated and fusiform, tapering distally until it resumes normal size. According to their location, the popliteal aneurysms may be divided into three types: (1) proximal, often multilobular, occupying the area behind the condyles of the femur; (2) medial, extending both proximally and distally around the knee joint space; and (3) distal, usually smaller than the preceding two forms.

Popliteal aneurysms, like the other lesions elsewhere, are associated with a high incidence of cardiovascular diseases, in which arterial hypertension is present in almost one out of two patients (Inahara and Toledo 1978). Preexisting occlusive arterial disease in approximately 60% of the involved limbs (acute and chronic thrombosis) is an important feature of this aneurysm. In most of these patients the nature of the occlusion is considered to be arteriosclerosis obliterans, but in some others it is difficult to determine whether the occlusion is an embolic complication from the aneurysm. One of the important features of this aneurysm is its bilaterality in a large percentage of cases. In addition, associated aneurysms in other locations of the arterial tree, such as abdominal or thoracic aorta, are not infrequent. Diagnosis of a popliteal aneurysm is usually easily made by physical examination. Arteriography is often necessary if the leg arteries appear to be occluded. Ultrasound scan in the diagnosis of these peripheral aneurysms has been used in recent years, as already mentioned earlier, and should be applied more frequently in the evaluation of the size of the aneurysm and the degree of thrombosis present in the sac.

Management of the femoral or popliteal aneurysms consists only of resection of the lesion, with reestablishment of continuity of the arterial tree, either with a prosthetic material or with a vein. The use of a bypass procedure, with ligation of the aneurysm above and below, is being used by a number of vascular surgeons, especially on smaller lesions. Occasionally, a lumbar sympathectomy may be indicated in the presence of associated occlusive disease of the leg. To be successful, surgery must be undertaken before the aneurysm becomes large and causes complications.

IV. Anastomonic Aneurysms

False aneurysms due to disruption of an anastomonic line of a graft or secondary to trauma, are a rather frequent occurrence (Fig. 5). The clinical manifestations vary with the location and the presence or absence of sepsis (SZILAGYI et al. 1975). In the septic group a false aneurysm is a rather early postoperative manifestation consisting of intermittent bleeding from the affected areas, formation of a hematoma, pus drainage, and lymphorrhea, all of which precede the appearance of

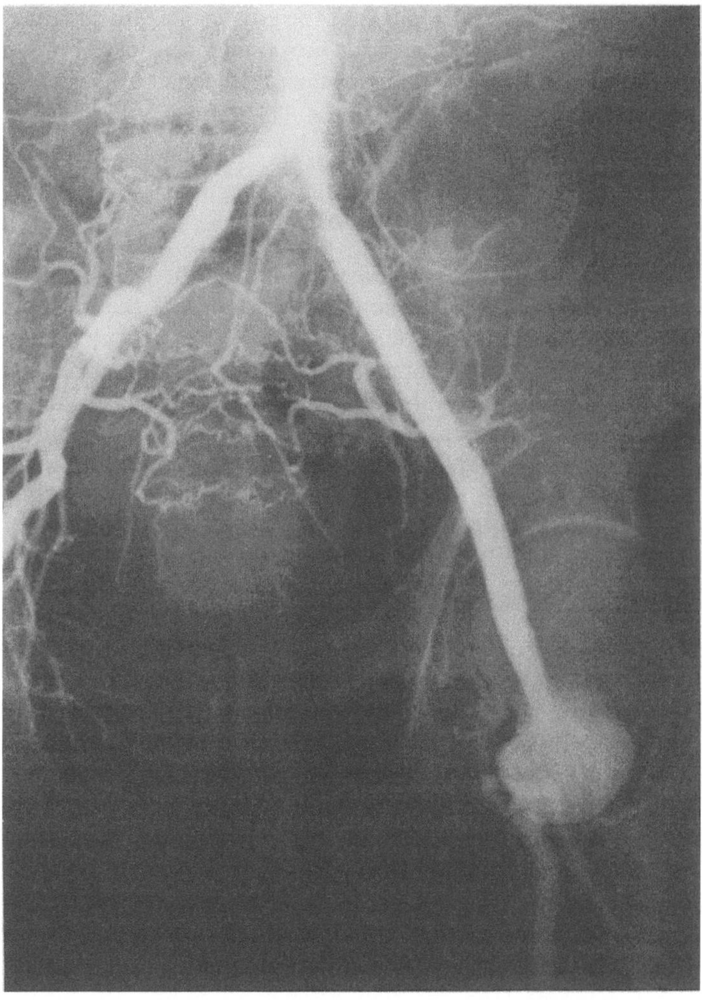

Fig. 5. Translumbar aortogram depicting a left iliofemoral Dacron bypass graft with an anastomotic aneurysm at the common femoral level. Note the presence only of the profunda femoris distal to the aneurysm. The superficial femoral had been occluded 6½ years prior to the original graft implantation. The patient underwent excision of this aneurysm with an end-to-end anastomosis between the proximal graft and the profunda femoris (HAIMOVICI 1976)

the aneurysm. Presence of sepsis is a very serious, if not ominous, prognostic factor. The exact incidence of anastomonic aneurysms is not entirely known, and has been variously estimated to range between 2.9% and 16%. Their management is somewhat more difficult than that of a spontaneous aneurysm of the popliteal arteries. It consists of either simple suture of the site of disruption of the edge of the arteriotomy, or excision of a distal portion of the graft and of the anastomotic area with regrafting from more proximal to distal levels. In infected false aneurysms, a bypass procedure around the septic area is indicated in order to overcome a most serious situation.

Whereas the gravest complications of abdominal aortic aneurysms are their rupture, in peripheral aneurysms the greatest hazard remains thrombosis with possible loss of limb. Both hazards are equally serious. They can be easily prevented by prompt diagnosis and management. Reconstructive arterial surgery has proven successful even in advanced age.

D. Acute Venous Thrombosis

Acute venous thrombosis affects primarily the deep veins of the lower extremity and very rarely those of the upper. It is one of the most common vascular conditions encountered particularly after the age of 40, and is seen with greater frequency in geriatric patients. The increased incidence in this latter group is related to a longer survival of critically ill patients, as well as after extensive surgical procedures. There is a great susceptibility to thromboembolism in both medical and surgical patients in the geriatric group. An anatomic risk factor in the elderly appears to be directly related to a progressive enlargement of the intramuscular calf veins, which occurs with advancing years (Hume et al. 1970).

I. Clinical Manifestations

There are several anatomic areas of predilection for the occurrence of thrombophlebitis in the lower extremities. One of the most common is the calf muscle veins referred to often as "sural thrombophlebitis." The venous thrombosis usually involves the *tibial veins* but often extends into the popliteal as well. It is most frequently seen as a postoperative complication or in patients bedridden as a result of a chronic ailment (infections, blood dyscrasias, neoplasms, cardiac decompensation) or during convalescence from a myocardial infarction. Occasionally, it may occur without any apparent cause (Moser et al. 1977).

Mild to moderate edema of the involved leg or ankle in the pretibial area is detectable. Cyanosis, usually mild, is most often absent. Engorgement of the superficial veins over the anterior surface of the leg is an unreliable diagnostic sign in most instances. Homans' sign, often credited as a reliable index of the presence of venous thrombosis of the calf, has been shown to be present in only a small percentage of cases. Therefore, the positive findings of calf thrombophlebitis are unfortunately not always conclusively demonstrable.

Under these circumstances, a presumptive diagnosis based on one's experience and comprehension of the problem is often the only alternative. This is especially

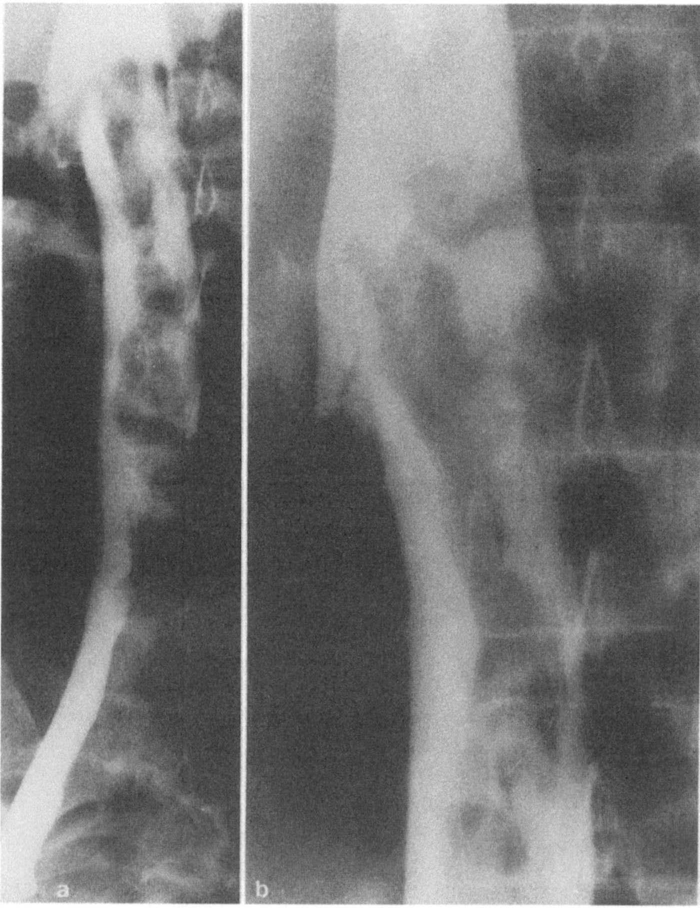

Fig. 6 a, b. Right transfemoral vein inferior vena cavagram. **a** Nonvisualization of the left common iliac vein due to acute thrombosis and presence of an intraluminal thrombus in the inferior vena cava. **b** Magnification of the inferior vena cava in **a,** depicting in its lumen a floating thrombus, which extends above the two renal veins. Thrombectomy of the left iliac vein and of the inferior vena cava prevented further pulmonary emboli that the patient had had prior to this procedure (HAIMOVICI 1982)

valid from a statistical standpoint in the postoperative state, during heart disease, anemia, carcinoma, very advanced age, obesity, or varicose veins. Because the clinical manifestations are often inconclusive, deep venous thrombosis of the calf has been the subject of great controversy. In recent years, however, noninvasive methods, in addition to contrast visualization of the veins, have been used more extensively to render the diagnosis more precise (see below).

The second commonest location of thrombophlebitis is the *iliofemoral segment*. In contrast to calf vein thrombosis, it usually offers no diagnostic problems because the clinical manifestations are more obvious. There is usually diffuse enlargement with swelling involving the entire lower extremity, including the thigh, along with general aching, mild cyanosis, tenderness of the upper thigh over the femoral vein, especially in the fossa ovalis, and engorgement of the superficial veins. Occasionally, arterial pulsations are decreased due to arteriospasm. This may account for the pain of the entire leg, some pallor, coolness, and even absence of arterial pulsations in the involved limb. As a result this clinical picture may occasionally be confused with an arterial embolism.

Thrombosis of the *inferior vena cava* (Fig. 6) may represent a primary condition, or extension of an iliofemoral thrombophlebitis. It may occur first on one side, especially on the left, then involve the inferior vena cava and the right side. The symptomatology and physical findings in inferior vena cava thrombosis are the same as for iliofemoral, except that they are bilateral.

Thrombophlebitis of the *superficial veins* in the lower extremity is simple to diagnose in most instances. It may involve the greater or lesser saphenous vein, whether normal or varicose. Occasionally, this diagnosis may have to be differentiated from acute cellulitis or lymphangitis. Most patients with lymphangitis, however, have a fever ranging from 101 °F to 104 °F, with a shaking chill at the onset. In contrast, with superficial thrombophlebitis there is practically no significant temperature elevation or chills, except if there is associated sepsis.

A frequently encountered superficial thrombophlebitis in the elderly is that affecting *varicose veins*. The diagnosis is usually simple. The only question is the extent of the process. Occasionally, the thrombosis extends toward the groin, or affects the communicating veins, linking the superficial to the deep venous system. Under these circumstances, thromboembolic manifestations may occur and may require urgent ligation of the saphenous veins at its junction with the femoral or popliteal veins, as the case may be.

II. Upper Extremity Thrombophlebitis

Venous thrombosis in the upper extremities is rare (ADAMS et al. 1965; COON and WILLIS 1966; HUGHES 1949; LORING 1952; SWINTON et al. 1968; TILNEY et al. 1970; VEAL and HUSSEY 1943). It may occur as a result of extension from superficial veins into the deep venous system in patients who have intrathoracic neoplasms or aneurysms compressing the subclavian vein, or following trauma. One of the most common known upper extremity venous thromboses is the so-called effort thrombosis which occurs as a result of trauma, stress, or injury involving the arm. Recently, PRESCOTT and TIKOFF (1979) presented a series of patients with both "stress" and "spontaneous" thrombosis on the left side, in six of the nine arms so affected. The etiology varied from congestive heart failure, cor pulmonale, lymphoma, coagulation abnormality, and quadriplegia with an associated polycythemia and thrombocytosis.

III. Precipitating Factors

There are many such precipitating events causing thrombophlebitis in the elderly. Any cause that leads to stasis and coagulation of blood in the calf veins or in the iliac system, is associated with an increased risk of pulmonary embolism and that risk increases with age. Bedrest is the most potent, immediate cause, and its incidence is known to rise with increasing length of immobility. Another major precipitating factor is operative trauma of tissues with its mobilizing clotting factors occurring mostly after exploratory laparotomies for gastric, biliary, and prostate operations, as well as in fractures of the lower limbs and pelvis.

The poor position of the bedridden patient often causes stasis and subsequent thromboembolic phenomena. Prophylaxis may be achieved by promoting venous drainage of the lower extremities in raising the foot of the bed, and using the head-down position. It has been calculated that a 10° head-down position promotes venous drainage of the legs at a rate almost double that in the horizontal position. In severe thrombophlebitis and edema, a 30°–40° elevation of the bed would be necessary to promote greater and faster drainage of the venous blood.

IV. Ischemic Venous Thrombosis

In contrast to the common form of iliofemoral thrombosis, referred to as "phlegmasia alba dolens," there are a certain number of cases in which the circulatory disturbances associated with acute thrombophlebitis may range from severe anoxemia of the tissues to gangrene (HAIMOVICI 1971). All these circulatory disturbances are secondary to venous thrombosis, without arterial participation. The dominant manifestations in these cases being ischemia of tissues, I have proposed the comprehensive term "ischemic venous thrombosis" for this entity, and subdivided it into two clinical forms: (a) *phlegmasia cerulea dolens,* or "blue thrombophlebitis," which is a reversible ischemic form, and (b) *venous gangrene,* in which the changes are, by definition, irreversible. These two forms are part of the same clinical pathologic entity, the distinction between them being a significant difference only of degree and extent of the underlying venous thrombosis. Recognition and management of phlegmasia cerulea dolens is of the utmost importance in order to prevent its progression to venous gangrene, the prognosis of which is not only loss of limb but often death of the patient.

1. Phlegmasia Cerulea Dolens

Phlegmasia cerulea dolens is characterized by a classic triad of pain, cyanosis, and edema. The pain is usually severe and is always present. Cyanosis is the pathognomonic sign, and is as striking as the severity of the pain. A sharp line seperates normal skin from the discoloration in some patients, lending the impression of a tourniquet-induced anoxemia with purpuric-like lesions. Usually pain and cyanosis are followed almost immediately by edema, which becomes quite pronounced and often has a characteristic woody or rubbery consistency. Arterial pulses at the initial stage of the acute syndrome may be felt only in the femoral or axillary arteries, but not distally to them. However, at the recovery stage all pulses become palpable.

If treated promptly, one may avoid pulmonary embolism and progression of the local condition to gangrene. The overall recovery in untreated and treated patients was 83% in a total series of 175 patients studied by the author. Seventeen percent died in the immediate acute phase after onset.

2. Venous Gangrene

Venous gangrene is characterized by three distinct phases: (1) phlegmasia alba dolens, (2) phlegmasia cerulea dolens, and (3) gangrene.

3. Management

In phlegmasia cerulea dolens, immediate administration of heparin and elevation of the limb are the major initial steps. Venous thromboectomy is sometimes indicated. If gangrene occurs, one should bear in mind that most often the lesion is superficial and self limiting, provided infection is avoided.

V. Diagnosis

The clinical recognition of a deep venous thrombosis is often difficult. False positive, or false negative signs occur quite often in these patients. Recent development of screening tests which can reveal venous thrombi before they become evident clinically has facilitated recognition of this process.

Noninvasive screening tests are being used extensively in many vascular centers. They consist of the ultrasonic technique, using the Doppler effect, radioactive-labeled fibrinogen, impedance plethysmography, and phleborheography (YAO et al. 1973). Most of these noninvasive techniques provide 80%–90% clear indications of the presence of deep thrombi. In the cases in which there is doubt as to the presence or absence of venous thrombi, venography remains the most accurate means for confirming the diagnosis and the extent of the disease.

Indeed, *contrast venography* will provide direct evidence of both occlusive and nonocclusive venous thrombi. The disadvantages of venography are that it usually requires movement of the patient to the X-ray table, which may result in local complications, such as thrombosis or pulmonary embolism.

Laboratory testing for hypercoagulability of the blood has been disapointing because it has been unable, routinely, to provide evidence for altered clotting factors responsible for this state. Indeed, most hematologists have denied existence of such a state of hypercoagulability, and only recently has the significance been acknowledged.

VI. Pulmonary Embolism

Pulmonary embolism is one of the most dreaded complications of acute venous thrombosis. Theoretically and ideally, pulmonary embolism should be prevented by immediate treatment of peripheral venous thrombosis. Unfortunately, clinical and necropsy studies have shown that about 85% of fatal emboli are not preceded by evidence of peripheral venous thrombosis. The exact incidence of pulmonary embolism is variable according to published reports, but it seems to have been increasing in recent years (DETAKATS 1968; VIAMONTE et al. 1980).

Based on autopsy series, about 85% of pulmonary emboli originate from thrombi in the calf veins, about 10% from thrombi in the pelvis, and about 5% from clots in the heart itself. The magnitude of the problem of emboli is reflected in the annual number of 50,000 deaths in the United States from this complication.

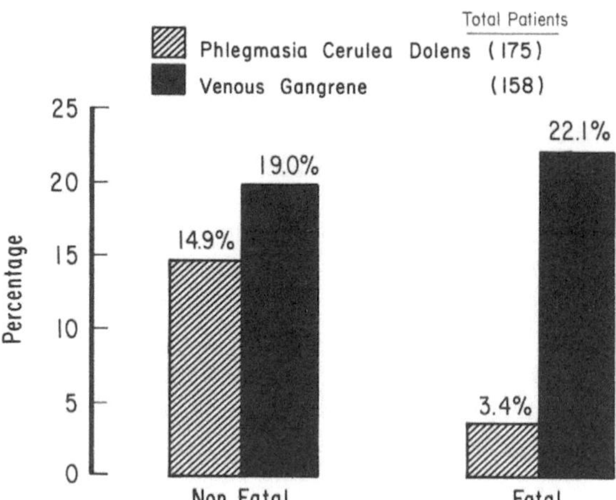

Fig. 7. Incidence of pulmonary embolism in ischemic venous thrombosis (HAIMOVICI 1982)

Figure 7 shows the incidence of pulmonary embolism in ischemic venous thrombosis. In the nonfatal pulmonary emboli, there is only a slightly higher incidence in the cases with gangrene than in the cases of phlegmasia cerulea dolens. In contrast, in the cases of fatal pulmonary emboli, the patients with phlegmasia cerulea dolens showed an incidence of only a 3.4%, while in the group of venous gangrene, it was 22.1%.

The clinical manifestations of pulmonary embolism depend on the size of the embolus in relation to the pulmonary aterial branch it obstructs. Four recognizable forms of pulmonary embolism occur, although transition from one form to another readily occurs. The four forms are: (1) fatal pulmonary embolus without no evidence of a source of thrombosis, (2) the massive sublethal pulmonary embolus which is still amenable to salvage if measures are taken without delay, (3) small pulmonary infarct, and (4) subclinical embolism. Diagnostic tests for pulmonary embolism do not always provide adequate information. Arterial oxygen determination is usually most useful. If it is 90 mm Hg or greater, the likelihood of a pulmonary embolism is remote. Pulmonary–perfusion scanning appears to be an accurate screening test. However, pulmonary angiography remains the most reliable means for diagnosing pulmonary embolism, and should be used as a last resort.

VII. Treatment of Thromboembolism

1. Medical Treatment

Superficial thrombophlebitis of an extremity rarely requires bedrest. In the absence of spreading thrombosis, simple application of moist heat may be all that is needed, together with an antiinflammatory medication [phenylbutazone (Butazolidin) or oxyphenbutazone (Tandearil)]. If the superficial thrombophlebitis extends above the knee or elbow, and has a definite tendency to spread to the groin or axilla, bedrest, elevation, anticoagulants, and possibly surgical ligation of the involved vein, especially in the groin, may be indicated. Pulmonary embolism associated with superficial thrombophlebitis is extremely rare, unless the thrombosis extends to the deep veins.

Deep venous thrombosis. Thrombophlebitis, involving the sural veins or the iliofemoral segment, may require the patient's hospitalization. Bedrest with elevation of the extremity and head-down position are essential in order to provide adequate venous drainage. If treated at home, the latter may best be accomplished by raising the foot of the bed by blocks 12"–15" high. If the head-up position is necessary because of cardiac decompensation with orthopnea, the leg should be in the horizontal position as a compromise solution.

Local application of moist, hot packs for the full length of the involved extremity is helpful at the acute stage. Hydration of the patient is important to prevent hemoconcentration, which predisposes to thrombosis of the veins. Lung scanning and chest X-rays should be carried out with the utmost care for fear of mobilizing floating thrombi, especially at the initial stage of the process.

2. Anticoagulant Therapy

In geriatric patients, especially undergoing surgical procedures, whether abdominal or hip fracture repair, it is often desirable to use anticoagulant drugs as a prophylaxis to venous thromboembolism. Under these circumstances, to minimize complications of the antiocagulant agents, small doses of heparin given subcutaneously have been recommended and appear generally effective (KAKKAR et al. 1975). Electric calf stimulation and both active and passive postoperative exercise, and graded compression stockings are other prophylactic measures recommended against deep vein thrombosis. Their effectiveness is mostly considered as adjunct to the anticoagulant therapy.

In established thromboembolism, however, heparin should be given intravenously by continuous infusion, using a loading dose of 2,000–4,000 units, and thereafter 1,000 units or more per hour. Intermittent administration of heparin, or by the subcutaneous route, is not desirable. Heparin should be administered for at least 1–2 weeks after the onset of the thromboembolic episode, and thereafter continued with oral anticoagulant therapy, using sodium warfarin (Coumadin). The initial dose of sodium warfarin ranges from 10–40 mg. Maintenance doses range from 0.5–10 mg/day, adjusted to the prothrombin time, between 2 or 3 times above normal. Oral therapy should be continued for 3–6 months, especially if the patient has a chronic condition predisposing to embolism.

Fibrinolysins have been used in recent years with variable degrees of effectiveness (NATIONAL COOPERATIVE STUDY 1974). Their usefulness is still questionable. Low-molecular weight dextran may likewise be administered in certain cases for 3–4 days. In the elderly it must be given cautiously to prevent cardiac overload.

3. Surgical Management

Surgical management (COON 1974; INAHARA 1968) is indicated only if anticoagulant therapy fails to prevent pulmonary embolism or in the presence of potentially bleeding conditions due to its use. Two modalities are then available: (1) vein interruption and (2) thrombectomy.

The rationale for vein interruption is that of a mechanical barrier provided to prevent extension of thrombosis and pulmonary emboli. Ligation, plication, or transvenous interruption of the inferior vena cava are variably indicated.

a) Plication

Plication may be achieved by suture, or by clips especially designed to divide the lumen of the cava into small compartments. *Complete ligation* of the inferior vena cava, although much simpler than plication, is fraught with certain disadvantages due to postligation venous stasis or distal extension of thrombosis or other sequelae. If ligation is to be carried out, the author prefers a stenosing ligation which is far safer, easier, and more expeditious. It is carried out around the tip of a Kelly clamp. The resulting vena cava lumen is approximately slightly more than the thickness of the tip of the clamp (HAIMOVICI 1971, 1976 d).

b) Transvenous Caval Interruption

Transvenous caval interruption by means of specially designed devices [Mobin-Uddin umbrella (MOBIN-UDDIN et al. 1977), Kim-Ray Greenfield filter (GOODALL and GREENAELD 1980) and the Hunter-Session balloon (HUNTER et al. 1977)] is indicated primarily in patients at high risk for plication or ligation. Morbidity and mortality appear to be reduced by this method, although pulmonary embolism is not entirely eliminated.

c) Venous Thrombectomy

Venous thrombectomy has been advocated both in phlegmasia alba dolens and phlegmasia cerulea dolens. Long-term results in the former for achieving venous patency have not been encouraging. Therefore, the majority of vascular surgeons feel that thrombectomy in the common form of iliofemoral thrombophlebitis is not useful (BARNER et al. 1969). In contrast, in phlegmasia cerulea dolens, thrombectomy may be indicated to prevent pulmonary emboli and further local extension of the thrombosis, which may actually lead to gangrene of the limb. To be successful, the procedure should be carried out in the first 2–3 days after onset (DRAPANAS and CURRAN 1966; HAIMOVICI 1971; LANSING and DAVIS 1968).

d) Pulmonary Embolectomy

Based on the most recent experience, indications for pulmonary embolectomy are confined to major embolism with shock, associated with central venous pressure exceeding 30 cm of saline, with an angiogram showing a filling defect in either or both pulmonary arteries and indicating more than 50% obstruction. If the patient's condition is very critical, partial venoarterial bypass in the groin improves the situation greatly and may thus render the patient operable.

Until a few years ago, before the use of cardiopulmonary bypass for pulmonary embolectomy, this procedure carried a forbiddingly high mortality. Even the current method of embolectomy with bypass is not an entirely benign procedure. The operative mortality for all patients undergoing pulmonary embolectomy is around, or above, 57%.

Recently, an alternative approach to open pulmonary embolectomy was suggested by GREENFIELD et al. (1974) consisting of a transvenous removal of pulmonary emboli. This procedure, however, is still at an experimental stage.

VIII. Postphlebitic Syndrome

One of the major sequelae of deep venous thrombosis is a later appearance of a clinicopathologic condition with a tendency to assume a chronic course. It is often neglected by both patient and physician and causes serious complications. It occurs as a result of an iliofemoral thrombophlebitis or deep venous thrombosis of the leg. The immediate cause is severe damage to the deep veins and their valves. The resulting valvular incompetency is in turn responsible for the chronic venous stasis. This initiates a chain of events starting with edema in the lower leg, leading to cellulitis, induration of the skin and subcutaneous tissue, pigmentation, dermatitis, and finally ulceration around the lower portion of the leg and ankle.

1. Venous Hemodynamics

The essential physiopathology of the postphlebitic syndrome is characterized by ambulatory venous hypertension in the area of the ankle, due to vavular incompetency. Measurements of the pressures at the ankle, both at rest and during exercise, have indicated conclusively that in the postphlebitic syndrome there is no fall of pressure on exercise in contrast to the normal leg, or even in patients with incompetence of primary superficial varicose veins. In the latter cases, although the pressure may rise on exercise, it falls immediately on cessation of motion.

In addition to the valvular incompetency of the deep veins, the ankle communicating veins between the superficial and deep system (ankle perforators) are credited by some investigators as also playing an important role in determining the local skin and subcutaneous changes.

Another factor in the pathogenesis of the postphlebitic syndrome is the presence of arteriovenous shunting in the lower leg and around the ankle as demonstrated by the author (HAIMOVICI 1976a). This contributes to the deprivation of the oxygenated blood in the capillaries, since it is shunted away through the precapillary channels. As a result, a degree of ischemia is also present in addition to the venous stasis, thus making this syndrome more complex than it is generally assumed.

The major *clinical components* of the postphlebitic syndrome are soft pitting edema at the early stage, later becoming indurated and less pitting. Inflammatory changes of the skin and subcutaneous tissues occur later, due to the persistent venous stasis on the medial side of the leg, and less often on the lateral. This location depends on whether the greater or shorter saphenous vein is involved. Pigmentation of the skin from the ankle may extend proximally to involve half of the leg. At an advanced stage, subcutaneous fibrosis or even calcification may take place and provide the hard texture already mentioned. The degree of edema varies considerably in these patients. In those with localized destruction of the valves in the calf veins and of those of the perforating branches, the edema may be minimal. However, in those patients who have complete postthrombotic destruction of the valves in the femoral, popliteal, and calf veins, edema may be a major complaint.

One of the symptoms accompanying this syndrome is what is described as "bursting pain." The patients usually complain of generalized aching pains in the leg and calf, which must be distinguished from that associated with an ulcer.

Enlargement of the calf is also a common finding. It is due to chronic intramuscular edema, which usually causes the symptom of aching at the end of the day, or after a period of prolonged standing. Nocturnal cramps are also a common component of the clinical picture.

Diagnosis of a postphlebitic syndrome is based on the past history of deep venous thrombosis associated with the symptoms as described above. Measurements of ambulatory venous pressure and venography would provide the necessary pathophysiologic criteria for the diagnosis. The venogram shows the enlarged valveless collateral veins, most often dilated with incompetent perforators in the lower leg and ankle.

One of the major findings, not necessarily always present, is the appearance of varicose veins. These are secondary to the venous obstruction and subsequent incompetence of the deep venous system. The secondary varicose veins should be distinguished from the primary type, which follow a more regular anatomic pattern than those observed after a postthrombotic syndrome.

2. Treatment

a) Nonsurgical Management

In an uncomplicated postphlebitic syndrome with only edema, elastic support during ambulation and nocturnal elevation of the lower extremity are helpful in controlling the chronic stasis insufficiency. The stockings should be fitted with a graded pressure from the ankle to the knee. Standard stockings are totally inadequate in such cases.

In the presence of cellulitis with lymphangitis, bedrest with leg elevation, and antibiotics, local warm compress application for a period of 1–2 weeks may be necessary for control of such complications.

b) Surgical Management

Surgical intervention (DALE 1980) may be necessary for two components of the syndrome: (1) secondary varicose veins and (2) leg ulceration.

Ligation and stripping of the secondary varicose veins should not be undertaken without a complete venographic evaluation of the deep venous system. Should the latter be patent, although incompetent, surgery can be useful in removing a source of stasis. On the other hand, if the deep venous system is still occluded, the excision of the varicose veins is contraindicated.

Ulcers, usually under adequate conservative management, may heal with bedrest, elevation and local treatment, bandages or Unna's boots. However, if recurrence or lack of healing persists, excision of the ulcers with skin grafting becomes necessary. The subfascial ligation of perforators, advocated in the past, is not universally accepted since the current concept of the pathophysiology attributes the stasis mainly to the deep major veins. In addition, after the excision of the ulcer and skin grafting, an adequate fitted elastic support will be necessary for the patient to wear for several years, or indefinitely.

Since the postphlebitic syndrome has a tendency to persist and show recurrences, it is mandatory that follow-up of the patients should be advised and carried out periodically.

References

Abbott WM, Abel RM, Beck CH, Fischer IE (1975) Renal failure after ruptured aneurysm. Arch Surg 110:1110

Adams JT, McEvoy RK, DeWeese JA (1965) Primary deep venous thrombosis of upper extremity. Arch Surg 91:29

Adiseshiah M, Bailey H (1977) Aneurysms of the femoral artery. Br J Surg 64:174

Alpert J, Bhaktan EK, Gielchinsky I (1976) Vascular complications of intra-aortic balloon pumping. Arch Surg 111:1190

Barabas AP, Offen DN, Meinhard EA (1973) The arterial complications of polycythemia vera. Brit J Surg 60:183

Barner HB, Willman VL, Hanlon CR (1969) Thrombectomy for iliofemoral venous thrombosis. JAMA 208:2442

Bernstein EF, Dilley RB, Goldberger LE, Gosink BB, Leopold GR (1976) Growth rates of small abdominal aortic aneurysms. Surgery 80:765

Bertelsen S, Mathiesen FR, Phlenschlaeger HH (1968) Vascular complications of cervical rib. Scand J Thorac Cardiovasc Surg 2:133

Blaisdell FW, Steele M, Allen RE (1978) Management of acute lower extremity arterial ischemia due to embolism and thrombosis. Surgery 84:822

Brener BJ, Couch NP (1973) Peripheral arterial complications of left heart catheterization and their management. Am J Surg 125:521

Bush HL Jr, LoGerfo FW, Weisel RD, Mannick JA, Hechtman HB (1977) Assessment of myocardial performance and optimal volume loading during elective abdominal aortic aneurysm resection. Arch Surg 112:1301

Byrnes G, MacGowan WAL (1975) The injury potential of Fogarty balloon catheters. J Cardiovasc Surg 16:590

Champion HR, Gill W (1973) Arterial embolus to the upper limb. Br J Surg 60:505

Chitwood WR, Stocks LH, Wolfe WG (1978) Popliteal artery aneurysms. Arch Surg 113:1078

Coon WW (1974) Operative therapy of venous thromboembolism. Mod Conc Cardiovasc Dis 43:71

Coon WW, Willis PW (1966) Thrombosis of axillary and subclavian veins. Arch Surg 94:657

Dale WA (1980) Surgery for chronic peripheral venous hypertension. Contemp Surgery 16:28

Daley R, Mattingly TW, Holt CL (1951) Systemic arterial embolism in rheumatic heart disease. Am Heart J 42:566

Danto LA, Fry WJ, Kraft RI (1971) Acute aortic thrombosis. Arch Surg 106:66

Darling RC, Austen WG, Linton RR (1967) Arterial embolism. Surg Gynecol Obstet 124:106

Darling RC, Raines JK, Brener BJ, Austen WG (1972) Quantitative segmental pulse volume recorder: A clinical tool. Surgery 72:873

Darling RC, Messina CR, Brewster DC, Ottinger LW (1976) Autopsy study of unoperated abdominal aortic aneurysms. Cardiovasc Surg 56:161

Davis RP, Neiman HL, Yao JST, Bergan JT (1977) Ultrasound scan in diagnosis of peripheral aneurysms. Arch Surg 112:55

DeTakats G (1968) Pulmonary embolism: A second look. J Cardiovasc Surg [Suppl] 9:3

DiGiovanni R, Nicholas G, Volpetti G, Berkowitz H, Banker C, Roberts B (1975) Twenty-one years experience with ruptured abdominal aortic aneurysms 141:859

Dotter CT, Judkins MP (1964) Transluminal treatment of atherosclerotic obstruction. Description of a new technique and a preliminary report of its application. Circulation 30:654, 670

Drapanas T, Curran WL (1966) Thrombectomy in the treatment of „effort" thrombosis of the axillary and subclavian veins. J Trauma 6:107

Edwards WS (1978) Arterial grafts. Arch Surg 113:1225

Eriksson I, Holmberg JT (1977) Analysis of factors affecting limb salvage and mortality after embolectomy. Acta Chir Scand 143:237

Ernst CB, Hagihara PF, Daugherty ME, Sachatello CR, Griffen WO Jr (1976) Ischemic colitis incidence following abdominal aortic reconstruction: A prospective study. Surgery 80:417

Farrar DJ, Malindzak GS Jr, Johnson G Jr (1976) Large vessel impedance in peripheral atherosclerosis. Cardiovasc Surg 56:171

Fitzgerald JF, Stillman RM, Powers JC (1978) A suggested classification and reappraisal of mortality statistics for ruptured atherosclerotic infrarenal aortic aneurysms. Surg Gynecol Obstet 146:344

Flory CM (1945) Arterial occlusions produced by emboli from eroded aortic atheromatous plaques. Am L Pathol 21:549

Fogarty TJ, Cranley JJ (1965) Catheter technic for arterial embolectomy. Ann Surg 161:325

Gensler SW, Haimovici H, Hoffert P (1965) Study of vascular lesions in diabetic nondiabetic patients. Arch Surg 91:617

Goodall RJR, Greenfield LJ (1980) Clinical correlations in the diagnosis of pulmonary embolism. Ann Surg 219:191

Greenfield LJ, Peyton MD, Brown PP, Elkins RC (1974) Transvenous management of pulmonary embolic disease. Ann Surg 180:461

Haimovici H (1950) Peripheral arterial embolism: A study of 330 unselected cases of embolism of the extremities. Angiology 1:20

Haimovici H (1959) Late arterial embolectomy. Surgery 46:775

Haimovici H (1960) Arterial embolism with acute massive ischemic myopathy and myoglobinuria: Evaluation hitherto unreported syndrome with report of two cases. Surgery 47:739

Haimovici H (1967a) Abdominal aortic aneurysm. NY State J Med 67:691

Haimovici H (1967b) Patterns of arteriosclerotic lesions of the lower extremity. Arch Surg 95:918

Haimovici H (1971) Ischemic forms of venous thrombosis, phlegmasia cerulea dolens, venous gangrene. Charles C. Thomas, Springfield, Illinois

Haimovici H (1976a) Abnormal arteriovenous shunts associated with chronic venous insufficiency. J Cardiovasc Surg 17:473

Haimovici H (ed) (1976b) Peripheral aneurysms. In: Vascular surgery. McGraw-Hill Book Comp, New York, Chap 30, p 505

Haimovici H (ed) (1976c) Femoropopliteal arteriosclerotic occlusive disease. In: Vascular surgery. McGraw-Hill Book Co, New York, Chap 25, p 422

Haimovici H (ed) (1976d) Vascular surgery: principles and techniques. McGraw-Hill Book Co, New York

Haimovici H (1977a) Atherogenesis: Recent biological concepts and clinical implications. Am J Surg 134:174

Haimovici H (1977b) Diseases of small arteries of the extremities. In: Hardy JD (ed) Rhoads textbook of surgery, principles and practice. JB Lippincott Co, New York, Chap 55, p 1827

Haimovici H (1979) Muscular, renal, and metabolic complications of acute arterial occlusions; myonephropathic-metabolic syndrome. Surgery 85:461

Haimovici H (1982) Vascular emergencies. Appleton-Century-Crofts, New York

Haimovici H, Steinman C (1969) Aortoiliac angiographic patterns associated with femoropopliteal occlusive disease: Significance in reconstructive arterial surgery. Surgery 65:232

Halsted WS (1916) An experimental study of circumscribed dilatation of an artery immediately distal to a particularly occluding band, and its bearing on the dilatation of the subclavian artery observed in certain cases of cervical rib. J Exp Med 124:271

Hertzer NR, Beven EG (1978) Ultrasound aortic measurement and elective aneurysmectomy. JAMA 240:1966

Hughes ESR (1949) Venous obstruction in the upper extremity (Paget-Schroeder's syndrome). Surg Gynec Obstet 88:89

Hume M, Sevitt S, Thomas DP (1970) Venous thrombosis and pulmonary embolism. Harvard University Press, Cambridge, Mass

Hunter JA, Dye WS, Jarid H (1977) Permanent transvenous balloon occlusion of the inferior vena cava: Experience with 60 patients. Am Surg 186:491

Inahara T (1968) Surgical treatment of „effort" thrombosis of the axillary and subclavian veins. Am Surg 34:479

Inahara T, Toledo AC (1978) Complications and treatment of popliteal aneurysms. Surgery 775

Jarrett F, Dacumos GC, Crummy AB (1979) Late appearance of arterial emboli: diagnosis and management. Surgery 86:898

Judy KL, Heyman RL (1972) Vascular complications of the thoracic outlet syndrome. Am J Surg 123:521

Kakkar VV, Carrigan TP, Fossard DP (1975) Prevention of fatal pulmonary embolism by low doses of Heparin. Lancet 2:45

Kazmier FJ, Sheps SG, Bernatz PE, Sayre GP (1966) Livedo reticularis and digital infarcts: A syndrome due to cholesterol emboli; arising from atheromatous abdominal aneurysms. Vasc Dis 3:12

Kempczinski RF (1979) Lower extremity arterial emboli from ulcerating atherosclerotic plaques. JAMA 241:807

Kohn RR (1977) Heart and cardiovascular system. In: Finch CE, Hayflick L (eds) The biology of aging. Van Nostrand Reinhold Co, New York, p 281

Lansing AM, Davis WM (1968) Five-year follow-up study of iliofemoral venous thrombectomy. Ann Surg 168:620

Loring WE (1952) Venous thrombosis in the upper extremities as a complication of myocardial failure. Am J Med 12:397

Martin J, Gaspard DJ, Johnston PW, Koh RD, Dietrick W (1976) Vascular manifestations of the thoracic outlet syndrome. Arch Surg 111:779

McKusick VA, Harris WS, Ottesen OE (1962) Buerger's disease: A distinct clinical and pathologic entity. JAMA 181:5

McNamara MF, Takaki HS, Yao JST, Bergan JJ (1978) A systematic approach to severe hand ischemia. Surgery 83:1

Mobin-Uddin K, Callard GM, Bolooki H (1972) Transvenous caval interruption with umbrella filter. New Engl J Med 286:55

Moser KM, Brach BB, Dolan GF (1977) Clinically suspected deep venous thrombosis of the lower extremities. JAMA 237:2195

National Cooperative Study (1974) The urokinasestreptokinase pulmonary embolism trial. JAMA 299:1606

Panum PL (1862) Experimentelle Beiträge zur Lehre von der Emboli. Virchows Arch Path Anat 25:308

Prescott SM, Tikoff G (1979) Deep venous thrombosis of the upper extremity: A reappraisal. Circulation 59:350

Raines JK, Darling RC, Buth J, Brewster DC, Austen WG (1976) Vascular laboratory criteria for the management of peripheral vascular disease of the lower extremities. Surgery 79:21

Raithel D (1973a) Ein neuartiger Katheter-Stripper zur Behandlung der akuten Gliedmaßenischämie. Chirurg 44:434

Raithel D (1973b) Surgical treatment of acute embolization and acute arterial thrombosis. J Cardiovasc Surg (Special issue, 11th World Congress Int Cardiovasc Soc, Barcelona, Sept 27–29) 61

Roach MR, Burton AC (1959) The effect of age on the elasticity of human iliac arteries. Can J Biochem Physiol 37:557

Salzman EW, Davies GC (1980) Prophylaxis of venous thromboembolism. Ann Surg 191:207

Savelyev VS, Zatevakhin II, Stepanov NV (1977) Artery embolism of the upper limbs. Surgery 81:367

Stamler J, Berkson DM, Lindberg HA (1971) Risk factors: Their role in the etiology and pathogenesis of the atherosclerotic diseases. In: Wissler RW, Geer JC (eds) The pathogenesis of atherosclerosis. Williams and Wilkins Co, Baltimore, p 41

Stokes J, Butcher HR Jr (1973) Abdominal aortic aneurysms. Arch Surg 107:297

Strong JP, Eggen DA, Oalmann MC (1971) The natural history, geographic pathology and epidemiology of atherosclerosis. In: Wissler RW, Geer JC (eds) The pathogenesis of atherosclerosis. Williams and Wilkins Co, Baltimore, Chap 2, p 20

Swinton NW, Edgett JW, Hall RJ (1968) Primary subclavian-axillary vein thrombosis. Circulation 38:737

Szilagyi DE, Smith RF, Elliott JP, Hageman JH, Dall'Olmo CA (1975) Anastomotic aneurysms after vascular reconstruction: problems of incidenc, etiology, and treatment. Surgery 78:800

Tilney NL, Griffiths HJG, Edwards EA (1970) Natural history of major venous thrombosis of the upper extremity. Arch Surg 101:792

Veal JR, Hussey HH (1943) Thrombosis of the subclavian and axillary veins. Am Heart J 25:355

Veith FJ, Moss CM, Fell SC, Rhodes BA, Haimovici H (1978) Comparison of expanded PTFE and vein grafts in lower extremity arterial reconstructions. J Cardiovasc Surg 19:341

Verta MJ Jr, Gross WS, Van Bellen B, Yao TST, Bergan JJ (1976) Forefoot perfusion pressure and minor amputation for gangrene. Surgery 80:729

Viamonte M Jr, Koolpe H, Janowitz W, Hildner F (1980) Pulmonary thromboembolism – update. JAMA 243:2229

Wiest JW, Traverso LW, Dainko EA, Barker WF (1980) Atrophic coarctation of the abdominal aorta. Ann Surg 191:224

Yao ST, Henkin RE, Conn T, Quinn JL III, Bergan JJ (1973) Combined isotope venography and lung scanning. Arch Surg 107:146

Central Nervous System

Cerebral Blood Flow, Electroencephalography, and Behavior

S. HOYER

A. Introduction

During recent decades, an old desire of mankind seems to be fulfilled: that of becoming older and older. Progress in medical and social areas has increased the life expectancy of the population, at least in the highly developed countries. Epidemiological projections have revealed that about 12% of the population of the United States was 65 years and older in 1980 (National Center for Health Statistics 1975). While in 1974 in West Germany about 13% of the population was 65 years and older (LAUTER 1974), this rate increased to about 16% by 1980 (Statistisches Bundesamt FRG 1981). Similar data were reported from the Soviet Union (ROUBAKINE 1975). If these developments continue along with a declining birth rate, which will further increase relatively the number of aged people in the population, people aged 60 years and older will account for about 10% of the world's population in the year 2000 (Technical Report of WHO 1972). The estimated number of inhabitants aged 65 years and older will be still 16% in West Germany by the year 2000 although the population will have decreased by 7% (Statistisches Bundesamt FRG 1981). According to ROTH (1980), there will be 20% more people aged 75, and the number of 85-year-old people will have increased by 60% in Great Britain by 1986.

The process of aging is often a problem of the aging brain. However, physiological cerebral aging should be strictly differentiated from pathological cerebral aging, i.e., dementia which is strongly age related (KATZMAN 1979). The prevalence of severe dementia in people aged 65 years and older was estimated at 4%–7% (KATZMAN 1976, 1979; KAY et al. 1964a, b; ROTH 1978; TERRY 1976; TOMLINSON 1980) increasing to more than 20% above the age of 80 years (KAY 1972; KAY et al. 1970). Mild to moderate forms of dementia were estimated at about 11% in people aged 65 years and over (KATZMAN 1976; TERRY 1976). No figures are known about the prevalence of presenile dementia, neither in severe nor in mild or moderate forms.

In the following, different aspects such as behavior, cerebral blood flow and metabolism, and electroencephalography (EEG) will be discussed in terms of normal cerebral aging and abnormal aging processes in the brain, i.e., dementia.

B. Normal Cerebral Aging

I. Behavior

Decreasing speed of reaction seems to show most sensitive changes with advancing age. BIRREN and BOTWINICK (1955) ivestigated the reaction times to an auditory signal in two different age groups. Reaction time was significantly higher in people aged 61–91 years as compared to a control group aged 18–36 years. With inclusion of complex word completion tests, it could be demonstrated that the determinants of behavior of young and old people are different. However, slowing of motor movements or peripheral sensitivity is only one aspect which occurs with advancing age. Slowness of cognitive abilities seems to be even more evident in the elderly (BIRREN et al. 1962, 1979). Intellectual abilities decline progressively with age after they have reached a culminating point in early adolescence (WECHSLER 1939, 1958). However, this generalization had not been accepted in this way by several other investigators. Differences in mean performance of the Wechsler subtests in aged individuals were reported by RABIN (1945) as well as MADONICK and SOLOMON (1947), who found that not all abilities measured by the Wechsler test were affected in an equal manner in people aged 60–85 years. FOX and BIRREN (1950) investigated 50 individuals restricted to 60–69 years of age and they found that the subtests concerning information, vocabulary, and comprehension showed least decline while those concerning block design, picture arrangements, and digit symbols had declined more. BOTWINICK (1967) described a more rapid decline in performance of nonverbal abilities than of verbal abilities with age. EISDORFER et al. (1959) investigated the relationship between verbal and performance IQs in 130 volunteers aged over 60 years and in 32 hospitalized patients. Verbal IQs were found to be higher than performance IQs in 94% of people with higher socioeconomic standard and in 72% of people with lower socioeconomic standard. These relationships could be found in both groups, the volunteers and the hospitalized patients. EISDORFER (1963) performed a second full-scale WAIS in a 3-year follow-up study in 165 volunteers (65–75 years old) from the Duke Geriatrics Project sample. As a result of the retest, he found only minor decline in scores and minor changes in test performance tending to the mean. THALER (1956) investigated the relationships among the different psychometric tests such as Wechsler-Bellevue Intelligence Scale, Weigl Color Form Sorting Test, and Rorschach Test in 116 normal volunteers ranging from 60 to 101 years of age with a mean age of 73 years deriving from middle and lower middle class socioeconomic standard. She found a decreased performance in the Wechsler subtests (vocabulary, information, block design, and digit symbol tests) with increasing age. Another finding which seems to be of importance is that of JARVIK et al. (1962), who investigated intellectual changes in 134 aged twins living in the community. Using the Wechsler-Bellevue Intelligence Scale and the Stanford-Binet-Test, they found improved scores in a retest 1 year later, which were attributed to "test wiseness."

A second retest 7 years later showed a significant decline in performance (tapping and digit symbols) while other subtests did not yield different results as compared to investigations performed before. The authors concluded that not all functions of intelligence decline with age but only some abilities. BIRREN (1968) retested 29 aged persons after an interval of 5 years. During this time, the result of the full-scale score of WAIS had decreased 9.6 points on average in 24 out of the 29 people. In the remaining five people, the score showed a small increase or did not change at all. From these studies and from the investigation of BIRREN et al. (1963), it thus becomes clear that a decline in intellectual functions occurs only over a period of normal cerebral aging lasting years. Furthermore, the intellectual changes in normal elderly people are subject to considerable individual variations.

II. Cerebral Blood Flow

A large number of well-documented relationships exists between cerebral blood flow on the one hand and oxidative metabolism of the brain [i.e., the cerebral metabolic rates (CMR) of both oxygen and glucose] on the other. Therefore, cerebral blood flow will be discussed along with CMR-oxygen and CMR-glucose.

In normal adults, cerebral blood flow is controlled by two main factors which also ensure the enormously high supply of the brain with blood and substrates. These factors are the cerebral perfusion pressure and the partial pressure of CO_2 in the arterial blood (pa CO_2). The cerebral perfusion pressure is calculated as the difference of mean arterial blood pressure and intracranial pressure. In the case of a normal intracranial pressure, only the relationship between mean arterial blood pressure and cerebral blood flow is of importance.

This pressure/flow relationship is well known as autoregulation of cerebral blood flow which remains unchanged within the ranges of mean arterial blood pressure of 50–150 mm Hg (BERNSMEIER 1963; CARLYLE and GRAYSON 1955; DINSDALE et al. 1974; EKSTRÖM-JODAL et al. 1972; HÄGGENDAL 1965; HARPER 1965, 1966; HOYER et al. 1974; JONES et al. 1975; LASSEN 1959, 1974; LASSEN and AGNOLI 1972; MILLER et al. 1972; RAPELA and GREEN 1964; STRANDGAARD et al. 1973, 1974, 1975; YOSHIDA et al. 1966). Within these ranges of mean arterial blood pressure, both the oxidative and energy metabolism of the brain seem to remain unchanged (HOYER et al. 1974; KAASIK et al. 1970; SIESJÖ and ZWETNOW 1970; SIESJÖ et al. 1971; ZWETNOW 1970).

Cerebral blood flow changes with pa CO_2. Blood flow of the brain falls in arterial hypocapnia, whereas it increases in arterial hypercapnia. This phenomenon is known as CO_2 reactivity of the cerebral vessels (ALBERTI et al. 1975; ALEXANDER et al. 1964, 1965, 1968a; GOTOH et al. 1965; HÄGGENDAL and JOHANSSON 1965; HARPER and GLASS 1965; HERRSCHAFT and SCHMIDT 1973; KETY and SCHMIDT 1946, 1948; LASSEN 1974; MEYER et al. 1962; PATTERSON et al. 1955; RAICHLE et al. 1970; REIVICH 1964; SEVERINGHAUS and LASSEN 1967; SHAPIRO et al. 1965, 1966; WOLLMAN et al. 1965, 1968).

Within the ranges of pa CO_2 of 15 to about 80 mm Hg, the cerebral metabolic rates of both oxygen and glucose remain constant and so does cerebral energy metabolism (ALBERTI et al. 1975; ALEXANDER et al. 1965, 1968b; COHEN et al. 1964, 1968; FOLBERGROVA et al. 1972; GOTTSTEIN et al. 1976, 1977; GRANHOLM and SIESJÖ 1969, 1971; GRANHOLM et al. 1969; SIESJÖ and MESSETER 1971).

Under normal conditions, the brain only uses glucose to obtain energy (GIBBS et al. 1942; GOTTSTEIN et al. 1963; HOYER 1970a). Glucose enters the brain by means of a facilitated transport mechanism across the blood-brain barrier. Only about 5% of the total amount of glucose metabolized in the brain diffuses across the blood brain barrier under normal conditions (ATKINSON and WEISS 1969; BACHELARD 1971a, b, 1975; BACHELARD et al. 1972, 1973; CRONE and THOMPSON 1970; NEMOTO et al. 1978; OLDENDORF 1971, 1976; PARDRIDGE and OLDENDORF 1977). In the brain cells, glucose is metabolized in the cytoplasm via the Embden-Meyerhof pathway and in the mitochondria via the tricarboxylic acid cycle, which is extended by a γ-aminobutyric acid (GABA) shunt and an amino acid pool with different compartments (SACKS 1957, 1965, 1969, 1976).

The problem as to whether autoregulation of cerebral blood flow or CO_2 reactivity of the cerebral vessels are unchanged or disturbed in normal cerebral aging is far from being resolved. No data on autoregulation of cerebral blood flow in aged normals can be found in the literature. Only scanty results on CO_2 reactivity of the cerebral vessels are available in normal elderly people. SCHIEVE and WILSON (1953) found that CO_2 reactivity of cerebral blood vessels in seven normal people aged 50–76 years did not differ from a normal young control group though the reaction of CO_2 was insignificantly reduced. These findings agree with the observation of DEKONINCK et al. (1975), who found normal responses of cerebral blood flow to both hypercapnia and hypocapnia in relatively healthy elderly people. YAMAMOTO et al. (1980) investigated 24 volunteers aged from 24 to 82 years without any cerebro- or cardiovascular disorders and risk factors. They found a significant reduction of vasodilatation response to hypercapnic CO_2 with advancing age, which was accounted for by an atrophy of cortical gray matter or cerebral arteriosclerosis or both.

Another question yielding conflicting results is whether advancing age will reduce cerebral blood flow and metabolism.

In 1956, KETY reviewed the results of 11 publications of different investigators. He concluded that there is a remarkable decline in both cerebral blood flow and oxygen uptake of the brain from childhood through adolescence, then followed by a more gradual but progressive reduction in senility. Corresponding to the reduction in blood flow and oxygen uptake of the brain, the cerebral vascular resistance increased with age. FAZEKAS et al. (1952) compared mentally normal people below and over the age of 50 years. Individuals younger than 50 years did not reveal any variations of blood flow and oxygen consumption of the brain as compared to a group of young healthy volunteers. Individuals over the age of 50 years, however, showed significant reductions in both brain blood flow and oxygen uptake. It is, however, remarkable that the individual data of cerebral blood flow and cerebral metabolic rate of oxygen scattered very much with age: low values were found as well as "normal" ones in both parameters. SCHEINBERG et al. (1953) investigated 32 people aged from 38 to 79 years with normal brain functions. They obtained a significantly lower cerebral blood flow as compared to a control group aged 18–36 years, but the cerebral metabolic rate of oxygen had not significantly changed. Individuals older than 56 years showed a significantly reduced cerebral blood flow as compared to a group aged 38–55 years. The cerebral metabolic rate of oxygen did not show any significant differences between these two groups. NARITOMI et al. (1979) investigated cerebral blood flow in 46 volunteers aged from 21 to 63 years, who were arbitrarily classified into two subgroups below and above 40 years of age. The investigators found a gradual reduction of gray matter flow with advancing age, which was attributed in part to neuronal atrophy and in part to cerebral arteriosclerosis. FRACKOWIAK et al. (1980) investigated cerebral blood flow and the cerebral metabolic rate of oxygen in cerebral gray matter as well as in cerebral white matter in 14 normal volunteers aged from 26 to 74 years. They showed reductions of both cerebral blood flow and cerebral metabolic rate of oxygen in cerebral gray matter with increasing age while no age-related changes could be observed in cerebral white matter.

Although these above-mentioned studies seem to demonstrate a clear relationship between advancing age and decreasing brain blood flow and metabolism, it would be necessary to regard it with certain reserve. For these studies are limited in that elderly individuals investigated were both volunteers living in the community and hospitalized patients. They were designated "normal" by exclusion of mental or vascular diseases, but mental normality was not proved by means of psychological test or EEG or both. LASSEN et al. (1960) studied cerebral blood flow and brain oxygen uptake bilaterally in young and aged normal subjects, whereby normality was demonstrated by several psychometric tests. Normal elderly subjects aged 66–79 years did not show any differences in cerebral blood flow as compared to a control group aged 22–29 years neither in the 10 min nor in the infinity values. However, brain uptake of oxygen was significantly reduced in the elderly to 2.72 ml/100 g min as compared to 2.98 ml/100 g min in the controls as calculated to infinity. The 10-min values did not show any difference in brain oxygen consumption between these two groups.

SCHIEVE and WILSON (1953) studied cerebral blood flow and cerebral metabolic rate of oxygen in a total of 29 healthy people at mean ages of 29, 40, and 64 years. They found no statistically significant difference in cerebral blood flow and brain oxygen consumption within these different age groups. DASTUR et al. (1963) investigated a total of 68 individuals in the 8th decade of their life. Twenty-six out of these, aged 71 years on average, were mentally and physically intact (BUTLER et al. 1965); the remaining suffered from arterial hypertension, arteriosclerosis, or both. Fifteen people aged 21 years served as controls. The investigators failed to demonstrate changes in the blood flow and oxygen consumption of the brain in the elderly healthy subjects as compared to the control group of young people. There was, however, a significant decrease in cerebral glucose consumption in healthy elderlies. This result could be confirmed in animal experiments. SMITH et al. (1980) demonstrated in the resting conscious rat that aging is associated with decreases in glucose utilization in specific regions of the brain.

In the study of DASTUR et al., 22 out of the 26 healthy old people showed normal EEG tracings; the other four people had mild diffuse slowing of EEG frequency, focal slow waves, or amplitude asymmetry (OBRIST et al. 1963).

It thus becomes evident that cerebral blood flow does not seem to decline with normal cerebral aging. Changes in the brain blood flow with age are therefore probably related to illnesses in age than to age per se (GOTTSTEIN and HELD 1979; HEDLUND et al. 1964; OLESEN 1974; SHENKIN et al. 1953). The small but significant reductions in the cerebral metabolic rates of oxygen (LASSEN et al. 1960) and of glucose (DASTUR et al. 1963; SMITH et al. 1980) might tentatively be accounted for by a progressive loss of cerebral cortical neurons, dendrites, and dendritic spines with physiological cerebral aging. BRODY (1955, 1978) described a decrease in neurons of approximately 40% by the 9th decade, particularly in frontal and temporal areas. COLON (1972) confirmed these findings in two cases of undemented people over 80 years of age. SHEFER (1973) reported a decrease of 22% in area 6, of 28% in area 10, and of 23% in area 21 with an average decrease of 20% for all regions. BALL (1977) calculated approximately 6% neuron loss per decade. It is well documented that the loss of cortical neurons with physiological aging is associated with a reduction in the number of dendrites and dendritic spines (SCHEIBEL 1978; SCHEIBEL and SCHEIBEL 1975; SCHEIBEL et al. 1975, 1976). It is speculated by BIRREN et al. (1979) that both the loss of neurons and the reduction in synapses might be the cause of the slowing of complex behavioral patterns.

III. Electroencephalography

As has been mentioned above, healthy elderly people show as well as normal EEG tracings with a mean frequency of 9.16 c/s, a mild diffuse slowing of EEG frequency, as focal abnormalities and amplitude asymmetry (Obrist et al. 1963). Busse et al. (1956) studied 223 healthy volunteers, of whom 153 underwent psychometric tests, which revealed no significant differences between them. Of the volunteers, 49% had normal EEG tracings as compared to EEG standards established for young adults. In 15% of the subjects, diffuse disturbances, i.e., diffusely slowed or diffusely fast or combined fast and slow records, could be observed. Thirty-five percent of the total of 223 volunteers demonstrated focal disturbances, of which all but two were localized temporally. These temporal focuses could be found on the left side in 78%. Reduction in alpha frequency seems to be a most common finding with age. In young adults, the mean alpha rhythm was found to be 10.2–10.5 c/s (Brazier and Finesinger 1944). In mentally healthy subjects between 60 and 90 years of age, alpha frequency fell from 9.7 to 9.0 c/s (Obrist and Busse 1965; Otomo 1966). Mundy-Castle et al. (1954) found a mean alpha rhythm of 9.4 c/s in a group of healthy individuals aged 75 years on average. Studying aged normal individuals, Obrist (1954) and Obrist et al. (1966) observed a mean alpha frequency of 9.1 c/s in the 7th and 8th decade of life, and a decrease to 8.6 c/s over the age ov 80 years. The progression of reduction of alpha rhythm was apparent in more than 50% of mentally healthy old people over a period of 15 years. Thaler (1956) reported that advancing age does not seem to correlate with any particular EEG classification. She found abnormal EEGs in 62% of 116 normal volunteers aged from 60 to 101 years. Comparing EEG changes between males and females with respect to normal aging, Obrist and Busse (1965) found significantly lower alpha frequencies in males than in females of comparable age.

Fast EEG activity was observed as low-voltage beta rhythm in about 50% of mentally healthy individuals with well-preserved intellect (Busse and Wang 1965; Obrist 1954). Diffuse slow activity under 7 c/s was found to be relatively rare among mentally normal volunteers aged 60–75 years. Obrist and Busse (1965) found such slow waves in only 6%–8% of the subjects investigated. After the age of 75 years, a significant increase of slow EEG frequency could be observed in more than 20% of the subjects (Silverman et al. 1955). As mentioned above (Busse et al. 1956), focal slow EEG activities could be found in 30%–40% of healthy community volunteers over the age of 60 years. Foci were predominant over the left anterior temporal area (Busse et al. 1954). They consisted mainly in the appearance of theta and delta rhythms, in marked amplitude asymmetries and occasionally in spikes and waves. The demonstration of such temporal foci seems to depend on the electrode placement (Silverman et al. 1955). Differences in EEG recording techniques may therefore lead to a failing of high incidence of temporal foci in mentally healthy elderly people (Obrist 1954; Sheridan et al. 1955). Evidence for focal temporal abnormalities were repeatedly reported and their significance discussed by Busse et al. (1956) and Busse and Obrist (1965). However, the exact origin of these temporal foci on the left side has still remained unclear. Several different reasons are discussed (Obrist 1976). These foci are most often clinically silent and do not show any relationship to cerebral dominance, aphasia, or seizures

(BUSSE and OBRIST 1963; FREY and SJÖGREN 1959; SILVERMAN et al. 1955). Longitudinal studies over a period of 3–4 years showed stability of the foci and absence of clinical symptoms (BUSSE and OBRIST 1963).

To summarize the influence of normal cerebral aging on behavior, blood flow, and oxidative metabolism of the brain and EEG, the following conclusions can be drawn:

Intellectual functions do not generally decline with aging. Age-related changes in intelligence are subject to considerable individual variations. If a reduction occurs, it is more noticeable in nonverbal performance than in verbal abilities.

In the EEG, alpha rhythm shifts to the slow side and shows a frequency of 8–9 c/s. Focal disturbances can be observed relatively often, predominantly over the left anterior temporal region.

Cerebral blood flow is not significantly reduced with normal cerebral aging. However, there is evidence that both oxygen and glucose consumption of the brain decrease to a smaller but significant extent with age.

As far as correlations between behavior, EEG, and/or cerebral blood flow and metabolism are concerned, OBRIST et al. (1962) failed to demonstrate any relation between intellectual function and EEG in normal senescence. After an interval of 3.5 years on average, WANG et al. (1970) found a decline in both verbal and performance abilities which was greater in subjects having temporal foci than in individuals without temporal foci. OBRIST (1975) could not find any differences between individuals with and without temporal focal EEG abnormalities with respect to learning ability, 48-h retention, memory scale performance, or intelligence test scores. When EEG on the one hand and brain blood flow and oxygen consumption on the other were compared, no relationship could be demonstrated. WANG et al. (1970) studied cerebral blood flow in 24 volunteers aged 79 years on average. Twelve years after the initial investigations, subjects having normal cerebral blood flow rates showed higher scores in both verbal and performance abilities than those individuals in whom cerebral blood flow had decreased. However, none of these differences was statistically significant. LASSEN et al. (1960) concluded from their bilateral study of cerebral blood flow and oxygen consumption that the beginning of intellectual decline with age may possible be associated with a mild reduction in oxygen consumption in the dominant hemisphere. This intriguing assumption is not inconsistent with the high rate of EEG abnormalities in the left temporal lobe.

If thus may be unequivocally stated that normal cerebral aging is associated with only minor slowness in behavior and EEG and only minimal reductions in the cerebral metabolic rates of both oxygen and glucose.

C. Abnormal Cerebral Aging

Dementia due to primary or secondary brain diseases is the most common cerebral illness in middle-aged and elderly people. Degenerative or cerebrovascular changes in brain tissue are responsible for primary dementias, while dementia symptoms associated with extracerebral diseases should be strictly distinguished in clinical and pathophysiological terms and should be designated as secondary dementia.

Degenerative changes in brain tissue cause dementia in about 60%–70%. Cerebrovascular disturbances (multi-infarct) alone are responsible for dementia in only 20%–30%, while both degenerative and cerebrovascular variations are present in 15%–20% (JELLINGER 1976; TOMLINSON 1980; TOMLINSON et al. 1970). Nosologically, "simple" senile dementia and both Alzheimer's senile and Alzheimer's presenile dementia may be regarded as variations of the same degenerative brain disease (ALBERT 1964; ARAB 1960; CONSTANTINIDIS 1978; KATZMAN 1976; LAUTER and MEYER 1968; NEWTON 1948; TERRY 1976, 1978). It has become evident that the cerebrovascular (multi-infarct) brain processes may be related to disturbances in cerebral microcirculation, which might lead to circumscribed nerve cell loss with gliosis (CORSELLIS 1969). From these findings, HACHINSKI et al. (1974) pointed out that "the use of the term ‚cerebral atherosclerosis' to describe mental deterioration in the elderly is probably the most common medical misdiagnosis." Arteriosclerosis or thrombosis of the larger arterial brain vessels would lead primarily to neurological disorders such as strokes and may therefore be of marginal relevance in the development of dementia symptoms.

I. Clinical Symptoms

Dementia comprises a global deterioration of higher mental functions and intellectual capacities. It may be defined as a global disturbance of "mental functioning in its intellectual, emotional, and cognitive aspects" (MAYER-GROSS et al. 1969). According to WEITBRECHT (1963) and HUBER (1972), it should be stressed that dementia can develop reversibly and irreversibly. McHUGH and FOLSTEIN (1979) defined dementia as a deterioration of cognitive functions including memory, abstract reasoning, attention, language, and perception without prominent disturbances in consciousness. Disturbances in mood with anxiety and depression, in affectiveness, paranoid symptoms, delusions, hallucinations, personality changes, and catastrophic reactions are also associated with dementia (BLESSED 1980; McHUGH and FOLSTEIN 1979). Different dementia syndromes can be well documented and classified in respect to severity as clusters by means and the AMP rating scale system (HELMCHEN 1975; SCHARFETTER 1972).

Differentiating degenerative from multi-infarct dementia due to primary brain diseases, ROTH (1978) pointed out that females show a marked higher predominance of degenerative dementia while multi-infarct dementia is found to be more frequent in men. Sudden appearance of neurological or psychological deficits such as aphasia, agnosia, or apraxia and emotional lability with depressive symptoms along with well-preserved intelligence and personality are more common and pronounced in multi-infarct dementia, the course of which is mostly intermittent and fluctuating ("stepwise downhill") (BLESSED 1980). Such clinical symptoms are almost invariably obscured in presenile and senile degenerative dementia. Its course is slowly progressive (BLESSED 1980) and shows general impairment of cognitive functions. BLESSED et al. (1968) studied demented patients and scaled their psychiatric symptoms. There was no support that degnerative changes in brain tissue had caused functional psychiatric disturbances or delirious states. However, a close correlation could be found between the number of senile plaques and scores for dementia and performance in psychological tests. By means of an ischemic score outlined by MAYER-GROSS et al. (1969), it is possible to differentiate between the two main dementia types, primary degenerative and multi-infarct dementia. Its usefulness was tested by HACHINSKI et al. (1975) and confirmed by HARRISON et al. (1979), ROSEN et al. (1980), and LOEB (1980). LOEB, however, stressed that a definite grouping between the two main types of dementia should be based upon additional investigations such as EEG and computerized tomography of the brain besides clinical and psychometric examinations.

Dementia due to extracerebral diseases or due to brain diseases, which cannot be accounted for by degenerative or multi-infarct brain processes, should be designated as secondary dementias. Cardiac or circulatory diseases, endogenous or exogenous intoxications, infections, traumas, oxygen, glucose, mineral, or vitamin deficiencies, blood diseases, etc., may produce dementia symptoms which are frequently characterized by delirious and clouded states (ROTH 1978). Differentiation between primary and secondary dementia should be based upon exact physical and neuropsychiatric examinations, psychometric tests, and laboratory investigations including blood chemistry, cerebrospinal fluid, ECG, EEG, computerized tomography of the brain, and other X-ray studies.

II. Cerebral Blood Flow and Metabolism

It has been well documented in numerous investigations that, irrespective of its cause, dementia is closely related to changes in brain blood flow and metabolism. FREYHAN et al. (1951) studied blood flow and oxygen consumption of the brain in patients suffering from psychoses of senility due either to cerebral arteriosclerosis or senile psychosis and they found reductions in both blood flow and oxygen consumption in both groups of patients. Differences between the two groups were not evident. In comparable groups of patients, reductions in cerebral blood flow and oxygen consumption, of the same degree, were reported by FAZEKAS et al. (1952, 1953), LASSEN et al. (1960), OBRIST et al. (1962), HEDLUND et al. (1964), BUTLER et al. (1965), MUNCK et al. (1968), INGVAR (1970), OBRIST et al. (1970), and GRUBB et al. (1977).

A close correlation between reduced cerebral oxygen consumption and intellectual impairment was demonstrated by LASSEN et al. (1957) and KLEE (1964). HAGBERG and INGVAR (1976) correlated psychometric findings with regional cerebral blood flow in presenile dementia. The abnormalities in regional cerebral blood flow with accentuation in posteriotemporal, parietal, and occipital areas correlated well with the type of reduction of cognitive functions. These findings had been outlined with more detailed psychological data by GUSTAFSON and RISBERG (1974), GUSTAFSON (1975), and GUSTAFSON and HAGBERG (1975). All these results mentioned above might support the assumption that dementia may be mainly associated with disturbances in global or regional cerebral blood flow which are mostly due to arteriosclerosis of the brain vessels. However, this assumption had to be dismissed after GOTTSTEIN et al. (1964) had described a decrease of the cerebral glucose consumption as the main variation. This was accompanied by normal or only slightly decreased cerebral blood flow and normal oxygen consumption. The findings of HOYER (1970b) confirmed the results of GOTT-

STEIN et al. In could furthermore be demonstrated that, in unclassified dementia, cerebral blood flow was predominantly decreased in about 20% of the patients investigated while in about 80% of the dementia patients disturbances in either oxygen consumption or glucose metabolism of the brain were the main derangements. It thus became evident that cerebral blood flow and metabolism were not uniformly varied in dementia but could be related to different dementia types in pathophysiological terms (HOYER 1969; HOYER and BECKER 1966). O'BRIEN and MALLETT (1970) and O'BRIEN (1972) studied cerebral blood flow in patients suffering either from primary neuronal degeneration or from dementia symptoms due to cerebrovascular disease. They found that the cortical perfusion rates and cerebrovascular resistance was different between the two groups. In primary neuronal degeneration, no change of blood flow could be observed as compared to dementia-free controls, and in patients with cerebrovascular disease brain blood flow was decreased. However, the primary neuronal group did not consist of a single pathological type. Based on the ischemic score outlined by MAYER-GROSS et al. (1969) (see above), HACHINSKI et al. (1975) confirmed this pattern in cerebral blood flow in pure dementia patients. They described a decrease of flow in patients suffering from multi-infarct dementia. In patients belonging to the primary degenerative type of dementia, cerebral blood flow was normal. There was no correlation between degree of dementia and cerebral blood flow in the primary degenerative group, but an inverse relationship could be found in the patients suffering from multi-infarct dementia. Studying regional cerebral blood flow pattern, INGVAR et al. (1978) reported on most marked flow decreases in postcentral regions in the occipito-temporal-parietal and in the frontal areas in Alzheimer's disease while in multi-infarct dementias flow was reduced without a notable lack of regional features. Additionally, LADURNER et al. (1977) found lower flow rates in the left cerebral hemisphere as compared to the right mainly in multi-infarct dementias, whereas in primary degenerative dementia there was only a trend in this direction. From a statistical point of view, different distribution curves of blood flow and oxygen consumption of the brain between the two main dementia types could be demonstrated. Mean global blood flow and mean oxygen consumption of the brain were low in multi-infarct dementia, but could be found to be unchanged on average in primary degenerative dementia. However, there was no correlation, but an overlap in cerebral glucose uptake between the two groups (HOYER et al. 1975a). As far as cerebral blood flow and cerebral oxygen consumption are concerned, DEKONINCK et al. (1977) confirmed these findings in patients with senile dementia either due to primary degenerative or due to multi-infarct brain processes. With respect to the course of both dementia types, HOYER (1978a, b, 1980) described the predominant disturbance as being that in cerebral glucose metabolism in the early stage of the dementias, whereas cerebral blood flow and oxygen consumption of the brain were found to be normal. It was presumed that the lack of glucose found in the degenerative type might be compensated by the combustion of subtrates other than glucose and that the "surplus" of glucose found in the multi-infarct type might not be used metabolically, but abnormally stored in the brain cells. In the further course of both dementia types, blood flow and oxygen and glucose consumption of the brain decline progressively to run into a final common path of a low functional level in the chronic phase of the dementias. Thus, significant differences might be observed between the two main dementia types with respect to blood flow and metabolism in the earlier stages of the dementia process. This distinction might be impossible in more advanced dementias (OBRIST 1978; OBRIST et al. 1975). When cerebral blood flow and metabolism were related to the psychiatric status as measured by means of the AMP rating scale system (see above), HOYER et al. (1979) could not find any correlation between the degree of psychiatric impairment and the reduced cerebral blood flow and metabolism as described by GUSTAFSON et al. (1972). HOYER et al., however, demonstrated a clear correlation between the functional state of the brain and its blood flow and metabolism, i.e., productive dementia symptoms seem to be associated with abnormally increased brain blood flow and metabolism if no brain atrophy exists, but brain blood flow and metabolism are significantly decreased if the brain has atrophied although the clinical symptomatology is productive. In nonproductive dementia, however, a close correlation between reduced mental impairment and brain blood flow and metabolism is present. This pattern of blood flow and metabolism becomes strikingly evident in patients suffering from Korsakow's syndrome as was pointed out by SIMARD et al. (1971) and HOYER and OESTERREICH (1980).

There are only scanty investigations on cerebral blood flow and metabolism in dementia with respect to autoregulation of cerebral blood flow and CO_2 reactivity of the brain vessels, respectively. SCHIEVE and WILSON (1953) found different effects of CO_2 on cerebral blood flow and thus suggested two types of dementia: one due to primary degeneration of brain parenchyma and the other due to diseases of the brain vessels. FAZEKAS et al. (1953) also demonstrated well-preserved reactions of cerebral blood flow and oxygen consumption under hypercapnia as well as under hypocapnia, which were confirmed by LASSEN et al. (1957). SIMARD (1971) and SIMARD et al. (1971) demonstrated that neither global nor focal abnormalities to vasoreactive functions such as hypo- or hypercapnia, arterial hypo- or hypertension were present in dementia. HACHINSKI et al. (1975) reported on a normal reactivity of blood vessels to hypocapnia in primary degenerative and in multi-infarct dementia although the reactivity was slightly less in the multi-infarct group as compared to the patients with primary degenerative dementia. Similar results were described by DEKONINCK et al. (1977). The vasoactive response to CO_2 due to hypercapnia was stronger in primary degenerative dementia than in multi-infarct dementia. There were, however, no statistically significant differences. On the other hand, YAMAGUCHI et al. (1980) found a reduced cerebral vasodilator response to carbon dioxide in multi-infarct dementia while the CO_2 reactivity of the cerebral vessels was normal in patients with Alzheimer's disease.

As far as secondary dementia is concerned, only those extracerebral diseases shall be referred to here which frequently produce severe changes in brain function, e.g., dementia. Secondary dementia is associated with various disturbances in brain blood flow and oxidative metabolism. KETY et al. (1948a) found blood flow and oxygen consumption of the brain to be decreased in patients suffering from a severe diabetic acidosis. The cerebral metabolic rate of oxygen was decreased to about 50% of normal in diabetic coma, but cerebral blood flow was increased. Reduction in cerebral oxygen consumption correlated well with a ketonemia in arterial blood. PAULSON et al. (1968) also described a decrease in the cerebral metabolic rate of oxygen in patients suffering from diabetes mellitus. GOTTSTEIN et al. (1971) showed a cerebral utilization of ketone bodies in diabetic patients: the cerebral uptake of ketone bodies depends on their arterial concentration. Arterial hypoglycemia below a critical level of 1.7 mM will also lead to functional disturbances of the brain since the carrier mediating the glucose transport across the blood-brain barrier is not sufficiently saturated and is thus reduced in its capacity (BACHELARD 1971 b, 1975). The cerebral metabolic rate of oxygen decreases beyond the threshold of arterial glucose concentration of 1.7 mM (GOTTSTEIN et al. 1977; KETY et al. 1948 b).

Cerebral blood flow and metabolism were described to be not uniformly varied in arterial hyperammonemia due to liver diseases. FAZEKAS and BESSMAN (1953), FAZEKAS et al. (1956), POSNER and PLUM (1960), and WECHSLER et al. (1954) found both decreases in blood flow and oxygen consumption of the brain in precoma and hepatic coma. BIANCHIPORRO et al. (1969) and MAIOLO et al. (1971) grouped their patients suffering from hepatic insufficiency into three: those having liver cirrhosis, hepatic encephalopathy, or hepatic coma. They reported normal cerebral blood flow rates in liver cirrhosis and hepatic encephalopathy, and in general also in coma regardless of its degree and duration. Oxygen consumption and glucose uptake of the brain were found to be within normal limits in liver cirrhosis. The cerebral metabolic rate of oxygen was decreased in patients suffering from hepatic encephalopathy and from coma, but the cerebral metabolic rate of glucose was described to be at a rather low but normal level. When the degree of coma was graded, cerebral blood flow was found to be slightly increased in the mildest form of neuropsychiatric involvement but it decreased proportionally to more severe coma grades. The cerebral metabolic rates of both oxygen and glucose behaved similarly. Separating acute from chronic cases, they found increased cerebral blood flow rates in acute and decreased rates in chronic in both hepatic encephalopathy and coma. In acute hepatic encephalopathy and coma, the oxygen consumption of the brain was described as within normal limits and the glucose uptake as slightly increased. In chronic hepatic encephalopathy and coma, marked reductions in the cerebral metabolic rates of both oxygen and glucose were observed. These investigators speculated whether the slightly increased cerebral glucose uptake would serve to bind and thus to detoxify ammonia in the brain, yielding glutamine, a reaction which was suggested by BESSMAN (1961), BESSMAN and BESSMAN (1955), and BESSMAN et al. (1954). In patients with hepatic encephalopathy, HOYER et al. (1975 b) found normal rates of blood flow and oxygen consumption of the brain but different changes in the cerebral metabolic rates of glucose. An increased glucose uptake was associated with a cerebral release of glutamate and glutamine. When cerebral glucose uptake was decreased, a delivery of glutamate and glutamine by the brain could not be measured. ERBSLÖH et al. (1958) found a significant decrease of cerebral glucose uptake correlating with increasing impairment of the liver. In precomatose patients due to hepatic insufficiency, GOTTSTEIN (1966, 1975) found significant reductions in blood flow, as well as oxygen and glucose consumption of the brain. In a catamnestic study, PAPENBERG et al. (1975) observed normal rates of cerebral blood flow and oxygen uptake and normal EEG in hepatoencephalic patients who were still alive 3 years after the first investigation. Patients suffering from hepatic encephalopathy of the same degree, but showing a decreased cerebral oxygen uptake and severe changes in EEG at the first investigation had died by that time.

In uremia, HEYMAN et al. (1951) and SCHEINBERG (1954) measured a reduction of the cerebral metabolic rates of oxygen and glucose. GOTTSTEIN et al. (1972) described a close correlation between the degree of disturbance of consciousness and the reduction of the cerebral parameters mentioned. In all studies, cerebral blood flow was not different from normal.

In different blood diseases, the abnormalities in cerebral blood flow and metabolism were different. In pernicious anemia, both oxygen and glucose consumption of the brain were found to be decreased though cerebral blood flow was increased (GOTTSTEIN 1979; SCHEINBERG 1951). In hypochromic anemia, cerebral blood flow is also increased but the cerebral metabolic rates of oxygen and glucose are normal. These cerebral metabolic rates are also unchanged as compared to normal in polycythemia, in which cerebral blood flow is decreased due to an increase in hematocrit, resulting in a deterioration of blood viscosity (GOTTSTEIN 1979).

In dementia due to chronic alcoholism, HOYER (to be published) described reductions in blood flow and oxygen and glucose consumption of the brain. The cerebral metabolic rate of oxygen was decreased most and thus confirmed the findings of BATTEY et al. (1953) and FAZEKAS et al. (1955). On the other hand, INGVAR et al. (1969) reported on increased, as well as normal and subnormal blood flow rates in patients with chronic alcoholism. No correlations with the type or degree of intellectual impairment were found. MARX et al. (1975) suspected a tendency to higher cerebral blood flow rates in delirious and postdelirious phases of delirium tremens.

III. Electroencephalography

In the previous chapter, it was outlined that the different types of dementia are associated mainly with reductions in cerebral blood flow and/or oxygen consumption and/or glucose uptake of the brain. Since it can be expected that the maintenance of the electrical activity of the brain depends on an adequate cerebral blood flow and metabolism (KRUPP 1966), changes in the latter should produce impairments in EEG. So OBRIST et al. (1963) reported on increasing slow activity in EEG along with reductions in cerebral blood flow and oxygen consumption. Similar correlations had been described by JOHANNESSON et al. (1977), who did not find a consistent relationship between EEG abnormalities and mean hemispheric blood flow, but there was a significant negative correlation between EEG variations and blood flow in occipital regions. In a more extensive study, SULG (1969) came to the same conclusion. Besides these correlations between cerebral blood flow and metabolism on the one hand and electrical activity of the brain on the other, the problem as to which EEG changes occur in dementia with respect to the different types and to the severity of the symptoms is of importance. McADAM and ROBINSON (1956) used a psychiatric rating scale to grade the degree of dementia which was compared with EEG. They found that the worse the EEG, the lower the psychiatric score, or, the lower the frequency, the lower the clinical score. In a subsequent study, McADAM and ROBINSON (1962) demonstrated correlations between the severity of dementia and the occurrence of theta and delta activities in the EEG. Along with the results of Mundy-Castle et al. (1954), Weiner and Schuster (1956), and Turton and Warren (1960), one might conclude that the slower the EEG activity, the greater the mental impairment. On the other hand, Liberson and Sequin (1945) concluded from their studies in arteriosclerotic and senile patients that mental disturbances such as anxiety, agitation, and delusions did not show marked abnormalities in EEG. Luce and Rothschild (1953) also failed to demonstrate any relationship between disturbances in the EEG and psychiatric symptoms such as delusions, hallucinations, or emotional derangement. In their study in almost 200 hospitalized elderly individuals, Barnes et al. (1956) found marked electroencephalographic differences. Patients suffering from organic brain disease showed generalized disturbances, mostly diffuse slow waves in 69%, while normal tracings in the EEG were identified in 17%. According to Luce and Rothschild (1953), normal EEG was generally associated with mild or moderate indications of mental deficit. Obrist et al. (1962) and Irving et al. (1970) confirmed these findings. The EEG is of great help in distinguishing between organic brain disease and functional psychiatric illness. In the latter, EEG was described as abnormal in only 9%–38% (Barnes et al. 1956; Luce and Rothschild 1953; Obrist and Henry 1958; Pampiglione and Post 1958). Patients suffering from organic brain disease and showing a high incidence of diffuse slow (delta and theta) wave activity remained hospitalized or died within a year. The majority of patients with functional brain disorders and normal EEG, however, were more likely to be discharged or transferred to convalescent homes (Obrist and Henry 1958; Pampiglione and Post 1958; Sheridan et al. 1955). In patients suffering from confirmed Alzheimer's disease, abnormalities in the EEG can be found in approximately 100%. These changes are characterized by generalized irregular, sometimes rhythmic, slow activity (2–7 c/s) and scanty or absent alpha activity (Gordon and Sim 1967; Letemendia and Pampiglione 1958; Liddell 1958; Swain 1959). In cerebrovascular disease, however, the background rhythm in EEG is generally well preserved, but it is also slow with a higher incidence of focal appearance of theta and delta activity (van der Drift and Kok 1972). Constantinidis et al. (1969) investigated EEG changes in cerebrovascular, degenerative, and mixed dementias. In patients suffering from Alzheimer type of dementia, the diffuse EEG slowing with predominant theta and delta activity was confirmed. In dementia due to cerebrovascular disease, a three times slower rhythm with 7–8 c/s and five times more theta and delta foci could be observed. In this way, the EEG might yield the possibility of improving the differential diagnosis of the two main dementia types.

D. Concluding Remarks

There are numerous well-documented findings in gerontology and gerontopsychiatry, which prove unequivocally the significant difference between normal and abnormal cerebral aging. The characteristics of normal cerebral aging differ from those of abnormal cerebral aging in behavior, as well as in cerebral blood flow and metabolism, and in EEG.

The most frequent clinical syndrome in abnormal cerebral aging is dementia, which sould be classified into primary and secondary dementias. Primary dementia is mainly due to degenerative and less due to cerebrovascular disturbances in brain tissue. Secondary dementia is produced by extracerebral diseases or by illnesses not primarily in brain tissue. The degenerative type of dementia is characterized clinically by an impairment of memory and intellect deteriorating slowly but progressively. The cerebrovascular or multi-infarct type shows more emotional lability in direction of depression. Its course is intermittent and fluctuating. In secondary dementia, delirious, and clouded states dominate the clinical picture.

Cerebral blood flow and the cerebral metabolic rates of both oxygen and glucose are not uniformly varied, neither in primary nor in secondary dementia. It has become evident that cerebral blood flow and obviously oxygen consumption of the brain are more deranged in multi-infarct dementia than in the degenerative type, in which disturbances in cerebral glucose metabolism seem to prevail. In secondary dementia, no clear-cut correlations with the changes of brain blood flow and metabolism are found except for the decreased cerebral oxygen consumption, which is associated with several extracerebral diseases.

General slowing of EEG activity along with a loss in alpha rhythm is described to be typical for primary degenerative dementia. In multi-infarct processes, however, a slow alpha rhythm along with frequent theta and delta foci seems to be the characteristic EEG variation.

Although our knowledge on normal and abnormal cerebral aging in the fields of psychology, physiology, and pathophysiology has increased during the past years, it appear necessary to work out more sensitive methods for easier and more exact differentiation between normal and abnormal cerebral aging, i.e., dementia on the one hand and the different dementia types on the other. It may be assumed that recently developed new techniques may be of great assistance (LENZI et al. 1978; SOKOLOFF et al. 1977).

References

Albert E (1964) Senile Demenz und Alzheimersche Krankheit als Ausdruck des gleichen Krankheitsgeschehens. Fortschr Neurol Psychiat 32:625–673

Alberti E, Hoyer S, Hamer J, Stoeckel H, Packschiess P, Weinhardt F (1975) The effect of carbon dioxide on cerebral blood flow and cerebral metabolism in dogs. Br J Anaesth 47:941–947

Alexander SC, Wollman H, Cohen PJ, Behar M (1964) Cerebrovascular response to pa CO_2 during halothane anesthesia in man. J Appl Physiol 19:561–565

Alexander SC, Cohen PJ, Wollman H, Smith TC, Reivich M, van der Molen RA (1965) Cerebral carbohydrate metabolism during hypocarbia in man. Studies during nitrous oxide anesthesia Anesthesiology 26:624–632

Alexander SC, Marshall BE, Agnoli A (1968a) Cerebral blood flow in the goat with sustained hypocapnia. Scand J Clin Lab Invest 22:Suppl 102, VII C

Alexander SC, Smith TC, Strobel G, Stephen GW, Wollman H (1968b) Cerebral carbohydrate metabolism of man during respiratory and metabolic alkalosis. J Appl Physiol 24:66–72

Arab A (1960) Unité nosologique entre démence sénile et maladie d'Alzheimer d'après une étude statistique et anatomo-clinique. Sist Nerv 12:189–201

Atkinson AJ, Weiss MF (1969) Kinetics of blood-cerebrospinal fluid glucose transfer in normal dogs. Am J Physiol 216:1120–1126

Bachelard HS (1971a) Specificity and kinetic properties of monosaccharide uptake into guinea pig cerebral cortex in vitro. J Neurochem 13:213–222

Bachelard HS (1971 b) Glucose transport and phosphorylation in the control of carbohydrate metabolism in the brain. In: Brierly JB, Meldrum BS (eds) Brain hypoxia. Heinemann, London, pp 251–260

Bachelard HS (1975) How does glucose enter brain cells? In: Ingvar DH, Lassen NA (eds) Brain work. The coupling of function, metabolism and blood flow in the brain. Munksgaard, Copenhagen, pp 126–141

Bachelard HS, Daniel PM, Love ER, Pratt OE (1972) The in vivo influx of glucose into the brain of the rat compared with the net cerebral uptake. J Physiol 222:149–150 P

Bachelard HS, Daniel PM, Love ER, Pratt OE (1973) The transport of glucose into the brain of the rat in vivo. Proc R Soc Lond (Biol) 183:71–82

Battey LL, Heyman A, Patterson JL (1953) Effects of ethyl alcohol on cerebral blood flow and oxygen consumption. JAMA 152:6–10

Bernsmeier A (1963) Durchblutung des Gehirns. In: Monnier M (ed) Physiologie und Pathophysiologie des vegetativen Nervensystems, Bd II. Hippokrates, Stuttgart, pp 607–640

Bessman SP (1961) Ammonia and coma. In: Folch-Pi J (ed) Chemical pathology of the nervous system. Pergamon, New York, pp 370–376

Ball MJ (1977) Neuronal loss, neurofibrillary tangles and granulovacuolar degeneration in the hippocampus with ageing and dementia. Acta Neuropath (Berl) 37:111–118

Barnes RH, Busse EW, Friedman EL (1956) The psychological functioning of aged individuals with normal and abnormal electroencephalograms. J Nerv Ment Dis 124:585–593

Bessman SP, Bessman AN (1955) The cerebral and peripheral uptake of ammonia in liver disease with a hypothesis for the mechanism of hepatic coma. J Clin Invest 34:622–628

Bessman SP, Fazekas JF, Bessman AN (1954) Uptake of ammonia by the brain in hepatic coma. Proc Soc Exp Biol Med 85:66–67

Bianchiporro G, Maiolo AT, Galli C, Polli EE (1969) Brain energy metabolism in hepatic coma. II. Int Meet Int Soc Neurochem

Birren JE (1968) Increments and decrements in the intellectual status of the aged. In: Simon A, Epstein LJ (eds) Aging in modern society. Psychiatric report 23. Am Psychiatr Assoc, Washington DC, pp 207–214

Birren JE, Botwinick J (1955) Age difference in finger, jaw, and foot reaction time to auditory stimuli. J Gerontol 10:429–432

Birren JE, Riegel KF, Morrison DF (1962) Age differences in response speed as a function of controlled variations of stimulus conditions: evidence of a general speed factor. Gerontologia 6:1–18

Birren JE, Butler RN, Greenhouse SW, Sokoloff L, Yarrow MR (1963) Interdisciplinary relationships: Interrelations of physiological, psychological, and psychiatric findings in healthy elderly men. In: Birren JE, Butler RN, Greenhouse SW, Sokoloff L, Yarrow MR (eds) Human aging: a biological and behavioral study. Government Printing Office, Washington DC, pp 283–305

Birren JE, Woods AM, Williams MV (1979) Speed of behavior as an indicator of age changes and the intergrity of the nervous system. In: Hoffmeister F, Müller C (eds) Brain function in old age. Evaluation of changes and disorders. Springer, Berlin Heidelberg New York, pp 10–44

Blessed G (1980) Clinical aspects of senile dementia. In: Roberts PJ (ed) Biochemistry of dementia. Wiley, Chichester New York Brisbane Toronto, pp 1–14

Blessed G, Tomlinson BE, Roth M (1968) The association between quantitative measures of dementia and of senile change in the cerebral grey matter of elderly subjects. Br J Psychiat 114:797–811

Botwinick J (1967) Cognitive processes in maturity and old age. Springer, Berlin Heidelberg New York

Brazier MAB, Finesinger JE (1944) Characteristics of the normal electroencephalogram. I. A study of the occipital cortical potentials in 500 normal adults. J Clin Invest 23:303–311

Brody H (1955) Organization of cerebral cortex. III. A study of aging in human cerebral cortex. J Comp Neurol 102:511–556

Brody H (1978) Cell counts in cerebral cortex and brainstem. In: Katzman R, Terry RD, Bick KL (eds) Alzheimer's disease: senile dementia and related disorders (Aging Vol 7). Raven, New York, pp 345–351

Busse EW, Obrist WD (1963) Significance of focal electroencephalographic changes in the elderly. Postgrad Med 34:179–182

Busse EW, Obrist WD (1965) Pre-senescent electroencephalographic changes in normal subjects. J Gerontol 20:315–320

Busse EW, Wang HS (1965) The value of electroencephalography in geriatrics. Geriatrics 20:906–924

Busse EW, Barnes RH, Silverman AJ, Shy GM, Thaler M, Frost LL (1954) Studies of the process of aging: factors that influence the psyche of elderly persons. Am J Psychiat 110:897–903

Busse EW, Barnes RH, Friedman EL, Kelty EJ (1956) Psychological functioning of aged individuals with normal and abnormal electroencephalograms. I. A study of non-hospitalized community volunteers. J Nerv Ment Dis 124:135–141

Butler RN, Dastur DK, Perlin S (1965) Relationships of senile manifestations and chronic brain syndromes to cerebral circulation and metabolism. J Psychiat Res 3:229–238

Carlyle A, Grayson J (1955) Blood pressure and the regulation of brain blood flow. J Physiol 127:15–16 P

Cohen PJ, Wollmann H, Alexander SC, Chase PE, Behar MG (1964) Cerebral carbohydrate metabolism in man during halothane anesthesia. Effects of pa CO_2 on some aspects of carbohydrate utilization. Anesthesiology 25:185–191

Cohen PJ, Alexander SC, Wollman H (1968) Effects of hypocarbia and of hypoxia with normocarbia on cerebral blood flow and metabolism in man. Scand J Clin Lab Invest 22:Suppl 102 IV A

Colon EJ (1972) The elderly brain: a quantitative analysis of cerebral cortex in two cases. Psychiat Neurol Neurochir 75:261–270

Constantinidis J (1978) Is Alzheimer's disease a major form of senile dementia? Clinical, anatomical, and genetic data. In: Katzman R, Terry RD, Bick KL (eds) Alzheimer's disease: senile dementia and related disorders (Aging Vol 7). Raven, New York, pp 15–25

Constantinidis J, Krassojevitch M, Tissot R (1969) Corrélations entre les perturbations électroencéphalographiques et les lésions anatomohistologiques dans les démences. Encephale 58:19–52

Corsellis JAN (1969) The pathology of dementia. Br J Hosp Med 3:695–703

Crone C, Thompson AM (1970) Permeability of brain capillaries. In: Crone C, Lassen NA (eds) Capillary permeability. Munksgaard, Copenhagen, pp 446–455

Dastur DK, Lane MH, Hansen DB, Kety SS, Butler RN, Perlin S, Sokoloff L (1963) Effects of aging on cerebral circulation and metabolism in man. In: Birren JE, Butler RN, Greenhouse SW, Sokoloff L, Yarrow MR (eds) Human aging. A biological and behavioral study. US Govt Print Off, Washington DC, pp 59–78

Dekoninck WJ, Collard M, Jacquy J (1975) Comparative study of cerebral vasoactivity in vascular sclerosis of the brain in elderly men. Stroke 6:673–677

Dekoninck WJ, Jacquy J, Jocquet Ph, Noel G (1977) Cerebral blood flow and metabolism in senile dementia. In: Meyer JS, Lechner H, Reivich M (eds) Cerebral vascular disease. Excerpta Medica, Amsterdam Oxford, pp 29–32

Dinsdale HB, Robertson DM, Haas RA (1974) Cerebral blood flow in acute hypertension. Arch Neurol 31:80–87

Eisdorfer C (1963) The WAIS performance of the aged: A retest evaluation. J Gerontol 18:169–172

Eisdorfer C, Busse EW, Cohen LD (1959) The WAIS performance of an aged sample: The relationship between verbal and performance IQs. J Gerontol 14:197–201

Ekström-Jodal B, Häggendal E, Linder L-E, Nilsson NJ (1972) Cerebral blood flow autoregulation at high arterial pressures and different levels of carbon dioxide tension in dogs. In: Fieschi C (ed) Cerebral blood flow and intracranial pressure. Karger, Basel München Paris London New York Sydney, pp 6–10

Erbslöh F, Bernsmeier A, Hillesheim HR (1958) Der Glukoseverbrauch des Gehirns und seine Abhängigkeit von der Leber. Arch Psychiat Z Ges Neurol 196:611–626

Fazekas JF, Bessmann AN (1953) Coma mechanisms. Am J Med 15:804–812

Fazekas JF, Alman RW, Bessman AN (1952) Cerebral physiology of the aged. Am J Med Sci 223:245–257

Fazekas JF, Bessman AN, Cotsonas NJ, Alman RW (1953) Cerebral hemodynamics in cerebral arteriosclerosis. J Gerontol 8:137–145

Fazekas JF, Albert SN, Alman RW (1955) Influence of chlorpromazine and alcohol on cerebral hemodynamics and metabolism. Am J Med Sci 230:128–132

Fazekas JF, Ticktin HE, Ehrmantraut WR, Alman RW (1956) Cerebral metabolism in hepatic insufficiency. Am J Med 21:843–849

Folbergrova J, MacMillan V, Siesjö BK (1972) The effect of moderate and marked hypercapnia upon the energy state and upon the cytoplasmatic $NADH/NAD^+$-ratio of the rat brain. J Neurochem 19:2497–2505

Fox Ch, Birren JE (1950) The differential decline of subtest scores of the Wechsel-Bellevue Intelligence Scale in 60–69-year-old individuals. J Genet Psychol 77:313–317

Frackowiak RSJ, Lenzi GL, Jones T, Heather JD (1980) Quantitative measurements of regional cerebral blood flow and oxygen metabolism in man using ^{15}O and positron emission tomography: Theory, procedure, and normal values. J Comput Ass Tomogr 4:727–736

Frey TS, Sjögren H (1959) The electroencephalogram in elderly persons suffering from neuropsychiatric disorders. Acta Psychiat Scand 34:438–450

Freyhan FA, Woodford RB, Kety SS (1951) Cerebral blood flow and metabolism in psychoses of senility. J Nerv Ment Dis 113:449–456

Gibbs EL, Lennox WG, Nims LF, Gibbs FA (1942) Arterial and cerebral venous blood. Arterial-venous differences in man. J Biol Chem 144:325–332

Gordon EB, Sim M (1967) The EEG in presenile dementia. J Neurol Neurosurg Psychiat 30:285–291

Gotoh F, Meyer JS, Tagaki Y (1965) Cerebral effects of hyperventilation in man. Arch Neurol 12:410–423

Gottstein U (1979) Cerebral blood flow, $CMR O_2$ and CMR of glucose in patients with hypo- and hyperchromic anemia and polycythemia. The effect of hemodilution on CBF, CMR and hematocrit. In: Meyer JS, Lechner H, Reivich M (eds) Cerebral vascular disease 2. Excerpta Medica, Amsterdam Oxford, pp 225–229

Gottstein U (1966) Zirkulation, Sauerstoff- und Glukosestoffwechsel des Gehirns bei den Encephalopathien. Verh Dtsch Ges Inn Med 72:185–198

Gottstein U (1975) Discussion of T.E. Duffy, F. Plum: α-ketoglutaramate in the CSF: Clinical implications in hepatic encephalopathy. In: Ingvar DH, Lassen NA (eds) Brain work. The coupling of function, metabolism, and blood flow in the brain. Munksgaard, Copenhagen, pp 293–294

Gottstein U, Held K (1979) Effects of aging on cerebral circulation and metabolism in man. Acta Neurol Scand 60:Suppl 72, 54–55

Gottstein U, Bernsmeier A, Sedlmeyer I (1963) Der Kohlenhydratstoffwechsel des menschlichen Gehirns. I. Untersuchungen mit substratspezifischen enzymatischen Methoden bei normaler Hirndurchblutung. Klin Wschr 41:943–948

Gottstein U, Bernsmeier A, Sedlmeyer I (1964) Der Kohlenhydratstoffwechsel des menschlichen Gehirns. II. Untersuchungen mit substratspezifischen enzymatischen Methoden bei Kranken mit verminderter Hirndurchblutung auf dem Boden einer Arteriosklerose der Hirngefäße. Klin Wschr 42:310–313

Gottstein U, Müller W, Berghoff W, Gärtner H, Held K (1971) Zur Utilisation von nicht veresterten Fettsäuren und Ketonkörpern im Gehirn des Menschen. Klin Wschr 49:406–411

Gottstein U, Held K, Sedlmeyer I, Steiner K, Haberland KU, Berghoff W (1972) Hirndurchblutung und cerebraler Stoffwechsel bei Kranken mit chronischer Niereninsuffizienz. Klin Wschr 50:594–602

Gottstein U, Zahn U, Held K, Gabriel FH, Textor Th, Berghoff W (1976) Einfluß der Hyperventilation auf Hirndurchblutung und cerebralen Stoffwechsel des Menschen. Untersuchungen bei fortlaufender Registrierung der arterio-hirnvenösen Glucosedifferenz. Klin Wschr 54:373–381

Gottstein U, Gabriel FH, Held K, Textor Th (1977) Continuous monitoring of arterial and cerebral venous glucose concentrations in man. Advantage, procedure, and results. In: Blood glucose monitoring. Methodology and clinical application of continuous in vivo glucose analysis. Thieme, Stuttgart, pp 127–135

Granholm L, Siesjö BK (1969) The effects of hypercapnia and hypocapnia upon the cerebrospinal fluid lactate and pyruvate concentrations and upon the lactate, pyruvate, ATP, ADP, phosphocretine, and creatine concentrations of cat brain tissue. Acta Physiol Scand 75:257–266

Granholm L, Siesjö BK (1971) The effect of combined respiratory and nonrespiratory alkalosis of energy metabolites and acid-base parameters in rat brain. Acta Physiol Scand 81:307–314

Granholm L, Lukjanova L, Siesjö BK (1969) The effect of marked hyperventilation upon tissue levels of NADH, lactate, pyruvate, phosphocreatine and adenosine phosphates of rat brain. Acta Physiol Scand 77:179–199

Grubb RL Jr, Raichle ME, Gado MH, Eichling JO, Hughes CP (1977) Cerebral blood flow, oxygen utilization, and blood volume in dementia. Neurology 27:905–910

Gustafson L (1975) Dementia with onset in the presenile period. Part I. Psychiatric symptoms in dementia with onset in the presenile period. Acta Psychiat Scand Suppl 257:9–35

Gustafson L, Hagberg B (1975) Dementia with onset in the presenile period. Part II. Emotional behavior, personality changes and cognitive reduction in presenile dementia: related to regional cerebral blood flow. Acta Psychiat Scand Suppl 257:38–71

Gustafson L, Risberg J (1974) Regional cerebral blood flow related to psychiatric symptoms in dementia with onset in the presenile period. Acta Psychiat Scand 50:516–538

Gustafson L, Hagberg B, Ingvar DH (1972) Psychiatric symptoms and psychological test results related to regional cerebral blood flow in dementia with early onset. In: Meyer JS, Reivich M, Lechner H, Eichorn O (eds) Research on the cerebral circulation. Thomas, Springfield, pp 291–300

Hachinski VC, Lassen NA, Marshall J (1974) Multi-infarct dementia. A cause of mental deterioration in the elderly. Lancet 2:207–210

Hachinski VC, Iliff LD, Zilkha E, Du Boulay GH, McAllister VL, Marshall J, Ross-Russell RW, Symon L (1975) Cerebral blood flow in dementia. Arch Neurol 32:632–637

Häggendal E (1965) Blood flow autoregulation of the cerebral grey matter with comments on its mechanism. Acta Neurol Scand 41, Suppl 14:104–110

Häggendal E, Johansson B (1965) Effects of arterial carbon dioxide tension and oxygen saturation on cerebral blood flow autoregulation in dogs. Acta Physiol Scand 66, Suppl 258:27–53

Hagberg B, Ingvar DH (1976) Cognitive reduction in presenile dementia related to regional abnormalities of the cerebral blood flow. Br J Psychiat 128:209–222

Harper AM (1965) The inter-relationship between ap CO_2 and blood pressure in the regulation of blood flow through the cerebral cortex. Acta Neurol Scand 41, Suppl 14:94–103

Harper AM (1966) Autoregulation of cerebral blood flow: Influence of the arterial blood pressure on the blood flow through the cerebral cortex. J Neurol Neurosurg Psychiat 29:398–403

Harper AM, Glass HJ (1965) Effect of alteration in the arterial carbon dioxide tension on the blood flow through the cerebral cortex at normal and low arterial blood pressure. J Neurol Neurosurg Psychiat 28:449–452

Harrison MJG, Thomas DJ, Du Boulay GH, Marshall J (1979) Multi-infarct dementia. J Neurol Sci 40:97–103

Hedlund S, Kohler V, Nylin G, Olsson R, Regnstrom O, Rothstrom E, Anstrom KE (1964) Cerebral blood circulation in dementia. Acta Psychiat Scand 40, Suppl 1:77–106

Helmchen H (1975) The AMP-system as a method in clinical pharmacopsychiatry. In: Hippius H (ed) Assessment of pharmacodynamic effects in human pharmacology. Schattauer, Stuttgart, pp 87–134

Herrschaft H, Schmidt H (1973) Die quantitative Messung der örtlichen Hirndurchblutung in Allgemeinnarkose unter Normo-, Hypo- und Hyperkapnia. Anaesthesist 22:442–456

Heyman A, Patterson JL, Jones RW (1951) Cerebral circulation and metabolism in uremia. Circulation 3:558–563

Hoyer S (1969) Cerebral blood flow in senile dementia. In: Brock M, Fieschi C, Ingvar DH, Lassen NA, Schürmann K (eds) Cerebral blood flow. Clinical and experimental results. Springer, Berlin Heidelberg New York, pp 235–236

Hoyer S (1970a) Der Aminosäurenstoffwechsel des normalen menschlichen Gehirns. Klin Wschr 48:1239–1243

Hoyer S (1970b) Der Hirnstoffwechsel und die Häufigkeit cerebraler Durchblutungsstörungen beim organischen Psychosyndrom. Dtsch Z Nervenheilk 197:285–292

Hoyer S (1978a) Blood flow and oxidative metabolism of the brain in different phases of dementia. In: Katzman R, Terry RD, Bick KL (eds) Alzheimer's disease: senile dementia and related disorders (Aging Vol 7). Raven, New York, pp 219–226

Hoyer S (1978b) Das organische Psychosyndrom. Überlegungen zur Hirndurchblutung, zum Hirnstoffwechsel und zur Therapie. Nervenarzt 49:201–207

Hoyer S (1980) Factors influencing cerebral blood flow, CMR-oxygen and CMR-glucose in dementia patients. In: Roberts PJ (ed) Biochemistry of dementia. Wiley, Chichester New York Brisbane Toronto, pp 252–257

Hoyer S (to be published) Veränderungen von Hirndurchblutung und Hirnstoffwechsel bei verschiedenen Formen exogener Psychosen. In: Beckmann H (ed) Fortschritte der Psychiatrie. Huber, Bern

Hoyer S, Becker K (1966) Hirndurchblutung und Hirnstoffwechselbefunde bei neuropsychiatrisch Kranken. Nervenarzt 37:322–324

Hoyer S, Oesterreich K (1980) Brain blood flow and metabolism in middle-aged and elderly patients with Korsakow's syndrome. In: Betz E, Grote J, Heuser D, Wüllenweber R (eds) Pathophysiology and pharmacotherapy of cerebrovascular disorders. Witzstrock, Baden-Baden Köln New York, pp 94–97

Hoyer S, Hamer J, Alberti E, Stoeckel H, Weinhardt F (1974) The effect of stepwise arterial hypotension on blood flow and oxidative metabolism of the brain. Pflügers Arch 35:161–172

Hoyer S, Oesterreich K, Weinhardt F, Krüger G (1975a) Veränderungen von Durchblutung und oxydativem Stoffwechsel des Gehirns bei Patienten mit einer Demenz. J Neurol 210:227–237

Hoyer S, Papenberg J, Berendes K, Peddinghaus WD (1975b) Störungen des Hirnstoffwechsels bei Leberkrankheiten. In: Holm E (ed) Ammoniak und hepatische Enzephalopathie. Biochemie, Elektrophysiologie, Toxikologie. Fischer, Stuttgart, pp 27–32

Hoyer S, Krüger G, Weinhardt F (1979) Brain blood flow and metabolism in relation to psychiatric status in patients with organic brain syndromes. In: Meyer JS, Lechner H, Reivich M (eds) Cerebral vascular disease 2. Excerpta Medica, Amsterdam Oxford, pp 151–154

Huber G (1972) Klinik und Psychopathologie der organischen Psychosen. In: Kisker KP, Meyer J-E, Müller M, Strömgren E (eds) Psychiatrie der Gegenwart, Bd II/2, 2. ed. Springer, Berlin Heidelberg New York, pp 71–146

Ingvar DH (1970) Cerebral blood flow in organic dementia. In: Meyer JS, Reivich M, Lechner H, Eichhorn O (eds) Research on the cerebral circulation. Thomas, Springfield, pp 199–204

Ingvar DH, Risberg J, Cronquist S, Zätterström U, Gustafson L, Ljungberg K (1969) Regional cerebral blood flow in chronic alcoholism. In: Brock M, Fieschi C, Ingvar DH, Lassen NA, Schürmann K (eds) Cerebral blood flow. Springer, Berlin Heidelberg New York, pp 231–234

Ingvar DH, Brun A, Hagberg B, Gustafson L (1978) Regional cerebral blood flow in the dominant hemisphere in confirmed cases of Alzheimer's disease, Pick's disease and multi-infarct dementia: Relationship to clinical symptomatology and neuropathological findings. In: Katzman R, Terry RD, Bick KL (eds) Alzheimer's disease: senile dementia and related disorders (Aging Vol 7). Raven, New York, pp 203–211

Irving G, Robinson RA, McAdam W (1970) The validity of some cognitive tests in the diagnosis of dementia. Br J Psychiat 117:149–156

Jarvik LF, Kallmann FJ, Falek A (1962) Intellectual changes in aged twins. J Gerontol 17:289–294

Jellinger K (1976) Neuropathological aspects of dementias resulting from abnormal blood and cerebrospinal fluid dynamics. Acta Neurol Belg 76:83–102

Johannesson G, Brun A, Gustafson L, Ingvar DH (1977) EEG in presenile dementia related to cerebral blood flow and autopsy findings. Acta Neurol Scand 56:89–103·

Jones JV, Strandgaard S, Mackenzie ET, Fitch W, Lawrie TDV, Harper AM (1975) Autoregulation of cerebral blood flow in chronic hypertension. In: Harper AM, Jennett WB, Miller JD, Rowan JO (eds) Blood flow and metabolism in the brain. Churchill Livingstone, Edinburgh London New York, pp 5.10–5.13

Kaasik AE, Nilsson L, Siesjö BK (1970) The effect of arterial hypotension upon the lactate, pyruvate, and bicarbonate concentrations of the brain tissue and cisternal CSF and upon the tissue concentrations of phosphocreatine and adenine nucleotides in anesthetized rats. Acta Physiol Scand 78:448–458

Katzman R (1976) The prevalence and malignancy of Alzheimer disease. Arch Neurol 33:217–218

Katzman R (1979) Introduction: Comments on epidemiological and socioeconomic implications. In: Katzman R (ed) Congenital and acquired cognitive disorders. Raven, New York, pp 1–4

Kay DWK (1972) Epidemiological aspects of organic brain disease in the elderly. In: Gaitz GM (ed) Aging and the brain. Plenum, New York, pp 15–27

Kay DWK, Beamish P, Roth M (1964 a) Old age mental disorders in Newcastle upon Tyne. Part I: A study of prevalence. Br J Psychiat 110:146–158

Kay DWK, Beamish P, Roth M (1964 b) Old age mental disorders in Newcastle upon Tyne. Part II: A study of possible social and medical causes. Br J Psychiat 110:668–682

Kay DWK, Foster EM, McKechnie AA, Roth M (1970) Mental illness and hospital usage in the elderly: a random sample followed up. Compr Psychiat 2:26–35

Kety SS (1956) Human cerebral blood flow and oxygen consumption as related to aging. J Chron Dis 3:478–486

Kety SS, Schmidt CF (1946) The effects of active and passive hyperventilation on cerebral blood flow, cerebral oxygen consumption, cardiac output and blood pressure of normal young men. J Clin Invest 25:107–119

Kety SS, Schmidt CF (1948) The effects of altered arterial tensions of carbon dioxide and oxygen on cerebral blood flow and cerebral oxygen consumption of normal young men. J Clin Invest 27:484–492

Kety SS, Polis D, Nadler CS, Schmidt CF (1948 a) The blood flow and oxygen consumption of the human brain in diabetic acidosis and coma. J Clin Invest 27:500–510

Kety SS, Woodford RB, Harmel MH, Freyhan FA, Appel KE, Schmidt CF (1948 b) Cerebral blood flow and metabolism in schizophrenia. The effects of barbiturate-seminarcosis, insulin coma and electroshock. Am J Psych 104:765–770

Klee A (1964) The relationship between clinical evaluation of mental deterioration, psychological test results, and the cerebral metabolic rate of oxygen. Acta Neurol Scand 40:337–345

Krupp P (1966) Cerebrale Durchblutung und elektrische Hirnaktivität. Schwabe, Basel Stuttgart

Ladurner G, Ott EO, Perry PJ, Stix P, Schreyer H, Wiedner F, Lechner H (1977) Bilateral measurement of regional cerebral blood flow in dementia. In: Meyer JS, Lechner FH, Reivich M (eds) Cerebral vascular disease. Excerpta Medica, Amsterdam Oxford, pp 10–13

Lassen NA (1959) Cerebral blood flow and oxygen consumption in man. Physiol Rev 39:183–238

Lassen NA (1974) Control of cerebral circulation in health and disease. Circ Res 34:749–760

Lassen NA, Agnoli A (1972) The upper limit of autoregulation of cerebral blood flow in the pathogenesis of hypertensive encephalopathy. Scand J Clin Lab Invest 30:113–115

Lassen NA, Munck O, Tottey ER (1957) Mental function and cerebral oxygen consumption in organic dementia. Arch Neurol Psychiat 77:126–133

Lassen NA, Feinberg J, Lane MH (1960) Bilateral studies of cerebral oxygen uptake in young and aged normal subjects and in patients with organic dementia. J Clin Invest 39:491–500

Lauter H (1974) Epidemiologische Aspekte alterspsychiatrischer Erkrankungen. Nervenarzt 45:277–288

Lauter H, Meyer JE (1968) Clinical and nosological concepts of senile dementia. In: Müller C, Ciompi L (eds) Senile dementia. Huber, Bern, pp 13–27

Lenzi GL, Jones T, McKenzie CG, Buckingham PD, Clark JC, Moss S (1978) Study of regional cerebral metabolism and blood flow relationships in man using the method of continuously inhaling oxygen-15 and oxygen-15 labeled carbon dioxide. J Neurol Neurosurg Psychiat 41:1–10

Letemendia F, Pampiglione G (1958) Clinical and electroencephalographic observations in Alzheimer's disease. J Neurol Neurosurg Psychiat 21:167–172

Liberson WT, Sequin CA (1945) Brain waves and senile mental patients. Psychosom Med 7:30–35

Liddell DW (1958) Investigations of EEG findings in presenile dementia. J Neurol Neurosurg Psychiat 21:173–176

Loeb C (1980) Clinical diagnosis of multi-infarct dementia. In: Amaducci L, Davison AN, Antuono P (eds) Aging of the brain and dementia (Aging Vol 13). Raven, New York, pp 251–260

Luce RA Jr, Rothschild D (1953) The correlation of electroencephalographic and clinical observations in psychiatric patients over 65. J Gerontol 8:167–172

Madonick MJ, Solomon M (1947) The Wechsler-Bellevue scale in individuals past sixty. Geriatrics 2:34–40

Maiolo AT, Bianchiporro G, Galli C, Sessa M, Polli EE (1971) Brain energy metabolism in hepatic coma. Exp Biol Med 4:52–70

Marx P, Neundörfer B, Potz G, Hoyer S (1975) Cerebral blood flow and aminoacid metabolism in chronic alcoholism. In: Harper AM, Jennett WB, Miller JD, Rowan JO (eds) Blood flow and metabolism in the brain. Churchill Livingstone, Edinburgh London New York, pp 11.31–11.35

Mayer-Gross W, Slater E, Roth M (1969) Clinical psychiatry. 3. ed. Bailliere, Tindall and Carssell, London

McAdam W, Robinson RA (1956) Senile intellectual deterioration and the electroencephalogram: A quantitative correlation. J Ment Sci 102:819–825

McAdam W, Robinson RA (1962) Diagnostic and prognostic value of the electroencephalogram in geriatric psychiatry. In: Blumenthal HT (ed) Medical and clinical aspects of aging. Columbia Univ Press, New York, pp 557–564

McHugh PR, Folstein MF (1979) Psychopathology of dementia: implications for neuropathology. In: Katzman R (ed) Congenital and acquired cognitive disorders. Raven, New York, pp 17–30

Meyer JS, Gotoh F, Tazaki Y, Hamaguchi K, Ishikawa S, Novailhat F, Symon L (1962) Regional cerebral blood flow and metabolism in vivo. Effects of anoxia, hyperglycemia, ischemia, acidosis, alkalosis, and alterations of blood p CO_2. Arch Neurol 7:560–581

Miller JD, Stanek A, Langfitt TW (1972) Concepts of cerebral perfusion pressure and vascular compression during intracranial hypertension. Progr Brain Res 35:411–432

Munck O, Bärenholdt O, Busch H (1968) Cerebral blood flow in organic dementia measured with the xenon-133 desaturation method. Scand J Lab Clin Invest 22, Suppl 102, XII:A

Mundy-Castle AC, Hurst LA, Beerstecher DM, Prinsloo T (1954) The electroencephalogram in senile psychoses. Electroenceph Clin Neurophysiol 6:245–252

Naritomi H, Meyer JS, Sakai F, Yamaguchi F, Shaw T (1979) Effects of advancing age on regional cerebral flow. Studies in normal subjects and subjects with risk factors for atherothrombotic stroke. Arch Neurol 36:410–416

National Center for Health Statistics (1975) The projection of the population of the US 1975–2050. In: Census Bureau Current Population Reports, Series P 25, No 601

Nemoto EM, Stezoski SW, MacMurdo D (1978) Glucose transport across the rat blood-brain barrier during anesthesia. Anesthesiology 49:170–176

Newton RD (1948) The identity of Alzheimer's disease and senile dementia and their relationship to senility. Br J Psychiat 94:225–249

O'Brien MD (1972) Some aspects of cerebral blood flow in dementia. In: Meyer JS, Reivich M, Lechner H, Eichhorn O (eds) Research on the cerebral circulatio. Thomas, Springfield, pp 287–290

O'Brien MD, Mallett BL (1970) Cerebral cortex perfusion rates in dementia. J Neurol Neurosurg Psychiat 33:497–500

Obrist WD (1954) The electroencephalogram of normal aged adults. Electroenceph Clin Neurophysiol 6:235–244

Obrist WD (1975) Cerebral physiology of the aged: Relation to psychological function. In: Burch N, Altshuler HL (eds) Behavior and brain electrical activity. Plenum, New York, pp 421–430

Obrist WD (1978) Noninvasive studies of cerebral blood flow in aging and dementia. In: Katzman R, Terry RD, Bick KL (eds) Alzheimer's disease: senile dementia and related disorders (Aging Vol 7). Raven, New York, pp 213–217

Obrist WD, Busse EW (1965) The electroencephalogram in old age. In: Wilson WP (ed) Applications of electroencephalography in psychiatry. Duke University Press, Durham, pp 185–205

Obrist WD, Henry CE (1958) Electroencephalographic findings in aged psychiatric patients. J Nerv Ment Dis 126:254–267

Obrist WD, Busse EW, Eisdorfer C, Kleemeier RW (1962) Relation of the electroencephalogram to intellectual function in senescence. J Gerontol 17:197–206

Obrist WD, Sokoloff L, Lassen NA, Lane MH, Butler RN, Feinberg J (1963) Relation of EEG to cerebral blood flow and metabolism in old age. Electroenceph Clin Neurophysiol 15:610–619

Obrist WD, Henry CE, Justiss WA (1966) Longitudinal changes in the senescent EEG: A 15-year study. Proceed 7 th Int Congr Geront Vienna, pp 35–38

Obrist WD, Chivian E, Cronquist S, Ingvar DH (1970) Regional cerebral blood flow in senile and presenile dementia. Neurology (Minneap) 20:315–322

Obrist WD, Thompson HK Jr, Wang HS, Wilkinson WE (1975) Regional cerebral blood flow estimated by ^{133}xenon inhalation. Stroke 6:245–256

Oldendorf WH (1971) Brain uptake of radiolabeled amino acids, amines and hexoses after arterial injection. Am J Physiol 221:1629–1639

Oldendorf WH (1976) Blood-brain barrier. In: Himwich HE (ed) Brain metabolism and cerebral disorders. Spectrum, New York, pp 163–180

Olesen J (1974) Cerebral blood flow. Methods for measurement, regulation, effects of drugs and changes in disease. Acta Neurol Scand 50, Suppl 57:1–134

Otomo E (1966) Electroencephalography in old age: Dominant alpha pattern. Electroenceph Clin Neurophysiol 21:489–491

Pampiglione G, Post F (1958) The value of electroencephalographic examinations in psychiatric disorders of old age. Geriatrics 13:725–732

Papenberg J, Lanzinger G, Kommerell B, Hoyer S (1975) Comparative studies of the electroencephalogram and the cerebral oxidative metabolism in patients with liver cirrhosis. Klin Wschr 53:1107–1113

Pardridge WM, Oldendorf WH (1977) Transport of metabolic substrates through the blood-brain barrier. J Neurochem 28:5–12

Patterson JL, Heyman A, Battey LL, Ferguson RW (1955) Threshold of response of the cerebral vessels of man to increase in blood carbon dioxide. J Clin Invest 34:1857–1864

Paulson OB, Bitsch V, Lassen NA (1968) The metabolism of glucose and other metabolites in the brain of patients with cerebral arteriosclerosis and of patients with diabetes mellitus. Acta Neurol Scand 44:183–199

Posner JB, Plum F (1960) The toxic effects of carbon dioxide and acetazolamide in hepatic encephalopathy. J Clin Invest 39:1246–1258

Rabin AJ (1945) Psychometric trends in senility and psychoses of the senium. J Genet Psychol 32:149–162

Raichle ME, Posner JB, Plum F (1970) CBF during and after hyperventilation. Arch Neurol 23:394–403

Rapela CE, Green HD (1964) Autoregulation of canine cerebral blood flow. Circulation Res 15, Suppl. I:205–211

Reivich M (1964) Arterial p CO_2 and cerebral hemodynamics. Am J Physiol 206:25–35

Rosen WG, Terry RD, Fuld PA, Katzman R, Peck A (1980) Pathological verification of ischemic score in differentiation of dementias. Ann Neurol 7:486–488

Roth, Sir Martin (1978) Diagnosis of senile and related forms of dementia. In: Katzman R, Terry RD, Bick KL (eds) Alzheimer's disease. Senile dementia and related disorders (Aging Vol 7). Raven, New York, pp 71–85

Roth, Sir Martin (1980) Aging of the brain and dementia: An overview. In: Amaducci L, Davison AN, Antuono P (eds) Aging of the brain and dementia (Aging Vol 13). Raven, New York, pp 1–21

Roubakine A (1975) Le problème de la vieillesse en Union Soviétique depuis la grande révolution socialiste d'octobre 1917. Bull Acad Med 159:547–551

Sacks W (1957) Cerebral metabolism of isotopic glucose in normal human subjects. J Appl Physiol 10:37–44

Sacks W (1965) Cerebral metabolism of doubly labeled glucose in humans in vivo. J Appl Physiol 20:117–130

Sacks W (1969) Cerebral metabolism in vivo. In: Lajtha A (ed) Handbook of neurochemistry, vol 1. Plenum, New York, pp 301–324

Sacks W (1976) Human brain metabolism in vivo. In: Himwich HE (ed) Brain metabolism and cerebral disorders. Spectrum, New York, pp 89–127

Scharfetter C (1972) Das AMP-System. 2. ed. Springer, Berlin Heidelberg New York

Scheibel AB (1978) Structural aspects of the aging brain: Spine systems and the dendritic arbor. In: Katzman R, Terry RD, Bick KL (eds) Alzheimer's disease: senile dementia and related disorders (Aging Vol 7). Raven, New York, pp 353–373

Scheibel ME, Scheibel AB (1975) Structural changes in the aging brain. In: Brody H, Harman D, Ordy JM (eds) Clinical, morphologic, and neurochemical aspects in the aging central nervous system (Aging Vol 1). Raven, New York, pp 11–37

Scheibel ME, Lindsay RD, Tomiyasu U, Scheibel AB (1975) Progressive dendritic changes in the aging human cortex. Exp Neurol 47:392–403

Scheibel ME, Lindsay RD, Tomiyasu U, Scheibel AB (1976) Progressive dendritic changes in the aging human limbic system. Exp Neurol 53:420–430

Scheinberg P (1951) Cerebral blood flow and metabolism in pernicious anemia. Blood 6:213–227

Scheinberg P (1954) Effects of uremia on cerebral blood flow and metabolism. Neurology (Minneap) 4:101–105

Scheinberg P, Blackburn J, Rich M, Saslaw M (1953) Effects of aging on cerebral circulation and metabolism. Arch Neurol Psychiat 70:77–85

Schieve JF, Wilson WP (1953) The influence of age, anesthesia and cerebral arteriosclerosis on cerebral vascular activity to CO_2. Am J Med 15:171–174

Severinghaus JW, Lassen NA (1967) Step hypocapnia to separate arterial from tissue p CO_2 in the regulation of cerebral blood flow. Circulation Res 20:272–278

Shapiro W, Wassermann AJ, Patterson JL (1965) Human cerebrovascular response time to elevation of arterial carbon dioxide tension. Arch Neurol 13:130–138

Shapiro W, Wassermann AJ, Patterson JL (1966) Human cerebrovascular response to combined hypoxia and hypercapnia. Circ Res 19:903–910

Shefer VF (1973) Absolute number of neurons and thickness of the cerebral cortex during aging, senile and vascular dementia, and Pick's and Alzheimer's disease. Neurosci Behav Physiol 6:319–324

Shenkin HA, Novak P, Goluboff B, Soffe AM, Bortin L (1953) The effects of aging, arteriosclerosis and hypertension upon the cerebral circulation. J Clin Invest 32:459–465

Sheridan FP, Yeager CL, Oliver WA, Simon A (1955) Electroencephalography as a diagnostic and prognostic aid in studying the senescent individual: A preliminary report. J Geront 10:53–59

Siesjö BK, Messeter K (1971) Factors determining intracellular pH. In: Siesjö BK, Sørensen SC (eds) Ion homeostasis of the brain. Munksgaard, Copenhagen, pp 244–262

Siesjö BK, Zwetnow NN (1970) The effect of hypovolemic hypotension on extra- and intracellular acid-base parameters and energy metabolism in the rat brain. Acta Physiol Scand 79:114–124

Siesjö BK, Nilsson L, Rokeach M, Zwetnow NN (1971) Energy metabolism of the brain at reduced cerebral perfusion pressures and in arterial hypoxaemia. In: Brierley JB, Meldrum BS (eds) Brain hypoxia. Heinemann, London, pp 79–93

Silverman AJ, Busse EW, Barnes RH (1955) Studies in the processes of aging: Electroencephalographic findings in 400 elderly subjects. Electroenceph Clin Neurophysiol 7:67–74

Simard D (1971) Regional cerebral blood flow and its regulation in dementia. In: Ross Russell RW (ed) Brain blood flow. Pitman, London, pp 322–326

Simard D, Olesen J, Paulson OB, Lassen NA, Skinhøj E (1971) Regional cerebral blood flow and its regulation in dementia. Brain 94:273–288

Smith CB, Goochee C, Rapoport I, Sokoloff L (1980) Effects of ageing on local rates of cerebral glucose utilization in the rat. Brain 103:351–365

Sokoloff L, Reivich M, Kennedy C, Des Rosiers MH, Patlak CS, Pettigrew KD, Sakurada O, Shinohara M (1977) The (^{14}C) deoxyglucose method for the measurement of local cerebral glucose utilization: theory, procedure, and normal values in the conscious and anesthetized albino rat. J Neurochem 28:897–916

Statistisches Bundesamt FRG 1981

Strandgaard S, Olesen J, Skinhøj E, Lassen NA (1973) Autoregulation of brain circulation in severe arterial hypertension. Br Med J 1:507–510

Strandgaard S, Mackenzie ET, Sengupta D, Rowan JO, Lassen NA, Harper AM (1974) Upper limit of autoregulation of cerebral blood flow in the baboon. Circulation Res 34:435–440

Strandgaard S, Sengupta D, Mackenzie ET, Rowan JO, Olesen J, Skinhøj E, Lassen NA, Harper AM (1975) The lower and upper limits for autoregulation of cerebral blood flow. In: Langfitt TW, McHenry LC Jr, Reivich M, Wollman H (eds) Cerebral circulation and metabolism. Springer, New York Heidelberg Berlin, pp 3–6

Sulg I (1969) The quantitative EEG as a measure of brain dysfunction. Scand J Clin Lab Invest 23, Suppl 109:1–155

Swain JM (1959) Electroencephalographic abnormalities in presenile atrophy. Neurology (Minneap) 9:722–727

Terry RD (1976) Dementia. A brief and selective review. Arch Neurol 33:1–4

Terry RD (1978) Aging, senile dementia and Alzheimer's disease. In: Katzman R, Terry RD, Bick KL (eds) Alzheimer's disease: senile dementia and related disorders (Aging Vol 7). Raven, New York, pp 11–14

Thaler M (1956) Relationships among Wechsler, Weigl, Rorschach, EEG findings, and abstract-concrete behavior in a group of normal aged subjects. J Gerontol 11:404–409

Tomlinson BE (1980) The structural and quantitative aspects of the dementias. In: Roberts PJ (ed) Biochemistry of dementia. Wiley, Chichester New York Brisbane Toronto, pp 15–52

Tomlinson BE, Blessed G, Roth M (1970) Observations on the brains of demented old people. J Neurol Sci 11:205–242

Turton EC, Warren PKG (1960) Dementia: a clinical and EEG study of 274 patients over the age of 60. J Ment Sci 106:1493–1500

van der Drift JH, Kok NK (1972) The EEG in cerebrovascular disorders in relation to pathology. In: Remond A (ed) Handbook of electroencephalography and clinical neurophysiology. Vol 14, Part A. Elsevier, Amsterdam, pp 12–64

Wang HS, Obrist WD, Busse EW (1970) Neurophysiological correlates of the intellectual function of elderly persons living in the community. Am J Psychiatry 126:1205–1212

Wechsler D (1939) The measurement of adult intelligence. Williams and Wilkins, Baltimore

Wechsler D (1958) The measurement and appraisal of adult intelligence. Williams and Wilkins, Baltimore

Wechsler RL, Crum W, Roth JLA (1954) The blood flow and O_2 consumption of the human brain in hepatic coma. Clin Res Proc 2:74

Weiner H, Schuster DB (1956) The electroencephalogram in dementia: some preliminary observations and correlations. Electroenceph Clin Neurophysiol 8:479–488

Weitbrecht HJ (1963) Psychiatrie im Grundriß. Springer, Berlin Göttingen Heidelberg
Wollman H, Alexander SC, Cohen PJ, Smith TC, Chase PE, van der Molen RA (1965) Cerebral circulation during anesthesia and hyperventilation in man. Thiopental induction to nitrous oxide and d-tubocurarine. Anesthesiology 26:329–334
Wollman H, Smith TC, Stephen GW, Colton ET, Gleaton HE, Alexander SC (1968) Effects of extremes of respiratory and metabolic alkalosis on cerebral blood flow in man. J Appl Physiol 24:60–65
World Health Organization (1972) Psychogeriatrics. Report of a WHO scientific group. Technical Report, Series NO 507, Geneva
Yamaguchi F, Meyer JS, Yamamoto M, Sakai F, Shaw T (1980) Noninvasive regional cerebral blood flow measurements in dementia. Arch Neurol 37:410–418
Yamamoto M, Meyer JS, Sakai F, Yamaguchi F (1980) Aging and cerebral vasodilator responses to hypercarbia. Responses in normal aging and in persons with risk factors for stroke. Arch Neurol 37:489–496
Yoshida K, Meyer JS, Sakamoto K, Handa J (1966) Autoregulation of cerebral blood flow. Electromagnetic flow measurements during acute hypertension in the monkey. Circ Res 19:726–738
Zwetnow NN (1970) The influence of an increased intracranial pressure on the lactate, pyruvate, bicarbonate, phosphocreatine, ATP, ADP, and AMP concentrations of the cerebral cortex of dogs. Acta Physiol Scand 79:158–166

Functional Consequences of Neurofibrillary Degeneration of the Alzheimer Type

D. R. Crapper McLachlan and U. De Boni

A. Introduction

Understanding neurofibrillary degeneration of the Alzheimer type is a key step in understanding the senile changes responsible for diminished intellectual function in the elderly. Neurofibrillary change restricted to the medial temporal lobes and hippocampus is remarkably common in the older human brain; however, when this change occurs in neurons of the neocortex there is usually an association with some degree of impairment in intellectual and other higher brain functions (Tomlinson et al. 1970). The ultrastructural subunits of neurofibrillary degeneration are paired helical filaments. This unique change is also found in neuronal processes surrounding the other hallmark of senile brain change; the senile plaques. However, animal models of senile plaques such as those found in mouse brain infected with scrapie agent (Bruce and Fraser 1975; Wisniewski et al. 1975), the "senile" plaques of aged animal brains and the plaques of Kuru and Jacob-Creutzfeld's disease lack paired helical filaments and therefore may have limited application to the study of senile brain disease. Elucidating the intracellular events responsible for paired helical filament formation and their aggregation into the dense bundles responsible for neurofibrillary degeneration is of the utmost importance in understanding the changes responsible for human brain aging. The purpose of this chapter is to summarize present understanding of neurofibrillary change and inquire into the possible significance of the change to human brain function.

B. Classification of Neurofibrillary Degeneration

When Alzheimer applied a silver stain, developed by his associate Bielschowski as a "neurofilament" stain, to the brain of a 51-year-old woman whose symptoms began with loss of memory and disorientation and who died 5 years later with profound dementia, he noted dark staining intracytoplasmic whirls of thickened filaments (Alzheimer 1907). The changes resembled black, twisted threads and became known as neurofibrillary tangles. A large number of degenerative and toxic brain conditions exhibit neurofibrillary degeneration and electron microscopic examination has revealed at least three different types of filaments.

I. Neurofibrillary Degeneration of the Alzheimer Type

Kidd (1963, 1964) examined neurofibrillary tangles from brains of patients with Alzheimer's disease with the aid of the electron microscope and interpreted the images to represent bundles of fibres, each fibre composed of two 10-nm filaments, twisted in a helix making one complete turn in 160 nm. The individual strands of the helix had a centre-to-centre separation of 15 nm. He later published negative-stained formalin-fixed neurofibrillary material also suggestive of two filaments paired into a helix (Kidd 1970). A resulting controversy involving the interpretation of the images as representing twisted tubules, twisted ribbons or pairs of 10 nm filaments in a helical array persisted until the application of an electron microscopic technique which employed a goniometer tilt stage revealed a series of images consistent with paired helical filaments (Wisniewski et al. 1976).

II. Neurofibrillary Degeneration of Supranuclear Palsy

In 1964, Steele et al. described a progressive condition associated with vertical gaze palsy and neurons in the brain stem exhibiting neurofibrillary degeneration. Subsequent ultrastructural examination revealed bundles of straight solid filaments of about 15 nm diameter (Tellez-Nagel and Wisniewski 1973). Although in this syndrome dementia is not a prominent feature, cases of dementia with brain stem neurofibrillary degeneration of the 15-nm type have been encountered. Furthermore, both paired helical filaments and 15-nm filaments have been observed in the same neuron in such a case (Seema and Crapper, unpublished work). The biochemical composition of the 15-nm filament is unknown, although two laboratory models of this change have been described (Crapper and De Boni 1980).

III. Experimentally Induced Neurofibrillary Degeneration

Two groups of agents induce neurofibrillary degeneration in experimental models: the antimitotic agents related to colchicine and the vinca alkaloid family of compounds, and the trace metals aluminum and cadmium. In the experimental models, however, bundles of single 10-nm solid filaments accumulate and the paired helical configuration of the Alzheimer type never occurs. Biochemical and immunohistological data indicate that the colchicine-induced filaments are chemically related to vimentin of molecular weight 52,000 (Lazarides 1980), whereas the aluminum-induced filaments have a chemical composition identical to the molecular weight of the peptide-triplet-forming neurofilaments: 68,000, 140,000, and 210,000 daltons (Selkoe et al. 1979). Considerable circumstantial evidence implicates the trace element aluminum as a possible toxic factor associated with neurofibrillary degeneration of the Alzheimer type (Crapper et al. 1973, 1976, 1978). Two laboratories employing different techniques have reported aluminum to be present in the nuclei of neurons with Alzheimer neurofibrillary degeneration (Crapper et al. 1976; Perl and Brody 1980). Employing atomic absorption spectroscopy, work in our laboratory revealed an increase in aluminum content in nuclei in brain regions associated with neurofibrillary degeneration (Crapper et al. 1980). In addition, Perl and Brody, employing the scanning microscope with emission spectroscopy, recently reported that neurons with neurofibrillary degeneration from patients with Alzheimer's disease and neurons with neurofibrillary degeneration from older-aged brains from patients without dementia had detectable aluminum within the nuclei, whereas neurons in the immediate vicinity, void of neurofibrillary degeneration, had no detectable aluminum in the nucleus. The possible role of aluminum in Alzheimer's disease has been discussed elsewhere and may represent an important neurotoxic factor associated with the basic metabolic deficits underlying Alzheimer's disease (CRAPPER et al. 1980).

IV. Occurrence of Neurofibrillary Degeneration Other than in Alzheimer's Disease

Neurofibrillary degeneration of the paired helical filament type occurs in a number of brain diseases in addition to senile and presenile dementia. WISNIEWSKI et al. (1979) has recently reviewed in detail those human conditions in which neurofibrillary degeneration has been reported.

Until recently, paired helical filaments were considered to be unique to human central nervous system pathology. However, several examples of paired helical filaments in animal neurons have been reported, although the period of the helix is different from that found in Alzheimer's disease. Detailed examination by WISNIEWSKI et al. (1973) of aged monkey brain revealed examples of paired helical filaments with a half-twist period of about 50 nm. Giant sensory neurons of the foreleg of a whip spider have been reported by FOELIX and HAUSER (1979) to contain dense bundles of 10-nm filaments wound in a helix with a half-turn period of 50 nm. After prolonged exposure to ethanol, neurons of dorsal root ganglia of rats have been found by VOLK (1980) to contain bundles of paired 10-nm-diameter filaments wound in a helical array with a half-turn period of about 35 nm. In contrast, rabbit fetal cerebral neurons and spinal cord neurons maintained in vitro exhibit paired 10-nm filaments wound in a helix with a period ranging between 160 and 50 nm when exposed to an extract prepared from Alzheimer affected brain (DE BONI and CRAPPER 1978, and unpublished work).

Considering the diverse human and animal conditions in which neurofibrillary degeneration composed of paired helical filaments is now known to occur, neurofibrillary degeneration may well represent a non-specific, cellular response to an unidentified pathological process. Since 10-nm filaments appear to have a cytoplasmic skeletal function, the helical array may represent a response to pathological processes related to collapse of intraneuronal space. Diseases associated with neurofibrillary degeneration are usually associated with neuron loss, cerebral atrophy and dendritic "dying back." Therefore, it is unlikely that neurofibrillary degeneration is directly related to any of the specific primary pathogenic events which cause the various diseases associated with neurofibrillary degeneration and is probably best considered a non-specific neuronal marker of a disease process. Whether this change defines the anatomical limits of a pathological process within the brain is unresolved.

C. Distribution of Neurofibrillary Degeneration in Alzheimer's Disease

The anatomical distribution of neurofibrillary degeneration is important to the understanding of the functional consequences of neurofibrillary degeneration upon brain function. Generally, large neurons with extensive dendritic trees are the most susceptible. Certain cells such as the cerebellar Purkinje cell, the motor neurons of the brain stem and spinal cord and dorsal root ganglion cells have not been reported to exhibit paired helical filaments in Alzheimer's disease.

However, certain brain stem nuclei exhibit a predilection for neurofibrillary degeneration. Ishii (1966) reported that nucleus dorsalis raphe and nucleus centralis superior were the most severely affected. Periaqueductal grey matter, reticular formation of pons and medulla oblongata, and the substantia nigra ranked next. Within the hypothalamus, nuclei tuberis, substantia innominata and nucleus mamillo-infundibularis were sites of predilection for tangles. Within the hippocampus there is a selective vulnerability to neurofibrillary degeneration. Quantatitive analysis of the topographical distribution of neurofibrillary tangles in hippocampal cortex by Ball (1978) revealed a predilection for certain regions. Ranked in decreasing order of density of neurofibrillary degeneration the distribution was: Entorhinal cortex > subiculum > H_1 > end-plate > presubiculum > H_2. Within the neocortex the distribution appears to be non-random as well. Brun and Gustafson (1976) reported the light microscopic distribution of cell loss, gliosis, neurofibrillary degeneration and senile plaques in seven cases of Alzheimer's disease ranging in age from 58 to 74 years. All manifestations of Alzheimer's disease were found to be most pronounced in the medial temporal areas, posterior cingulate gyrus and over the lateral hemispheres in a zone expanding from the posterior inferior temporal areas to the adjoining portions of the parietal and occipital lobes. The parietal lobes were involved to a lesser degree and the primary sensory and motor areas of the frontal parietal and occipital lobe were spared or the least involved. Unpublished observations from our laboratory indicate that while neurofibrillary degeneration of sufficient magnitude to be detected by the light microscope rarely occurs in the calcarine cortex (Brodman area 17), electron microscopic examination reveals paired helical filaments in processes surrounding senile plaques in area 17 and in myelinated axons in this region. The biological origin of this peculiar distribution of neurofibrillary degeneration in Alzheimer's disease is unknown but the pattern of distribution within the brain appears to be related to the pattern of deficits which patients exhibit (Brun and Gustafson 1976).

D. Survival Time of Neurons with Neurofibrillary Degeneration

Neurofibrillary degeneration is usually associated with neuron loss and it is sometimes assumed that neurofibrillary degeneration is a sign of dying neurons. Suitable methods have not been developed to measure precisely the survival time of neurons with neurofibrillary degeneration. Based upon experimentally induced aluminum neurofibrillary degeneration, neurons survive at least 90 days but not more than 1,000 days (Crapper 1973, 1974). To obtain an estimate of survival time of neurons affected with tangles, we examined in detail the brains of two men of similar anthropomorphic type, racial background and life style. Both men were modest social drinkers, had no history of head injury or serious systemic illness prior to death. One died suddenly of myocardial infarction with no intellectual impairment at the age of 64 and the other of Alzheimer's disease at the age of 65.

Histological criteria were established for classifying cortical cells and neuron counts were made in radial columns in cerebral cortex. The histometric techniques are given in detail elsewhere (CRAPPER et al. 1975). At death the control brain was estimated to have 1.2×10^{10} cortical neurons based on sample counts from four neocortical areas corresponding approximately to Brodman areas 11, 21, 17, and 19. The calculation was based on the mean number of neurons in a column oriented radial to the cortical surface and $1\ mm^2$ in surface area multiplied by the mean total neocortical surface area as published by HENNEBERG (1910). The brain of a patient with an 8-year or 3,000-day history of progressive dementia of the Alzheimer type had an estimated 0.9×10^{10} neurons. Assuming the cortex of both the control and Alzheimer affected brains contained about the same number of neurons at the onset of Alzheimer's disease, the Alzheimer affected brain lost 3×10^9 neurons or 1×10^6 neurons per day over the 8-year course. At death the Alzheimer affected brain had 3% of neocortical neurons involved by neurofibrillary degeneration, or 270×10^6 neurons. Assuming the percentage of neurons affected by neurofibrillary degeneration and the survival time of affected neurons remained constant throughout the 8-year history of the disease, then a neuron would be expected to survive about 270 days or 9 months for the patient under consideration. While this estimate is based upon assumptions which cannot yet be adequately tested, the estimated survival time falls within the range of the experimentally induced aluminum tangle.

E. Molecular Origin of Neurofibrillary Degeneration

Although neurofibrillary degeneration is not unique to the senile brain or Alzheimer's disease, understanding the chemical composition and origin of the ultrastructural subunits of the paired helical filaments may offer important insight into the primary pathogenic events which initiate the senile process. Since the subunit structure of neurofibrillary degeneration is the accumulation of helically wound pairs of single filaments, an important question concerns the origin of the filamentous proteins. The paired helical configuration may represent a cellular modification of existing gene products to neuronal structural alterations induced by the primary pathogenic events or the paired helical filament may represent new gene products perhaps foreign to the human neuron.

Significant advances in defining the polypeptide composition of naturally occurring 10-nm intermediate filaments has recently been achieved. Five chemically distinct classes of intermediate filaments are now identified within the eukaryotic cell and each class of filaments tends to be characteristic of a particular cell type (LAZARIDES 1980). Neuronal axons contain 10-nm filaments composed of a triplet of polypeptides of molecular weight 68,000, 150,000, and 200,000 Daltons (ANDERTON et al. 1978; SCHLAEPFER 1978; MICKO and SCHLAEPFER 1978). Glial 10-nm filaments are of 51,000 molecular weight. Despite initial confusion, most workers now agree that the 51,000-molecular-weight peptides originally considered to be neurofilaments are of glial origin. Neurofilaments were probably lost in the initial preparations of YEN et al. (1976) due to their solubility in solutions of low ionic strength. Certain epithelial cells contain a family of fibrinous proteins, the keratins, ranging in molecular weight from 40,000 to 70,000 Daltons. Cells of mesenchymal origin contain 10-nm filaments of 52,000 molecular weight called vimentin. This protein is identical to that which forms perinuclear bundles following exposure to colchicine, a finding which originally prompted the erroneous belief that the filaments were degradation products of microtubules. A fifth type of intermediate filament, desmin, occurs in muscle, predominantly smooth muscle, and has a molecular weight of about 50,000 Daltons.

Neurons presumably carry the genome for each of these filaments although only neurofilaments so far have been identified within normal central nervous system neurons. Neuroblastoma cells contain both neurofilaments and vimentin, and glia appear to contain both glial acidic 51,000-molecular-weight fibrinous proteins and vimentin. Muscle cells have been reported to contain both vimentin and desmin while epithelial cells may contain both keratin and vimentin. Within the epithelial cells the peptide composition of intermediate filaments varies considerably and in the liver hepatocyte there is both vimentin and keratin.

The remarkable feature of neurofibrillary degeneration is the perinuclear or proximal dendritic distribution of paired helical filaments. Dendrites are not as rich in 10-nm filaments as are axons and at present it is unknown whether axonal and dendritic filaments are of the same peptide composition.

The chemical composition of Alzheimer paired helical filaments has been examined by Iqbal et al. (1978). Unfortunately, the interpretation of the results is uncertain. Their technique involved the preparation of neuron-enriched fractions from Alzheimer affected brains which were also enriched in neurons with neurofibrillary degeneration. While these workers did not publish the percentage of neurons in the enriched fraction which exhibited either light or electron microscopic evidence of neurofibrillary degeneration, our experience with this technique indicated that preparations usually contain about 3%–5% of cells which exhibit Congo red birefringence and preparations are rare where 12% of cells with neurofibrillary degeneration are achieved. The next step in isolation involved homogenation and removal of nuclei with the paired helical filaments remaining in the postmitochondrial supernatant after centrifugation. Paired helical filaments were then solubilized in 1% SDS after heating for an unspecified length of time. In the experience of this laboratory, the paired helical filaments are remarkably resistant to boiling for 10 min in 1% SDS and this procedure may not completely solubilize the paired helical filaments. Iqbal et al. (1974) have also reported that the paired-helical-filament-enriched proteins contain an unique band corresponding to a molecular weight of about 50,000 daltons. Trypsin digestion of this 50,000-molecular-weight peptide indicated fragments related to β-tubulin and neurofilaments. Shelanski (1978) has challenged this work on the grounds that a central hypothesis was that neurofilaments were composed of a single group of polypeptides of 51,000 molecular weight. However, this polypeptide was probably of glial origin and since the neurofibrillary enriched fraction came from gliosed brain it may represent a contaminant. He emphasized that a completely homogenous preparation of paired helical filaments has not yet been achieved and therefore the chemical composition cannot be ascertained.

Attempts to employ immunological labelling of the neurofibrillary tangle have also been inconclusive. Grundke-Iqbal et al. (1979) have reported that antibodies raised against the proteins of twice-recycled microtubules stain neurofibrillary tangles at the light microscopic level. RUNGE et al. (1979) have presented evidence that twice-cycled tubulin preparations contain both microtubular accessory proteins and a subunit of the neurofilament, the 68,000-molecular-weight moiety. It is therefore uncertain whether the tubulin antibody preparations stained the paired helical filaments, the proteins trapped among the aggregates of paired helical filaments or one of the microtubular associated proteins. It is difficult to conclude on the evidence available that the paired helical filament peptides are related to tubulin. Furthermore, an antigen raised against chick brain "neurofilaments" of molecular weight 54,000 daltons has been reported by GAMBETTI et al. (1979) to stain human brain neurofilaments, Alzheimer neurofibrillary tangles and aluminum-induced neurofibrillary tangles. Finally, ISCHII et al. (1979) employed the YEN et al. (1976) method for preparing filamentous proteins and purified a 50,000-molecular-weight protein. An antibody raised to this protein decorated both glial filaments and Alzheimer neurofibrillary tangles. Despite great effort, the chemical identity of the peptides involved in the filaments of the paired helical array cannot be considered as known at this time. The technical difficulties of purification must be surmounted before the chemical composition of paired helical filaments of the Alzheimer type is known with certainty, a step which is critical in understanding the cellular origin of neurofibrillary degeneration.

F. Neurofibrillary Degeneration and Altered Function

I. Human Brain

An enquiry into the functional significance of neurofibrillary degeneration implies that this morphological change is indeed associated with some unique contribution to altered brain function and the clinical state. In conditions such as the parkinsonism-dementia complex of Guam, dementia pugilistica or the experimental aluminum encephalopathy in cats and rabbits, in which neurofibrillary degeneration is the only morphological change, this position may be defensible. However, considerable circumstantial evidence suggests that neurofibrillary degeneration may be an epiphenomenon in a special group of neurons in response to a pathogenic event. Therefore, function may be altered in other types of brain cells even in the absence of structural change. The difficulty is componded by the complex nature of neuron–neuron interactions. Altered function may exist in morphologically normal-appearing neurons through such physiological mechanisms as disinhibition, disfacilitation, or alterations in modulatory or trophic factors. Techniques have yet to be developed which will permit rigorous examination of these possibilities in human brain disease; for the present only indirect evidence from clinicopathological studies and animal dementia models permit a correlation between altered function and neurofibrillary degeneration.

In Alzheimer's disease, the relation between altered function and tangles is obscured by various other types of brain pathology associated with the condition. In particular, senile plaques appear to be regions in which synaptic terminals are affected and may result in defective synaptic transmission. Employing a psychiatric evaluation instrument and subsequent histopathological examination, Roth et al. (1966) concluded that dementia was present when the number of senile plaques exceeded an average density of ten per field. These workers counted senile plaques in 60 low-power fields of 1.3 mm diameter taken from twelve 25-µm-thick sections of frontal, temporal, parietal, and occipital lobes for each brain. In the report of Blessed et al. (1968), 73% of a group considered not to have cognitive deficits had plaque counts under two per field and 9% of brains of patients with dementia had average plaque counts of under two per low-power field. In a group of brains from individuals considered to be intellectually normal old people, Tomlinson et al. (1968) reported that widespread neocortical plaques in low density together with neurofibrillary change and granulovacuolar degeneration restricted to the hippocampus or hippocampal cortex may even be accompanied by several small or one to two considerable cerebral infarcts with slight or no mental deterioration.

II. Experimental Animal Models of Neurofibrillary Degeneration

Considering the difficulty in assigning accurately altered function to one of several histopathological changes which occur in aging human brain, it would seem reasonable to consider the physiological alterations associated with an animal model in which neurofibrillary degeneration occurs. No satisfactory animal model of neurofibrillary degeneration composed of paired helical filaments exists; however, aluminum-induced neurofibrillary degeneration has served as a useful model of a dementia process (Crapper and Dalton 1973 a, b; Crapper 1973, 1976). In susceptible species a single, intracranial aluminum injection is followed by an asymptomatic period of several days, which in turn is then followed by a progression of signs beginning with minor changes in learning-memory performance and motor control, which subsequently terminate with profound motor deficits and status epilepticus. Several observations indicate that it is the neurofibrillary degeneration and not the mere presence of aluminum which correlates well with altered function. First, in animal species, such as cat and rabbit, which develop neurofibrillary degeneration in response to aluminum there is an accompanying encephalopathy. In contrast, despite high brain aluminum content, animals such as rat, mouse and monkey do not exhibit histological evidence of neurofibrillary degeneration and do not develop a progressive encephalopathy or altered learning-memory performance. Second, in susceptible species such as rabbit, injection of aluminum by slow infusion into one cerebral cortex resulted in a progressive decline in visual evoked potentials whereas the contralateral cortex exhibited no alteration in evoked potentials (Crapper 1973). The distribution of neurofibrillary degeneration was asymmetrical and the hemisphere with the highest density of tangles was associated with the most marked changes in evoked potentials. Third, employing spike train analysis of the discharge pattern of neurons in the visual cortex of cat, aluminum-treated animals lacked a group of neurons which discharged with a mean spontaneous frequency of greater than seven spikes per second (Crapper and Tomko 1975). Specifically, in the untreated control group of animals, 10% of neurons had spontaneous frequencies between seven and ten spikes per second, and these were recorded at cortical depths corresponding to the supra- and infragranular layers. Light microscopic counts of tissues stained by the Bielschowsky method from the recording site of these aluminum-treated animals revealed that 10%–15% of neurons had neurofibrillary degeneration. The percentage of neurons with neurofibrillary degeneration in the aluminum-treated cats was approximately the same as the number of neurons in the untreated cats with spontaneous mean frequencies of between seven and ten. Furthermore, based on evidence that the majority of cells with mean spontaneous frequencies of spike discharge around ten per second have complex receptive fields and that complex cells are pyramidal in shape, usually in layer 5, it is highly probable that the functionally absent group of cells were the pyramidal-shaped neurons which exhibited neurofibrillary degeneration. Finally, an associative relationship exists between the density of neurofibrillary degeneration and the acquisition of a conditioned avoidance response task. The brains of seven cats employed in experiments designed to measure the acquisition of conditioned avoidance responses were examined histologically (CRAPPER and DALTON 1973 b). The animals received aluminum chloride in the ventral hippocampi and extensive neurofibrillary degeneration was always encountered in that region. However, acquisition performance and density of neocortical neurofibrillary degeneration both varied. To evaluate a possible relationship, the density of neurofibrillary degeneration in the neocortex and entorhinal cortex were ranked according to density and distribution from a minimum of three Bielschowsky-stained sagittal sections about 4–8 mm lateral to the midline of each brain. Utilizing the most difficult criteria of acquisition performance available, namely, the number of trials to make 15 correct avoidances in a row, the data revealed that the more neurofibrillary degeneration was present, the more trials the animals required to attain criterion performance. The animal with the lowest density of neurofibrillary degeneration reached criteria in about 15 trials while the animal with the highest density of tangles required 45 trials to reach criterion performance.

Recent work by FARNELL et al. (1980), employing the in vitro hippocampal slice prepared from control and aluminum-treated rabbits, indicates more precisely the manner in which neuronal function is altered in the aluminum encephalopathy. The first alteration noted in slices removed from aluminum-treated animals is related to long-lasting potentiation of a population spike evoked from hippocampal CA-1 pyramidal-shaped neurons. A conditioning stimulus of 100-Hz pulses for 1 s applied to the stratum radiatum input of CA-1 neurons was employed. The criteria for potentation was a population spike showing an increase of at least 25% baseline response for 30 min after tetanization. The percentage of slices meeting this criteria was 68% for untreated and sodium lactate treated controls, 50% for 5-day, 35% for 10-day, 30% for 25-day, and 20% for 20-day post-aluminum-treated animals. Furthermore, input–output studies relating stimulus strength to input fibre prepotential, population excitatory postsynaptic potentials (EPSPs) and population CA-1 spike potential revealed a significant reduction in the CA-1 spike potential. No alteration in either the pre- or postsynaptic potentials was noted at this early stage in the encephalopathy.

These investigations suggest that an early manifestation of aluminum toxicity is a functional disconnection between postsynaptic potentials and the spike-generating zone of the neurons. It is of interest that the CA-1 neurons do not exhibit light microscopic evidence of neurofibrillary degeneration at the time of recording although neurofibrillary degeneration is present in other brain areas of the animals. Further work will be necessary to establish whether the dissociation between postsynaptic potentials and spike generation in hippocampal neurons without neurofibrillary degeneration is a result of a loss of some trophic or modulatory factors from cells already affected by neurofibrillary degeneration, or an early manifestation of the aluminum-induced metabolic disorder which will eventually manifest itself as neurofibrillary degeneration. However, this study emphasizes that altered neuronal function may occur in hippocampal neurons, which do not themselves exhibit neurofibrillary degeneration. An analogous disorder and dysfunction may occur in morphologically normal-appearing neurons in the human brain when neurofibrillary degeneration affects other neurons in the population.

The next major alteration in neuronal functional properties involves loss of postsynaptic potentials when examined as population responses evoked by either the visual or transcallosal pathways (Crapper 1973). The decreased voltage amplitude in the population response appears related to the density of neurofibrillary degeneration. The final stage of the aluminium encephalopathy is characterized by an alteration in neuron membrane properties which result in prolonged somadendritic depolarization and high frequency axonal spike discharges. This is associated with status epilepticus or myoclonic jerks. The alteration in electrophysiological properties of neurons with neurofibrillary degeneration has been described in detail elsewhere (Crapper 1973, 1976; Crapper and Tomko 1975).

How useful a prediction of the functional consequences of neurofibrillary degeneration the aluminum model will serve for human diseases such as Alzheimer senile dementia cannot be ascertained at present. However, neurons with Alzheimer-type neurofibrillary degeneration contain intranuclear aluminum, as localized by both the electron probe and atomic absorption methods. Furthermore, some regions of Alzheimer affected brain which have high densities of tangles also have concentrations of aluminum which are closely similar to those found lethal to cats and rabbits (Crapper et al. 1980; Perl and Brody 1980). In addition, human cerebral fetal neurons in explant cultures are as susceptible to the toxic effects of aluminum as are cat and rabbit cerebral neurons; hence there is strong circumstantial evidence to indicate that aluminum may exert a toxic role in Alzheimer's disease as a secondary consequence of the primary pathogenic events which initiate the Alzheimer degenerative process (De Boni et al. 1980; Crapper McLachlan and De Boni 1980).

One major difference between the aluminum-induced experimental encephalopathy and Alzheimer's disease is the terminal state of status epilepticus which occurs in the experimental encephalopathy. In the experimental model, a single lethal dose of aluminum is injected and this results in altered function in a large population of cells simultaneously. In Alzheimer's disease, the increase in aluminum probably occurs as a result of a metabolic defect which occurs over a period of many years. Thus, synchronous neurophysiological changes in large numbers of neurons do not occur. It is unlikely that a few widely separated neurons in the human brain passing through a hyperexcitable state would trigger an epileptic seizure. It is therefore speculated that the asynchronous manner in which neurofibrillary degeneration occurs in Alzheimer's disease may explain the difference in terminal states between these two conditions.

G. Summary

In conclusion recent work indicates:

1. The ultrastructural subunit of neurofibrillary degeneration, the paired helical filament, is not unique to human brain disease but may occur in animal brain, both in aging and under certain experimental conditions. Moreover, it is important to note that the period of the helix in animals differs from that found in Alzheimer's disease.

2. Neurofibrillary degeneration is probably an epiphenomenon, a response of an unidentified class of intermediate filaments to the disorganization of intracellular space. Such a disorganization may be precipitated by the primary pathogenic events which underlie the various diseases in which neurofibrillary degeneration is present.

3. Neurofibrillary degeneration is probably a marker for a degenerative process but several lines of evidence indicate that altered function is not restricted to only those neurons which exhibit neurofibrillary degeneration.

4. The unique anatomical distribution of neurofibrillary degeneration within a brain probably determines the distribution of neuronal failure within the brain and this in turn correlates approximately with the pattern of deficits which the individual exhibited during life.

5. The sequence of alterations in neuronal function associated with aluminum-induced neurofibrillary degeneration so far documented is the following:

One of the first observed changes is a loss of long-lasting potentiation of the population spike in CA-1 hippocampal neurons in the absence of changes in amplitude of either the evoked presynaptic volley or the postsynaptic potential. Next, a decrease in the amplitude of the spike potential to single stimuli in the absence of amplitude changes in pre- or postsynaptic potentials. This change is followed by a decrease in postsynaptic potential amplitude with the inhibitory postsynaptic potential more severely affected than the excitatory postsynaptic potential. This stage is followed by a hyperexcitable state in which there are prolonged depolarizations of the somadendritic membrane with multiple spike firing from the neuronal axons, associated with status epilepticus and myclonic jerks.

6. The survival time of neurons with neurofibrillary degeneration in a brain of an individual with an 8-year history of Alzheimer's disease was estimated to be about 270 days.

References

Alzheimer A (1907) Über eine eigenartige Erkrankung der Hirnrinde. Allg Z Psychiat 64:146–148

Anderton BH, Ayers M, Thorpe R (1978) Neurofilaments from mammalian central and peripheral nerve share certain polypeptides. FEBS Letters 96:159–163

Ball MJ (1978) Topographic distribution of neurofibrillary tangles and granulovacuolar degeneration in hippocampal cortex of aging and demented patients. A quantitative study. Acta Neuropath (Berl) 42:73–80

Blessed G, Tomlinson BE, Roth M (1968) The association between quantitative measures of dementia and of senile change in the cerebral grey matter of elderly subjects. Br J Psychiat 14:797:811

Bruce MA, Fraser H (1975) Amyloid plaques in the brains of mice injected with scrapie: morphological variation and staining properties. Neuropath Appl Neurobiol 1:189–202

Brun A, Gustafson L (1976) Distribution of cerebral degeneration in Alzheimer's disease. A clinical-pathological study. Arch Psychiatr Nervenkr 223:15–33

Crapper DR (1973) Experimental neurofibrillary degeneration and altered electrical activity. Electroenceph Clin Neurophysiol 35:575–588

Crapper DR (1974) Dementia: recent observations on Alzheimer's disease and experimental aluminium encephalopathy. In: Seeman P, Brown GM (eds) Frontiers in neurology and neuroscience research, Parkinson foundation. Symposium No 1 of the Neuroscience Institute of the University of Toronto. University of Toronto, pp 97–111

Crapper DR (1976) Functional consequences of neurofibrillary degeneration. In: Gershon S, Terry RD (eds) Functional consequences of neurofibrillary degeneration. Raven Press, New York, pp 405–432

Crapper DR, Dalton AJ (1973a) Alterations in short term retension, conditioned avoidance response acquisition and motivation following aluminum induced neurofibrillary degeneration. Physiol Behav 10:925–933

Crapper DR, Dalton AJ (1973b) Aluminum induced neurofibrillary degeneration, brain electrical activity and alterations in acquisition and retention. Physiol Behav 10:935:945

Crapper DR, De Boni U (1980) Models for the biochemical study of dementia. In: Roberts PH (ed) Biochemistry of Dementia. John Wiley and Sons Ltd, New York, pp 53–68

Crapper McLachlan DR, De Boni U (1980) Aluminum in human brain disease – an overview. Neurotoxicol 1:3–16

Crapper DR, Tomko GJ (1975) Neuronal correlates of an encephalopathy induced by aluminum neurofibrillary degeneration. Brain Res 97:253–364

Crapper DR, Krishnan SS, Dalton AJ (1973) Brain aluminum distribution in Alzheimer's disease and experimental neurofibrillary degeneration. Science 180:511–513

Crapper DR, Dalton AJ, Skopitz M, Scott JW, Hachinski VC (1975) Alzheimer degeneration in Down syndrome: electrophysiological alterations and histopathology. Arch Neurol 32:618–623

Crapper DR, Krishnan SS, Quittkat S (1976) Aluminum, neurofibrillary degeneration and Alzheimer disease. Brain 99:67–79

Crapper DR, Karlik S, De Boni U (1978) Aluminum and other metals in senile (Alzheimer) dementia. In: Katzman R, Terry RD, Bick KL (eds) The neurobiology of aging, vol VII. Raven Press, New York, pp 477–491

Crapper DR, Quittkat S, Krishnan SS, Dalton AJ, De Boni U (1980) Intranuclear aluminium content in Alzheimer's disease, dialysis encephalopathy and experimental aluminium encephalopathy. ActaNeuropath 50:19–24

De Boni U, Seger M, Crapper McLachlan DR (1980) Functional consequences of chromatin bound aluminum in cultured human cells. Neurotoxicol 1:65–81

Farnell B, De Boni U, Crapper McLachlan DR (1980) Electrophysiological correlates of aluminum neurotoxicity in the absence of neurofibrillary degeneration. Soc Neurosc, abstract 248.10, 6:741

Foelix RF, Hauser M (1979) Helically twisted filaments in giant neurons of a whip spider. Eur J Cell Biol 19:303–306

Gambetti P, Velasko ME, Dahl D, Bignami A, Roessmann U (1979) Neurofibrillary tangles in Alzheimer's disease. An immunological study. Abstract. International Society for Neurochemistry, Florence, p 10

Grundke-Iqbal I, Johnson A, Wisniewski M, Term RD, Iqbal K (1979) Evidence that Alzheimer neurofibrillary tangles originate from neurotubules. Lancet 1:578–580

Henneberg R (1910) Messung der Oberflächenausdehnung der Großhirnrinde. J Psychol Neurol 17:144

Iqbal K, Wisniewski HM, Shelanski ML, Brostoff S, Liwnicz, Terry RD (1974) Protein changes in senile dementia. Brain Res 77:337–343

Iqbal K, Grundke-Iqbal J, Wisniewski M, Terry RD (1978) Chemical relationship of the paired helical filaments of Alzheimer's dementia to normal neurofilaments and neurotubules. Brain Res 142:321–332

Ishii T (1966) Distribution of Alzheimer's neurofibrillary changes in the brain stem and hypothalamus of senile dementia. Acta Neuropath 6:181–187

Ishii T, Haga S, Tokutake S (1979) Presence of neurofilament protein in Alzheimer's neurofibrillary tangles (ANT). Acta Neuropath (Berl) 48:105–112

Kidd M (1963) Paired helical filaments in electron microscopy of Alzheimer's disease. Nature (Lond) 197:192–193

Kidd M (1964) Alzheimer's disease – an electron microscopical study. Brain 87:307–319

Kidd M (1970) Neurofibrillary changes in conditions related to Alzheimer's disease. In: Wolstenholme GE, O'Connor M (eds) Alzheimer's disease and related conditions. J and A Churchill, London, pp 202–203

Lazarides E (1980) Intermediate filaments as mechanical integrators of cellular space. Nature 283:249–256

Micko S, Schlaepfer WW (1978) Protein composition of axons and myelin from rat and human peripheral nerves. J Neurochem 30:1041–1049

Perl DP, Brody AR (1980) Alzheimer's disease: X-ray spectrometric evidence of aluminum accumulation in neurofibrillary tangle-bearing neurons. Science 208:297–299

Roth M, Tomlinson BE, Blessed G (1966) Correlation between scores for dementia and counts of senile plaques in cerebral gray matter of elderly subjects. Nature 209:109–110

Runge MS, Dietrich H, Williams RC (1979) Identification of the major 68,000 dalton protein of microtubule preparations as a 10 nm filament protein and its effects on microtubule assembly in vitro. Biochemistry 18:1689–1698

Schlaepfer WW (1978) Observations on the disassembly of isolated mammalian neurofilaments. J Cell Biol 76:50–56

Selkoe DJ, Liem RKH, Yen S, Shelanski M (1979) Biochemical and immunological characterization of neurofilaments in experimental neurofibrillary degeneration induced by aluminum. Brain Res 163:235–252

Shelanski ML (1978) Discussion. In: Katzman R, Terry RD, Bick KL (eds) Alzheimer's disease: senile dementia and related disorders. Raven Press, New York, pp 425–426

Steele JC, Richardson JC, Olszewski J (1964) Progressive supranuclear palsy. Arch Neurol 10:333–359

Tellez-Nagel I, Wisniewski H (1973) Ultrastructure of neurofibrillary tangles in Steele-Richardson-Olszewski syndrom. Arch Neurol 29:324–327

Tomlinson BE, Blessed G, Roth M (1968) Observations on the brains of now-demented old people. J Neurol Sci 7:331–356

Tomlinson BE, Blessed G, Roth M (1970) Observations on the brains of demented old people. J Neurol Sci 11:205–242

Volk B (1980) Paired helical filaments in rat spinal ganglia following chronic alcohol administration: an electron microscopic investigation. Neuropath Appl Neurobiol 6:143–153

Wisniewski HM, Ghetti B, Terry RD (1973) Neuritic (senile) plaques and filamentous changes in aged rhesus monkeys. J Neuropath Exp Neurol 32:566–584

Wisniewski HM, Bruce MA, Fraser H (1975) Infectious etiology of neuritic (senile) plaques in mice. Science 190:1108–1110

Wisniewski H, Narang H, Terry RD (1976) Neurofibrillary tangles of paired helical filaments. Neurol Sci 27:173–181

Wisniewski K, Jervis GA, Moretz RC, Wisniewski H (1979) Alzheimer neurofibrillary tangles in diseases other than senile and presenile dementia. Ann Neurol 5:288–294

Yen SH, Dahl D, Schachner M, Shelanski ML (1976) Biochemistry of the filaments of brain. Proc Natl Acad Sci USA 73:529–533

Neurochemistry of the Aging Brain

W. Meier-Ruge

A. Introduction

A number of reviews have appeared on the neurochemistry of the aging brain (Bürger 1957; Samorajski and Ordy 1972; Timiras 1972; Ordy and Kaack 1975; Domino et al. 1978; Bowen and Davison 1978, Frolkis and Bezrukov 1979). These have dealt excellently with the literature up to about 1973 and there is therefore no need to cover this ground again in this chapter. Most investigations on human brain aging, however, have appeared in the last 10 years.

B. Nucleic Acids and Protein Biosynthesis

It is now regarded as proven that the control of cell function is embodied in the genetic code in the cell nucleus. Nuclear DNA exerts its control over cell function by synthesis of RNA. The latter, in turn, synthesises membrane proteins and enzymes which regulate the chemical activity of the cell.

We now know that there are three main types of RNA: messenger RNA (mRNA), ribosomal RNA (rRNA), and transfer RNA (tRNA). Precursors of mRNA are: heterogeneous nuclear RNA (hnRNA) and premessenger RNA (pmRNA). Messenger RNA is synthesised in the cell nucleus and is believed to transcribe the genetic code in the nucleus and convert the instructions for synthesis of the protein structure into the actual synthesis of a polypeptide on rRNA (Wulf et al. 1967).

The key role of protein metabolism and protein biosynthesis in the aging process was recognized as early as 1956 in a review by Bürger. In the sixties neurochemists became increasingly interested in neuronal RNA metabolism, since the studies by Hydén (1967) suggested that a specific protein might be formed in memory storage. No entirely plausible explanation has, as yet, been put forward to explain how RNA might play a part in the transfer and storage of information.

Hydén's theory of memory storage aside, nucleic acid and protein metabolism is also of particular interest since it is of fundamental importance for the maintenance of cell compartments and for energy and transmitter metabolism. Although protein metabolism appears to play a key role in the development of senile brain disorders, particularly senile dementia, very few studies have so far been undertaken in pursuance of this line of research.

Frolkis and Bezrukov (1979) regard altered protein synthesis (damage to DNA, loss of RNA-encoding DNA, reduced RNA synthesis and changed protein synthesis) as the pathogenetic basis underlying age-related impairment of nerve-cell function. If a way could be found of activating the genetic apparatus and stimulating protein synthesis pharmacologically, this would offer a causal treatment of age-related brain disorders.

Reviews in the literature of investigations on nucleoprotein and protein metabolism over the last decade have been published by Herrmann (1971), Frolkis (1973 a, b), Cutler (1976), Finch (1977), and Kanungo (1980).

I. Deoxyribonucleic Acid

NABER and DAHNKE (1979) observed no age-related reduction in the DNA content of the human brain. But also in laboratory animals has no major decrease of DNA been found. Cytophotometric estimates of DNA have revealed hyperploidy and, occasionally, tetraploidy of neuronal nuclear DNA (KRYGIER et al. 1977).

Studies of the molecular biological aspects of age-related changes in DNA point to decreased DNA methylation (KUDRYASHOVA and VANYUSHIN 1976) and histone methylation (LEE and DUERRE 1974). Other investigations dealing with the physicochemical properties of DNA have shown that the temperature at which DNA undergoes thermal denaturation increases progressively with age, this being attributed to stabilisation of the DNA helix (KURTZ and SINEX 1967).

A loss of genes which encode ribosomal RNA in the cell nucleus has actually been demonstrated in human hippocampal gyrus and somatosensory cortex (STREHLER and CHANG 1979). The brains of aging humans (STREHLER and CHANG 1979) display a progressive age-related decrease in hybridisable rDNA.

Changes such as these in the genetic material suggest that age-related alteration of DNA plays a key role in the aging process.

II. Chromatin and Histone

Various molecular-biological papers in recent years have adduced further proof for the hypothesis that the regulation of the genetic activity of the nerve cell (template activity) is linked with the interaction between chromatin and histone (DE BONI and CRAPPER-MCLACHLAN 1980; FROLKIS and BEZRUKOV 1979).

The metabolic activity of chromatin-bound histone declines with increasing age (ERMINI and REICHLMEIER 1976; ERMINI et al. 1978).

A typical sign of aging is the decreased ability of chromosomal histone in nerve cell nuclei to undergo phosphorylation (ERMINI and REICHLMEIER 1976).

Chromatin-bound histone 4 derived from isolated human corticocerebral neurons and separated by electrophoresis displays a 50% lower rate of incorporation of phosphate in old individuals, indicating an age-related increase in the degree of condensation of the chromatin (ERMINI et al. 1978).

These findings also suggest that with increasing age the nucleoproteins undergo a change of conformation. This probably results in declining genetic activity, which would explain many of the age-related changes in brain cells. Thus DE BONI and CRAPPER-MCLACHLAN (1980) regard a change in the conformation of neuronal chromatin as the aetiological step responsible for the development of senile dementia.

III. Ribonucleic Acid

Determination of *age-related changes in the RNA content of the brain* yields very limited information since, for example, the RNA content might remain constant despite an age-related decline in RNA turnover.

Neuronal RNA levels determined by the cytophotometric method in different regions of the human brain (Table 1) likewise indicate an age-related reduction in

Table 1. Cytophotometric RNA measurements in the aging brain

Species	Age	Tissue	RNA content	Reference
Man	2 y→91 y	Dentate nucleus Hippocampus	} −15%–30%	MANN et al. (1978)
		Olivary nucleus	−60%	
Man	1/66 y→ >80 y	Prefrontal gyrus	−34%	UEMURA and HARTMANN (1978a)
Man	1/49 y→92 y	Hypoglossal nucleus	−48%	UEMURA and HARTMANN (1978b)
Man	Normal elderly →senile dementia	Locus coeruleus Substantia nigra Thalamus Motor. nuclei III, IV, VIII, XII	} −10%	MANN et al. (1977)
		Betz cells Hippocampus h_1 Motor. nucleus V	} −20%	
		Purkinje cells Nucl. dentatus Nucl. olivae Hippocampus h_3, h_5 Motor. nucleus	} −30%	
		Hippocampus h_2, h_4	−44%–51%	
Man	Normal elderly →senile dementia	Cerebellum (Purkinje cells)	−28%	MANN and SINCLAIR (1978)
		Hippocampus	−33%	
Man	Normal elderly →Alzheimer's disease	Locus coeruleus Subst. nigra	−21% − 4%	MANN et al. (1980)
Man	Normal elderly →arteriosclerosis	Locus coeruleus Subst. nigra	− 4% − 6%	

y, years; →, in comparison with

RNA (MANN and YATES 1974; UEMURA and HARTMANN 1978a, b; MANN et al. 1978). Biochemical assays of RNA in human brain have merely revealed a decrease in the RNA/DNA ratio (SMITH 1978) or have failed to show any age-related change in RNA content (NABER and DAHNKE 1979) (Table 2).

Cytophotometric assays of RNA in the brains of patients with senile dementia showed that RNA content of the neurons was greatly reduced, although there was much individual variation (MANN et al. 1977; UEMURA and HARTMANN 1978a, b).

It is noteworthy that similar investigations on the hippocampal gyrus revealed an increase in RNA, coinciding with the occurrence of neurofibrillary tangles which are believed by these authors to be associated with pathological change in RNA synthesis (UEMURA and HARTMANN (1979a). Normally neurons with neurofibrillary tangles have a reduced RNA content (UEMURA and HARTMANN 1979b). Findings by O'BRIEN et al. (1980), who discovered structures containing rRNA in

Table 2. Changes in the nucleic acid content of the brain in normal old people and in patients with senile dementia

Age		DNA	RNA	RNA/DNA	Reference
46–68 y→70–90 y (normal aging)	Putamen	(↑)	±0	(↓)	Samorajski and Rolsten (1973)
	Caudate nucleus	(↑)	(↑)	(↑)	
	Frontal cortex	(↓)	(↑)	(↑)	
16 y→91 y (normal aging)	Thalamus Putamen Caudate nucleus Cerebellum Frontal cortex	±0	±0	±0	Naber and Dahnke (1979)
Normal elderly →senile dementia	Temporal lobe	±0	±0		Bowen et al. (1977)
Normal elderly →senile dementia	Temporal lobe			Decrease	Smith (1978)

y, years; →, in comparison with; ( ), non-significant trend; (↓), decrease; (↑), increase

Hirano bodies in the hippocampus from patients with senile dementia, also support the view that there might be a relationship between impaired RNA synthesis and the occurrence of neurofibrillary tangles.

Our knowledge of receptor synthesis and its posttranslational modification is still very limited. Mendez et al. (1980) were the first to identify the mRNA which induces the synthesis of acetylcholine receptor peptides. De Baetselier et al. (1980) found a marked age-related increase in relative translations of mRNA which transmits the synthesis code for isotubulin. This increased translation of mRNA is believed to be responsible for the increased variation in chemical structure of the tubulins in old age.

These more recent papers also illustrate the importance of nucleic acid metabolism for the maintenance of functional integrity. They afford an explanation of how such disturbances, if they affected a sufficiently large number of nerve cells, could give rise to a host of metabolic regulatory defects. It is also conceivable that brain disorders of old age, such as Alzheimer's disease, might arise in this way.

IV. Protein Biosynthesis in the Brain: The Investigation of Free Amino Acid Levels

In the aging brain *cytoplasmic protein synthesis* is generally reduced. However, in order to make a reliable assessment of protein synthesis, each cell compartment must be examined separately. Thus with increasing age the quantity of neuronal protein, S-5 and S-6 (neuronin), decreases, whereas the quantity of the glia-specific protein S-100 is significantly raised (Perez and Moore 1970; Bowen et al. 1976).

Low protein values have been found in various brain structures of old people (Naber and Dahnke 1979), and bands 2 and 4 of the soluble proteins separated by polyacrylamide-gel electrophoresis show an age-related decrease (Kaneko et al. 1979).

Table 3. Age-dependent changes in the protein content of the human brain

Age	Tissue	Protein	Neuronin (S–5) (S–6)	Reference
16 y→91 y	Thalamus	−15%		NABER and
	Putamen	− 8%		DAHNKE (1979)
	Caudate nucleus	− 9%		NABER et al. (1979)
	Cerebellum	−13%		
	Frontal cortex	− 5%		
17/49 y→80/89 y	Frontal pole	± 0		BERLET and VOLK (1980)
Normal elderly →senile dementia	Temporal lobe	± 0	Neuronin S–6 −83% Neuronin S–5 ±0	BOWEN et al. (1977)
Normal elderly →senile dementia	Temporal lobe	−21%		DAVISON (1978)
Normal elderly →senile dementia	Grey matter	−40%		KANEKO et al. (1979)

y, years; →, in comparison with

In the geriatric brain disorder *Alzheimer's disease* soluble proteins show changes only in a few brain areas (see Table 3). Total proteins are reported by some authors to be unchanged (OP DEN VELDE and STAM 1976; BOWEN et al. 1977), while others have found a reduction in total proteins (KANEKO et al. 1979). When the soluble proteins are separated by polyacrylamide-gel electrophoresis, protein bands 2 and 4, which in the normal way show an age-related decrease, are almost totally lacking (HARIGUCHI 1978; KANEKO et al. 1979).

The soluble protein of the hippocampus from brains of patients with Alzheimer's disease is found to contain a new band of proteins with a molecular weight of 50,000. This band is a characteristic feature of the disease and corresponds in weight to the protein of the twisted tubules (IQBAL et al. 1974; MINER et al. 1976). In the temporal lobes of brains from patients with Alzheimer's disease neuronin S-6 and the protein content of the light mitochondrial fraction are significantly reduced (BOWEN et al. 1977).

V. Proteins of the White Matter and Extracellular Space

Glycoproteids consist of a polypeptide and oligosaccharide side chain. The glycoproteids were previously also known as glycoproteins. Proteids are fairly readily cleaved compounds with a protein moiety and a non-protein component. Where a non-protein component is firmly bound to a protein moiety and forms an integral part of the molecule, such a substance is known as a protein.

The properties of glycoproteids resemble those of proteins. The carbohydrate component of the glycoproteids accounts for 10%–25% of the molecular weight and may be sialic acid, glucosamine, galactosamine, fucose, mannose or galactose. Usually only a few oligosaccharide groups are linked to the protein chain. The glycoproteids form a group with few functional or structural characteristics, and no uniform terminology has been devised to describe them. Glycoproteids are frequently classified according to where they occur, rather than according to their chemical nature. They owe their importance mainly to their role as transport or membrane proteins.

The total quantity of cerebral glycoproteids is reduced in old age, but the composition of these membrane proteins remains unchanged (BERRA and BRUNNGRABER 1975).

With increasing age, changes occur in the *basic protein of myelin in the white matter*. In elderly people the basic protein component of myelin is reduced by as much as 45% (ANSARI and LOCH 1975). BERLET and VOLK (1980) observed only a trend to lower levels of basic protein in elderly people. Basic proteins from old and young people displayed no qualitative differences. The reduction in basic protein is probably due to a decrease in the total quantity of myelin (ANSARI and LOCH 1975; see Table 4).

The total protein content of the white matter and myelin (frontal lobes, corpus callosum) remains unchanged with increasing age (BERLET and VOLK 1980). TOEWS and HORROCKS (1976) are the only investigators who reported a drop (8%) in protein concentration in the 60–83 year age group compared with the 15–60 year age group. No age-related change is observed in the activity of 2′3′-cyclic nucleotide-3′-phosphohydrolase (CNP), the characteristic enzyme of the myelin sheath.

Most findings on changes in myelin glycoproteids point to an age-related reduction in the glycoproteids characteristic of myelin.

C. Lipids of the Central Nervous System

A few general remarks are needed concerning the lipids of the central nervous system (Table 5) since confusion may easily arise owing to the large number of components which go to form the lipids of the brain. But also the use of different lipid classifications may be confusing.

In the past, lipids of the brain were differentiated into phosphatides (phosphatidic acids, lecithins, cephalins, inositphosphatides, acetalphosphatides, sphingomyelins), cerebrosides and gangliosides.

Today a classification is preferred, the distinguishing feature of which is the presence of the main alcohol moiety:

1. Glycerophospholipids (diglycerides)

    a) Phosphatidic acids
    b) Lecithins
    c) Cephalins
    d) Inositphosphatides
    e) Acetalphosphatides

2. Sphingolipids (*N*-acylsphingosines)

    a) Sphingomyelins
    b) Cerebrosides
    c) Sulphatides
    d) Gangliosides

Cerebrosides, sulphatides and gangliosides are classified as glycolipids on the basis of their sugar component.

Reviews of the neurochemistry of the lipids have been published by BURTON (1971) and BOWEN et al. (1974).

Table 4. Changes in the protein content of the white matter in the aging brain

Species	Age	Tissue	Protein	Basic protein	Mitochondrial light proteins	References
Man	55 y→76 y	White matter of frontal brain		−45%		ANSARI and LOCH (1975)
Man	15/60 y→61/63 y	White matter		− 8%		TOEWS and HORROCKS (1976)
Man	16 y→91 y	White matter	−7%			NABER and DAHNKE (1979) NABER et al. (1979)
Man	17/49 y→80/89 y	White matter of frontal brain	(↓)			BERLET and VOLK (1980)
		Corpus callosum	(↓)			
Man	Normal elderly→senile dementia	Temporal lobe			−45%	BOWEN et al. (1977)
Man	Normal elderly→Alzheimer's disease	White matter	Decrease			KANEKO et al. (1979)

y, years; →, in comparison with; ( ), non-significant trend; (↓), decrease; (↑), increase

Table 5. Changes of the lipid content of the aging brain

Species	Age	Tissue	Total content of				Reference
			Lipid	Phospho-lipid	Myelin	Gangli-oside	
Man	30 y→98 y	Total brain	−19%	±0 (↑)	(↓)	−80%	ROUSER and YAMAMOTO (1968) YAMAMOTO and ROUSER (1973)
Man	17 y→89 y	White matter (frontal pole)			−30%		BERLET and VOLK (1980)
		Corpus callosum			−30%		
Man	Normal elderly→senile dementia	Temporal lobe				−44%	BOWEN et al. (1977)
						−28%	DAVISON (1978)

y, years; →, in comparison with; ( ), non-significant trend; (↓), decrease; (↑), increase

I. Fatty Acid Metabolism

Studies of fatty acids in the aging brain are difficult to evaluate unless it is borne in mind that the length of the carbon chain of the fatty acids may vary in different lipids. Gangliosides are characterized by C_{20} or higher fatty acids and cerebrosides by C_{24} and higher fatty acids.

Studies of changes in the fatty acid composition of myelin in old age have mainly been carried out on the human brain. Yamamoto and Rouser (1973) observed a decrease in free fatty acids and a reduction in total lipid content in brains from old people. The ethanolamine-containing phosphoglycerides of myelin have been found to have an increased content of fatty acids C 18:1 and C 20:1, only the polyunsaturated fatty acids C 20:4, C 22:4, and C 22:6 showing a significant decrease with age (Rouser and Yamamoto 1969).

The fatty acid content of cerebrosides and sulphatides shows no change in the aging brain. However, there is a decrease in C 24:1 fatty acids and an increase in C 18:0 fatty acids in the single myelins (Samorajski and Rolsten 1973; Heipertz et al. 1977).

II. Gangliosides of the Aging Brain

The fatty acid content of the gangliosides, which are a characteristic feature of the grey matter, increases with age (Mansson et al. 1978) (Table 5).

Accordingly there is an age-related decrease in the ganglioside content of the grey matter in man (Berra and Brunngraber 1975; Bowen et al. 1977). The reduction in ganglioside levels is particularly pronounced in Alzheimer's disease (Suzuki and Chen 1966; Cherayil 1969; op den Velde and Hooghwinkel 1975; Bowen et al. 1977). In presenile dementia of the Jacob-Creutzfeld type the fall in ganglioside level was particularly marked and correlated with the degree of severity of the disease (Suzuki and Chen 1966).

The concentration of the D 20-sphingosine component of the gangliosides in the white matter decreases only slightly in old age in human subjects (Mansson et al. 1978).

III. Lipids of the Myelin Sheath

Few studies have been carried out on changes in the myelin of the white matter in old age. The work that has been done points mainly to a reduction in 2',3'-cyclic-nucleotide-3'-phosphohydrolase activity (CNP) (Smith 1978; Berlet and Volk 1980). Toews and Horrocks (1976) failed to find any age-related change in CNP activity.

The actual myelin content appears to decrease with increasing age, according to analyses carried out on human brain tissue obtained at autopsy (Berlet and Volk 1980) (Table 5). According to Sun and Sun (1979), aging is associated with qualitative changes in the lipid constituents of myelin. Prominent among these are an increase in ethanolamine and plasmalogen (acetalphosphatides) and a decrease in the polyunsaturated acyl groups of the membrane phosphoglycerides which are important for myelin function.

D. Carbohydrate Metabolism of the Aging Brain

I. Glucose Uptake and Utilisation

Since the fundamental work by GOTTSTEIN et al. (1964, 1972) and SOKOLOFF (1966, 1975), we know that the glucose consumption of the brain in normal old people is 23% lower than in young adults (Table 6), despite the fact that the oxygen consumption of the brain remains within normal limits (SOKOLOFF 1975). GOTTSTEIN et al. (1972) observed that the brains of old people metabolise increased quantities of ketones and may thus require less glucose.

In senile dementia there is a further massive reduction in glucose consumption, which falls to nearly half the values for young adults (Table 6) (SOKOLOFF 1975).

II. Glycolysis and the Metabolic Activity of the Citric Acid Cycle

Glycolysis is one of the most fundamental energy-producing metabolic processes in the brain. In recent years glycolysis has attracted increasing interest in connection with age-related metabolic changes. A number of studies have shown that the aging brain has a reduced glycolytic capacity and consequently the efficiency of the neurons is impaired (MEIER-RUGE et al. 1978; FROLKIS and BEZRUKOV 1979; IWAN-GOFF et al. 1979, 1980; MEIER-RUGE et al. 1979, 1980).

It should be emphasised that not all the glycolytic enzymes display reduced activity as a result of advanced cerebral aging processes. Only the key enzymes in the glycolytic process, such as hexokinase and phosphofructokinase, display reduced activity in old age (MEIER-RUGE et al. 1978; IWANGOFF et al. 1979).

The reduction in energy-producing capacity probably has a significant adverse effect on the ability of the neurons to meet increased demands, in particular in connection with active ion transport for repolarisation of excitatory and inhibitory neurons and for the maintenance of cell membrane potentials (FROLKIS 1970; FROLKIS and BEZRUKOV 1979; MEIER-RUGE et al. 1979, 1980). Evidence that this is the case was recently published by SYLVIA and ROSENTHAL (1978 b, 1979 a, b).

In Alzheimer's disease the temporal lobes not only show greatly depressed phosphofructokinase and increased soluble hexokinase activity, but also a significant reduction in phosphoglycerate mutase, aldolase, phosphoglucose-isomerase and triose-phosphate-isomerase activity. There were no significant changes in the activities of any of the other glycolytic enzymes (IWANGOFF et al. 1980). In severe cases of Alzheimer's disease, OP DEN VELDE and STAM (1976) found that lactate dehydrogenase and acid phosphatase activity tended to be depressed.

The activity of the citric acid cycle enzyme, SDH, was depressed by 37% in the temporal lobes of patients with senile dementia (BOWEN et al. 1977). Other investigators observed an increase in malate dehydrogenase activity (OP DEN VELDE and STAM 1976).

III. Oxidative Phosphorylation and Oxygen Consumption in the Aging Brain

In normal individuals no decrease in cerebral oxygen consumption is observed up to the age of 60 (SOKOLOFF 1966, 1975). An approximately 20% decrease in oxygen

Table 6. Age-related changes in cerebral glucose uptake, carbohydrate metabolism and respiration rate

Species	Age	Tissue	Glucose consumption	Glycolysis	Respiration O_2 consumption	Reference
Man	20 y→71 y	Normal brain	−23%		6% n.s.	Sokoloff (1966, 1975)
Man	21 y→72 y	Chronic senile brain syndrome	−40%		−23%	Sokoloff (1975)
Man	21 y→91 y	Cortex; Putamen		Soluble hexokinase +46% Phosphofructokinase −56% Aldolase −19% n.s. Phosphoglycerate mutase −26% n.s. All other glycolytic enzymes ±0		Meier-Ruge et al. (1978, 1979) Iwangoff et al. (1979)
Man	Normal elderly →senile dementia	Temporal lobe		Soluble hexokinase +61% Phosphofructokinase −88% Phosphoglycerate mutase Aldolase Phosphoglucose Isomerase Triosephosphate Isomerase } −25%–50%		Iwangoff et al. (1980)
Man	Normal elderly →senile dementia	Temporal lobe		Decrease >55%		Bowen et al. (1979)

y, years; →, in comparison with; n.s., non-significant

consumption is observed only in organic psychoses associated with degeneration of the brain in elderly people (GOTTSTEIN et al. 1964; SOKOLOFF 1966, 1975).

Convincing evidence obtained by non-invasive and invasive methods in laboratory animals has been presented by SYLVIA and ROSENTHAL (1979a), confirming the hypothesis that the inability of the aging brain to meet increased energy requirements may be due to inhibition of glycolytic key enzymes (FROLKIS and BEZRUKOV 1979; MEIER-RUGE et al. 1979, 1980).

During heightened metabolic demands, cytochrome a and a_3 levels are transiently reduced (SYLVIA and ROSENTHAL 1978a, b, 1979a, b).

Metabolic studies of synaptic and non-synaptic mitochondria have revealed a reduction in state 3 and 4 respiration (DESHMUKH et al. 1980; DESHMUKH and PATEL 1980). However, the NAD/NADH redox response remains unchanged in old age (SYLVIA and ROSENTHAL 1978b). Under resting conditions respiratory chain oxidation in the CNS is unchanged in old age (SYLVIA and ROSENTHAL 1978a).

Broadly speaking the energy-producing metabolism of the aging brain reflects a progressive decline.

E. Age-Related Changes in Various Enzymes Unrelated to Transmitter Production

Enzymes involved in neurotransmitter metabolism, such as AChE, MAO, GAD, CAT, GABA, TH etc. as well as transmitter-dependent metabolic systems such as adenylcyclase, phosphodiesterase, protein-kinase, cAMP, cGMP, etc. have been excluded from this chapter, since they are dealt with in the chapter on neurotransmitters in normal aging.

I. Oxidoreductases

The enzymes of this group catalyse oxidation–reduction processes. It is the first main group in the International Enzyme Nomenclature and comprises dehydrogenases, reductases, transhydrogenases, oxidases, which reduce oxygen directly, oxygenases, which introduce the oxygen molecule into the substrate, peroxidases having H_2O_2 as their hydrogen acceptor and catalases.

All the oxidoreductases which have been investigated in connection with age-related changes in glycolysis and the respiratory chain have already been dealt with (see Sect. D).

In recent years superoxide-dismutase has attracted increasing attention in connection with aging processes in the central nervous system. TOLMASOFF et al. (1980) failed to find any age-related changes in cerebral superoxide-dismutase not only in man, but also in several primate species and two rodent species. They merely noted that superoxide-dismutase activity was greater in long-lived species.

II. Age-Related Changes in the Hydrolases

Hydrolases are enzymes which bring about the cleavage of esters, acid amides, glycosides and acid anhydrides with addition of water. These hydrolases are located in lysosomes. Lysosomal hydrolases include acid phosphatase, cathepsins, ribonuclease, glucuronidase, esterase, lipase, amylase, nucleosidase, and leucine-aminopeptidase. The ATP-splitting phosphatases also belong to the hydrolase group.

In the brain of normal elderly people, no significant changes are found in the lysosomal enzymes β-galactosidase, β-glucosidase, α-mannosidase, hexosamini-dase, and acid phosphatase (Brun and Hultberg 1975). Acid phosphatase activity tends to increase only in severe forms of dementia (Op Den Velde and Stam 1976).

Phosphohydrolase characteristic of medullated axons shows approximately a 37% decrease in activity in the temporal region of the brain in old people. However, β-glucuronidase, which is characteristic of cerebral glial cells, remains unchanged (Bowen et al. 1977).

The overall activity of ATPases involved in the cleavage of energy-rich phosphates remains largely unchanged with increasing age in the human brain (Sun and Samorajski 1975).

Iwangoff et al. (1979, 1980) arrived at similar results for brain tissue from old people.

Sun and Samorajski (1975) observed that synaptosomal Na^+/K^+ ATPase was inhibited by alcohol to a greater extent in old than in young human brains.

III. Lyases

The lyases are the fourth enzyme group in the International Enzyme Nomenclature. They split functional groups from their substrate in non-hydrolytic reactions. Examples are dehydratases, which split off water, and decarboxylases, which split off CO_2.

The only lyase investigated for changes with increasing age in human brain is carbonic anhydrase. Studies of brain tissue obtained at autopsy have yielded varying results. Bowen et al. (1977) found no significant reduction in carbonic anhydrase activity in temporal lobes from patients with senile dementia. On the other hand, systematic investigations of normal age changes in human brain showed that there was a significant age-related reduction in carbonic anhydrase activity in the cerebral cortex and corpus striatum and that the difference became significant from the age of 70 onwards. Carbonic anhydrase activity was reduced by 17% in the cerebral cortex and 25% in the corpus striatum (Reichlmeier et al. 1977, 1978 a, b; Iwangoff et al. 1979).

The age-related reduction in carbonic anhydrase activity probably correlates with the reduced glucose metabolism and oxygen turnover in the aging brain.

References

Ansari KA, Loch J (1975) Decreased myelin basic protein content of the aged human brain. Neurology 25:1045–1050
Berlet HH, Volk B (1980) Age-related microheterogeneity of myelin basic protein isolated from human brain. In: Amaducci I et al. (eds) Aging of the brain and dementia. Raven Press, New York, pp 81–90
Berra B, Brunngraber EG (1975) Glycopeptide composition, ganglioside patterns and glycosaminoglycan content of human cerebral grey matter at different ages. Biochem Exp Biol 11:401–405
Bowen DM, Davison AN (1978) 3. Biochemical changes in the normal ageing brain and in dementia. In: Isaacs B (ed) Recent advances in geriatric medicine. Churchill-Livingstone, Edinburgh London New York, pp 41–59

Bowen DM, Davison AN, Ramsey RB (1974) The dynamic role of lipids in the nervous system. In: Goodwin TW (ed) Biochemistry series one, vol 4. Butterworths, London, University Park Press, Baltimore, pp 142–179

Bowen DM, Smith CB, White P et al. (1976) Neurotransmitter-related enzymes and indices of hypoxia in senile dementia and other abiotrophies. Brain 99:459–496

Bowen DM, Smith CB, White P et al. (1977) Chemical pathology of the organic dementia. I. Validity of biochemical measurements on human post-mortem brain specimens. Brain 100:397–426

Bowen DM, Spillane JA, Curzon G et al. (1979) Accelerated ageing or selective neuronal loss as an important cause of dementia? Lancet 1:11–14

Brun A, Hultberg B (1975) Regional study of acid hydrolases and lysosomal membrane properties in the normal human brain at various ages. Mech Age Developm 4:201–213

Bürger M (1956) Das Altern des Zentralnervensystems. Experientia Suppl 4:101–111

Bürger M (1957) Die chemische Biomorphose des menschlichen Gehirns. Abh. Sächs. Akad. Wiss. Leipzig. Math Naturwiss Klasse 45 No 6:1–62

Burton RM (1971) The turnover of lipids. In: Lajtha A (ed) Handbook of neurochemistry. Plenum Press, New York London, pp 199–214

Cherayil GD (1969) Estimation of glycolipids in four selected lobes of human brain in neurological diseases. J Neurochem 16:913–920

Cutler RG (1976) Nature of aging and life maintenance processes. Interdiscipl Topics Geront 9:83–133

Davison AN (1978) Biochemical aspects of the ageing brain. Age Ageing 7 (Suppl):4–11

De Baetselier A, Gozes J, Littauer UZ (1980) Translation in vitro of rat brain mRNA coding for a variety of tubulin forms. Arch Int Physiol Biochim 88:B 72–B 73

De Boni U, Crapper-McLachlan DR (1980) Senile dementia and Alzheimer's disease: A current view. Life Sci 27:1–14

Deshmukh DR, Patel MS (1980) Age-dependent changes in glutamate oxidation by nonsynaptic and synaptic mitochondria from rat brain. Mech Age Developm 13:75–81

Deshmukh DR, Owen OE, Patel MS (1980) Effect of aging on the metabolism of pyruvate and 3-hydroxybutyrate in nonsynaptic and synaptic mitochondria from rat brain. J Neurochem 34:1219–1224

Domino EF, Dren AT, Giardina WJ (1978) Biochemical and neurotransmitter changes in the aging brain. In: Lipton MA (eds) Psychopharmacology: A generation of progress. Raven Press, New York, p 1507–1515

Ermini M, Reichlmeier K (1976) Studies on age-related structural changes in chromatin of postmitotic cells by means of in vitro-phosphorylation of the histones. 29th Ann Meeting Gerontol Soc New York, Oct 13–17 (Abstr 42)

Ermini M, Moret ML, Reichlmeier K et al. (1978) Age-dependent structural changes in human neuronal chromatin. Aktuel Gerontol (GF) 8:675–680

Finch CE (1977) Neuroendocrine and autonomic aspects of aging. In: Finch CE, Hayflick L (eds) Handbook of the biology of aging. Van Nostrand Reinhold Comp, New York, pp 262–280

Frolkis VV (1970) Regulation, adaptation, and aging. Nauka, Moscow

Frolkis VV (1973a) Functions of cells and biosynthesis of protein in aging. Gerontology 19:189–202

Frolkis VV (1973b) Protein biosynthesis and hyperpolarization of cells. Experientia 29:1492–1494

Frolkis VV, Bezrukov VV (1979) Aging of the central nervous system. Interdiscipl Topics Gerontol 16:1–131

Gottstein U, Bernsmeier A, Sedlmeyer I (1964) Der Kohlenhydratstoffwechsel des menschlichen Gehirns. II. Untersuchungen mit substratspezifischen enzymatischen Methoden bei Kranken mit verminderter Hirndurchblutung auf dem Boden einer Arteriosklerose der Hirngefäße. Klin Wochenschr 42:310–313

Gottstein U, Held K, Müller W et al. (1972) Utilization of ketone bodies by the human brain. In: Meyer JS, Reivich M, Lechner H (eds) Research on the cerebral circulation. Thomas CC, Springfield, Ill, pp 137–145

Hariguchi S (1978) Biochemical studies on the ageing of the human brain. Changes in the brain water-soluble proteins of demented patients and the aged. Osaka Daigaku Igaku Zasshi 30:407–430

Heipertz R, Pilz H, Scholz W (1977) The fatty acid composition of sphingomyelin from adult human cerebral white matter and changes in childhood, senium, and unspecific brain damage. J Neurol 216:57–65

Herrmann RL (1971) Aging. In: Lajtha A (ed) Handbook of neurochemistry, vol V, part B. Plenum Press, New York London, pp 481–487

Hyden H (1967) RNA and brain cells. In: Quarton, Melnechuk, Schmitt (eds) Neuroscience. Rockefeller University Press, New York, pp 248–266

Iqbal K, Wisniewski HM, Shelanski ML et al. (1974) Protein changes in senile dementia. Brain Res 77:337–343

Iwangoff P, Reichlmeier K, Enz A et al. (1979) Neurochemical findings in physiological aging of the brain. Interdiscipl Topics Gerontol 15:13–33

Iwangoff P, Armbruster R, Enz A et al. (1980) Glycolytic enzymes from human autoptic brain cortex: Normally aged and demented cases. In: Roberts PJ (ed) Biochemistry of dementia. John Wiley and Sons Ltd, Chichester, pp 258–262

Kaneko Z, Nishimura T, Hariguchi S et al. (1979) Changes in brain proteins in senile dementia. In: Orimo H, Shimada K, Jrki M et al. (eds) Recent advances in gerontology. Internat Congr Series No 469. Excerpta Medica, Amsterdam Oxford Princetown, pp 171–172

Kanungo MS (1980) Biochemistry of ageing. Academic Press, London New York Toronto Sydney San Francisco

Krygier Stojalowska A, Kulczycki J, Madej M et al. (1977) DNA content in neurons and glial cells of human brain assayed by a cytophotometric method. Neuropatol Pol 15:349–356

Kudryashova IB, Vanyushin BF (1976) Methylation of nuclear DNA from different rat organs in vitro: Tissue and age differences in acceptor capacity of DNA. Biokhimiya 41:1106–1115

Kurtz DI, Sinex FM (1967) Age related differences in the association of brain DNA and nuclear protein. Biochim Biophys Acta 145:840–842

Lee TC, Duerre JA (1974) Changes in histone methylase activity of rat brain and liver with ageing. Nature 251:240–242

Mann DMA, Sinclair KGA (1978) The quantitative assessment of lipofuscin pigment, cytoplasmic RNA and nucleolar volume in senile dementia. Neuropathol Appl Neurobiol 4:129–135

Mann DMA, Yates PO (1974) Lipoprotein pigments – their relationship to ageing in the human nervous system. I. The lipofuscin content of nerve cells. Brain 97:481–488. II. The melanin content of pigmented nerve cells. Brain 97:489–498

Mann DMA, Yates PO, Barton CM (1977) Cytophotometric mapping of neuronal changes in senile dementia. J Neurol Neurosurg Psychiat 40:299–302

Mann DMA, Yates PO, Stamp JE (1978) The relationship between lipofuscin pigment and ageing in the human nervous system. J Neurol Sci 37:83–93

Mann DMA, Lincoln J, Yates PO et al. (1980) Changes in the monoamine containing neurones of the human CNS in senile dementia. Br J Psychiat 136:533–541

Mansson JE, Vanier MT, Svennerholm L (1978) Changes in the fatty acid and sphingosine composition of the major gangliosides of human brain with age. J Neurochem 30:273–275

Meier-Ruge W, Hunziker O, Iwangoff P et al. (1978) Alterations of morphological and neurochemical parameters of the brain due to normal aging. In: Nandy K (ed) Senile dementia a biomedical approach. Series: Development of neuroscience, vol 3. Elsevier/North Holland Biomed Press, New York Amsterdam, pp 33–44

Meier-Ruge W, Gygax P, Emmenegger H et al. (1979) Pharmacological aspects of ergot alkaloids in gerontological brain research. In: Cherkin A, Finch CF, Kharasch N et al. (eds) Physiology and cell biology of aging, Series: Aging vol 8. Raven Press, New York, pp 203–221

Meier-Ruge W, Iwangoff P, Reichlmeier K et al. (1980) Neurochemical findings in the aging brain. In: Goldstein M, Calne DB, Lieberman A et al. (eds) Ergot compounds and brain function, Series: Adv biochem psychopharm vol 23. Raven Press, New York, pp 323–338

Mendez B, Valenzuela P, Martial JA et al (1980) Cell-free synthesis of acetylcholine receptor polypeptides. Science 209:695–697

Miner GD, Trapp GA, McSwigan J et al. (1976) Alzheimer's disease: Human brain protein 13.7. J Neurochem 26:605–607

Naber D, Dahnke HG (1979) Protein and nucleic acid content in the aging human brain. Neuropath Appl Neurobiol 5:17–24

Naber D, Korte U, Krack K (1979) Content of water-soluble and total proteins in the aging human brain. Exp Gerontol 14:59–63

O'Brien I, Shelley K, Towfighi J et al. (1980) Crystalline ribosomes are present in brains from senile humans. Proc Natl Acad Sci USA 77:2260–2264

Op Den Velde W, Hooghwinkel GJM (1975) The brain ganglioside pattern in presenile and senile dementia. J Am Geriatr Soc 23:301–303

Op Den Velde W, Stam FC (1976) Some cerebral proteins and enzyme systems in Alzheimer's presenile and senile dementia. J Am Geriatr Soc 24:12–16

Ordy JM, Kaack B (1975) Neurochemical changes in composition, metabolism, and neurotransmitters in the human brain with age. In: Ordy JM, Brizzee KR (eds) Neurobiology of aging. Plenum Press, New York London, pp 253–285

Perez VJ, Moore BW (1970) Biochemistry of the nervous system in aging. Interdiscipl Topics Gerontol 7:22–45

Reichlmeier K, Schlecht HP, Iwangoff P (1977) Enzyme activity changes in the aging human brain. Experientia 33:R 798

Reichlmeier K, Ermini M, Schlecht HP (1978 a) Altersbedingte enzymatische Veränderungen im menschlichen Großhirncortex. Akt Gerontol 8:441–448

Reichlmeier K, Enz A, Iwangoff P et al. (1978 b) Age-related changes in human brain enzyme activities: A basis for pharmacological intervention. In: Roberts J, Adelman RC, Cristofalo VJ (eds) Pharmacological intervention in the aging process, Series: Adv exper med biol vol 97. Plenum Press, New York London, pp 251–252

Rouser G, Yamamoto A (1968) Curvilinear regression course of human brain lipid composition changes with age. Lipids 3:284–287

Rouser G, Yamamoto A (1969) Lipids. In: Lajtha A (ed) Handbook of neurochemistry, vol 1. Plenum Press, New York, pp 121–169

Samorajski T, Ordy JM (1972) Neurochemistry of aging. In: Gaitz CM (ed) Aging and the brain. Plenum Press, New York London, pp 41–61

Samorajski T, Rolsten C (1973) Age and regional differences in the chemical composition of brains of mice, monkeys, and humans. Progr Brain Res 40:253–265

Smith CB (1978) Studies on biochemical changes in aging brain. In: Nandy K (ed) Senile dementia: A biomedical approach, Series: Developm neurosc, vol 3. Elsevier/North-Holland Biomedical Press, New York Amsterdam, pp 45–60

Sokoloff L (1966) Cerebral circulatory and metabolic changes associated with aging. Res Publ Assoc Res Nerv Ment Dis 41:237–254

Sokoloff L (1975) Cerebral circulation and metabolism in the aged. In: Gershon S, Raskin A (eds) Genesis and treatment of psychologic disorders in the elderly, Series: Aging, vol 2. Raven Press, New York, pp 45–54

Strehler BL, Chang MP (1979) Loss of hybridizable ribosomal DNA from human post-mitotic tissue during aging: II Age-dependent loss in human cerebral cortex-hippocampal and somatosensory cortex comparison. Mech Age Developm 11:379–382

Sun AY, Samorajski T (1975) The effects of age and alcohol on $(Na^+ + K^+)$-ATPase activity of whole homogenate and synaptosomes prepared from mouse and human brain. J Neurochem 24:161–164

Sun AY, Sun GY (1979) Neurochemical aspects of the membrane hypothesis of aging. Interdiscipl Topics Gerontol 15:34–53

Suzuki K, Chen G (1966) Chemical studies on Jakob-Creutzfeldt disease. J Neuropath Exp Neurol 25:396–408

Sylvia AL, Rosenthal M (1978 a) The effect of age and lung pathology on cytochrome a,a$_3$ redox levels in rat cerebral cortex. Brain Res 146:109–122

Sylvia AL, Rosenthal M (1978 b) Age-related changes in brain energy metabolism with electrical activity. Fed Proc 37, Abst 3488:878

Sylvia AL, Rosenthal M (1979 a) Effects of age on brain oxidative metabolism in vivo. Brain Res 165:235–248

Sylvia AL, Rosenthal M (1979 b) Aging and brain energy metabolism in vivo. In: Orimo H, Shimada K, Irki M et al. (eds) Recent advances in gerontology. Proceedings of the XI Int. Congress of Gerontology Tokyo August 20–25, 1978: Internat Congr Series, vol 469. Excerpta Medica, Amsterdam Oxford Princeton, pp 141–142

Timiras PS (ed) (1972) Developmental physiology and aging. Macmillan Comp, New York Toronto London

Toews AD, Horrocks LA (1976) Developmental and aging changes in protein concentration and 2′,3′ cyclic nucleoside monophosphate phosphodiesterase activity (EC 3.1.4.16) in human cerebral white and gray matter and spinal cord. J Neurochem 27:545–550

Tolmasoff JM et al. (1980) Superoxide dismutase: Correlation with life-span and specific metabolic rate in primate species. Proc Natl Acad Sci USA 77:2777–2781

Uemura E, Hartmann HA (1978 a) Age-related changes in RNA content and volume of the human hypoglossal neuron. Brain Res Bull 3:207–211

Uemura E, Hartmann HA (1978 b) RNA content and volume of nerve cell bodies in human brain. I. Prefrontal cortex in aging normal and demented patients. J Neuropathol Exp Neurol 37:487–496

Uemura E, Hartmann HA (1979 a) RNA content and volume of nerve cell bodies in human brain. Exp Neurol 65:107–117

Uemura E, Hartmann HA (1979 b) Quantitative studies of neuronal RNA on the subiculum of demented old individuals. Brain Res Bull 4:301–305

Wulf VJ, Samis HV, Falzone JA (1967) The metabolism of ribonucleic acid in young and old rodents: In: Strehler BL (ed) Advances in gerontological research, vol 2. Academic Press, New York London, pp 37–76

Yamamoto A, Rouser G (1973) Free fatty acids of normal human whole brain at different ages. J Gerontol 28:140–142

Neuronal Lipofuscin and Its Significance

K. NANDY

A. Introduction

The term "lipofuscin" was introduced in the literature by BORST (1922), although the pigment was first demonstrated by HANNOVER (1842). The name was derived from a Greek word *lipo* (meaning fat) and a latin word *fuscus* (meaning brown). The deposition of the pigment in the cytoplasm of the neurons is one of the consistent age-related cytological changes, although it is found in myocardium and skeletal muscle as well. Various investigators demonstrated the pigment and used different names, such as chromolipid, age pigment, and ceroid (BONDAREFF 1957; DUNCAN et al. 1960; PEARSE 1964; SAMORAJSKI et al. 1964). The genesis of lipofuscin has been investigated by a number of workers, but the results are inconclusive (DE-DUVE 1963; ESSNER and NOVIKOFF 1960; FRIEDE 1962; GOLDFISCHER et al. 1966; BARKA and ANDERSON 1963; NANDY 1968; SULKIN 1953; WHITEFORD and GETTY 1966). In this chapter, an attempt is made to discuss the pertinent literature on lipofuscin and its possible significance.

B. Distribution and Properties

Lipofuscin pigment formation is a continuous process starting early in life and increasing progressively as age advances. The distribution of the pigment in the neurons of CNS in various animals including humans have been studied in different laboratories using histochemical, fluorescence, and ultrastructural methods. The neurons in the CNS exhibit a variable pattern of pigmentation in their cytoplasm. Lipofuscin pigment is generally not detected in the neurons of very young animals, including man. The pigment is rather diffuse in its distribution at first and gradually appears to develop clumps, perinuclear or polar, as age advances. The percentages of nerve cells showing heavy (clumpy) and moderate (diffuse) pigmentation among the Purkinje cells of cerebellum and pyramidal cells of cerebral cortex appear to increase progressively with age.

The staining properties of the pigment appear to vary in different ages. While Sudan black B and PAS stains visualize the pigments in the young, pigments in the old are more easily stained by Nile blue and ferricferricyanide methods. A difference in the fluorescence properties is also noted in these two types of pigment. Upon activation at a wave length of 3650 Å the pigment in younger animals gives mostly a green-yellow fluorescence with an emission spectrum of 2400–4200 Å and an intensity peak at 3400 Å. The autofluorescence of the lipofuscin in older animals is mostly orange yellow with an emission spectrum of 3400–4000 Å and a peak at 3800 Å. The pigments in brain of young animals are partially dissolved by trypsin, lipase, and lipid solvents.

C. Isolation and Quantitation

SIAKOTOS et al. (1970) isolated lipofuscin from frozen postmortem human brain samples to study both the quantitative and qualitative changes as a function of age. Five brain samples were collected for each decade and frozen at $-25\,°C$. The samples were thawed overnight at $4\,°C$ and blended for 5–10 s in sucrose solution (0.4 M) containing 0.05 M Tris base. The homogenates were disrupted with nitrogen at 900 psi in a Parr cell decompression bomb and centrifuged at 7,000 g. The supernatant was centrifuged at 27,000 g for 30 min and the light-brown floating layer of fat were resuspended in a 0.4 M sucrose and filtered through a 420 mesh nylon filter. The packed lipofuscin concentrate was then scraped and resuspended on 5% NaCl and centrifuged at 170,000 g for 30 min. The resulting brown top layer was collected by aspiration and purified further by centrifuging on freshly prepared continuous gradients of water to 20% NaCl at 110,000 g for 60 min. The last procedure was repeated two to three times and the top brown band was examined by phase contrast, fluorescence, and electron microscopy to judge the purity of the samples.

The concentration or pool size of lipofuscin material per brain was relatively uniform until 16.8 years of age and thereafter the pool size increased progressively as a function of age. Electron micrography of the isolated preparations of the pigment exhibited a large number of lipid bodies or lipid-filled lysosomes enclosed by a membrane with occasional electron dense lipofuscin-like areas relative to the globular granules. As brains of progressively older individuals were examined, isolated materials showed higher proportions of electron dense pigment. Although the procedure was able to isolate and quantitate lipofuscin in fairly pure form from the human brains, the possibility of losses during the isolation procedure cannot be ruled out. The study, however, confirms the observation by others on the age-related increase in lipofuscin in human brain by morphological methods (SIAKOTOS et al. 1977).

D. Origin of Lipofuscin

Despite numerous reports on the lipofuscin pigment in the literature, knowledge of its mode of origin is suprisingly lacking. Although the pigment might be derived from one or more of the organelles within the cells, the association of the pigment formation with lysosomes is generally favored by most investigators. The strong acid phosphatase activity and the striking ultrastructural similarity between the two are the major evidence for this hypothesis (NANDY 1971; SAMORAJSKI et al. 1964; NANDY 1978c). Biochemical isolation of the pigment from the brain samples followed by electron microscopy provides further support in this matter.

Some arguments have also been made in favor of the possible origin of the pigment from the mitochondria (HESS et al. 1958). The areas of pigment formation in the neurons of the mesencephalic nucleus of the trigeminal nerve have been correlated with high concentration of the mitochondria (HASAN and GLEES 1972). It has been suggested that the pigment formation may be preceded by an increased concentration and clumping of mitochondria resulting in the disturbance of normal metabolic activity. This latter condition might lead to the accumulation of insoluble fatty acids which are introduced in the pigment formation (GOPINATH and GLEES 1974). These authors have further extended the work in the lipofuscin formation in dorsal root ganglion cells in culture with similar observations.

The possible origin of the pigment for Golgi apparatus and endoplasmic reticulum has also been suggested. The evidence in favor of the origin of the lipofuscin from Golgi apparatus mainly came from the Sudanophilic and osmiophilic properties of both the organelle and the pigment (BONDAREFF 1962). Although there is no direct evidence of the association of the pigment to the striations of the cardiac muscle (STREHLER 1964), a decreased level of cytoplasmic RNA in the neurons of aged human brain has been considered in favor of this argument (MANN and YATES 1974). It is difficult at present to make any precise statement on the origin of this pigment. The association of the pigment with lysosomes, the frequent presence of lysosomal vacuoles in the pigment particle, and strong activity of acid phosphatase in the pigment mass offer stronger support for the lysosomal origin than from other organelles. It is also possible that the origin of the pigment may take place from a variety of intracellular organelles and cell membranes which have undergone wear and tear and deterioration during aging. The final breakdown might take place in the lysosomes where these are segregated in an attempt to metabolize or dispose the materials.

Observations were made in a group of mutant mice who appeared to have a condition of premature aging. The animals usually died within 8 weeks of age and lipofuscin pigment in quantities comparable to that in neurons of 12-month-old mice was found in neurons with some evidence of degeneration (O'STEEN and NANDY 1970).

E. In Pathological States

Lipofuscin pigment in excessive amounts in neurons has been observed in a number of pathological conditions of the brain.

In Batten-Vogt syndrome, also known as neuronal ceroid-lipofuscinosis, an excessive amount of lipofuscin-like pigment in the neurons has been described (ZEMEN 1971). Subsequently, SIAKOTOS et al. (1970) succeeded in isolating pigment from English Setters with the same disease. The pigment was described as ceroid and the chemical analysis of the isolated pigment revealed some difference from the typical lipofuscin. Of the two pigments ceroid contained a higher concentration of acidic lipid polymer, iron, calcium, and copper (SIAKOTOS et al. 1977). Histochemical study of ceroid revealed that the material is more easily extractible in the unfixed state with acidified or alkalized chloroform-methanol mixtures than lipofuscin (ELLENDER 1977). However, recent studies by WEST (1979), using the section of autopsied brains of patients with Down's Syndrome, phenylketonuria, and progeria, did not demonstrate any significant difference between the lipofuscin content in the neurons of inferior olivary nucleus and lateral geniculate bodies and those in normal people of the same age.

F. Significance of Lipofuscin

There are numerous reports in the literature indicating that lipofuscin is found in the nondividing cells, which are more likely to show the effects of aging (NANDY 1971; SAMORAJSKI et al. 1964; HASAN and GLEES 1972; BRODY and VIJAYASHANKAR 1977; BRODY 1960; HASAN et al. 1974 a, b; SPOERRI and GLEES 1973). Recent studies in our laboratory using neuroblastoma cells in culture have provided further evidence in favor of a close relationship between cell differentiation and lipofuscin formation. These cells are capable of dividing indefinitely in tissue culture, but exhibit properties of normal neurons if division is inhibited by chemicals such as papaverine. It has been observed that the differentiated neuroblastoma cells age like normal neurons in animals and develop lipofuscin pigment. It was possible to alternately increase or reduce the pigment formation by alternately inducing differentiation and division in these cells. Although lipofuscin pigment appears to be a property of aging postmitotic cells, the mechanism underlying its formation is not clear. It may, however, be speculated that the cells in the young animals may have the special ability to metabolize the products of intracellular wear and tear in order to reutilize them, and this property might be lost during aging. This might lead to the accumulation in the old neurons of partially digested or undigested cellular residue or "garbage" as lipofuscin pigment. Future studies along these lines might appear promising.

Our understanding of the functional significance of the pigment in the neurons is even more lacking. While some investigators think that the pigment might be harmful to the cells, others are in favor of its beneficial effects. NANDY (1978 a, b) showed a significant improvement of learning and memory in mice following centrophenoxine treatment and this was also associated with a reduction in lipofuscin in the neurons of cerebral cortex and hippocampus. On the other hand, LAL et al. (1973) demonstrated that rats subjected to a vitamin E deficient diet showed a deterioration of learning and memory as well as an increase in the lipofuscin pigment in the neurons of the cerebral cortex and hippocampus. The possibility of a positive correlation between lipofuscin formation and neuronal function cannot be ruled out. Although lipofuscin might not be directly harmful or toxic to the cells, the process of wear and tear underlying pigmentogenesis might still be detrimental to the cellular functions. Lipofuscin may, therefore, represent the product after damage rather than a causative factor. On the other hand, the accumulation of large amounts of pigment occupying a substantial part of the cell soma might also interfere with the functional machinaries within the cells.

G. Summary

Lipofuscin pigment appears to be one of the most consistent changes in the neurons associated with mammalian aging. The pigment is easily visualized by its histochemical, fluorescence and ultrastructural characteristics. Numerous studies using different animals including humans indicate that the pigment formation is a continuous process beginning early in life and thereafter increasing progressively as a function of age. Recent studies tend to indicate that lipofuscin probably develops in early and late stages, differing in its histochemical, fluorescence, and ultrastructural properties. The early stage, predominant in younger age, is more easily stained by PAS and Sudan black B methods and has a greenish-yellow fluorescence. The late stage, on the other hand, is more frequently encountered in older age. This is more easily stainable with Nile blue and ferric-ferricyanide methods, and has an orange-yellow fluorescence. The pigment in the brain has been isolated and quantitated by biochemical methods from human and animal brains and a progressive increase with age was noted. The pigment has been demonstrated to be a property of differentiated cells using neuroblastoma cells in culture. The possible origin of the pigment from various cell organelles has been discussed and it appears that lysosomes appear to play an important role in its development. Although the functional significance of the pigment is not clearly understood, treatment with centrophenoxine was associated with improved learning and memory and reduction of lipofuscin in the neurons. Although there is no direct evidence for a precise functional relation of the pigment, the age-associated wear and tear within the cells underlying pigment formation could still be detrimental to the cells.

References

Barka T, Anderson PJ (1963) Histochemistry: Theory, practice and bibliography. Harper and Row, Inc Hoeber Div, New York, pp 190–193

Bondareff W (1957) Genesis of intracellular pigment in the spinal ganglia of senile rats. An electron microscope study. J Gerontol 12:364–369

Bondareff W (1962) Distribution of Nissl substance in neurons of rat spinal ganglia as a function of age and fatigue. In: Shock NW (ed) Biological aspects of aging. Columbia University Press, New York, pp 147–154

Borst M (1922) Pathologische Histologie. Vogel, Leipzig

Brody H (1960) The deposition of aging pigment in the human cerebral cortex. J Gerontol 15:258–261

Brody H, Vijayashankar N (1977) Anatomical changes in the nervous system. In: Finch CE, Hayflick L (eds) Handbook of the biology of aging, vol I. Van Nostrand Reinhold Company, New York, pp 241–261

DeDuve C (1963) The lysosomes concept. In: deReuck AVS, Cameron MP (eds) Lysosomes. Little, Brown and Company, Boston, pp 1–31

Duncan D, Nall D, Morales R (1960) Observations on the fine structure of old age pigment. J Gerontol 15:366

Ellender M (1977) So-called neuronal ceroid-lipofuscinosis. Acta Neuropath 39:117–122

Essner E, Novikoff AB (1960) Human hepatocellular pigments and lysosomes. J Ultrastruct Res 3:374–391

Friede RL (1962) The relation of the formation of the lipofuscin pigment to the distribution of the oxidative enzymes in the human brain. Acta Neuropath 2:113–125

Goldfischer S, Villarverde H, Forschirm R (1966) The demonstration of acid hydrolase, thermostable reduced diphosphopyridine nucleotide tetrazolium reductase and peroxidase activities in human lipofuscin pigment granules. J Histochem Cytochem 14:641–652

Gopinath G, Glees P (1974) Mitochondrial genesis of lipofuscin in the mesencephalic nucleus of the V nerve of the aged rats. Acta Anat 89:14–20

Hannover A (1842) Videnskappsselsk Math Afth (Copenhagen) 10:1
Hasan M, Glees P (1972) Genesis and possible dissolution of neuronal lipofuscin. Gerontology 18:217
Hasan M, Glees P, Spoerri PI (1974a) Dissolution and removal of neuronal lipofuscin following dimethylaminoethyl p-chlorophenoxyacetate administration to guinea pigs. Cell Tissue Res 150:369
Hasan M, Glees P, El-Ghazzawi E (1974b) Age-associated change in the hypothalamus of the guinea pig: Effect of dimethylaminoethyl p-chlorophenoxyacetate. An electron microscopic and histochemical study. Exp Gerontol 9:153
Hess R, Scarpelli DG, Pearse AG (1958) Cytochemical localization of oxidative enzymes. II. Pyridine nucleotide-linked dehydrogenases. J Biophys Biochem Cytol 4:753–760
Lal H, Pogacar S, Daly PR, Puri SK (1973) Behavioral and neuropathological manifestations of nutritionally induced central nervous system aging in the rat. In: Ford D (ed) Neurobiological aspects of maturation and aging. Elsevier, New York, pp 129–140
Mann DMA, Yates PO (1974) Lipofuscin pigments – their relationship to aging in the human nervous system. I. The lipofuscin content of nerve cells. Brain 97:481–488
Nandy K (1968) Further studies on the effects of Centrophenoxine on the lipofuscin pigment in the neurons of senile guinea pigs. J Gerontol 23:82–92
Nandy K (1971) Properties of lipofuscin pigment in neurons. Acta Neuropath 19:25–32
Nandy K (1978a) Centrophenoxine: Effects on aging brain. J Am Geriatr Soc 26 (No. 2):74–81
Nandy K (1978b) Experimental studies on Centrophenoxine in aging brain. In: Nandy K (ed) Geriatric psychopharmacology. Elsevier North Holland, Inc, New York
Nandy K (1978c) Morphological changes in aging brain. In: Nandy K (ed) Senile dementia: A biomedical approach. Elsevier North Holland, Inc, New York
O'Steen KW, Nandy K (1970) Lipofuscin pigment in neurons of young mice with a hereditary central nervous system defect. Am J Anat 128:359–365
Pearse AGE (1964) Histochemistry, theoretical, and applied. Little, Brown and Co, Boston, pp 661–675
Samorajski T, Keefe JR, Ordy JM (1964) Intracellular localization of lipofuscin age pigments in the nervous system. J Gerontol 19:262–276
Siakotos AN, Watanaba I, Siato A, Flesicher S (1970) Procedure of the isolation of two distinct lipopigments from human brain: Lipofucsin and ceroid. Biochem Med 4:361–375
Siakotos AN, Armstrong D, Koppang N, Muller J (1977) Biochemical significance of age pigment in neurons. In: Nandy K, Sherwin I (eds) The aging brain and senile dementia. Plenum Press, New York
Spoerri PE, Glees P (1973) Neuronal aging in culture: An electron microscopic study. Exp Gerontol 9:259
Strehler BL (1964) Advances in gerontological research. In: Strehler BL (ed) Advances in gerontological research, vol 1. Academic Press, New York
Sulkin NM (1953) Histochemical studies of the pigment in human anatomic ganglion cells. J Gerontol 8:435–448
West C (1979) A quantitative study of lipofuscin accumulation with age in normals and individuals with Down's syndrome, phenylketonuria, progeria, and transneuronal atrophy. J Comp Neurol 186:109–116
Whiteford R, Getty R (1966) Distribution of the lipofuscin in the canine and porcine brain as related to aging. J Gerontol 21:31–44
Zemen W (1971) The neuronal ceroid-Lipofuscinosis-Batten-Vogt Syndrome: A model for human aging? In: Strehler BL (ed) Adv Gerontol Res 3:147–169

Neurotransmitters in Normal Aging

E. G. McGeer and P. L. McGeer

A. Introduction

Aging is associated with physiological changes, such as a short sleep span, flattening of mood, decreased total motor activity, altered endocrine function and declining mental acuity. Such physiological changes occur both prematurely and in increased amount in cases of senile dementia or Alzheimer's disease. It has been difficult to correlate the lipofuscin deposits and other age-induced phenomena seen in pathological examination of brains with the functional deficits of aging. In the past decade there have been an increasing number of studies indicating marked changes in specific neurotransmitter systems with normal aging and further specific deficits in senile dementia or Alzheimer's disease. These may be correlatable with changes both in function and in sensitivity to various psychoactive drugs. In this chapter we will review the literature comparing adult with normal aged systems in humans; the considerable, generally supporting, data from animal studies are not included. Most neurotransmitter indices in the postnatal period show rapid increases in most brain areas coincident with synaptic development. In this chapter we are interested in the other end of the continuum – where losses in neurotransmitter indices may reflect losses of neurons or reduction in their synaptic numbers and functions.

Studies on humans are, of course, of particular interest but also involve particular difficulties. Experience has indicated that the sex of the individual or delays of 2–48 h between death and autopsy have surprisingly little effect on many neurotransmitter indices measured. The immediate premortem condition and certain drugs have, however, been found to be of great importance; persons dying after prolonged coma or unconsciousness, for example, show extremely low levels of several of the indices which have been studied and such cases must often be excluded (P. L. McGeer and McGeer 1976).

All laboratories studying human brains have encountered more scattered data than from corresponding animal experiments. This is not surprising in view of the extreme disparity in both genetic makeup and environmental factors. Individual variation may be a particularly difficult factor in aging studies since the genetic clock presumably runs at different rates for different people. And species differences may render work with other animals difficult to interpret in terms of human aging. Nevertheless, there is evidence from a number of laboratories and species that catecholaminergic, cholinergic, and possibly GABAergic neuronal activities probably decline with age in certain brain regions. The situation with regard to serotonergic systems is unclear and there are few data on any other biochemically defined neuronal types. It does seem clear from the available evidence that it is just as important to specify the region as the system under study. The activity of a given neuronal type may decline significantly with age in one brain area while it is not significantly affected in other areas. This is a point which will be stressed in the discussion of specific systems, and it is for this reason that brief comments on the anatomy of the various systems are included.

It is also very important to understand the nature and validity of the various indices that have been used to assess specific neurotransmitter systems. Almost all of the available information on humans – and much of the data on other species – concerns the levels of the transmitters themselves and the activities of neurotransmitter synthetic and degradative enzymes. The enzymes are usually preferred since they are generally easier to analyse on small tissue samples and seem somewhat less subject to post-mortem changes and pharmacological manipulation. The synthetic enzymes are particularly valuable as specific neuronal markers. They are generally localized only in neurons of a given neurotransmitter type and are good indices of the integrity of those neurons; degradative enzymes, on the other hand, tend to be more generally distributed (E.G. McGeer and McGeer 1980). They are therefore not very good indices. It is well established, however, that changes in the release and turnover of a neurotransmitter need not be accompanied by changes in the more static levels of either the neurotransmitter itself or the synthetic enzyme. Thus, these indices give poor insight into possible short-term changes. One or two attempts have been made to study turnover of the aromatic amines in aged animals in comparison with younger ones but the available data are, so far, very few. The methods do not lend themselves to human study. Similarly, high affinity uptake of transmitter or precursor, which is another possible index of synaptosomal activity, cannot be applied to human post-mortem tissue because of the lability of the transport systems.

Recently, work has begun to appear on changes with age in the number or properties of binding ("receptor") sites for various neurotransmitters in brain. Measurements of binding sites have the advantage of very good post-mortem stability. On the other hand, Na^+-independent binding sites are postsynaptic and hence do not give direct information on the integrity and functional activity of neurons of a defined biochemical type which are presynaptic to the receptors. Presynaptic and postsynaptic sites respond very differently in disease. For example, the dramatic change in Parkinson's disease is loss of presynaptic dopaminergic nerve endings; therapy is based on stimulation of postsynaptic receptor sites which are not lost. There may be many similar dichotomies in aging. Information is not yet available.

It has been suggested that Na^+-dependent binding of GABA (ROBERTS et al. 1978) or glutamate (VINCENT and McGEER 1980) might provide a measure of presynaptic transport (uptake) sites as opposed to postsynaptic receptor sites for evaluation of human post-mortem tissue where other indices are lacking. The validity of these suggestions has not yet been tested. The situation is complicated because it is becoming apparent that there may be both Na^+-dependent and Na^+-independent binding sites for some neurotransmitters on glia and other structural elements apart from synaptic membranes. Despite these difficulties we have included literature on changes with age in binding sites, but the data must be regarded with caution at this stage.

B. Specific Neuronal Systems

I. Catecholamine Systems and Aging

These have been more intensively studied than any other system in aging humans and data are available on levels, related enzyme activities and receptors. There are also data indicating specific losses in the numbers of catecholaminergic cells with age in the human brain.

There are three catecholamines in mammalian brain, dopamine, noradrenaline and adrenaline, but the adrenergic systems are relatively minor and little known, may be easily confused with the more extensive noradrenergic systems and are not of particular importance for this review (McGeer et al. 1978). All three catecholamines tend to be primarily in long-axonal neurons originating in circumscribed brain stem nuclei and spreading widely to innervate diffusely many more rostral areas. Noradrenergic and dopaminergic projections are also known to descend caudally to the spinal cord. Major dopaminergic systems originate in the substantia nigra and adjacent A 10 (ventral tegmental area of Tsai) region to innervate densely the caudate, putamen and nucleus accumbens, and, more sparsely, the amygdala, septal area, hippocampus, frontal cortex, and various other areas. A relatively short dopaminergic tract runs from the arcuate nucleus to the median eminence of the hypothalamus. There are, additionally, dopaminergic interneurons in the brain stem, superior cervical ganglia, retina, olfactory bulb and carotid body but these are not of particular concern for this review.

Noradrenergic systems arise in the locus coeruleus and immediately adjacent (but less well-defined) areas and innervate the cerebellum, spinal cord and a wide variety of forebrain areas. Noradrenergic terminals are particularly concentrated in the hypothalamus.

1. Catecholamine Levels and Aging

Significant declines with age in the dopamine content of the caudate and putamen in humans have been found by a number of investigators (Bertler et al. 1966, Carlsson and Winblad 1976). Adolfsson et al. (1979) also reported significant decreases with age in the caudate, globus pallidus, hippocampus, mesencephalon, and entorhinal cortex but not in the putamen, hypothalamus, pons, medulla, thalamus, cerebellum or five other cortical areas. Robinson et al. (1977) found no loss in dopamine with age in the caudate, substantia nigra or globus pallidus but did show a slight negative correlation in the thalamus and hypothalamus. In their study the noradrenaline content of the hypothalamus and hippocampus showed a significant negative correlation with age and there appeared to be a similar trend in all areas except the substantia nigra. Mackay et al. (1978 b), however, found no significant correlation with age for dopamine, noradrenaline or any of their metabolites (Eq. 1) in the 20 areas of ten human brains which they studied (age range 46–74 years).

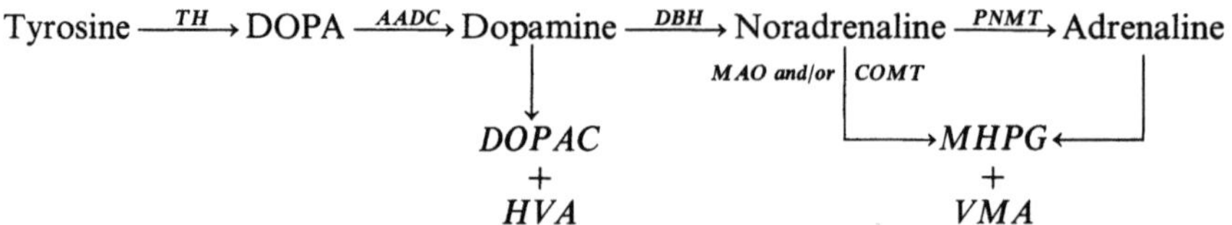

Equation 1. Synthesis and metabolism of the catecholamines. *TH*: tyrosine hydroxylase; *AADC*: L-aromatic amino decarboxylase (*DOPA* decarboxylase); *DBH*: dopamine-β-hydroxylase; *PNMT*: phenylethanolamine-N-methyl-transferase; *MAO*: monoamine oxidase; *COMT*: catecholamine-O-methyltransferase; *DOPAC*: dihydroxyphenylacetic acid; *HVA*: homovanillic acid; *VMA*: vanillylmandelic acid; *MHPG*: methoxyhydroxyphenylglycol

In histofluorescent studies on sympathetic ganglia from humans 57–75 years of age, Hervonen et al. (1978) found a marked decrease in formaldehyde-induced fluorescence with age and, indeed, no such fluorescence was visible in the oldest patients studied. Such fluorescence is attributable to an accumulation of catecholamines.

2. Catecholamine Enzymes and Aging

The catecholaminergic transmitters, dopamine, nonadrenaline, and adrenaline, are synthesized and metabolized by the routes shown in Eq. 1. Of the six enzymes involved in synthesis and metabolism, five have been studied to some extent in both human and animal brain tissue as a function of age. The general results are the following: Sharp declines in age have been found for tyrosine hydroxylase (TH) and L-aromatic amino acid decarboxylase (AADC) in some brain regions. The situation is unclear with regard to dopamine-β-hydroxylase (DBH), catecholamine-0-methyltransferase (COMT) and phenylethanolamine-N-methyltransferase (PNMT). Monoamine oxidase (MAO) appears to increase with age.

Tyrosine hydroxylase (TH) is limited to catecholamine neurons in the central nervous system and catalyzes a rate-controlling step in the synthesis of the catecholamines. In our study of brains from 28 neurologically normal humans aged 5–87 years of age, TH activity in six areas of the brain was found to correlate significantly with age (Fig. 1) (E.G. McGeer and McGeer 1976). There were, however, 11 areas where five or more samples were analysed which showed no significant correlation between TH activity and age, although the trend always seemed to be downwards; these areas were the hippocampus, anterior perforating substance, septal area, olfactory tubercle, anterior globus pallidus, hypothalamus, substantia nigra, locus coeruleus, and red nucleus.

The declines of TH activity with age in the caudate, putamen and nucleus accumbens were the most striking examples of age-related changes found in our entire study. Others have indicated a decline in the substantia nigra as well (Cote and Kremzner 1974), but Robinson et al. (1977) found no statistically significant relation between TH and age in a study of nine brain areas (including the caudate) in a series of 39 humans ranging in age from 4 to 83 years. Grote et al. (1974) and

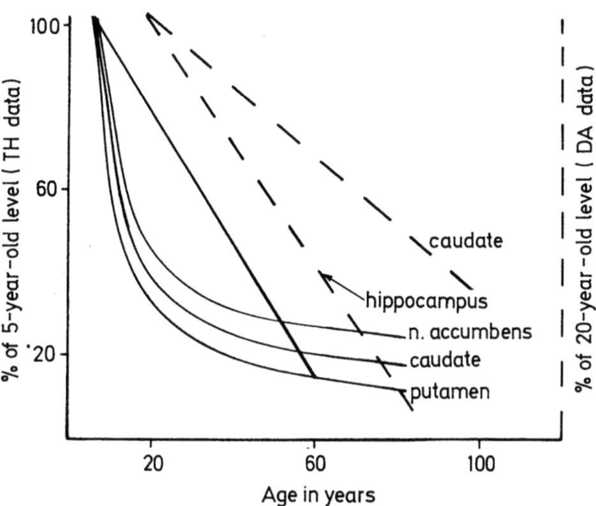

Fig. 1. Representative calculated lines of significant correlation between TH activity or dopamine (DA) levels *(dashed lines)* and age in various regions of human brain. Most of the TH curves reflect equations of the form: $TH = a + b/age$. Data on TH are from E.G. McGeer and McGeer (1976) while those on DA are from Adolfsson et al. (1979)

Mackay et al. (1978a) also failed to find any decline of TH with age but this may have been because their youngest cases were over 30 while the most rapid decline seems to be in the prior 3 decades.

Consistent with a rapid decline in young humans is the "strong inverse" correlation between age and CSF HVA concentrations found in children by Seifert et al. (1980); in this study no significant effects were observed for MHPG levels in the CSF.

L-Aromatic amino acid decarboxylase [dopa decarboxylase; 5-HTP-decarboxylase (AADC)] occurs in serotonergic as well as catecholaminergic neurons and, at least in animals, occurs in great excess. It is found in brain capillary endothelium (Bertler 1961). These factors make it a less sensitive indicator than the specific enzyme (TH) of the functional integrity of the catecholamine neurons. Moreover, the human enzyme appears to be relatively unstable and particularly subject to the effect of premortem coma (P.L. McGeer and McGeer 1976). Although the results obtained in human tissue have been more variable than with enzymes such as TH, studies done both by ourselves (E.G. McGeer and McGeer 1976) and by Lloyd and Hornykiewicz (1972) in human tissue indicate substantial and significant declines of this decarboxylase with age in many areas (Fig. 2). Only a few areas (olfactory tubercle, preoptic area, anterior globus pallidus and hypothalamus) showed no significant decrease of AADC with age in our study and all showed a definite trend, which was rendered insignificant by the great variability of the data. This variability was probably a factor in the failure of Mackay et al. (1978a) to find any relationship between age and AADC activity in the smaller series of human brains which they studied.

There is a very large excess of AADC in animal brains and presumably in young humans (who show levels comparable to those found in animals) (Lloyd and Hornykiewicz 1972; E.G. McGeer and McGeer 1976), so that age-related declines in AADC are not apt to be as physiologically significant as declines in TH. The clinical benefits of L-dopa therapy in many cases of parkinsonism, a condition where

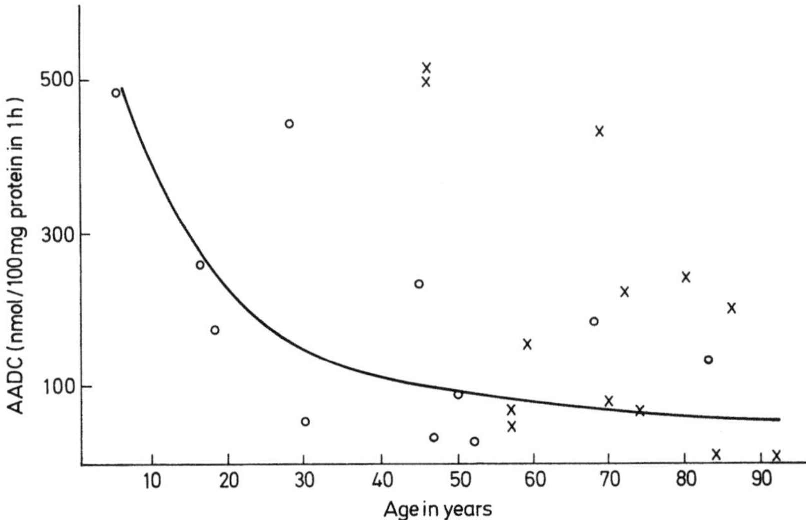

Fig. 2. AADC activity in human caudate as a function of age. The *x(s)* are individual data of Lloyd and Hornykiewicz (1972); *o(s)* and calculated line of correlation of the form: AADC = a + b/age are from the data of E.G. McGeer and McGeer (1979)

AADC activity is abnormally low, support the view that the levels of decarboxylase activity even in aged brains are probably sufficient for the needs.

Dopamine-β-hydroxylase (DBH) catalyses the last and one of the rate-limiting steps in noradrenaline synthesis (Eq. 1). In two studies of its activity in various areas of the brains of humans ranging in age from 33 to 74 years, no correlation between age and activity was found (Grote et al. 1974; Mackay et al. 1978a). It should be noted that the locus coeruleus was not included in either of these studies. One might expect this to have the highest activity of any region of brain and to be perhaps the most sensitive to age in view of Brody's report (1976) of cell loss in the locus coeruleus with aging. DBH is a relatively unstable enzyme post-mortem, and this inevitably leads to a wide variation from case to case.

In a study of the activity of DBH in cerebrospinal fluid from 59 psychiatric patients, Lerner et al. (1978) reported a small, but statistically significant positive correlation between activity and age ($r = 0.38$). On the other hand, the data given in the initial report demonstrating the existence of DBH activity in human CSF (Goldstein and Cubeddu 1976) show a significant negative correlation with age [activity = 576 − (3.5 × age), $r = 0.57$]. Whether or not a correlation exists and whether it is positive or negative, therefore, remains uncertain.

Phenylethanolamine-N-methyltransferase (PNMT) converts noradrenaline to adrenaline (Eq. 1). Although adrenaline is quantitatively much less important in the mammalian central nervous system than either dopamine or noradrenaline, it is now clear that there are adrenergic neurons and that they do contain PNMT (McGeer et al. 1978). There are, however, as yet no reports on the possible relationship of brain PNMT activity to age in humans.

Monoamine oxidase (MAO) is the enzyme of primary importance in metabolizing the catecholamines and serotonin (Eqs. 1 and 2).

$$\text{Tryptophan} \xrightarrow{\;TrH\;} \text{5-Hydroxytryptophan} \xrightarrow{\;AADC\;} \text{Serotonin}$$
$$\downarrow MAO$$
$$\text{5-Hydroxyindoleacetic acid}$$

Equation 2. Synthesis and neuronal metabolism of serotonin. TrH: tryptophan hydroxylase

It differs from TH, AADC, DBH, and PNMT in that a very large fraction of the MAO in brain appears to be extraneuronal in location. Several groups have reported an increase with age in humans of MAO activity in brain (COTE and KREMZNER 1974; GROTE et al. 1974; NIES et al. 1973; ROBINSON 1975; ROBINSON et al. 1972; SAMORAJSKI and ROLSTEN 1973) and serum (TRYDING et al. 1972). MACKAY et al. (1978a), however, found no significant correlation in various brain regions. One complication may be that brain MAO is believed to exist in two forms (A and B) and GOTTFRIES et al. (1974) found that the rise in brain MAO activity with advancing age was observed with β-phenylethylamine (preferred by MAO-B) as substrate, but not with tryptamine (substrate for both MAO-A and B). MACKAY et al. (1978a) used tyramine which is also a substrate for both enzymes. ROBINSON et al. (1977), however, reported significant correlations with age in humans using both benzylamine (an MAO-B substrate) and tryptamine. In addition, they found significantly higher activity in women than in men. This is one of the few neurotransmitter-related enzymes where activity seems to be related to sex, not only in brain but in human serum (TRYDING et al. 1972) and platelets. The percentage change found with age varied markedly from region to region in brain. In the 20–30 age group compared to the 50–60 age group, the change found was about 160% in the hypothalamus and only 20% in the globus pallidus. The best correlations between age and activity seemed to be in the globus pallidus, hippocampus, substantia nigra, and some cortical areas (GOTTFRIES et al. 1974; ROBINSON et al. 1977). ADOLFSSON et al. (1978) reported positive correlations of decreasing magnitude in the putamen, pallidum, frontal cortex, caudate, hippocampus, cingulate gyrus, medulla, thalamus, hypothalamus, pons, and mesencephalon; in their study the only area showing a non-significant correlation was the occipital cortex.

Catecholamine-O-methyltransferase (COMT) is another enzyme which can metabolize the catecholamines (Eq. 1) but is not as important as MAO. Treatment of animals with MAO inhibitors results in marked increases in catecholamine (and serotonin) levels but treatment with COMT inhibitors does not have much effect. COMT, moreover, is not located within catecholamine neurons but is either on glial cells or on the surface of dendritic elements of the postsynaptic neurons. It is perhaps not surprising, therefore, that there is little evidence that COMT activity declines with age. In humans, GROTE et al. (1974) found no relation between COMT activity and either age or sex and ROBINSON et al. (1977) found none except in the hippocampus where there was a significant decline with age.

3. Catecholamine Receptors and Aging

Binding assays are now a popular method of measuring "receptors" and considerable data have already been gathered on age-related changes in animals. Relatively few data are available, however, from human studies. Maggi et al. (1979) found significant (50%) age-related reductions in β-adrenergic binding sites in human cerebellum. Decreased concentrations of β-adrenergic receptors have also been demonstrated in aged human lymphocytes (Schocken and Roth (1977), suggesting that the loss of these receptors with age may be a general phenomenon which is not limited to specific brain areas; it may explain the generally reduced ability of aged tissue to respond to adrenergic stimuli.

4. Catecholamine Cell Counts and Aging

The most consistent finding emerging from the literature cited in the preceding sections is the marked decline of dopaminergic activity in the striatum. The cell bodies for these dopaminergic neurons lie in the substantia nigra. Cell counts in the substantia nigra in a series of control human brains showed that there was a significant decrease in number with age (Fig. 3a) (McGeer et al. 1977). At birth there are

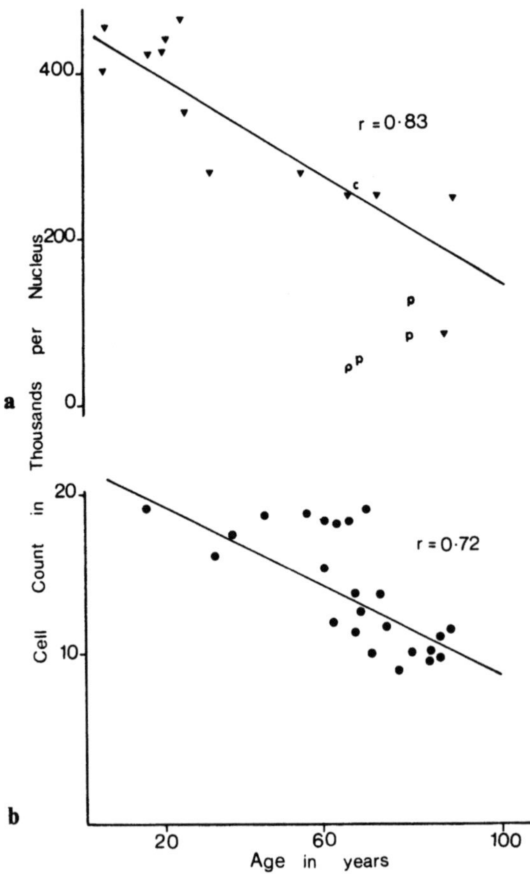

Fig. 3 a–c. Cell counts in human substantia nigra (a; McGeer et al. 1977), locus coeruleus (b; Brody 1976), and putamen (c, Bugiani et al. 1978) as a function of age. ▼ (s), ● (s), ■ (s) and calculated lines of regression are for data on neurologically normal individuals. The $p(s)$ in a are cases of Parkinson's disease while the c is a single case of Huntington's chorea. The correlation is more significant for the putamen data if semilog plots are used

about 400,000 dopaminergic cells in each human substantia nigra. By age 60, the number has dropped to about 250,000. In Parkinson's disease (designated by the symbol p in Fig. 3a), cell counts ranged from 60,000–120,000. The symptoms of the disease result from loss of these substantia nigra cells. But obviously many cells can disappear before decompensation occurs. The only stigmata may be the shuffling gait and stooped posture often seen in the very elderly.

BRODY (1976) found a similar cell loss in noradrenergic cells of the locus coeruleus (Fig. 3b). The calculated lines of regression are significant in both cases although the rate of loss is greater in the substantia nigra than in the locus coeruleus. As Brody points out, such losses are exceptional, for most brain stem nuclei show no detectable decrements in cell number (BRODY 1976; BUGIANI et al. 1978; HSU and PENG 1978; VIJAYASHANKAR and BRODY 1977).

Catecholamine cells therefore appear to be particularly prone to the effects of aging although losses in other types of cells may also occur. BUGIANI et al. (1978), for example, found a significant loss of both small and large cells in the putamen of humans (Fig. 3c). These cells are certainly not catecholaminergic since no catecholamine-containing perikarya are found in the putamen; they might be neurons using acetylcholine, GABA, substance P or enkephalin as a transmitter since such

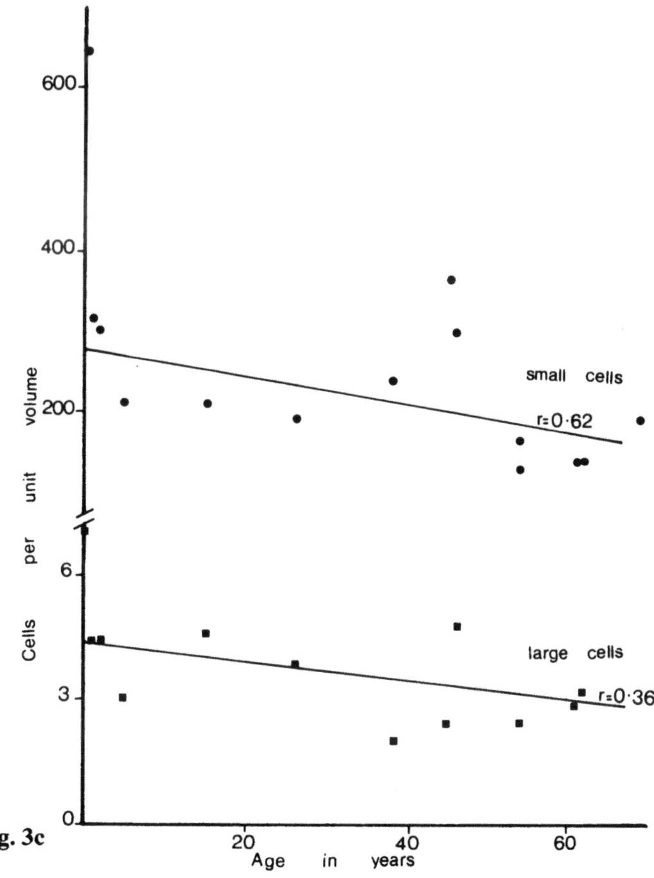

Fig. 3c

neurons are found in the putamen (McGeer et al. 1978). Equally, some or all of them might use some as yet unidentified transmitter. Bugiani et al. (1978) suggest that the loss of these putamen cells may help to keep some balance in the extrapyramidal system despite the severe age-related losses in dopaminergic input.

Even without actual cell death there may be a loss in cell vitality with consequent reductions in the numbers of synapses a given cell can maintain. The decrease in adrenergic axon sprouting seen in the septal area of senescent rats (Scheff et al. 1978) is consistent with such a view, as are the changes with age in the appearance of dopaminergic cells. Youthful human substantia nigra cells seen in the light microscope are plump with a clear cytoplasm. Older cells often appear shrunken and blackened by the melanin pigment which begins to appear between the ages of 5 and 15. During this period there seems to be a remarkable loss in TH levels in the neostriatum where the nerve endings are located (Fig. 1). The sharp decline in this period must reflect a loss of activity of individual cells rather than a decrease in the actual number of cells. It must be remembered that each cell, and particularly the dopaminergic cells which show such severe synaptic losses of TH activity with age, have an enormous number of boutons to serve. Bouton counts in the human caudate and putamen suggest bout 6×10^{11}/cc or about 150×10^{11} per caudate and putamen. If approximately 10% of these are dopaminergic, as suggested for the cat and rat, this would mean that each of the dopaminergic cells in the substantia nigra would have about 5×10^6 dopaminergic boutons in the caudate and putamen. With such a number to serve, it may not be surprising that these cells seem particularly prone to wear out. It is highly possible that the accumulation of melanin in catecholamine cells may gradually poison the cell and/or that free radicals, superoxides or quinones formed from the easily oxidized catecholamines are neurotoxic.

II. Serotonin Systems and Aging

Serotonergic systems also arise in the brain stem – in the raphe nuclei – and spread broadly. There is considerable parallelism between serotonergic and noradrenergic systems, not only in their diffuse innervation of the spinal cord and most areas of brain but in the particularly rich innervation of the hypothalamus by both of these amines.

The effects of age on serotonergic indices have been less studied than the effects on the catecholamines and the available reports are more contradictory. In humans, Mackay et al. (1978b) found a significant negative correlation between the age of the patient and the serotonin concentration in the pons, hypothalamus, substantia nigra and amygdala in a study of 19 brain areas from ten neurologically normal individuals, aged 46–74 years. The finding of a significant relationship between serotonin and age was particularly notable because no significant correlation with age was found for dopamine, noradrenaline or their various metabolites in this limited number of brains. Robinson et al. also initially (1972) reported a small but statistically significant decline with age of serotonin in the caudate and hind brain. But the same group later reported relatively little loss of serotonin from 25 to over 70 years of age (Nies et al. 1973). Decreases in serotonin levels with age could merely reflect increased MAO activity since this is the enzyme which metabolizes serotonin (Eq. 2), but the inverse correlation between 5-HIAA concentrations and age reported by SEIFERT et al. (1980) in humans aged 1 week to 45 years suggests some age-related decline in brain serotonin turnover.

Changes in the number and properties of serotonin binding sites with age in human cortex have been recently reported (SHIH and YOUNG 1978; CHENG and SHIH 1979). Two binding sites were found in the cortex from humans aged 23–29 years while only one type of binding site was found in humans aged 61–70 years. Although the total number of bindings sites (B_{max}) per milligram of protein was greater in the older brain than in the younger, the greatly decreased affinity for serotonin in the older brains meant that, at concentrations of serotonin ranging from 5–60 nM, there was significantly less binding in the aged cortices than in the young. As with all binding experiments, these data do not tell us anything about the integrity or state of activity of the serotonergic neurons but do suggest that the aged human might be subsensitive to physiological concentrations of serotonin or serotonergic agonists.

A handicap in studying serotonergic systems in humans has been the inability to demonstrate activity of the synthetic enzyme, tryptophan hydroxylase (TrH, Eq. 2) in post-mortem human tissue; this failure is perhaps understandable in view of the relatively low levels and instability reported for this enzyme in animal brains (PETERS et al. 1968). More information on serotonergic systems in human aging would clearly be desirable and might, in particular, cast light on the neuronal changes involved in age-related disturbances in hypothalamic functions.

Although the situation with regard to serotonergic systems is not completely clear, it does seem probable that they are less vulnerable to aging than are the catecholamine systems and it has been frequently suggest that the resultant changes in hypothalamic catecholamine to serotonin ratios may be related to changes in temperature regulation, sleep and hormonal function (MEITES et al. 1979).

III. Acetylcholine Systems and Aging

These are receiving particular attention at the moment because of the exciting reports of specific defects in senile dementia and Alzheimer's disease. There are indications that losses similar in kind but lesser in extent to those seen in dementia also occur in normal aging, that central cholinergic pathways may be involved in human age-related memory degeneration and that choline agonists may help restore some aspects of memory in aged, normal individuals (DAVIS and YAMAMURA 1978; DRACHMAN et al. 1979; DRACHMAN and LEAVITT 1974; SITARAM et al. 1978; BARTUS 1979).

The anatomy of cholinergic systems has not been worked out in the detail available for the aromatic amine neurons. Acetylcholine and its synthetic enzyme, choline acetyltransferase (CAT) (Eq. 3), are particularly concentrated in the caudate,

$$\text{Choline} + \text{Acetyl-Coenzyme A} \xrightarrow{\ CAT\ } \text{Acetylcholine}$$

$$\xrightarrow{\ AChE\ } \text{Acetic Acid} + \text{Choline}$$

Equation 3. Synthesis and metabolism of acetylcholine. *CAT*: choline acetyltransferase; *AChE*: acetylcholinesterase

Table 1. Relative[a] levels of CAT and GAD found in some representative areas of brains from neurologically normal humans aged 20–84 (average age 53)

Area	Activity as percent of that in caudate (Mean $\pm$ SE)	
	CAT	GAD
Motor cortex	6.0 $\pm$ 1.0	136 $\pm$ 12
Parietal cortex	3.2 $\pm$ 0.7	131 $\pm$ 20
Temporal tip	5.9 $\pm$ 0.8	113 $\pm$ 29
Hippocampus	8.1 $\pm$ 0.7	66 $\pm$ 4
Amygdala	20 $\pm$ 3	59 $\pm$ 4
Caudate	100 by definition	
Putamen	105 $\pm$ 10	107 $\pm$ 7
Globus pallidus	13 $\pm$ 3	163 $\pm$ 11
Hypothalamus	7.3 $\pm$ 0.8	141 $\pm$ 11
Medial geniculate	4.8 $\pm$ 1.0	85 $\pm$ 10
V.L. thalamus	5.2 $\pm$ 0.8	74 $\pm$ 9
Substantia nigra	6.8 $\pm$ 1.0	214 $\pm$ 20
Locus coeruleus	14 $\pm$ 1	97 $\pm$ 22
Cerebellar cortex	3.4 $\pm$ 0.6	99 $\pm$ 14

[a] Absolute mean caudate activities in µmol/h/100 mg protein were 4.51 $\pm$ 0.53 for GAD and 10.71 $\pm$ 0.92 for CAT (P.L. McGeer and McGeer 1976). These compare with TH activities of the order of 10–20 nmol/h/100 mg protein

putamen and parts of the limbic system, but substantial levels are found in almost every brain region (Table 1).

Cholinergic neurons are therefore presumably widespread but few have been precisely localized. There is reasonably good evidence that the very intense cholinergic activities of the caudate, putamen and nucleus accumbens are almost entirely in interneurons. Long-axoned cholinergic neurons, arising in the septal area, diagonal band of Broca, preoptic area and substantia innominata, probably provide some or all of the cholinergic innervation of the hippocampus, entorhinal cortex, interpeduncular nucleus, amygdala and frontal cortex. Approximately half of the cholinergic innervation of the frontal cortex seems to be derived from so far unidentified neurons which lie elsewhere than in the substantia innominata. Some of the mossy fibres to the cerebellum also appear to be cholinergic (P.L. McGeer and McGeer 1979). The successful application of immunohistochemical procedures based on specific antibodies to CAT may shortly provide more detailed information on central cholinergic systems (Kimura et al. 1981; Kan et al. 1980).

Acetylcholine is subject to rapid post-mortem changes so that the only index of the integrity of cholinergic neurons which can be used in human post-mortem tissue is the activity of the enzyme CAT (Eq. 3). In our series of 28 brains of neurologically normal humans 5–87 years of age (E.G. McGeer and McGeer 1976), almost a third of the areas examined showed a significant correlation between CAT activity and age. In contrast to TH, DDC, and GAD, the declines in CAT activity with age were particularly notable in cortical areas and less so in extrapyramidal

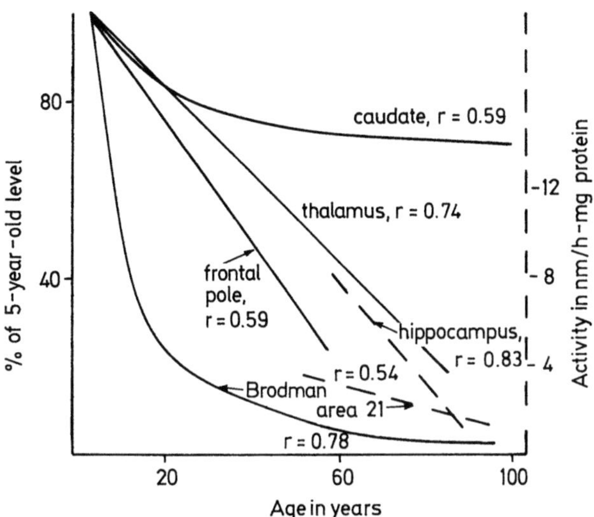

Fig. 4. Representative calculated lines of correlation for CAT activity in various regions of human brain: *solid lines* (and *left axis*) are from the data of *E.G. McGeer* and McGeer (1976), while the *dashed lines* (and *right axis*) are from the data of Perry et al. (1977). The solid curves for Brodman area 21 and the caudate reflect equations of the form: CAT = a + b/age

and rhinencephalic structures (Fig. 4). In our series, CAT activity in the hippocampus was not significantly correlated with age. Perry et al. (1977), however, recently reported on CAT activity in a series of 60 normal brains from humans aged 60–90 years of age and found a significant linear correlation in both area 21 of the cortex and the hippocampus; their lines of correlation are indicated in Fig. 4 along with representative lines calculated from our data. Davies (1979) also reported that controls aged 76–93 (mean 87 years) had much lower average CAT activities in the hippocampus (down to about 30%) and various cortical areas (down to about 10%) than found in controls aged 46–70 (mean 58 years).

Neither Davies (1979) or Perry et al. (1977) found a significant correlation between age and CAT activity in the caudate and putamen. In our series the caudate showed the least decline of any of the areas in which there was a statistically significant correlation while the decline in the putamen did not reach significance; a similar result in human putamen was reported by Bird and Iversen (1974).

No statistically significant correlation between age and CAT activity was noted in normal human frontal cortex by White et al. (1977) or by Mackay et al. (1978 a) in any of the 20 areas of brain studied in 10 neurologically and psychiatrically normal humans, age 46–74 years. The limited number of cases and age range involved in this latter series may account for the lack of statistical correlation.

Acetylcholinesterase (AChE) is the enzyme which metabolizes acetylcholine (Eq. 3). Like MAO, it is present in excess and is not limited to neuronal locations. Hence, it is not as satisfactory an index of neuronal vitality as is the synthetic enzyme. In our series, relatively few regions showed a significant correlation between AChE and age and in only about half of these cases were they areas which showed

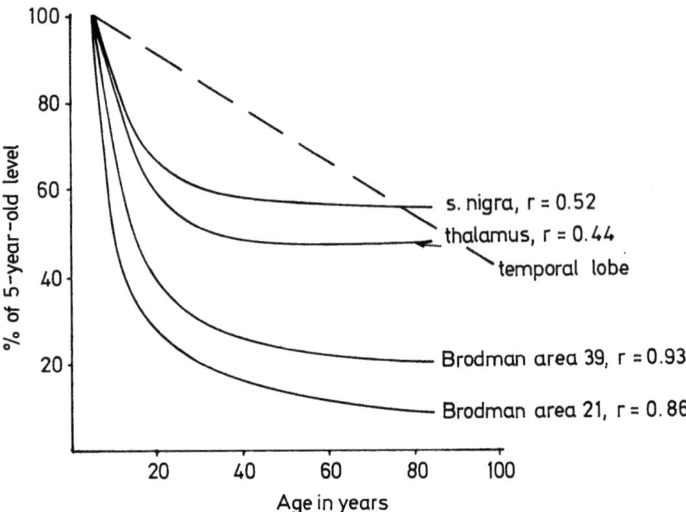

Fig. 5. Representative calculated lines of correlation for AChE activity in various regions of human brain. *Solid curves* reflect equations of the form: AChE = a + b/age (E.G. McGeer and McGeer 1976). *Dashed line* is from the data of Bowen et al. (1977b); an identical line (with a correlation coefficient $r = 0.61$) was given for the data of E.G. McGeer and McGeer (1976) on the temporal tip (Brodman area 38)

significant correlations between CAT activity and age (E.G. McGeer and McGeer 1976). Figure 5 shows some representative calculated lines of correlation. The small but significant loss in the substantia nigra with age may be an example of the difficulty in interpreting changes in AChE levels since in this structure much of the AChE appears to be in dopaminergic neurons (P.L. McGeer and McGeer 1979). Figure 5 also shows the significant correlation with age found by Bowen et al. (1977b) for AChE activity in the temporal lobe of humans.

MacKay et al. (1978a), in their study of ten humans, found no significant correlation between age and AChE levels in various brain regions, and AChE staining in human sympathetic ganglia was found to be unaffected by age (Hervonen et al. 1978).

In a recent study, Davies and Verth (1977) reported no evidence for age-related changes in the concentration of muscarinic acetylcholine receptors in a number of areas of 13 neurologically normal humans between 46 and 79 years of age. White et al. (1977), however, reported a significant negative correlation ($r = 0.49$) between age and cortical density of muscarinic receptors in humans.

It is interesting that the areas (cortex and hippocampus) which appear to show the greatest tendency towards cholinergic decrements with "normal" aging are also the areas showing specific losses in dementia. Some may be tempted to speculate that the particularly notable decline of CAT in the cortex with age may be related to the drop out of cortical cells reported by Brody (1976) and others but it now appears probable that most if not all of the cholinergic activity in the cortex is derived from subcortical afferents (Kimura et al. 1981; P.L. McGeer and McGeer 1979). CAT in the hippocampus is almost certainly in cholinergic nerve endings of the septohippocampal tract. Losses in cholinergic activity may well reflect loss of presynaptic nerve endings attaching to the atrophic dendrites which have been shown to occur in the hippocampus and cortex of animals and humans (SCHEIBEL et al. 1975, 1976).

It might be hypothesized that many age-related declines in neuronal activity, where actual cell loss is minimal, may involve a primary decrease in axonal transport with subsequent degeneration, first of the poorly supplied nerve endings and second of the deafferentated dendritic spines. If decreased axonal transport were an important factor, one might predict that areas richly innervated by long-axoned neurons might show the earliest and most severe losses. The losses of catecholamines and TH from forebrain areas and of CAT from the cortex and hippocampus are consistent with such a prediction. It is also consistent that MARCHI et al. (1980) recently reported data suggesting that the activities of both CAT and AChE, as well as acetylcholine levels, decline during aging more rapidly and more markedly in peripheral (ganglion) cholinergic terminals than in the cholinergic cell bodies.

IV. GABA Systems and Aging

GABA and its synthetic enzyme, glutamic acid decarboxylase (GAD) (Eq. 4), are very widely and rather evenly distributed in the grey matter of brain (Table 1).

Glutamic Acid $\xrightarrow{\;GAD\;}$ $GABA$

$\xrightarrow{GABA\text{-}T}$ α-Ketosuccinic Acid

Equation 4. Synthesis and metabolism of $GABA$. GAD: glutamic acid decarboxylase; $GABA\text{-}T$: gaba transaminase

There appear to be extensive systems of GABA interneurons in most brain regions but there are probably also many long-axoned GABAeric systems. Among the few such tracts which have been tentatively identified are the striatonigral, entopeduncular-habenular, nigrothalamus, nigrocollicular, and Purkinje cell systems (P.L. McGEER and McGEER 1980).

GAD is specifically located in GABAergic neurons and has been the most frequently used indice of such neurons in studies of the possible effects of age. In our series of 28 "normal" human brains, there were 56 areas in which 5 or more samples were analysed for GAD and almost half showed a significant correlation between GAD activity and age (E.G. McGEER and McGEER 1976). This was almost always of a curvilinear nature so the loss was more severe in the younger age groups (Fig. 6). The dashed line in Fig. 6 is taken from the data of BOWEN et al. (1977a), who found a significant correlation in humans between age and GAD activity in the temporal lobe. It was particularly noteworthy in our series that the areas showing the most significant and greatest losses in TH or CAT were not the same as those showing the most severe losses in GAD. In general, the thalamic areas showed the greatest declines in GAD, followed by cortical and rhinencephalic areas. The basal ganglia showed relatively little loss of GAD with age. PERRY et al. (1979) very recently reported a significant negative correlation between age and GABA levels in human thalamus but not in the nucleus accumbens, while Spokes et al. (1979) found a negative correlation in the putamen for GABA levels but not for GAD.

Mackay et al. (1978a) found no significant correlation between GAD and age in various human brain areas. It seems probably that the difference lies in the fact that their ten humans were between 46–74 years of age and, as evident in Fig. 6, the sharpest declines in GAD appeared to have occurred before these age ranges. The same factor may explain why Perry et al. (1977) found no change in GAD in human cortex over the 7th to the 10th decades.

In a preliminary publication some years ago, Cote and Kremzner (1974) reported falls in GAD in the caudate and putamen with age but Bird and Iversen (1974) found no significant decline of GAD in the human putamen with age.

One problem in assaying GAD activity in human brain is that this enzyme seems particularly sensitive to premortem coma (P.L. McGeer and McGeer (1976) and may also be affected by antibiotics used for treatment of pneumonia, which is frequently the terminal condition in the aged (Iversen et al. 1978).

V. Other Neurotransmitter Systems and Aging

One of the major problems facing researchers in the field of neurotransmitters in aging is that almost all previous work has been concentrated in a few neurotransmitter systems (dopamine, noradrenaline and serotonin, with a few reports on GABA and acetylcholine). This focussing on the aromatic amines has been determined largely by the fact that the anatomy of their pathways has been well established and assay methods available. Taken together, however, the aromatic amine systems probably account for less than 1%–2% of the neurons in the brain. It is thus evident that the field has barely been touched. There are at least 20 compounds that are now tentatively accepted as putative neurotransmitters (or neuromodulators) in the brain, including, for example, histamine, glutamate, aspartate, adrenaline, glycine, and various peptides, such as substance P, enkephalin, neurotensin, VIP, and somatostatin. No research on possible changes in these systems as a function of normal and pathological aging in humans has yet appeared. Some scattered animal studies are now appearing but, in many cases, the techniques necessary for a study in humans have still to be established.

C. Conclusions

Clearly much remains to be done in determining what changes in neuronal activity accompany normal aging. The available data suggest that any changes may vary according to region and biochemical type of neuron, so that more attention must be given to such specificity. Moreover, there are many indications that physiological functions such as sleep, movement (McGeer et al. 1977) or hormonal secretion (Simpkins et al. 1977) may depend as much upon the balance between various neurotransmitters in a given brain region as on the absolute level of any single neurotransmitter. Even the very limited data that are so far available suggest mech-

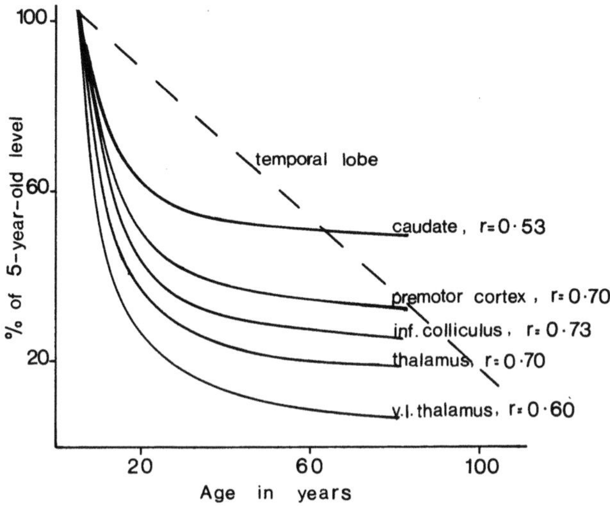

Fig. 6. Representative calculated lines of correlation for GAD activity in various regions of human brain. *Solid curves* reflect equations of the form: GAD = a + b/age (E.G. McGeer and McGeer 1976). *Dashed line* is from the data of Bowen et al. (1977a)

anisms for the functional deficits in drug sensitivity seen in aging (Beck 1978; Bender 1970; Kent 1976) and imply that the aging process might be ameliorated by agents which alter neurotransmitter metabolism (Cotzias et al. 1977; Samorajski 1977).

An even more fundamental question that needs to be addressed is why losses should occur at all. The progress of medicine is leading to an ever-increasing life span and, as it does, new physiological problems are unmasked. In the case of aging, there is an enormous cost to society of maintaining individuals whose mental and neurological capacities have slipped below the threshold necessary for independence. From the sorts of data reviewed here, temporary measures may be found to alleviate some of the symptoms, as with L-dopa therapy of parkinsonism, but the real problem remains unanswered until we can understand the mechanisms which make particular neuronal systems seem especially vulnerable to age-induced decay. As discussed in the section on catecholamine and acetylcholine systems, some of the losses may be related to actual cell death but more seem to depend upon decreases in cell vitality and in divergence number. It has been postulated that declining axonal transport may be an important factor. Even if further data are consistent with this supposition, more fundamental work will be needed to answer the basic question of why neurons lose their vitality and die.

References

Adolfsson R, Gottfries CG, Oreland L, Roos BE, Winblad B (1978) Reduced level of catecholamines in the brain and increased activity of monoamine oxidase in platelets in Alzheimer's disease: therapeutic implications. In: Katzman R, Terry RD, Bick KL (eds) Aging, vol 7. Raven Press, New York, pp 441–451

Adolfsson R, Gottfries CG, Roos BE, Winblad B (1979) Post-mortem distribution of dopamine and homovanillic acid in human brain, variations related to age, and a review of the literature. J Neural Trans 45:81–106

Bartus RT (1979) Physostigmine and recent memory: effects in young and aged nonhuman primates. Science 206:1087–1089

Beck CHM (1978) Functional implications of changes in the senescent brain: a review. Can J Neurol Sci 5:417–424

Bender AD (1970) The influence of age on the activity of catecholamines and related therapeutic agents. J Am Geriatr Soc 18:220–232

Bertler A (1961) Occurrence and localization of catecholamines in the human brain. Act Physiol Scand 51:97–107

Bertler A, Falck B, Owman C, Rosengrenn E (1966) The localization of monoaminergic blood-brain barrier mechanisms. Pharm Rev 18:369–385

Bird ED, Iversen LL (1974) Huntington's chorea – post-mortem measurement of glutamic acid decarboxylase, choline acetyltransferase and dopamine in basal ganglia. Brain 97:457–472

Bowen DM, Smith CB, White P, Godhardt MJ, Spillane JA, Flack RHA, Davison AN (1977a) Chemical pathology of the organic dementias. Part I. Validity of biochemical measurements in human post-mortem brain specimens. Brain 100:397–426

Bowen DM, Smith CB, White P, Flack RHA, Carrasco LH, Gedye GE, Davison AN (1977b) Chemical pathology of the organic dementias. Part II. Quantitative estimation of cellular change in post-mortem brains. Brain 100:427–453

Brody H (1976) An examination of cerebral cortex and brain stem in aging. In: Terry AD, Gershon S (eds) Neurobiology of aging, vol 3. Raven Press, New York, pp 177–181

Bugiani O, Salvarani S, Perdelli F, Mancardi GL, Leonardi A (1978) Nerve cell loss with aging in the putamen. Eur Neurol 17:286–291

Carlsson A, Winblad B (1976) Influence of age and time interval between death and autopsy on dopamine and 3-methoxytyramine levels in human basal ganglia. J Neural Trans 38:271–276

Cheng SC, Shih JC (1979) Photoaffinity labeling of serotonin binding proteins decreased in aged human brains. Int Soc Neurochem 9:273

Cote LJ, Kremzner LT (1974) Changes in neurotransmitter systems with increasing age in human brain. Trans Am Soc Neurochem 5:83

Cotzias GC, Miller ST, Tang LC, Papavasiliou PS (1977) Levodopa, fertility, and longevity. Science 196:549–551

Davies P (1979) Neurotransmitter-related enzymes in senile dementia of the Alzheimer type. Brain Res 171:319–327

Davies P, Verth AH (1977) Regional distribution of muscarinic acetylcholine receptor in normal and Alzheimer's-type dementia brains. Brain Res 138:385–392

Davis KL, Jamamura HI (1978) Cholinergic underactivity in human memory disorders. Life Sci 23:1229–1234

Drachman DA, Leavitt JL (1974) Human memory and the cholinergic system: a relationship to aging? Arch Neurol 30:113–121

Drachman DA, Noffsinger D, Sahakian BJ, Kurdziel S, Fleming P (1979) Aging, memory and cholinergic system: A study of dichotic listening. Ann Neurol 6:157–158

Goldstein DJ, Cubeddu XL (1976) Dopamine-β-hydroxylase activity in human cerebrospinal fluid. J Neurochem 26:193–195

Gottfries CG, Oreland L, Wiberg A, Winblad B (1974) Brain levels of monoamine oxidase in depression. Lancet 2:360–361

Grote SS, Moses SG, Robins E, Hudgens RW, Croninger AB (1974) A study of selected catecholamine metabolizing enzymes: a comparison of depressive suicides and alcoholic suicides with controls. J Neurochem 23:791–802

Hervonen A, Vaalasti A, Partanen M, Kanerva L, Hervonen H (1978) Effects of aging on the histochemically demonstrable catecholamines and acetylcholinesterase of human sympathetic ganglia. J Neurocytol 7:11–23

Hsu HK, Peng MT (1978) Hypothalamic neuron number of old female rats. Gerontology 24:434–440

Iversen LL, Spokes E, Bird E (1978) Agonist specificity of GABA binding sites in human brain and GABA in Huntington's disease and schizophrenia. In: Krogsgaard-Larsen P, Scheel-Kruger J (eds) GABA neurotransmitters. Alfred Benzon Symposium XII. Munksgaard, Copenhagen, pp 170–190

Kan K-S, Giolli RA, Chao L-P (1980) Immunohistochemical localization of choline acetyltransferase in forebrain. Am Soc Neurochem 11:203

Kent S (1976) Neurotransmitters may be weak link in the aging brain's communication network. Geriatrics 31:105–111

Kimura H, McGeer PL, Peng F, McGeer EG (1981) The central cholinergic system studied by immunohistochemistry in the cat. J Comp Neurol 200:151–201

Lerner P, Goodwin FK, Van Kammen DP, Post RM, Major LF, Ballenger JC, Lovenberg W (1978) Dopamine-β-hydroxylase in the cerebrospinal fluid of psychiatric patients. Biol Psychiatry 13:685–694

Lloyd KG, Hornykiewicz O (1972) Occurrence and distribution of aromatic L-amino acid (L-DOPA) decarboxylase in the human brain. J Neurochem 19:1549–1559

Mackay AVP, Davies P, Dewar AJ, Yates CM (1978 a) Regional distribution of enzymes associated with neurotransmission by monoamines, acetylcholine and GABA in the human brain. J Neurochem 30:827–839

Mackay AVP, Yates CM, Wright A, Hamilton P (1978 b) Regional distribution of monoamines and their metabolites in the human brain. J Neurochem 30:841–848

Maggi A, Schmidt MJ, Ghetti B, Enna SJ (1979) Effect of aging in neurotransmitter receptor binding in rat and human brain. Life Sci 24:367–374

Marchi M, Hoffman DW, Giacobini E (1980) Aging alters acetylcholine metabolism in autonomic terminals. Am Soc Neurochem Abstr 11:84

McGeer EG, McGeer PL (1976) Neurotransmitter metabolism in the aging brain. In: Terry RD, Gershon S (eds) Neurobiology of aging, vol 3. Raven Press, New York, pp 389–403

McGeer EG, McGeer PL (1980) Biochemical mapping of specific neuronal pathways. In: Federoff S, Hertz L (eds) Advances in cellular neurobiology, vol 1. Academic Press, New York, pp 347–372

McGeer PL, McGeer EG (1976) Enzymes associated with the metabolism of catecholamines, acetylcholine, and GABA in human controls and patients with Parkinson's disease and Huntington's chorea. J Neurochem 26:65–76

McGeer PL, McGeer EG (1979) Central cholinergic pathways. In: Barbeau A, Growdon JH, Wurtman RJ (eds) Nutrition and the brain, vol 5. Raven Press, New York, pp 177–199

McGeer PL, McGeer EG (1980) Amino acid neurotransmitters. In: Siegel GJ (ed) Basic neurochemistry, 3rd ed. Little Brown Comp, Boston

McGeer PL, McGeer EG, Suzuki JS (1977) Aging and extrapyramidal function. Arch Neurol 34:33–35

McGeer PL, Eccles JC, McGeer EG (1978) Molecular neurobiology of the mammalian brain. Plenum Press, New York

Meites J, Simpkins JW, Huang HH (1979) The relation of hypothalamic biogenic amines to secretion of gonadotropins and prolactin in the aging rat. Aging 8:87–94

Nies A, Robinson DS, Davis JM, Ravaris L (1973) Changes in monoamine oxidase with aging. In: Eisdorfer C, Fann WE (eds) Psychopharmacology and aging: advances in behavioral biology. Plenum Press, New York, pp 41–54

Perry EK, Perry RH, Gibson PH, Blessed G, Tomlinson BE (1977) A cholinergic connection between normal aging and senile dementia in the human hippocampus. Neurosci Lett 6:85–89

Perry TL, Kish SJ, Buchanan J, Hansen S (1979) γ-Aminobutyric acid deficiency in brain of schizophrenic patients. Lancet 1:237–239

Peters DAV, McGeer PL, McGeer EG (1968) The distribution of tryptophan hydroxylase in cat brain. J Neurochem 15:1431–1435

Roberts E, Wong E, Svenneby G, Degener P (1978) Sodium-dependent binding of GABA to mouse brain particles. Brain Res 152:614–619

Robinson DS (1955) Changes in monoamine oxidase and monoamines with human development and aging. Fed Proc 34:103–109

Robinson DS, Nies A, Davis JN, Bunney WE, Davis JM, Colburn RW, Bourne HR, Sahw DM, Coppen AJ (1972) Aging, monoamines, and monoamine oxidase levels. Lancet 1:290–291

Robinson DS, Sourkes TL, Nies A, Harris LS, Spector S, Bartlett DL, Kaye IS (1977) Monoamine metabolism in human brain. Arch Gen Psychiatry 34:89–92

Samorajski T (1977) Central neurotransmitter substances and aging: a review. J Am Geriatr Soc 25:337–348

Samorajski T, Rolsten C (1973) Age and regional differences in the chemical composition of brains of mice, monkeys, and humans. In: Ford DH (ed) Progress in brain research, vol 40. Elsevier Press, Amsterdam, pp 253–265

Scheff SW, Bernardo LS, Cotman CW (1978) Decrease in adrenergic axon sprouting in the senescent rat. Science 202:775–778

Scheibel ME, Lindsay RD, Tomiyasu U, Scheibel AB (1975) Progressive dendritic changes in aging human cortex. Exp Neurol 47:392–403

Scheibel ME, Lindsay RD, Tomiyasu U, Scheibel AB (1976) Progressive dendritic changes in aging human limbic system. Exp Neurol 53:420–430

Schocken DD, Roth GS (1977) Reduced β-adrenergic receptor concentrations in aging man. Nature 267:856–858

Seifert WE Jr, Foxx JL, Butler IJ (1980) Age effect on dopamine and serotonin metabolite levels in cerebrospinal fluid. Ann Neurol 8:38–42n

Shih JC Young H (1978) Alteration of serotonin binding sites in aged human brain. Life Sci 23:1441–1448

Simpkins JW, Mueller GP, Huang HH, Meites J (1977) Evidence for depressed catecholamine and enhanced serotonin metabolism in aging male rats: possible relations to gonadotropin secretion. Endocrinology 100:1672–1678

Sitaram N, Weingartner H, Caine ED, Gillin JC (1978) Choline-selective enhancement of serial learning and encoding of low imagery words in man. Life Sci 22:1555–1560

Spokes EGS, Garrett NJ, Iversen LH (1979) Differential effects of agonal status on measurements of GABA and glutamate decarboxylase in human postmortem brain tissue from Huntington's chorea subjects. J Neurochem 33:773–778

Tryding N, Tufvesson G, Ilsson S (1972) Aging, monoamines, and monoamine oxidase levels. Lancet 1:489

Vijayashankar N, Brody H (1977) Aging in the human brainstem: a study of the nucleus of the trochlear nerve. Acta Anat 99:169–172

Vincent SR, McGeer EG (1980) A comparison of sodium-dependent glutamate binding with high affinity glutamate uptake in rat striatum. Brain Res 184:99–108

White P, Goodhardt MJ, Keet JP, Hiley CR, Carrasco LH, Williams IEI, Bowen DM (1977) Neocortical cholinergic neurons in elderly people. Lancet 1:668–671

Neuroimmunology of the Aging Brain*

A. BALDINGER and H. T. BLUMENTHAL

A. Introduction

For some years now we have been developing the concept that there may be a direct link between biological and pathological aging (BLUMENTHAL and BERNS 1964; BLUMENTHAL 1978; BLUMENTHAL 1981). In general this concept holds that aging-related errors in the synthesis of structural, hormonal, enzymal, and antibody proteins are capable of directly generating disease, independent of environmental factors. This concept also recognizes that there are mechanisms which serve to compensate for or correct such errors including enzymes which selectively degrade misspecified proteins, DNA repair mechanisms, and immune responses which either inactivate or destroy faulty proteins. On the other hand, failure of these corrective mechanisms may also be characteristic of aging, thus facilitating the emergence of disease. The appearance of a variety of autoimmune phenomena associated with aging may reflect such failure on the part of the immune system.

Neurons of the CNS differ from most other cells in that they are postmitotic, and as ORGEL (1963) has pointed out "error catastrophe" may have greater impact on cells of this type than on those with a capacity to undergo mitotic division and thus "dilute" the effects of errors. It has been proposed that certain of the immunological manifestations of aging in the brain may derive from misspecifications which occur in neurons (BLUMENTHAL 1976). Heretofore, however, there has been less consideration as to the applicability of the above concept to disorders of the CNS than to those of other organ systems. In this chapter we discuss the status of information on CNS diseases associated with immune phenomena as well as some immune phenomena associated with aging.

B. Diseases of the Nervous System with Immune Components

BEHAN and CURRIE (1978) point out that there is now an impressive body of knowledge relating both to immunological factors underlying naturally occurring neurological diseases, and to experimental disorders affecting central and peripheral nervous systems and muscle. This includes a number of viral and bacterial diseases which infect the nervous system, some primarily (lymphocytic choriomeningitis, kuru, and Jakob-Creuzfeldt's disease), and some as extensions from infections in other areas; several acute and chronic demyelinating diseases such as acute hemor-

---

* From the Aging and Development Program, Department of Psychology, Washington University, St. Louis, Missouri, United States

rhagic leukoencephalitis and multiple sclerosis; polyneuritic syndromes; autoimmune disorders such as myasthenia gravis; the CNS involvement in connective tissue disorders of autoimmune origin such as systemic lupus and rheumatoid arthritis; and neurological disorders associated with neoplasms, particularly those in which CNS basic proteins have been demonstrated (FIELD and CASPARY 1970) as well as a neuron-binding antibody (ZEROMSKI 1970). There are, in addition, several primary disorders of the CNS which may have immune features [e.g., ataxia-telangiectasia and senile dementia of the Alzheimer type (SDAT)].

BEHAN and CURRIE (1978) divide these disorders into two categories, allergic and immune deficiency disorders, but point out that this is largely arbitrary since immune disturbances are complex. An important relevant consideration is the fact that an imbalance of T- and B-cell function underlies both aging of the immune system and several of these neurological disorders. These aging changes of the immune system may permit the activation of "latent" viruses, but they have also been linked with the emergence of a variety of autoimmune phenomena associated with aging.

For the most part the techniques that have been employed to demonstrate antibodies which bind to CNS components in some of these neurological disorders fall into two categories as shown in Table 1. In virtually every instance, however, antibody is also present in the serum of some small percent of normal subjects. For example, ALLERAND and YAHR (1964) demonstrated serum immunoglobulins (Igs) which bind to glial structures from subjects without evidence of a neurological disorder, and WHITAKER and ENGEL (1974) were not able to confirm the observations of MARTIN et al. (1974) regarding the specificity of ANA associated with myasthenia gravis. Similarly SOTELO et al. (1980) obtained positive binding of Ig to neurofilamentous structures in senile dementia as well as in normal subjects, while WHITTINGHAM et al. (1970) were unable to confirm the presence of a cytoplasmic neuron-binding antibody (NBA) in senile dementia. Further confounding these studies are the observations that antibodies to certain types of streptococci may cross react with neuronal cytoplasm (HUSBY et al. 1976) and that in some diseases there may be serum Igs which bind to several different target structures (D'ANGELO and D'ANGELO 1975; KAUFMAN and MILLER 1977). It therefore would appear to be important to determine the extent to which aging may play a role in the appearance of these antibodies.

C. Neuron-Binding Antibody and Aging

In this section we discuss the relationship between aging and the antibody which binds to neuronal cytoplasm. The reasons for this choice is that this antibody-binding characteristic has been associated with some seven neurological disorders as listed in Table 1, and that NBA has been studied more extensively in respect to aging than any of the other antibodies represented in Table 1. Much of the information presented here is tentative since it derives from ongoing studies, some of which are incomplete.

In by far the majority of studies on cytoplasmic NBA, the indirect immunofluorescence or immunoperoxidase technique has been used. Since in the

Table 1. Antibody and target associated with nervous system disease

Technique	Antigen (antibody target)	Disease	Reference
Serological	Encephalitogenic protein	Multiple sclerosis	ASBURY and LISAK (1980) FIELD et al. (1963) LEVIN and BOSHES (1969)
		Carcinomatous neuropathy	FIELD and CASPARY (1970)
		Schizophrenia	KOLYASKINA and KUSHNER (1969)
		Senile dementia	SKALICKOVA et al. (1962)
	Cholinergic receptors	Myasthenia gravis	LENNON (1976)
Immunocyto-chemical	Glial cells	Demyelinating disorders	EDDINGTON and DELASSIO (1970)
		Ataxia-telangiectasia	KAUFMAN and MILLER (1977)
	Nucleus (ANA)	Schizophrenia	HEATH and KRUPP (1967)
		Myasthenia gravis	MARTIN et al. (1974)
	Neuronal cytoplasm	Lupus and epilepsy	DIEDERICKSON and PYNDT (1968)
		Chorea	HUSBY et al. (1976)
		Cerebrovascular disease	MOTYKA and JEZKOVA (1975) SAVENKO and POLIENKO (1975)
		Carcinomatous neuropathy	ZEROMSKI (1970)
		Senile dementia	SKALICKOVA et al. (1962) KALTER and KELLY (1975) D'ANGELO and D'ANGELO (1975) MAYER et al. (1976) NANDY (1978)
		Chronic brain syndrome	INGRAM et al. (1974)
		Ataxia-telangiectasia	KAUFMAN and MILLER (1977)
	Neural filaments	Creutzfeldt-Jakob disease Kuru	SOTELO et al. (1980)

technique serum from the subject being tested is applied to a substrate brain section or spread of cell suspension prior to the application of labeled anti-Ig, we have designated this an in vitro technique. The reason for this is that the presence of an antibody in serum does not necessarily indicate that the antibody is actually bound to neurons of the subject being tested; this consideration is particularly applicable to the use of the term "neuron reactive antibody" (NANDY 1977, 1978). On the other hand, the direct technique in which the labeled anti-Ig is applied directly to sections from a series of brains provides evidence for in vivo binding, and the data presented here deriving from our own studies have been obtained, for the most part, with the use of this technique.

If the direct immunoperoxidase technique is applied to a series of human brains over a wide range of ages, a variety of structures can be seen to bind the labeled anti-Ig, including neuronal cytoplasm and nucleus, fibrillar cytoplasmic structure of neurons, glial cell cytoplasm and nucleus, blood vessels, corpora amylacea, choroid plexus cells, and concretions within choroidal vessels. Some of these observations are illustrated in Figs. 1–5, which show sections from cases over 60 years of age without evidence of neurological or psychiatric disorders. Except for neuronal cytoplasm, the specificity of binding of these structures remains to be determined. In the case of neuronal cytoplasm it has been observed that the application of similarly labeled albumin does not give evidence of binding, and that the application of unlabeled anti-Ig can saturate the binding sites and thus inhibit the binding of the corresponding labeled Ig.

Because, as discussed below, the implications of such binding may depend on the Ig class of the antibody and whether or not there is evidence of complement fixation, we have compared the binding of Igs, M, G, and A and have ascertained that peroxidase labeled anti-C_3 is also bound to some neurons which bind Ig. Sections from various regions were obtained from each brain, and binding intensity subjectively graded on a scale of + to + + +, representing a range of color from light brown to black. The highest grade for any neuron was recorded as the binding intensity for the region represented in the section. The data thus obtained have been analyzed in two ways: (1) The determination of the mean intensity for each

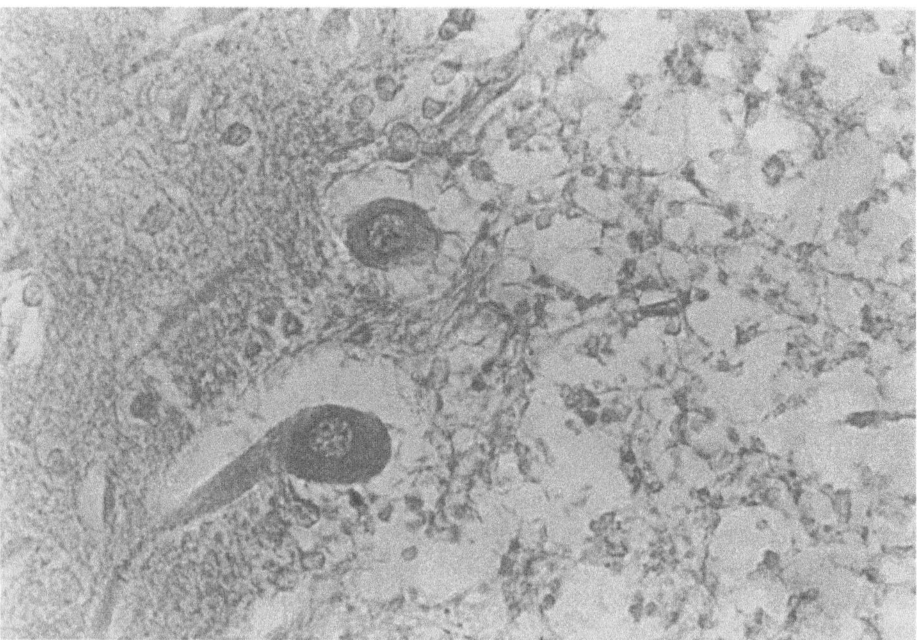

Fig. 1. Neurons at the edge of an area of encephalomalacia. Cytoplasm stains dark brown with peroxidase-tagged goat antihuman IgM, while axon is slightly lighter. Nucleus shows a stippled pattern of staining. × 250, reduced to 75%

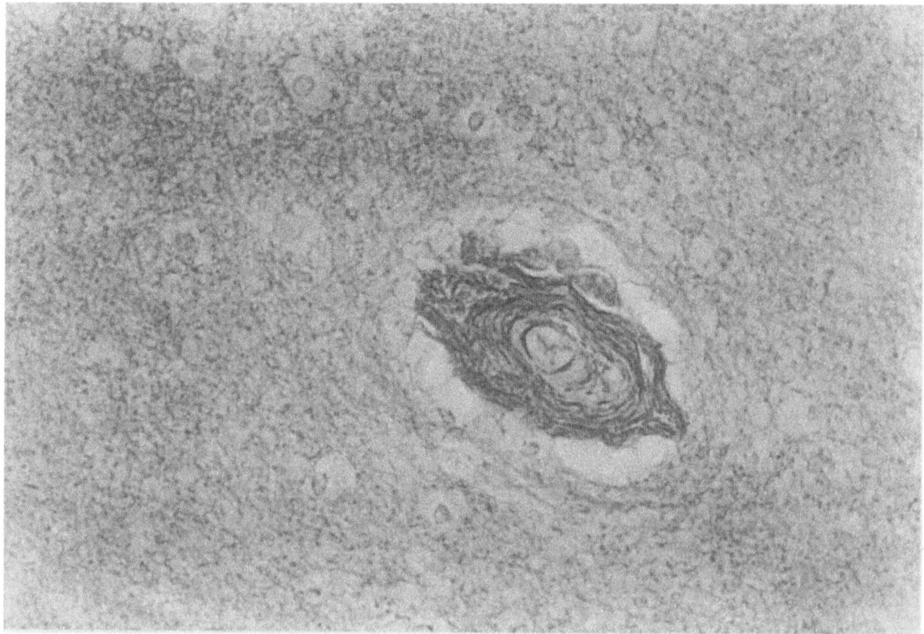

Fig. 2. Single neuron (in the center) showing a fibrillar pattern of staining with peroxidase-tagged goat antihuman IgG. The nucleus does not stain. × 400, reduced to 75%

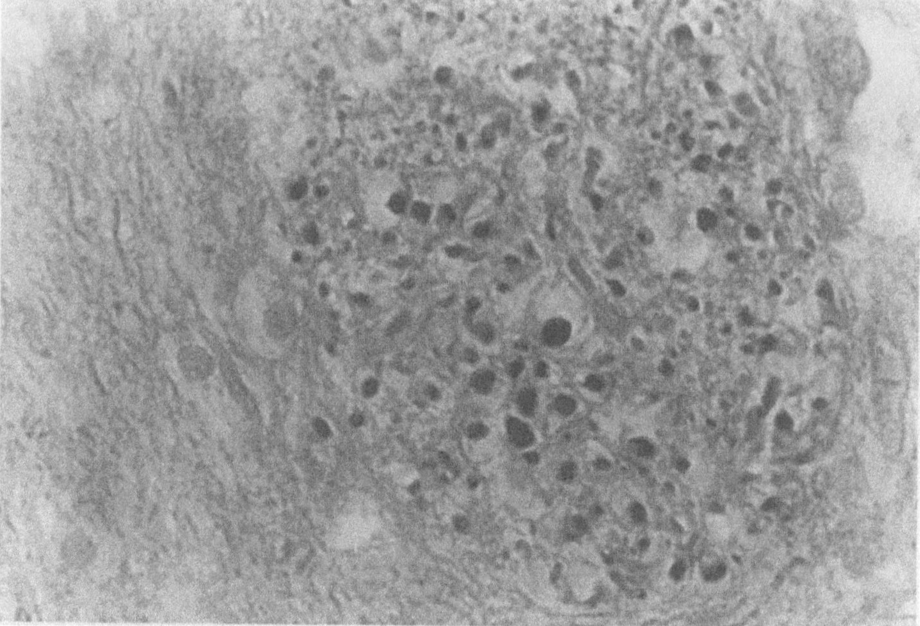

Fig. 3. Cross section of a nerve trunk which shows intense black staining of axons with peroxidase-tagged goat antihuman IgG. × 400, reduced to 75%

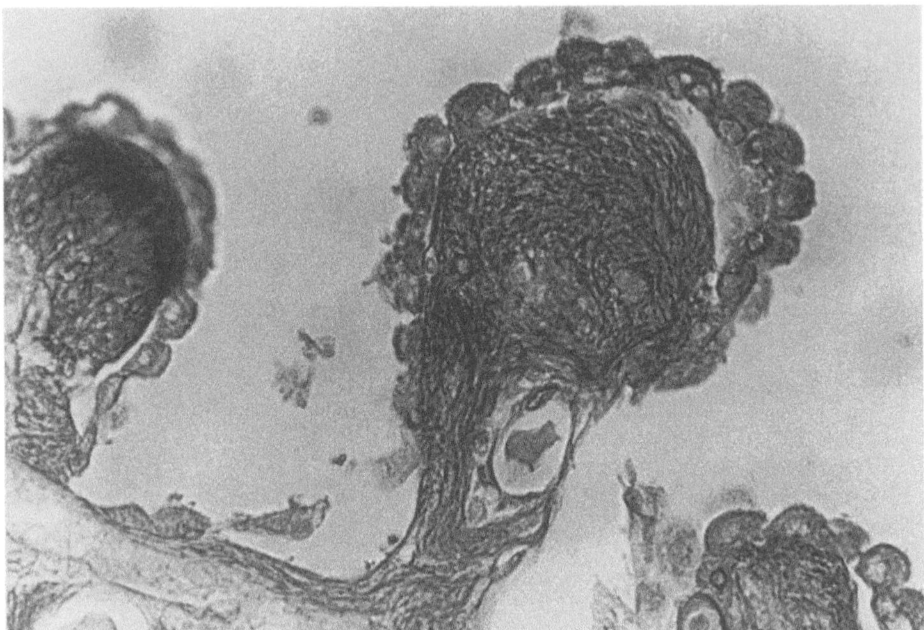

Fig. 4. Section through a portion of the choroid plexus stained with peroxidase-tagged goat antihuman IgG. It shows intense staining of laminated concretions and of ependymal cells surrounding the concretions. × 400, reduced to 75%

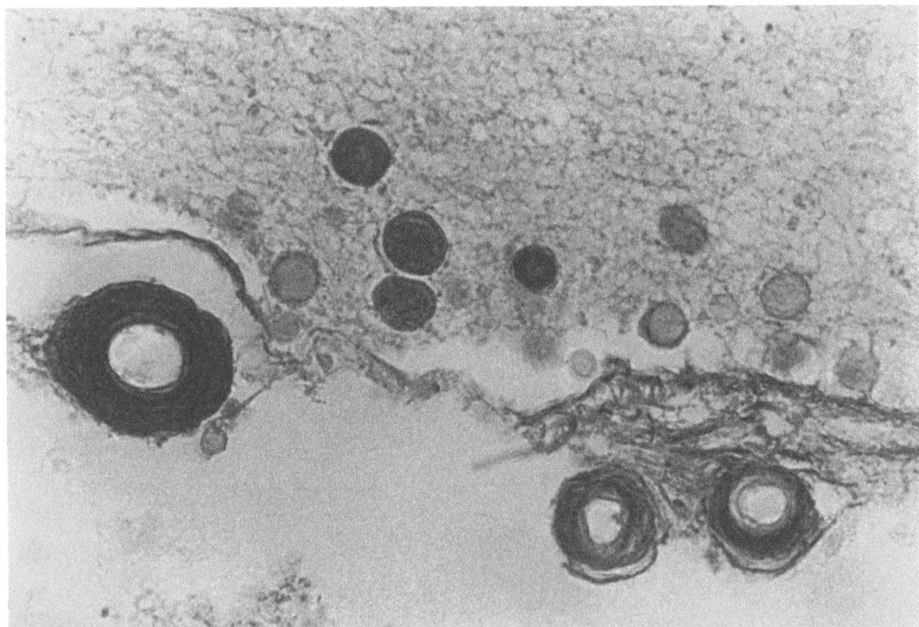

Fig. 5. Section through the superficial cortex stained with peroxidase-tagged antihuman IgM. Some concretions and thick-walled vessels show an intense black color. × 400, reduced to 75%

Table 2. Relation of age to mean NBA intensity in nonneurological, non psychiatric cases

Age group	Sex	Number	IgM	IgG	IgA
0–30	M	4	1.0	0.7	0.8
	F	5	0.7	0.3	0.5
Combined		9	0.8	0.5	0.6
31–50	M	6	1.2	1.4	0.9
	F	7	1.2	1.0	0.9
Combined		13	1.2	1.2	0.9
51–69	M	14	1.8	1.3	1.4
	F	10	1.1	1.0	1.1
Combined		24	1.6	1.2	1.3
70 and over	M	8	1.2	1.3	1.3
	F	8	1.4	1.2	0.8
Combined		16	1.3	1.3	1.1

Table 3. Relation of age to maximum NBA-binding intensity in nonneurological, nonpsychiatric cases

Age group	number	Per cent of cases		
		IgM	IgG	IgA
I. Criterion – + + or greater binding intensity				
0–30	9	56	11	22
31–50	13	62	77	88
51–69	24	58	71	88
70 and over	16	75	88	75
II. Criterion – + + + or greater binding intensity				
0–30	9	11	0	0
31–50	13	15	8	15
51–69	24	8	0	0
70 and over	16	75	38	25

brain and (2) the determination of the percent of cases with + + or greater, or + + + or greater binding intensity in any one region. It should be noted here in respect to these determinations that the pattern of binding is quite variable, not only from region to region of the same brain, but also within a single region. Where there are clusters of neurons the range of binding may sometimes vary from as much as 0 to + + +.

Table 2 presents the changes with age in mean NBA intensity for the three Ig classes. An analysis of variance showed that for IgG the mean intensity of the 0–30 age group was significantly lower than for the other three age groups ($P < 0.01$). For IgM and IgA the only significant differences were between the 0–30 and the 51–69 age groups (IgM, $P < 0.05$; IgA, $P < 0.05$). Table 3 shows the results of an-

Table 4. Comparison between in vivo and in vitro condition

Age group	In vivo IgG		In vitro IgG	
	Mean intensity	% + + and over	Mean intensity	% + + and over
I. Based on total brain [a]				
0–30	0.5	11	0.1	12
31–50	1.2	77	0.4	24
Over 50	1.2	80	2.1	74
II. Based on examination of hypothalamus [b]				
0–30	0	0	1.7	12
31–50	1.7	50	1.6	16
51–69	1.4	36	1.9	58
70 and over	2.1	75	1.6	40

[a] This comparison has used the in vitro data of Ingram et al. (1974)
[b] There were 28 cases examined under the in vivo and 140 cases under the in vitro conditions

alyses based on maximum rather than mean NBA intensity. If the criterion is set at + + intensity then there is an initially high incidence of IgM binding which then levels off and rises again in the oldest age group; by contrast, IgG and IgA have an initially low incidence but rise significantly in the 31–50 age group. The incidence of maximum IgG binding rises again in the oldest age group, but the incidence of IgA falls somewhat. If + + + is set as the criterion all three Ig classes show an initial low incidence, particularly IgG and IgA, but the incidence rises in the oldest age group, and this is most marked in respect to IgM.

It would appear that these observations confirm those of other studies based on the indirect (in vitro) technique. The latter include studies on mice (Threatt et al. 1971), on rats (Miller and Blumenthal 1978; Feden et al. 1979), on primates (Felsenfeld and Wolf 1972), and on human subjects (Felsenfeld and Wolf 1972; Ingram et al. 1974). However, we carried out comparisons of our results with those of Ingram et al. (1974), although immunofluorescence was used in the latter study, as well as with hypothalamus as tissue substrate in which both the in vitro and in vivo studies utilized the immunoperoxidase technique. The results are shown in Table 4. In the comparison with the data from Ingram et al., both in vivo and in vitro components show an aging effect, but there are also differences. The differences are even more pronounced in the hypothalamus study where there is no in vitro aging effect when mean intensity is the criterion. A comparison in respect to the pattern of regional binding (Table 5) also shows differences between in vivo and in vitro findings.

A study has also been undertaken regarding in vivo binding in affective disorders primarily for purposes of comparison with the several studies on senile dementia listed in Table 1. Thus far we have examined some 27 cases, which include a variety of affective disorders including a few cases of senile dementia. The affective disorders show significant differences from normal subjects only in the 0–30 age group, where they show a higher mean intensity of binding of all three Ig classes. Specifically in respect to senile dementia, a preliminary study comparing the

Table 5. In vivo – in vitro comparison of rank order of regional mean NBA intensity

In vivo	In vitro
Hippocampus	Occipital lobe
Parietal lobe	Hippocampus
Frontal lobe	Temporal lobe
Occipital lobe	Parietal lobe
Temporal lobe	Frontal lobe

Table 6. Comparison of mean NBA intensity with intensity of senile plaque formation

Number of cases	Plaque intensity	Mean NBA intensity		
		IgM	IgG	IgA
3	+ + +	1.5	2.0	1.0
5	+ +	1.4	1.4	1.2
3	+	1.8	1.3	1.3

intensity of senile plaque formation with Ig binding was carried out. As shown in Table 6, there is a correlation between intensity of plaque formation and intensity of IgG binding. This may be comparable to the observations by SOTELO et al. (1980); the latter reported that the antibody which binds to neurofibrillary elements of neurons is an IgG and not an IgM or IgA.

D. Effects and Potential Targets of Neuron-Binding Antibodies

According to HOLBOROW (1973), it was von PIRQUET who first pointed out in 1906 that antibodies may be beneficial, harmful, or neutral. This remains a relevant consideration, particularly since more recent studies (MACKAY et al. 1977) show that in many cases with aging-related autoantibodies there is no evidence of disease of the target organ, and this may also hold for NBA, particularly in those studies in which the antibody has only been identified in serum by the indirect technique.

Nevertheless NANDY (1977, 1978) has proposed that NBA may be responsible for the aging-related loss of neurons of the CNS. The observation by CHAFFEE et al. (1978) that human serum contains an Ig which is cytolytic for cultured neuroblastoma cells when complement is added to the testing system, would appear to support this proposal. However, CHAFFEE et al. found a peak incidence at 20–25 years, an observation which is not consonant with an aging phenomenon, and it remains to be determined whether or not similar results would be obtained with mature neurons as substrate.

With the exception of the study by SOTELO et al. (1980), in which the antibody binding to the neurofilamentous structures of neurons was determined to be an IgG and not an IgM or IgA, there have heretofore been no analyses of the Ig classes in respect to NBA. The peak incidence at 20–25 years in the study by CHAFFEE et al., noted above, when compared with the intensity levels of Ig binding at 0–30 years in Table 3, suggests that the cytolytic effect on neuroblastoma cells may be an IgM; CHAFFEE et al. did not study cases over age 65 when there might have been a second peak in the incidence curve. Several reports indicate that IgM levels are high early in life and then decline (WALFORD 1970; CASSIDY et al. 1974; RADL et al. 1975). There is, however, an increase in the serum level of Igs with age which is principally represented by IgG. While the aging-associated in vivo binding of IgG and IgA to neuronal cytoplasm follows a pattern similar to that of serum levels, the changes in IgM are most striking and may reflect some serum levels observed by RADL et al. (1975), who noted a particularly striking increase in the variation in the levels of IgM in elderly subjects.

WALFORD (1970) notes further that IgGs are protective in respect to graft rejection and enhancing in respect to tumor growth. On the other hand IgMs are the most primitive and are the first antibodies produced in the immune response (BEHAN and BEHAN 1979). They usually fix complement and enhance opsonization and destruction of microorganisms, and HELLSTROM (1970) notes that in patients with sarcoma there is an IgM complement-fixing antibody which correlates with a better clinical status. These observations suggest either that there is an IgM response to some continuous antigenic stimulus which is then converted into an IgG response, or that the IgM and IgG response are separate, or both. If the IgM and IgG responses are not related to one another, then the IgM may elicit a cytolytic effect while the IgG may be protective. There are a number of examples in which more than one antibody may be directed at a particular structure. In myasthenia gravis the immune response against the acetylcholine receptor involves a range of antibodies, each specific to a different molecular configuration or determinant on the receptor (LEWIN 1981); and there are a number of antibodies directed against thyroid cell structures, some of which may be destructive of thyroid tissue, while others may enhance the secretion of thyroid hormones as in Graves' disease (SOLOMON and KLEEMAN 1977). It appears likely, therefore, that our findings reflect several types of immunological effects on neurons.

Despite the narrow base of information reflected in the foregoing discussion, studies have already been carried out on behavioral effects which might be attributable to immune phenomena involving the CNS. RAPPORT and KARPIAK (1978) have reported studies in animals in which antisera containing antibodies against synaptic antigens were passively transferred to the brain. Epileptiform activity was elicited, and there were changes in passive avoidance behavior and in maze performance. EISDORFER et al. (1978) have reported studies on human subjects in which attempts were made to correlate various measures of cognition with serum IgM, G, and A levels. In these studies there was no demonstration that any of these Igs were directed against CNS components, and it is possible that their findings reflect a loss of immune capacity associated with aging as well as with various affective disorders. They report a significant correlation between IgM levels and better learners, but this may be a reflection of the fact that the latter subjects had better immune capacities than those of the poorer learners.

The problem of determining the target(s) against which NBA may be directed is indeed a formidable one. It has been estimated that the brain contains about 10^{11} neurons (HUBEL 1979; WEISS 1970), and despite certain common structural features, there is a considerably greater diversity of neurons than of the functional cells of other organs. Each neuronal circuit consists of cellular units which distinguish them from the components of other circuits. In the embryonal development of neural circuits, neurons often migrate over great distances. When they reach their definitive locations they generally aggregate with cells of similar kind. This selective aggregation which they exhibit is probably due to specific classes of large surface molecules which serve to "recognize" cells of the same type; these molecules are highly specific for each major type of cell (COWAN 1979).

Neurons also differ in respect to the chemical transmitters which they synthesize and which serve to transmit the electrical signals across the synapse. There are now some 30 different substances definitively identified as transmitters or suspected of serving this function (IVERSEN 1979). In respect to neurons with an endocrine function, there are hormonal peptides which certain neurons share with hormone-producing cells of the gastrointestinal tract and with other endocrine glands. Many neurons also possess hormone receptors which they have in common with cells of certain other organs. And there are enzymes common to almost all cells of the body, as well as some which are neuron specific (SCHMECHEL et al. 1978). In addition, neurons possess a distinctive protein designated 14-3-2 (CICERO et al. 1972), as well as proteins in common with other cells. Among the latter are the cell surface (HLA) antigens and the proteins of the neurotubular-neurofilamentous system.

This brief overview of the diversity of neurons is particularly relevant to certain aspects of aging of the brain, including immune phenomena which may be associated with aging of this organ. From a gross perspective aging appears to have a diffuse uniform effect manifested principally by an evenly distributed weight loss along with a uniform widening of sulci and flattening of gyri. It might be argued that this reflects surface and subsurface changes, and not alterations of deeper brain structures. However, BRODY's (1978) studies show that neuron loss is most marked in certain areas of the cortex, but is not uniform throughout the cortex. Other nonuniform changes associated with aging include lipofuscin accumulation (BRIZZEE et al. 1974), and the formation of neurofibrillary tangles and senile plaques. Even quantitative changes in 14-3-2 protein associated with aging have a regionally selective distribution pattern (CICERO et al. 1972). Our studies thus far in respect to NBA also appear to show a nonuniform distribution pattern, although it remains to be determined whether or not the latter conforms to the distribution of any of the other aging changes.

E. A Consideration of Immune Privilege

Such terms as "autonomous," "protected," and "privileged" have been applied to the unique status of the brain. Such terms are intended to express the fact that the brain is provided with privileges not "enjoyed" by other organs which, in a teleonomic sense, perhaps serve to protect the vital centers and homeostatic regulators critical to the maintenance of life. There are several well-known categories of this privileged status. While the brain constitutes only about 2% of total body weight, oxygen consumption of the brain represents 20%–25% of total body consumption. Moreover, there is an adaptive mechanism by which blood is shunted to the brain under conditions of oxygen deprivation. There is also a mechanism by which the brain is protected under conditions of starvation. As Ho et al. (1980) have noted, the weight of the brain changes only slightly despite wide fluctuations in body weight between emaciation and obesity. A third category is that of immunological privilege. Tissues and organs possessing such privilege are shielded from attack by the immune system.

The evidence usually offered in support of immune privilege for the brain is that allografts transplanted to it do not evoke a rejection reaction and therefore flourish. However, such privilege may be relative rather than absolute since GEYER and GILL (1979) have been able to elicit an immune response to skin transplanted into the brain of inbred rats "across different genetic disparities in the major histocompatibility complex," although intracerebral sensitization required at least two grafts, indicating an antigenic dose requirement. At any rate, the mechanism often invoked is that the blood-brain-barrier (BBB) provides this protection, although the absence of lympatic drainage has also been proposed (BARKER and BILLINGHAM 1977).

BEHAN and BEHAN (1979) reiterate what probably remains prevalent opinion regarding the nature of the immunological privilege of the brain as follows: "Immune processes within the CNS are modified by the BBB, which restricts the entry of antibody and antigen. The CNS has few indigenous lymphocytes and no lymphoid structures. However, inflammation of the CNS will allow access to it of the components which mediate both humoral and cellular responses." Nevertheless, they also note that in certain neurological disorders "antibodies are produced by lymphoid cells within the CNS itself."

NANDY (1972) evidently accepts this concept of the mechanism by which immune privilege is maintained, but proposes that the BBB progressively weakens with age, thus permitting NBA in serum to reach neurons. However, there is, as yet, no direct evidence for such an aging-related weakening (MILLER and BLUMENTHAL 1978); nor would it account for in vivo Ig-binding by neurons in patients under age 30. His hypothesis that NBA may be responsible for the aging-related loss of neurons also does not take into account that a cytolytic antibody is most likely to be of the IgM class, particularly since his studies have not analyzed the Ig classes of the serum-binding antibody. IgM is present in serum as a pentamer – 5 identical units jointed together by disulphide linkeages; it is considerably larger than IgG or IgA with a molecular weight of 900,000 Daltons, and it cannot cross the placenta whereas IgG can. One therefore has to account for the fact that in both the study on ataxia-telangiectasia (KAUFMAN and MILLER 1977) and in the data presented here IgM appears to be the principal antibody which binds to neuronal cytoplasm.

There is, however, evidence that the CNS may possess an immune compartment which may function independent of the systemic immune system. It has been proposed that the system of cerebrospinal canals may be analogous to the systemic lymphatic system, and the cerebrospinal fluid analogous to lymph (Editorial 1975). On the other hand PRINEAS (1979) presents evidence that "the thin-walled channels observed in perivascular spaces of unaffected CNS tissue" are indistinguishable from lymphatic capillaries in other tissues "in terms of both their structure and content," and he cites studies which support the view that these spaces serve to same function in the CNS as lymphatic vessels serve in other tissues." PRINEAS concludes: "... it is not unreasonable to view the presence of lymphocyte containing channels in the perivascular spaces in the CNS as evidence that lymphocytes normally circulate through these channels, possibly in the same manner and in the same numbers as lymphocytes circulate in other tissues, and that this may constitute the basis of immunological surveillance in the CNS."

Others (BLUMENTHAL 1976; OEHMICHEN 1978) have also proposed that the CNS may have elements of an independent immune compartment. In his review of the evidence supporting such a concept, BLUMENTHAL cites evidence that the CNS is capable of mounting both a primary and secondary immune response, as well as a capacity for independent Ig synthesis. He also cites reports that lymphomas develop exclusively or predominantly within the CNS in patients receiving immunosuppressive drugs, and this supports the view that there may be cells with lymphoid characteristics indigenous to the CNS which may undergo malignant transformation.

OEHMICHEN (1978) designates four sites in the CNS which may provide cells with a capacity for developing into mononuclear phagocytes; some of the same sites might also provide lymphoid cells. These include "progressive microglia," perivascular cells of intracerebral vessels, free subarachnoid cells, and epiplexus cells. Perivascular cells are also usually associated with vascular amyloid limited to the brain (BLUMENTHAL 1976), suggesting that such cells may be stem cells capable of differentiation into lymphocytes and synthesizing the Igs in amyloid.

The concept of an independent CNS immune compartment does not exclude a role for the BBB. We have emphasized here the potential for antibodies which may cross-react with neuronal elements, including antibodies against microorganisms, peptide hormones, enzymes, structural cell proteins, and cell surface antigens such as the Thy-1 antigen, which both neurons and glial cells share with T-lymphocytes (CAMPBELL et al. 1979). The BBB may serve to shield the CNS from such potentially damaging cross-reactivity. On the other hand, there may be antigenic changes such as those deriving from aging-related somatic mutations within the nervous system to which the systemic immune system would not have access. Teleonomically, a separate immunological compartment within the CNS would be immunologically poised to react to such antigenic changes. In the final analysis, therefore, it may be that the immunological privilege of the CNS resides as much in its possession of a separate immune compartment as in its exclusion from the systemic immune system.

F. Conclusion

As with immune phenomena associated with aging and disease of some other organs, there are antibodies to neuronal structures which appear to be associated with both aging and certain neurological diseases. In this chapter we have dealt particularly with Igs which bind to neuronal cytoplasm (NBA), and in an in vivo context we have demonstrated that they are at least of three classes, IgM, G, and A.

There is a parallel which can be drawn between NBA and islet cell antibody (ICA). Both bind to cytoplasm, and although ICA has been linked with insulin-dependent diabetes, it binds to all types of islet cells, while NBA appears to bind to all types of neurons. There are cases in which ICA fixes complement; and others in which it does not, and the same probably holds for NBA. ICA is also present in a small percent of apparently normal subjects (Doniach and Bottazzo 1977), although data on the age distribution in the latter have not been published. In vivo studies on ICA comparable to those discussed here have also not yet been reported.

Although it is common in respect to aging to find two or more autoantibodies in the same subject, even in the absence of associated disease, studies have not yet been carried out to determine the concomitancy of other antibodies which may be associated with NBA. At any rate, it appears likely that in some instances NBA may be associated with aging in the absence of CNS disease and in other instances disease may be present. A particularly confounding problem in respect to NBA is the possibility that many antibodies targeted primarily at other moieties have at least a potential for cross-reacting with neuronal constituents.

Also discussed here is the possibility that different classes of Igs may have different effects. IgM, particularly if complement is fixed with it, may be cytolytic, while IgG may be protective. It also appears that there may be an association between senile plaque formation and IgG-binding to neurons.

Finally, we have also discussed the so-called immune privilege of the brain usually attributed to the BBB, as well as the possibility that the CNS may have an independent immune compartment. It has been proposed that the BBB may serve to shield the brain from potentially cross-reacting antibodies; if so, it would explain the differences observed here between in vitro and in vivo binding. On the other hand, an independent immune compartment would be poised to react to antigens restricted to the brain which could not traverse the BBB in the other direction. The latter would be particularly relevant to aging since it would apply to aging-related misspecification of proteins of the CNS.

Acknowledgments. We are grateful for the technical assistance of Pearl N. Baum, and H. T. Briggs.

References

Allerand CD, Yahr MD (1964) Gamma-globulin for normal human tissue of the central nervous system. Science 144:1141–1142
Asbury AE, Lisak RP (1980) Demyelinative neuropathy and myelin antibodies. New Engl J Med 303:638:639
Barker CF, Billingham RE (1977) Immunologically privileged sites. Adv Immunol 25:1–54
Behan PO, Behan WMH (1979) Possible immunological factors in Alzheimer's disease. In: Glen AIM, Whalley LJ (eds) Alzheimer's disease. Early recognition of potentially reversible deficits. Churchill Livingstone, Edinburgh London New York, pp 33–35

Behan PO, Currie S (1978) Clinical neuroimmunology. WB Saunders Co Ltd, Philadelphia London Toronto

Blumenthal HT (1976) Immunological aspects of the aging brain. In: Terry RD, Gershon S (eds) Neurobiology of aging. Raven Press, New York, pp 313–334

Blumenthal HT (1978) Aging: Biologic or pathologic? Hospital Practice 13:127–137

Blumenthal HT (ed) (in press 1982) Handbook of diseases of aging. Van Nostrand Reinhold, New York

Blumenthal HT, Berns AW (1964) Autoimmunity in aging. In: Strehler BL (ed) Advances in gerontology research, vol 1. Academic Press, New York, pp 289–342

Brizzee KR, Ordy JM, Kaack B (1974) Early appearance and regional differences in intraneuronal and extraneuronal lipofuscin accumulation with age in the brain of a nonhuman primate (Macaca mullata). J Gerontol 29:366–381

Brody H (1978) Cell counts in cerebral cortex and brainstem. In: Katzman R, Terry RD, Bick KL (eds) Alzheimer's disease. Senile dementia and related disorders (Aging vol 7). Raven Press, New York, pp 11–14

Campbell DG, Williams AF, Bayley FM, Reid KBM (1979) Structural similarities between Thy-1 antigen from rat brain and immunoglobulin. Nature 282:341–342

Cassidy JT, Nordby GL, Dodge HJ (1974) Biologic variation of human serum immunoglobulin concentrations: Sex-age specific effects. J Chron Dis 27:507–518

Chaffee J, Hervat N, Robin S (1978) Cytotoxic autoantibody to brain. In: Nandy K (ed) Senile dementia: A biomedical approach. Elsevier/North Holland, Amsterdam, pp 61–72

Cicero TJ, Ferrendelle JA, Suntzeff V, Moore BW (1972) Regional changes in CNS levels in S-100 and 14-3-2 proteins during development and aging in the mouse. J Neurochem 19:2119–2125

Cowan WM (1979) The development of the brain. Sci Am 241:112–133

D'Angelo C, D'Angelo DB (1975) Possibility of an autoimmune pathogenesis of some histologic alterations, characteristics in presenile and senile dementia. In: Környey ST, Tariska St, Gosztonyi G (eds) Proc VII th Internat Congr Neuropath, vol II. Excerpta Medica, Amsterdam Oxford, pp 131–134

Diedericksen H, Pyndt IC (1968) Antibodies against neurons in patients with systemic lupus erythematosus, cerebral palsy and epilepsy. Brain 93:402–412

Doniach D, Bottazzo GF (1977) Autoimmunity and the endocrine pancreas. In: Ioachim HL (ed) Pathobiology annual. Appleton-Century-Crofts, New York, pp 327–346

Eddington TS, Delassio DJ (1970) The assessment of immunofluorescence methods of humoral and antimyelin antibodies in man. J Immunol 105:248–255

Editorial (1975) Cerebrospinal fluid: The lymph of brain? Lancet 2:444–445

Eisdorfer C, Cohen D, Buckley CE III (1978) Serum immunoglobulins and cognition in the impaired elderly. In: Katzman R, Terry RD, Bick KL (eds) Alzheimer's disease and related disorders (Aging vol 7). Raven Press, New York, pp 401–407

Feden G, Baldinger A, Miller-Soule D, Blumenthal HT (1979) An in vivo and in vitro study of an aging-related neuron cytoplasmic binding antibody in male Fischer rats. J Gerontol 34:651–660

Felsenfeld G, Wolf RF (1972) Relationship of age and serum immunoglobulins to autoantibodies against brain constituents in primates. I. A study in apparently healthy man, Macaca mullata and Erythrocebus pates. J Med Primatol 1:287–296

Field EJ, Caspary EA (1970) Lymphocyte sensitization: An in vitro test for cancer? Lancet 2:1337–1341

Field EJ, Caspary EA, Ball EJ (1963) Some biological properties of a highly active encephalitogenic factor isolated from human brain. Lancet 2:11–13

Geyer SJ, Gill TU III (1979) Immunogenetic aspects of intracerebral skin transplantation in inbred rats. Am J Path 94:569–584

Heath RG, Krupp IM (1967) The biological basis of schizophrenia. An autoimmune concept. In: Walaas O (ed) Molecular basis of some aspects of mental activity. Academic Press, New York, pp 313–344

Hellstrom KE (1970) Discussion in „Routes of escape from surveillance." In: Smith RT, Landry M (eds) Immune surveillance. Academic Press, New York, pp 506–507

Ho K, Roessmann U, Straumfjord JV (1980) Analysis of brain weight. I. Adult brain weight in relation to sex, race and age. II. Adult brain weight in relation to body height, weight and surface area. Arch Path Lab Med 104:635–645

Holborow EJ (1973) An ABC of modern immunology. Little Brown and Co, Boston

Hubel D (1979) The brain. Sci Am 241:44–53

Husby C, Riji IVE, Zabriskie JB, Abdin KM, Williams RC (1976) Antibodies reacting with cytoplasm of subthalamic and caudate nuclei neurons in chorea and acute rheumatic fever. J Exp Med 144:1094–1110

Ingram CR, Phegan KJ, Blumenthal HT (1974) Significance of an aging-linked neuron binding gamma globulin fraction of human sera. J Gerontol 29:20–27

Iversen LL (1979) The chemistry of the brain. Sci Am 241:134–149

Kalter S, Kelly S (1975) Alzheimers disease: Evaluation of immunologic indices. NY State J Med 75:1220–1225

Kaufman DB, Miller HC (1977) Ataxia telangiectasia: An autoimmune disease associated with a cytotoxic antibody to brain and thymus. Clin Immunol and Immunopath 7:288–299

Kolyaskina GI, Kushner SG (1969) Principles governing appearance of anti-brain antibodies in serum of schizophrenics. Neuropath Psychiatr (USSR) 69:1679–1682

Lennon VA (1976) Immunology of acetylcholine receptors. Immunol Commun 5:323–344

Levin JM, Boshes LD (1969) Autoimmunity and the central nervous system. Dis Nerv Syst 30:273–279

Lewin R (1981) Research news. Myasthenia gravis under monoclonal scrutiny. Science 211:38–42

Mackay IR, Whittingham SF, Mathews JD (1977) The immunoepidemiology of aging. In: Makinodan T, Yunis E (eds) Immunology and aging. Plenum Med Books Co, New York, pp 35–50

Martin I, Herr JC, Wanamaker BAW, Kornguth (1974) Demonstration of specific antineuronal nuclear antibody in sera of patients with myasthenia gravis. Indirect and direct immunofluorescence. Neurology 24:680–684

Mayer PP, Chughtai MA, Cape RDT (1976) An immunological approach to dementia in the elderly. Age Ageing 5:164–170

Miller DT, Blumenthal HT (1978) Neuron-thymic lymphocyte binding of serum IgG of 90- and 500-day-old female Wistar albino rats. J Gerontol 33:129–136

Motyka A, Jezkova A (1975) Autoantibodies and brain ischemia topography. Cas Lek Ces 114:1455–1457

Nandy K (1972) Neuronal degeneration in aging and after experimental injury. Exp Gerontol 7:303–311

Nandy K (1977) Immune reactions in aging brain and senile dementia. In: Nandy K, Sherwin I (eds) The aging brain and senile dementia. Plenum Press, New York, pp 181–196

Nandy K (1978) Brain-reactive antibodies in aging and senile ementia. In: Katzman R, Terry RD, Bick KL (eds) Alzheimers disease and related disorders (Aging, vol 7). Raven Press, New York, pp 401–407

Oehmichen M (1978) Mononuclear phagocytes in the central nervous system. Springer-Verlag, Berlin Heidelberg New York

Orgel LE (1963) The maintenance of the accuracy of protein synthesis and its relevance to aging. Proc Natl Acad Sci USA 49:517–521

Prineas JW (1979) Multiple sclerosis: Presence of lymphatic capillaries and lymphoid tissue in the brain and spinal cord. Science 203:1123–1125

Radl J, Sepers JM, Skvarii P, Morell A, Hijmans W (1975) Immunoglobulin patterns in humans over 95 years of age. Clin Exp Immunol 22:84–90

Rapport MM, Karpiak SE (1978) Immunological perturbation of neurological functions. In: Nandy K (ed) Senile dementia: A biomedical approach. Elsevier/North Holland Biomed Press, New York, pp 73–88

Savenko SN, Polienko EM (1975) Autoimmune factors in cerebral circulatory disorders. Zh Neuropatol Psikhiat V 75:3–7

Schmechel D, Marangos PJ, Zis AP, Brightman M, Goodwin PK (1978) Brain enolases as specific markers of neuronal and glial cells. Science 199:313–315

Skalickova O, Jezkova Z, Slavickova V (1962) Immunological aspects of psychiatric gerontology. Rev Czech Medicine 8:264–275
Solomon DH, Kleeman KE (1977) Concepts of pathogenesis of Graves' disease. Adv Internal Med 22:273–299
Sotelo J, Gibbs CJ Jr, Gajdusek DC (1980) Autoantibodies against axonal neurofilaments in patients with kuru and Creutzfeldt-Jakob disease. Science 210:190–193
Threatt J, Nandy K, Fritz R (1971) Brain reactive antibodies in serum of old mice demonstrated by immunofluorescence. J Gerontol 26:316–323
Walford RL (1970) Discussion in „Routes of escape from surveillance." In: Smith RT, Landry M (eds) Immune surveillance. Academic Press, New York, pp 277–278
Weiss PA (1970) Whither life science? Am Sci 58:156–163
Whitaker JM, Engel WK (1974) A search for antibodies in the serum of patients with myasthenia gravis. Neurology 24:61
Whittingham S, Lennon V, Mackay IR, Davies GV, Davies B (1970) Absence of brain antibodies in senile dementia. Brit J Psychiatry 116:447–448
Zeromski J (1970) Immunological findings in sensory carcinomatous neuropathy. Application of peroxidase labelled antibody. Clin Exp Immunol 6:633–637

Senile Dementia

H.H. Wieck†, J.U. Brückmann, C. Lang, and L. Blaha

A. Etymology, Historical, and Contemporary Use of the Term "Senile Dementia"

The interest in what is called senile dementia (SD) has risen in the past decades for different reasons: Progress in neurochemistry, clinical psychology, psychometry, geriatrics, and noninvasive technology for the morphological assessment of the brain has opened new insights; traditional views and classifications have become more and more insufficient facing this new material; and an ever-increasing longevity has meant a larger proportion of the population are struck with age-correlated diseases.

I. Historical Understanding

During Roman antiquity "de-mentia" marked a state of not having all one's wits about one and of lack of good sense, which if it started during old age was called "dementia senilis." A current view was that the process of aging was pathological in itself (Cicero: "Senectus ipsa morbus est," cited according to Burstein 1946) and in terms of humoral pathology due to a cooling down of the brain. Up to now the discussion is still great as to whether the process of aging in itself is a disease and SD only an acceleration and accentuation of it (Pick 1958) or whether the view of an only age-correlated disease which is by no means an inevitable consequence of a sufficiently long life comes closer to reality, a view, that meanwhile is unanimously favored (Lauter and Meyer 1968; Kral 1972; Miller 1974).

A division between SD and normal aging had already been postulated by Esquirol (1827), who characterized the "confusion of the elderly" as a mental disease taking its course without crisis and having an infaust prognosis. While during most of the nineteenth century the summing up of all mental disorders manifesting themselves during senium and showing a progressive intellectual or personality depravation as SD or senile psychosis was common (Fürstner 1889), Griesinger (1876) was one of the first to differentiate between sundry forms of underlying cerebral diseases when he in his book *Pathologie und Therapie der psychischen Krankheiten* under the heading „Der apathische Blödsinn" (the apathetic imbecility) wrote: „In der hier geschilderten extremen Weise endigt sowohl die senile Gei-

The commission to take part in this book originally was addressed to our joint teacher H.H. Wieck. After his sudden and untimely death, his former pupils indebted to the ideas he developed, have tried to complete this article in his sense.

stesschwäche, als manche ihr sehr analoge Zustände in früheren Lebensaltern, welche auch auf Gehirnatrophie, zum Theil mit Arteriendegeneration, zum Theil ohne solche beruhen." But it was left to ALZHEIMER to show senile plaques and neurofibrillary tangles (1907) to be the histopathological substrate of primary brain atrophy in adult life. This allowed him to make a distinction between the then dominating three forms of dementia, senile, arteriosclerotic, and luetic, on a histological basis. KRAEPELIN later on (1910) in honour of its discoverer argued in favor of a dichotomy into a presenile (MA) and senile (SD) form although already CLOUSTON (1884) had voted against an age mark as a constituting sign of the disease. Efforts of the following years were directed toward search for an etiologically or histopathologically well-defined nosological entity on the one hand, and for a clinically useful syndrome on the other hand.

This latter branch of efforts was mainly descriptive and initiated – among others – by MAUDSLEY (1868), who divided "chronic insanity" into three groups characterized by delusion, incoherence, and almost complete extinction of mind – the dementia sensu strictiori.

At the turn of the century there was consensus on at least two forms, one rather benign and marked by lack of initiative, mnemonic disturbances, and confusion – dementia senilis simplex – and a rather malignant form with loss of memory, increase of initiative, fear, depression, and delusion. Some contemporary authors adhere to this classification (HOFF 1956; HAASE 1971; HUBER 1976). Even the ninth revision of the international classification of diseases (ICD) distinguishes between simple, depressive, paranoid, and confusional dementia. Others widened the spectrum by adding abulic, alogical, aggressive, euphoric, dysphoric, affective incontinent, structural, logorrheic, amnesic, confabulatory, and delirious dementias (ALSEN 1981).

One variety extracted from the simplex type of SD by WERNICKE and KAHLBAUM has found wide acceptance and application: The presbyophrenic dementia or presbyophreny was defined as a serene and friendly variety of SD not affecting the primary personality or only slightly (FISCHER 1910, 1912; GRÜNTHAL 1936; HUGHES 1959). This clinical cross-sectional splitting is legitimate as long as it does not presume to indicate a specific pathomorphological substrate, to permit a valid prognosis, or to constitute nosological entities (ALEXANDROWSKAYA 1965). MIGNOT (1950) and WELLS (1971) pointed out that subdivisions of this kind are nothing but a typology and even by further subdivision can hardly do justice to a possible continuum of atrophying dementias.

Nevertheless serious investigation is necessary whether the dementia defined by the criteria of ALZHEIMER does not constitute a whole group of dementias of manifold etiology and pathogenetic mechanisms (ZWANGWILL 1964; BERGENER 1980).

On the other hand diagnostic lumping by combining an abundance of heterogenous and etiopathogenetically different elements into a nonspecific "diagnostic lumber-room" (LIEPMANN 1915) or "diagnostic waste-basket" (EASTMAN 1978) has its own risks at least as long as together with differential diagnosis differential therapy remains undone.

Scientifically, both procedures – the minute subdivision as well as the unscrupulous expansion – are equally doubtful when, as is the case with SD in default of a clearly outlined etiology, we are forced to operate on a syndromic level. The advantage of a restrictive definition, the reduction of heterogeneity of the term dementia, is counterbalanced by a reduction of precision within the category constituted by the higher term (TODOROV et al. 1975). One can understand why LEWIS (1946), cited according to ALEXANDER (1972) complained bitterly about the terminological status quo.

II. Contemporary Understanding

A superior possibility of reducing heterogeneity and of bringing into accordance symptomatology and pathology of SD is given by consideration of diachronia since it has long been known that chronological criteria such as speed of manifestation and course can be of considerable diagnostic and prognostic value. This knowledge had already been applied by LEVERT (1907) when he differentiated between acute and chronic, and reversible and irreversible dementias. An as yet unsolved ambiguity rose by use of the term dementia independently of its *Verlaufsgestalt*, i.e., its reversibility. WEITBRECHT (1962), BERGERON and HANUS (1964), BERGENER (1969), BOWER (1971), WELLS (1977), FOERSTER and REGLI (1980), and LAUTER (1980) are advocates of a cross-sectional definition of dementia and therefore speak of reversible and irreversible dementias while other authors – whom we join – reserve the term dementia for irreversible courses (BLEULER 1915; ROTHSCHILD 1941; SCHNEIDER 1966). Since the question of reversibility is tightly bound to therapeutic progress, it is understandable that, for example, STENGEL (1964b) argued only unsuccessfully treated cases of progressive palsy are dementias, and FOERSTER and REGLI (1980) returned to a pragmatically oriented classification of dementing syndromes in:
1. Dementia with (still) unknown etiology
2. Dementia with unknown and not yet treatable etiology
3. Dementia with known and treatable etiology.

It is clear from what was said that the last group cannot be regarded as dementia in our opinion. But it is indisputable that in severe organic damage of the CNS, a point of no return can be reached after which even without further continuation of the causal noxa a complete recovery is impossible. According to the theory developed by WIECK, substantial damage to the structural metabolism can at best be compensated for and leads to a defect syndrome *(Defektsyndrom)*, whereas a disorder of the functional metabolism leads to a fully reversible syndrome, the function psychosis *(Funktionspsychose)*. Both forms are unspecific with regard to etiology as BONHOEFFER (1917) pointed out: "There are typical psychic reaction patterns rather independent of special kinds of noxious agents."

That these considerations are shared by a number of other authors, even if they do not adhere to our nomenclature, is documented by terms like "irreversible organic mental disintegration syndrome" (HUBER 1962, 1980), "coarse organic mental syndrome with structural damage" (BERZEWSKI and SELBACH 1970), "intrinsic chronic late-onset severe brain failure" (ISAACS and CAIRD 1976), or "chronic organic brain syndrome" (KAY 1970; KENT 1977) in denominating SD. Other unspecified terms like "senile psychosis" (see above), "brain failure" (LIVESLEY 1976; LANGLEY 1977; ROBINSON 1977), and "organic brain syndrome" – related to the

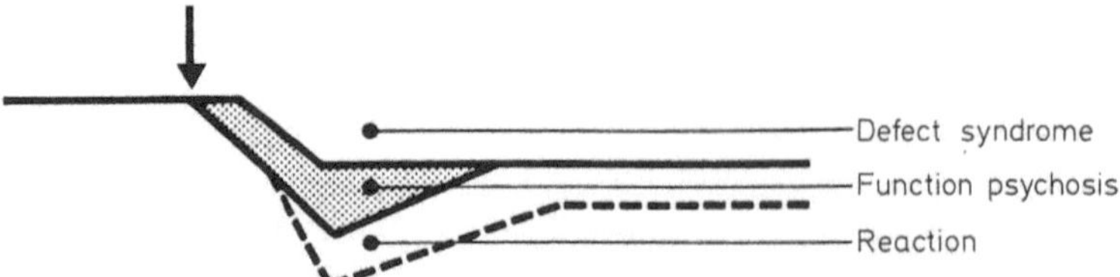

Fig. 1. Function psychosis, defect syndrome, and psychic reaction can combine to a complex symptomatology leading to persistent mental deterioration; →, onset of organic brain disease

"organic syndrome" by Bleuler (1975) – are in our opinion and also in that of others (Kolk 1978) useless in this context.

These considerations may explain the division of "organic psychoses" *(körperlich begründbare Psychosen)* (Schneider 1966) into "function psychoses" and "defect syndromes" (Wieck 1956, 1962, 1972, 1980a) which was recently restated by Kinzel (1972, 1979) and Lungershausen (1980). Naturally both forms, together with psychic reactions to these organic disorders, can combine to a more complex symptomatology, sometimes leading to rapid mental decline and episodes of partial recuperation (Fig. 1).

At this point the question rises whether the criterion of irreversibility is sufficient or whether only progressive courses should be called dementias. Spatz (1938) and later Huber (1972) have already proposed a distinction between stationary and progressive syndromes in connection with brain disease. Kinzel (1973) consequently established a "process syndrome" *(Prozeßsyndrom)* when he dealt with Pick's syndrome.

While to our present knowledge there is agreement about intellectual deficits in SD, consensus is lacking with regard to the symptomatological range. Gruhle (1956), Huber (1976), and Alsen (1980) would like to have disorders of personality and judgment separated from dementia, which they see as predominantly a disorder of memory, perception, and intelligence, because in their opinion there is no firm correlation between the two phenomena. In contrast we would like to include both under the term SD, since isolated personality disorders mostly occur at the beginning of the process when they escape attention of relatives and can be grasped only retrospectively. But because personality changes are obligatory for the advanced stages of SD, we keep to Lauter's definition of "all severe forms of cognitive incapacitation *and* organic personality changes."

III. Own Definition

Summarizing, we speak of SD if there is a progressive syndrome characterized by personality changes (behavioral functions), decrease of intellect (higher cognitive functions), and memory (mnestic functions) which manifests itself during senium. Morphological substrate is a widespread predominantly symmetrical and cortical brain atrophy. All reversible syndromes that are transversely similar do not belong here (Scheid 1962). This definition is conscientiously restrictive and is intended to make discussion and research in the field of gerontopsychiatry more precise and homogeneous, hoping that one day SD might be defined as part or group of (a) clinically and neuropathologically clearly outlined nosological entity(ies).

In the following we refer to this definition. With regard to the contents we essentially follow numerous original contributions, reviews, and proceedings of the last 2 decades, especially those of ALLISON (1962), MÜLLER and CIOMPI (1968), WOLSTENHOLME and O'CONNOR (1970), WELLS (1971), LAUTER (1972), CIOMPI (1972), PEARCE and MILLER (1973), MILLER (1977), NANDY and SHERWIN (1977), SMITH and KINSBOURNE (1977), KATZMAN et al. (1978a), NANDY (1978), TORACK (1978), KAPLAN (1979), and BERGENER (1980).

B. Clinical Semeiology

I. Psychopathology and Course of Senile Dementia

SD means a progressive deficit of personality, memory, and intelligence acquired during senium (KINZEL et al. 1979; SCHNEIDER 1966). However, its limits are not clearly defined. As to the age, the 7th decade is commonly accepted. But we do not have a commonly accepted definition of intelligence and its supporting structures. "The whole of thinking structures and thinking acts and their application to the practical and theoretical tasks of life" (SCHNEIDER 1966) serves us as a preliminary agreement. Practically, intelligence is a construct of what is demanded in the test applied (KAPLAN 1979). Memory and perception actually are not necessarily parts of the intelligence construct (SCHNEIDER 1966; JASPERS 1973) but are important as to the results if we want to quantify intelligence as a performance. Additionally, clinical experience shows that in diseases leading to dementia, memory and perception as psychic functions are implied early (BRÜCKMANN 1980).

The deterioration of mind and personality as the other component of SD results in an accentuation of preexisting characteristics and at the same time in a decline of distinguished "higher" properties of the individual. There is a narrowing of feelings, poverty of affective modulation, up to a loss of appropriate behavior and compassionate feelings. So-called more subtle ethical emotions in general are lacking. Here it shows that actually deterioration of personality is closely connected with intellectual deterioration. Still one or the other component can be pronounced in a single case, eventually depending on an accentuated affection of white or gray matter (HUBER 1962; PEREZ et al. 1975; FEIGENSON 1978).

The deterioration of power of judgment as the core symptom of dementia (SCHNEIDER 1966) not only refers to logical thinking and judging but also to the ability of a higher judgment and the ability to criticize and judge one's self (PAULEIKHOFF in WEITBRECHT 1962). SCHELLER (1965) calls this a decline of the person in being *(Abbau des Person-Seins)*, a loss of self-presentment, and ZUTT (1964) calls this a loss of reflexion ability.

The increasing intellectual decline begins with light memory losses, which not only present as "forgetting" details or actions of the actual day. The Gestalt psychological view implies the entire conscious mind *(Erleben)* with the consequence of a progressing "destructurization of the pattern of present mind" *(Entstaltung des aktuellen Erlebensfeldes)* (CONRAD 1947a, b). The availability of single elements in a mind primarily rich in patterns, with the possibility of a permanent gestalt relation to the mind's traces, narrows. As long as life goes on in habitual ways, judging ability stays intact for a long time. New ways, if possible, are avoided. Otherwise, through deteriorated possibilities of perception and processing, a lack of adaptiveness and the tendency to keep old patterns of reaction appear. In the terminology by CATTELL (1963) this process would act upon the "fluid intelligence", what SAVAGE (1977) in his reflexions about cognitive functioning calls "learning ability." This would primarily affect the ultra-short- and short-term memory. Memory is especially important in cognition deficits in general besides orientation, attention, and abstraction (McHUGH and FOLSTEIN 1979). AJURIAGUERRA et al. (1979) have developed a concept of disintegration of imagination in senile dementia in analogy to PIAGET's developmental psychology of the child.

They postulate a disturbance of anticipation of the course of an eventment rather than that of moving objects or static states. The clinical course of senile dementia is marked by continuous progression. First there is an uncharacteristic picture with an increase in irritability, emotional lability, sadness, lack of concentration, and functional paresthesias. HUBER (1980) has named this a "pseudoneurasthenic syndrome." Only later is a correct diagnosis possible. In verifying cognitive disturbances by psychopathometric methods, a psychosis of somatic origin becomes probable.

When the "core symptoms" (PFEIFFER 1978) appear, the actual dementing disease begins: Disorientation, disturbance of the short-term memory, disturbed memory of spatial relations, disturbed time lattice, decreased possibilities in performing a number of cognitive tasks, and finally also a disturbance of the long-term memory. Facultative symptoms can hide the actual disease. They represent the attempt of the individual to cope with the disease. There are depressive moods, paranoid disorders, increase in timidity up to panic states, and bursts of aggression. A denial of the disease, confabulations, avoidance behavior, negativism, perseverations, and distraction maneuvers, according to PFEIFFER (1978) and WEINSTEIN and KAHN (1955), indicate a process under way for at least 1 year. By this time the core symptoms dominate more and more, so that the correct diagnosis is obvious. Disorientation as to time and place are observed, family members are not recognized, and aphasic symptoms occur. The so-called *Werkzeugstörungen* are characteristic for advanced SD and therefore are presented as a whole in this paper. FEIGENSON (1978) empasizes that neuropsychological disturbances can appear in the early stages and sometimes are misinterpreted as exclusive cognitive-intellectual losses.

During the final states of the disease the handling of fire, gas, electricity, and the disorientation lead to self-endangerment by the patient. The treating physician and the relatives will then have to urge the patient to undergo treatment in a hospital. Sometimes forensic steps are necessary. They diverge in different countries, so we do not enlarge on this point here. Under further progress of the disease, the patient not only loses his intellectual but also his physiological adaptability.

Control of bowel and bladder diminishes together with motoric control of intended movements. Feebleness increases and bronchopneumonia usually leads to death.

This state of total dementia has been described by HUGHLINGS JACKSON (1834–1911) (in TORACK 1978): "Here the negative mental affection is greatest, is indeed total; there is dementia. There are no positive symptoms; there is no mind or consciousness ... In this depth there is no person but only a living creature."

II. Neuropsychology

Focal symptoms in the form of neuropsychological disorders or *Werkzeugstörungen* are an important part of the semeiology of SD. During the 4 years after ALZHEIMER (1907) had made his famous observations, 13 more cases were communicated of whom nine had an aphasia, eight an apraxia, five an agnosia, and four cerebral fits. SJÖGREN et al. (1952) in their investigation of MA found anomia in 100%, sensory aphasia in 83%, alexia in 77%, and perseveration in almost every case; LAUTER and MAYER (1968) reported on *Werkzeugstörungen* in 85% of their senile demented patients.

While this symptomatology was regarded as an essential part of at least the advanced stages of SD (KRAEPELIN 1910; BERTELSEN and WIMMER 1919; ALBERT 1964a; JACOB 1969; McDONALD 1969), some authors in the presence of focal disorders spoke of "Alzheimerization" (LAUTER 1972) or SDAT while in their absence they used the term "pure" or "simplex" SD.

As a rule during the course of SD, psychiatric symptoms precede the neuropsychological and neurological symptoms with a wide range of overlapping (ALBERT 1964a). Neuropsychological signs in the initial stage of SD or MA are rare (WECHSLER 1977). There is a similar hierarchy within neuropsychological disorders: Although, for instance, the language dissolution process of course is no true return to child language (TRUEBLOOD 1935) a "retrogenetic," "retroevolutive," or "devolutive" (TORACK 1978) line can be observed, during which ontogenetic earlier organizational levels as well as primitive and physiologically disappeared behavioral patterns come forth. This devolution is partial only, has its own quality, and is different from the normal senile involution. Furthermore stereotype and novel functional disorders arise.

More often than not the vagueness of the focal disorders is pointed out. This has to be explained by the diffuseness of the underlying brain atrophy and by the interaction of some of the "classical" neuropsychological syndromes – aphasic-agnosic-apraxic or AAA syndrome according to BERGENER 1980 – as well as by the cross-linking with psychiatric and subcortical disorders.

This makes categorization difficult. CRITCHLEY (1964), in attempting to do justice to the combination of thought and language disorders in dementing processes, proposed the term "dyslogia" instead of "dysphasia." It is evident that the separate treatise of different forms of neuropsychological disorders is done on account of clearness and better orientation and not to stress their peculiarity.

For a synopsis of neuropsychological symptomatology in four stages we advise the reader to consult AJURIAGUERRA et al. (1963).

1. Aphasia, Agraphia, and Alexia

Language disturbances are a very striking feature of SD and because they are relatively easy to register and quantify are used as an indicator of dementing incapacitation. The earliest observations of aphasia in SD were reported by WILLE (1873), GÜNTZ (1874), PICK (1892), and HEILBRONNER (1900). All four of them emphasized the existence of perseverations, echo, and iterative phenomena in contrast to vascular aphasias. Almost regularly anomia (amnestic aphasia) is to be found, which because of the preceding memory disturbances bears its name with peculiar justification. Vocabulary becomes impoverished, word finding difficulties arise, which are more common in propositional speech than in confrontation naming (BENSON 1979), the performance in synonym and antonym tests worsens (ACKELSBERG 1944), and categorizing and category-bound association are disturbed (STENGEL 1964b; IRIGARAY and DUBOIS 1966; BENSON 1979). In a task requiring the naming of unfamiliar objects without demonstration of object use, senile demented patients are easily separated from healthy elderly people if not only from the raw score of mistakes but also from the reaction times (LAWSON and BARKER 1968).

Iterative phenomena, such as verbigeration, palilalia, logoclonia (TISSOT et al. 1967), periphrastic sentences, and verbal paraphasias make the speech sound empty and vain. Even if the patient succeeds in approaching a preconceived semantic concept, the paraphasias seem to be improvised, a fact that was interpreted in terms of lack of speech and error consciousness and intellectual impairment (STENGEL 1964a, b). These improvisations have something in common with those in disorders of consciousness or in endogenous psychotic states. Semantic connections are more and more replaced by superficial associations; and assonance, clichés, and neologisms abound.

For the lexical disturbances it is characteristic that especially auxiliary verbs and verbs, pronouns, and conjunctions prevail while the frequency of proper names, nouns, and adjectives diminishes (FELDMAN and CAMERON 1944/45; FERRARO 1967; IRIGARAY 1973). From a statistical point of view rare words are used even more infrequently; at the same time frequent words are preferred. The language modalities are affected differently insofar as spontaneous speech vocabulary suffers more than writing vocabulary and this more than reading vocabulary (CRITCHLEY 1964), spontaneous writing being usually more impaired than writing to dictation or copying of printed material (ALLISON 1962; STENGEL 1964a, b).

The disintegration of the semantic field precedes phonemic disintegration (AJURIAGUERRA and TISSOT 1968). Finally formal and semantic structures are contaminated, leaving syntactical patterns intact for a long time. Frequently a conversational situation is readily recognized, but dialogue is reduced to stereotype communication or vocal pseudodialogue, a phenomenon called *Dialogslalie* by SPOERRI (1965). This is possible through preservation of prosody, which does not disappear until the final stage of the process, together with the appearance of dysarthria, anarthria, and mutism (GROSCH 1948). Along with interruption of speech initiative, gestural, and pantomimic compensation cease (ALLISON 1962).

ALBERT (1964b, 1965, 1968), whose longitudinal studies of SD are still authoritative, discerned four different stages of language dissolution:
a) anomia (amnestic aphasia) as the almost obligatory initial stage
b) transcortical sensory aphasia (mixed transcortical aphasia) marked by excellent (echolalic) repetition
c) cortical-sensory or Wernicke's aphasia (cf. BLEULER 1975) and mixed aphasia (ALLISON 1962) still met with in most of the cases
d) total or global aphasia as the final stage.

It has often been observed that even in the more advanced stages intermittent stereotype faultless instantaneous utterances are not unusual (GROSCH 1948; ALBERT 1965). The communicative defect in SD is judged as loss of abstraction, increasing syncretism, concretism, and egotism (STENGEL 1964b; IRIGARAY and DUBOIS 1966), and incapacity to generate or receive new information or to establish new relations (IRIGARAY 1967, 1973). In contrast to aphasia of vascular origin, language therapy in these cases is of no use (WALLACE 1971).

2. Apraxia

Apraxic and agnosic disturbances are less likely to be detected in the early stages of SD than aphasic ones, but are nevertheless well suited for detection by neuropsychological testing and selection of senile demented people out of a group of the same age (CALTAGIRONE et al. 1970). Early observations of apraxia in SD were made by MARCUSE (1904) and PICK (1906). Because memory disorders seemed to influence also apraxic behavior, MARCUSE named it "amnestic" apraxia while AJURIAGUERRA et al. (1960) doubt such influence. In this field iterative phenomena are also common.

The hierarchical dissolution process goes from constructional apraxia to ideomotor and ideational apraxia (GROSCH 1948; ALLISON 1962; AJURIAGUERRA et al. 1960; AJURIAGUERRA and TISSOT 1968). Constructional apraxia is found relatively early and reflects a visuospatial disorder manifesting itself by impaired drawing and copying (GROSSI et al. 1978; GAINOTTI et al. 1980), loss of perspective, directions, and topological relationships. Right-left disorientation occurs. Disturbances of dressing as a rule emerge sooner than those of undressing and are caused by complex mechanisms such as spatial dyskinesia, asomatognosis, serial disorders, and agnosia for reflected images (AJURIAGUERRA et al. 1960). Very characteristic is ideational apraxia, met mostly during the stage of transcortical-sensory aphasia (AJURIAGUERRA et al. 1965).

First, there are occupational restlessness and tendency of order, then disorder, bodily neglect, echopraxia, sometimes even oral apraxia (ERNST et al. 1970b, c) and automatisms, and finally a complete inability for appropriate action appears.

3. Agnosia and Acalculia

Arithmetical problems are not uncommon in the earlier stages of SD, since they are highly dependent on memory and spatial imagination (ERNST et al. 1970c; WELLS 1977). Not different from MA, visual agnosia is more common than tactile agnosia (astereognosis). Also common are color agnosia and cortical blindness, which are sometimes mistaken as a severe disturbance of confrontation naming (GROSCH 1948; ALLISON 1962; ALBERT 1968). If there is faulty recognition of some aspects of objects like edibility and danger independent of input modality, the term "semantic agnosia" is applied (TORACK 1978). Auditive agnosia (cortical deafness) is often discovered by inability to recognize and reproduce tonal and rhythmical patterns (HORENSTEIN 1971a). Autotopagnosia (asomatognosis and finger agnosia) plays an important role in dressing apraxia (AJURIAGUERRA and TISSOT 1968).

Testing of operational level according to PIAGET-INHELDER yielded a subsequent loss of the ability to name parts of the own mirror image, to comprehend the fact of reflection at all, and recognize oneself in the mirror (Ajuriaguerra and Tissot 1968).

4. Neurological Aspects

Neurological disorders are as a rule observed during the final stage of a complete senile dementing process. As it was outlined for the neuropsychological disorders, automatisms, atavistic, and stereotype behavior emerge, following destruction of higher inhibitory mechanisms (Paulson 1977). Oral tendencies increase; in some cases an abortive Klüver-Bucy Syndrome can be seen (Pilleri 1961 a; Sourander and Sjögren 1970; Torack 1978; Lauter 1980); and sucking, snouting, oral seeking, opposition hypertonia, grasping (Pilleri 1961 b), synkinesias, motor stereotypies, postural perseveration, proprioceptive clinging, gazing, and model imitation appear (Ajuriaguerra and Tissot 1968). Very common is hypermetamorphosis as a disturbance of selective attention and endeavour to devote oneself to and to touch everything. This behavior influences food uptake, which is characterized by defective initial saturation, stereotyped absorption of food (Torack 1978; Meyer et al. 1980), and fluctuation between anorexia and polyphagia.

Frequently, labioauricular (Hachinski 1977), linguomental, and palmomental reflexes can be elicited, often being an early sign of SD but unspecific and without firm correlation with psychopathological findings (Demeurisse et al. 1979). Due to participation of subcortical ganglia and nigrostriatal degeneration symptoms of parkinsonism-like tremor, especially of hands and jaw, parapatetic gait, reduced synkinesis of arms, asthenocoria, increase of repetitive movements, and rigor proceeding as far as decerebration may arise.

Disorders of cross modality run into sensory deficits, such as olfactory insensibility (Waldton 1974). Cerebral fits were observed in some cases. As a consequence of vegetative diencephalic disorder massive sleep disturbances with reversal of diurnal rhythms (Wever 1975), hypersalivation, hyperthermia, and micturition and defecation difficulties occur before in the long run inevitable internal complications lead to the final stage.

C. Additional Diagnostic Findings

I. Psychometry and Psychopathometry

Psychological testing according to Horenstein (1971 b) may attain one or more of five goals:
1. Quantification of a presumed deficit in intelligence, whether developmental or acquired
2. Definition and differentiation of cognitive, agnosic, aphasic, and amnestic elements
3. Documentation of the resolution, dissolution, or progression of the behavioral consequences of an illness
4. Assistance in planning follow-up or comprehensive care of individual patients, particularly by identifying interests and aptitudes

5. Separation of dementing symptoms from others related to premorbid personality or emotional response to illness.

Psychometry means evaluation and differentiation of performance, aptitudes, interests, and personality traits in normals and diseased, reflecting particularly points 1., 2. ("differentiation"), 4., and 5. of the above list, whereas psychopathometry is designed to measure the degree of pathological behavior as validated by causal external criteria or clinical diagnosis without much time consumption or need of personnel (WIECK 1973), thus reflecting points 2. ("definition") and 3.

Psychopathometry is preferably carried out by short and homogeneous single tests while psychometric testing is preferably carried out by test batteries. Progress in this area was rapid during the past decade and partially invalidates ALEXANDER'S (1972) complaint: "... there is almost complete lack of valid and reliable measures suitable for the longitudinal analysis of change." But it still cannot be overlooked that testing demented patients may be very difficult to virtually impossible through opposition, indifference, increased distractability, and lack of concentration power and attentiveness.

1. Psychophysiological Tests

Psychophysiological tests are valuable in evaluation of fundamental behavioral responses without much help from the patient: reaction time (FERRIS et al. 1976), particularly in a multiple-choice setting (MCGHIE 1969), critical flicker frequency, processing temporal information by bringing intervals of different duration into a serial order, pairwise comparison of intervals (HIBBARD et al. 1975), orienting reflex and habituation (MCGHIE 1969; JONSSON et al. 1976), and eyelid reflex (JONSSON et al. 1977). Performance in most of the tests is clearly reduced in senile demented patients, some of them (e.g., orienting and eyelid reflexes) seeming to have a certain degree of correlation with mental deterioration.

2. Memory Tests

They are of particular importance since memory deficits are among the most prominent signs of SD: One class of tests uses mainly verbal material, such as the subtest digit repetition of the WAIS (HAWIE) (CANTONE et al. 1978), nonsense-syllable program (PEREZ et al. 1978), or synonym-learning test (LARNER 1977), while another class uses mainly pictorial material to avoid language influences, such as the Bender gestalt test (BENDER 1938), recurring-figures test (KIMURA 1963; ERNST 1970a; MILLER and LEWIS 1977), pictorial paired associate learning task (GEDYE et al. 1972), Bildertest (MÜLLER 1975), picture recognition (DIESFELDT 1978), random-visual-shapes program (PEREZ et al. 1978), and Corsi's block-tapping task (CANTONE et al. 1978). In some both kinds of requirements are combined as in the Wechsler Memory Scale (PEREZ et al. 1975), Syndrom-Kurz-Test (ERZIGKEIT 1977), and Funktionspsychose-Skala-B (LEHRL et al. 1977).

In SD, abilities for digit repetition and paired-associate learning are reduced (KASZNIAK et al. 1979), recognition is impaired by more liberal criterion and greater loss of encoding characteristics (LARNER 1977), less correct answers, and more mistakes than in depression (MILLER and LEWIS 1977). Patients affected by

SD have a worse overall memory than patients with MID or vertebrobasilar insufficiency, and they are impaired in perception, attention, and recall, while Korsakov and depressive patients show disturbances in at most two of these functions (NEVILLE and FOLSTEIN 1979).

There is evidence that function psychosis and defect syndrome can be separated (LEHRL et al. 1980).

3. Intelligence Tests

These tests aim at the very heart of the dementia syndrome: Well installed are the Wechsler Adult Intelligence Scale (WAIS) (WECHSLER 1956; PEREZ et al. 1975; FULD 1978), Raven's Progressive Matrices Test, a nonverbal test (EYSENCK 1945; ORME 1957; FULD 1978), and the Reduzierter Wechsler-Intelligenz-Test für psychiatrisch Kranke, derived from the WAIS and especially suitable for the psychiatrically ill (DAHL 1972). More recent developments are the purely verbal Mehrfachwahl-Wortschatz-Test (LEHRL 1977) and the Wide Range Achievement Test (JASTAK 1965; FULD 1978). Except for the purely verbal tests a distinct deterioration of performance can be expected.

4. Neuropsychological Tests

Neuropsychological tests are very helpful in evaluating the course of SD: Goldstein-Scheerer-Battery for abstract and concrete behavior (HORENSTEIN 1971a), Weigl's sorting test (WEIGL et al. 1945), Benton-Test (BENTON and SPREEN 1972), Kew's cognitive map (MCDONALD 1969), Reitan's Trail Making Test (HORENSTEIN 1971a), and constructional apraxia test (GROSSI et al. 1978). Language abilities are assessed by reaction time in naming (LAWSON and BARKER 1968), Eisenson's Examining for Aphasia (WALLACE 1971), Halstead-Wepman-Aphasia-Screening-Test (HORENSTEIN 1971a) and the Token Test (DERENZI and VIGNOLO 1962; ERNST 1970a) – a review was given by LANG (1981).

Luria's method achieves the widest neuropsychological range possible (ERNST 1970b), a German adaptation was carried out by HAMSTER et al. (1980).

It was only by some of these tests that the importance of visuospatial disorders in SD and their selection value could be demonstrated (KASZNIAK et al. 1979).

5. Questionnaires, Rating Scales, and Inventories

The Minnesota Multiphasic Personality Inventory (SPREEN 1963), Zung Self-Rating Depression Scale (STEUER et al. 1980), Short Portable Mental Status Questionnaire (PFEIFFER 1975), Mini-Mental-Status (FOLSTEIN et al. 1975), Inpatient Multidimensional Psychiatric Scale (LORR et al. 1963), Dokumentationssystem der Arbeitsgemeinschaft für Methodik und Dokumentation in der Psychiatrie (ANGST et al. 1969), and Mental Status Questionnaire and Grade Assessment Questionnaire (KAPLAN 1979) were all applied in SD. One obstacle is that demented patients are often not able to fill in self-rating scales.

6. Recent Developments for Senile and Demented People

KAHN et al. (1960) communicated an indirect rating scale comprising ten questions; more elaborate are the Dementia Rating Scale (MATTIS 1976) and Organic Mental Syndrome Screening Examination (MATTIS 1976), and especially refined is the Automatic Behavioral Assessment System by PEREZ et al. (1977). The purposes of detecting and documenting SD are fulfilled by the Plutchik Geriatric Rating Scale (PLUTCHIK et al. 1976), London Psychogeriatric Rating System (HERSCH et al. 1978), Crichton Geriatric Behavior Rating Scale (HARE 1978), Dokumentationssystem der Arbeitsgemeinschaft für Geronto-Psychiatrie (CIOMPI and KANOWSKI 1977), Psychological Abilities Scale for Seniles (KAPLAN 1979), Senility Rating Scale (BERGER 1980), Nürnberger Alters-Inventar (OSWALD 1980) and the Zahlen-Verbindungs-Test for older patients (OSWALD and ROTH 1978; OSWALD and FLEISCHMANN to be published).

With the aid of the Mental Deterioration Battery, CALTAGIRONE et al. (1970) were able to select 71%–91% of demented people out of control groups of the same age.

The Dementia Test by TOMLINSON et al. (1970), examining mainly memory and orientation, said to differentiate between Alzheimer's Disease (MA) and multi-infarct dementia (MID) and correlated with the density of neurofibrillary tangles and senile plaques, and the Hachinski Score (HACHINSKI 1978), separating vascular from degenerative dementia, have found wide acceptance.

Finally HERSCH et al. (1980) developed a prognostic index for time of discharge from hospital.

II. Instrumental Findings

Anamnestic and clinical findings are completed by additional examinations with technical instruments. They aim at excluding other, mainly curable, dementing processes.

In electroencephalography since OBRIST (1951), a slowing and spread of alpha activity are looked upon as normal in older persons. Additionally, focal changes like theta and delta activity especially in the temporal lobe are age related (BUSSE and OBRIST 1963; KOOI et al. 1964). These changes are observed in vascular as well as in degenerative diseases. The hypothesis that focal EEG disturbances could indicate an imminent vascular crisis was not confirmed in controlled investigations (BUSSE and OBRIST 1963; OBRIST 1972). The EEG is especially important in differentiating between senile dementia of Alzheimer's type (SDAT), Creutzfeldt-Jacob disease (CJD), and Huntington's disease (SISHTA 1974). In SD 31%–46% show normal EEG findings (MUNDY-CASTLE et al. 1953; SHERIDAN et al. 1954; BARNES et al. 1956). Even severe cases of SD in routine EEG sometimes show improvement (SHERIDAN et al. 1954). There is a statistically significant correlation between argyrophile dystrophy in SD and a slowing down of alpha rhythm in EEG as seen in semiquantitative morphometry (DEISENHAMMER and JELLINGER 1971). Computer analysis of sensory-evoked responses by acoustic and optic stimulation has recently shown diverging responses in both hemispheres. Therefore GERSON et al. (1976) assume a coordination deficit of the brain in SD.

The possibilities of computerized axial tomography in investigating degenerative cerebral diseases are not yet fully realized. First normal aging populations were studied, establishing indices of normal brain measurements (Huckman et al. 1975; Synek et al. 1976; Gyldensted and Kosteljanitz 1975; Barron et al. 1976; Reisner et al. 1980; Yamaura et al. 1980). Then classifications of pathological findings were presented. According to Meese and Grumme (1980) about 20% of cerebral atrophies could be due to normal aging if this atrophy is light to moderate and equal in all parts of the brain. Asymmetrical atrophies, in SD accentuated in the parietal or frontotemporal region, resulted in an increase of pathological EEG findings and of psychopathological deficiencies.

Cerebral blood flow and regional cerebral blood flow (CBF, rCBF) in SD are mainly found to be normal; only in advanced cases are they decreased. Investigations of cerebral metabolism have shown that while CMR glucose (cerebral metabolism rate for glucose) in the early stages is already markedly decreased, CMR oxygen is normal. Hoyer (1980) interpretes these findings as a result of oxidation of cerebral substrate, due to a degenerating disease.

Radioactive albumin or indium served in studies of CSF dynamics in SDAT and NPH. There are certain differential diagnostic problems resulting in the meningeal fibrosis often seen in SDAT, which can result in an inversion of CSF flow into the periventricular tissue (Coblentz 1973). This explains the success sometimes observed after shunt operation in cases of SDAT (Shenkin et al. 1973).

D. Epidemiology

Epidemiological investigations of senile dementia meet with several methodological difficulties. Therefore the results of the few thorough studies which have appeared so far are only conditionally comparable.

The main problems consist of the choice of a suitable population and of the exact diagnostic categorization of every proband. In many cases it is not easy to determine exactly the beginning of the disease and to calculate its course up to the date of investigation. Roth (1978a) in this context describes a "threshold effect," which shows in clinical observation of the disease. The same opinion is put forward by Kleemeier (1962) and Jarvik (1978). Nevertheless the Newcastle-upon-Tyne study has shown that, after 2–4 years of observation of 711 patients over 65 years of age, 30 had developed senile dementia, only six of which were classed as suspect cases at the initial examination (Kay et al. 1964; Roth 1978a).

Roth's (1955) criteria were accepted by most investigators classifying the clinical appearances of their geriatric patients. Others like Peck et al. (1978) used the diagnostic criteria of the American Psychiatric Association, Diagnostics and Statistics Manual. Here a diffuse and global impairment of cerebral function is assumed.

Akesson (1969) very clearly describes the investigator's difficulties in judging every single case. He decided for a better separation of vascular disease from senile dementia to regard only the cases with a severe and irreversible symptomatology. Other investigators (Hagnell 1970, Gruenberg 1978; Brückmann 1981), also indicate diagnostic problems. Therefore Gruenberg (1978) proposes a sequence of screening processes for a better diagnostic separation of the senile dementia cases from vascular diseases. Autoptic investigations (BLESSED et al. 1968) have shown that there is an overlapping, nevertheless. In Newcastle-upon-Tyne a ratio of 50% purely parenchymatous cases to 20% mixed to 30% purely vascular diseases was found.

1. Prevalence

KAY (1972) estimates the prevalence of senile dementia at 5%–10% among the general population over 65 years of age. The ratio of men/women is 1.7/4.1 in the age group 65–74 years and 4.4/9.3 over 75 years (ROTH 1978b). Surveying the literature, we found data in this respect to vary strongly. AKESSON (1969) found the by far lowest prevalence of 0.74% ± 0.13%. He investigated the population of two large islands off the Swedish coast and took for the above reasons only the severe cases, none being younger than 70 years. BOLLERUP (1975) found 1.3% among the 70-year-olds in nine Kopenhagen suburbs. STERNBERG and GAWRILOWA (1978) found 2.8% in Moskow, 1.1% for men and 3.8% for women. MAYER-GROSS et al. (1969) transduced his 4.4% prevalence among the population over 65 years of age to 3.3% for the general population. KAY et al. (1964) in Newcastle-upon-Tyne found a prevalence of 4.2% among those living at home, 2.9% being light cases, and 1.3% severe. ROTH (1978b) reported a prevalence of 5% among his 309 patients of the early cohort, which after further investigations was corrected to 6.2%. So today 60% of the old living in Newcastle's nursing homes are estimated to suffer from senile dementia. Several investigators, such as ESSEN-MÖLLER (1956), who found 3.9%, and PRIMROSE (1962), who found 5%, were able to confirm the results of the Newcastle group. NIELSEN (1962), however, found a prevalence of 18.5% on the island of Samsö, taking into account that among his severe cases there were some with a vascular disease. In 1957 he found a prevalence of 7.4% and in 1962 10.6% for all of Denmark. ESSEN-MÖLLER'S (1956) patients from Lundby were reinvestigated after 10 years by HAGNELL (1970). The prevalence mounted from 5.5% in 1956 to 16.1% in 1970, due to an increasing prevalence with age. This relationship between prevalence of senile dementia and age not only showed in Lundby but also in New York State (GRUENBERG 1961), Newcastle-upon-Tyne (KAY et al. 1964; KAY 1970), Sweden (AKESSON 1969; HAGNELL 1970), Denmark (NIELSEN 1962), and Missouri (TORACK 1978).

All comparable studies mentioned above show an increasing morbidity with increasing age up to 90 years. This tendency is visible despite different methods and material of the investigators. Above 90 years of age TORACK (1978) could not find a further increase. His results rather indicate a decrease but his number of patients is too small for proof.

LARSSON et al. (1963) also did not observe a further increase of morbidity above 90 years. This tendency is also supported by the age distribution given in the autoptic studies of FULLER (1911), UYEMATSU (1923), ROTHSCHILD (1937), CORSELLIS (1962), McMENEMEY (1968), PERESS et al. (1968), and TOMLINSON et al. (1970). Here the prevalence sinks already in the age group of 85–90 years. Therefore TORACK (1978) indicates "an intriguing resistance to dementia after the age of 90."

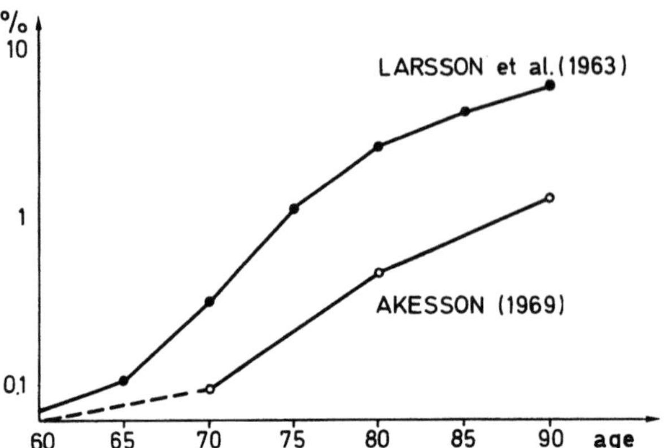

Fig. 2. Incidence of senile dementia as a percentage of the age-matched population

2. Incidence

As to the incidence there are less numerous results. Roth (1978 b) from the basis of the results of his group in Newcastle-upon-Tyne reports an average yearly incidence of 1.4% after 4–5 years of investigation. Akesson (1969) only found 0.38%, under the above-mentioned conditions. Age dependence of incidence acts similar to that of prevalence of senile dementia. The rate of new diseases mounts with age (Larsson et al. 1963; Akesson 1969; Torack 1978) (Fig. 2). It sinks again among those above 90, according to the results of Torack (1978) in St. Louis. Only 2% of his 24 probands above 90 became senile dements. Earlier investigations did not report age data sufficiently exact to support these results. According to Larsson et al. (1963) there was no increasing morbidity risk during the 30-year period he studied.

3. Mortality

All patients suffering from senile dementia must be aware of a very short life expectation as compared to age-matched controls. Among Roth's (1955) patients 58% were dead half a year and 82% 2 years after hospitalization. Those with cerebrovascular disease only amounted to 33% and 73%. Consecutively the author reports a life expectation of 30% of the age-related average. Larsson et al. (1963) found only 50% for men and 55% for women as compared to the age-related average. One year after hospitalization it sinks to 40%. The relative increase of the mortality rate amounts to 130% for men and 90% for women. In the age groups over 80 this high mortality rate sinks again (Larsson et al. 1963). Akesson (1969) reports a life expectation quotient (life expectation of patients investigated by life expectation of the age-matched general population) of 0.63% after 3 years of observation. This result is based on only 40 patients. On the other hand 15 out of 78 probands lived longer than 3 years.

4. Course

68% of Akesson's (1969) patients were first taken into other hospitals because of some somatic disease. 72% of these were transferred to a psychiatric hospital or dismissed within half a year. In the state of medium to severe dementia these patients were 79.5 years old on average. Thirteen percent of them had a course of 1 year after the first psychotic symptoms, 31% up to 2 years, 28% up to 3 years, and 28% over 3 years (AKESSON 1969). In the very large population of LARSSON et al. (1963) the symptoms of senile dementia began at an average of 73.4 years for men and 75.3 years for women. The range was 56–92 years. Hospitalization occurred at an average of 76.4 years for men and 78.4 years for women. At an average of 2.1 years later death occurred for both sexes. This means a life expectation of about 5 years after the first symptoms are noted. Similar results were published by KAY (1972). 81% of his patients finally reached a state of total dementia and 19%, severe dementia.

Memory loss seems to be an important prognostic factor. A reinvestigation of the patients of KAY et al. (1964) after 4 years (KAY et al. 1966) showed that light senile memory losses were a highly significant predictor of death 4 years later. BERGMANN (1976) confirms this result; EPSTEIN et al. (1964) reported death at an average of 6 years after the initial symptomatology. In a very thorough neurological, neuroradiological, neurophysiological, and neuropsychological investigation of 47 hospitalized patients these prediction criteria were stated more accurately (KASZNIAK et al. 1978): The degree of impairment of cerebral function seems to be more important as to life expectation than the degree of cerebral atrophy shown by the CAT scan. Additionally, the authors think they can predict the short-term life expectation very exactly by examining the cognitive functions. A deficit of expressive language is said to indicate a very bad survival prognosis (see C.II).

The autoptic investigations gave few results on the exact death cause (TOMLINSON et al. 1970; BERGMANN 1976). Therefore the cause of death is an "interesting mystery" (ROTH 1978 b). Several authors, however, underlined the importance of bronchopneumonia (KAY 1972; PARKER 1972; VARSAMIS et al. 1972; PECK et al. 1978). Regarding several factors as possible causes of death seems to offer the best possibilities for improving the bad prognosis according to our current state of knowledge (ROTH 1978 b). GOLDFARB (1969) and WANG (1978) have already indicated this view. They postulated a relationship between somatic disease and impaired cerebral function according to the concept of function psychosis (WIECK 1978). On the other hand an impaired cerebral function prepares the way for still more complications due to physical neglect such as malnutrition, vulnerations, hypoventilation, or aspiration, e.g., following a necessary sedation because of psychomotor agitation and infections of the urinary tract. Finally, an increasing irreversible damage of the circulatory system and the brain, provokes death. This opinion is supported by the results of BRODY et al. (1975). So the patient's care for his own body and the physician's judgment of cardiac function are of special prognostic importance.

5. Sociological Factors

The socioeconomic status has no influence on the occurrence of senile dementia. Single persons, however, have a higher hospitalization risk, according to AKESSON (1969). The increasing number of hospitalizations due to senile dementia, reported from all over the western hemisphere, according to Larsson et al. (1963), are a result of changes in population structure with respect to size and age.

6. Genetics

Since Meggendörfer (1925), a hereditary factor in senile dementia has been known. Sjögren et al. (1952) in their investigations on family members of 36 in part histologically confirmed cases found 30 secondary cases of Alzheimer's senile dementia. The morbidity age varied strongly. Larsson et al. (1963), investigating 374 families with 3,426 members, found 60 secondary cases of senile dementia. There was no difference compared to the sick probands of the study with respect to age at the beginning of the disease, symptomatology, and course. Therefore the authors discuss a monohybrid dominant mode of inheritance. The morbidity risk for parents and sibs is about 4.3 times above the average of the general population. According to Jarvik (1978) the morbidity risk in the general population is well under 1%, for sibs of Alzheimer patients about 3.8%, and for parents about 10%. Kallmann (1956) reported a concordance of senile dementia morbidity of 42.8% for monozygote twins and of 8% for dizygote twins. His investigations on 108 twin's families showed a morbidity risk of 3.4% for parents and of 6.5% for sibs. This resulted in his concept of a heterogene inheritance, which was also put forward by Zerbin-Rüdin (1972). Constantinidis et al. (1965) and Constantinidis (1978) in reviewing the literature observed an occurrence of presenile Alzheimer's dementia over two or more generations, which would favour a dominant mode of inheritance. However, familiar senile cases normally occur in only one generation of sibs, which would favor a recessive mode. The latest results by Constantinidis (1978) show an intrafamiliar concordance of two-thirds as to an inheritance of the presenile or senile form, a discordance of one-third. Additionally the female sex seems to be predominant in the higher age groups, contrary to those under 65 years. Altogether Constantinidis (1978) proposes a nosological entity of senile and presenile dementia of the Alzheimer type. He discusses a multifactorial etiopathogenetical concept where constitutional factors are related with several genes. Slater and Cowie (1971) express a similar opinion. Lauter (1968), however, proposes a dominant mode of inheritance.

Jarvik (1978) presented the results of the only twin study initiated by Kallmann (1956). She emphasizes the prognostic importance of the cerebral function quantified by psychological tests. In this context she recalls the "critical loss" phenomenon described earlier (Jarvik and Blum 1971). This confirms Kleemeier's (1962) hypothesis, called "terminal drop." Jarvik (1978) further reports a hypodiploidy in aged women with senile dementia as opposed to women in the same age with cerebrovascular insufficiency. These findings are supported by the results of Nielsen (1968). However, Bergener and Jungklaass (1970) found hyperdiploid cores in two cases of Alzheimer's disease but not in cases of senile dementia. Explication of these findings is not yet possible. Similarly a conclusive interpretation of the connections between serum immunoglobulins, vocabulary scores, and chromosome losses is so far not possible. It is striking, however, that the rate of hypodiploidy in young and old men is equal. In fact, senile dementia is found mainly in women (Jarvik 1978; Brückmann 1981).

E. Differential Diagnosis

1. Introduction

Differential diagnosis of a psychopathological syndrome like SD must predominantly aim at discovering etiologically defined and treatable diseases before palliative and symptomatic measures are used (BERGERON and HANUS 1964).

Refined means of assessment have disclosed more and more preventable and treatable causes of dementia-like function psychoses; FOX et al. (1975) were able to treat 12% of their patients with the initial diagnosis of SD successfully. This is why commitment to this severe diagnosis should be made only after exhaustion of all reasonable diagnostic procedures; LAUTER (1980) has given a checklist for that purpose.

The diseases that have to be taken into account are mentioned below except for the ones which usually cause no serious trouble in differential diagnosis (see Table 1). The percentage in brackets after some of the diseases stem from BERGER (1979) and indicate the relative frequency with which they were met in a sample of 222 demented elderly patients.

2. The Diseases

Atrophying cerebral processes (51%) are one of two groups to be most likely confused with SD. For the case of *MA (presenile dementia, Alzheimer's syndrome)* the necessity of differentiation has been disputed by many.

Alzheimer's (1907) opinion, that he had described a special form the SD, was endorsed by many of his followers (MARCHAND et al. 1942; ANGEL 1977). Some researchers stated that MA and SD were to be easily separated on clinical and neuropathological grounds and therefore to be regarded as two different diseases (KRAEPELIN 1910; GRÜNTHAL 1936), a view that presently is at least in part supported by SOURANDER and SJÖGREN 1970; RABINOWICZ 1972; ERBSLÖH and KOHLMEYER 1974; TODOROV et al. 1975. The exceptional position of MA is substantiated by earlier onset, higher intensity and faster progression (AJURIAGUERRA and TISSOT 1968), focal symptoms, and dominant heredity (TODOROV et al. 1975, see epidemiology). In contrast to this the bulk of geriatricians maintain that there is no reason for a discrimination of adult dementia before and after the 65th year of life neither on clinical nor pathological grounds (TORACK 1978). This view is favored by NEWTON 1948; RASKIN and EHRENBERG 1956; ARAB 1960; ALBERT 1964b; CONSTANTINIDIS 1968, 1978; TISSOT 1968; WEISS 1968; JACOB 1969; BARSTEIN 1970; LAUTER 1972, 1980; CIOMPI 1973; TERRY 1976; KATZMAN and KARASU 1975; MULDER 1976; ANGEL 1977; BRAIN 1977; KATZMAN et al. 1978b; PEREZ et al. 1978; WELLS 1978; BERGER 1979; and BERGENER 1980. That MA and SD have to be considered a disease and not a physiological involution or "senium praecox" (KRAEPELIN) is almost unanimously accepted.

Those scholars who lay stress on focal symptoms prefer the term SDAT (senile dementia of Alzheimer type) as proposed by the nosology commission of the workshop conference on MA/SD (KATZMAN et al. 1978b), while others (ALBERT 1964a, b; BARSTEIN 1970; REDLICH and FREEDMAN 1976, BERGENER 1980) do not make this difference.

Table 1. Differential diagnosis of senile dementia

I. *Cerebroatrophic processes*
  1. MA (Alzheimer's disease)
     (Katzman et al. 1978a)
  2. Temporal lobe atrophy
     (Shibayama et al. 1978)
  3. MP (Pick's syndrome)
     (Jakob 1979)
  4. Dementia-parkinsonism
     syndrome with Lewy bodies
     (Kosaka and Mehraein 1979;
     Ikeda et al. 1980)
  5. Dementia-parkinsonism complex
     of Guam (Jacob 1969)
  6. Parkinson's syndrome (Bowen
     and Davison 1975)
  7. Huntington's chorea (Chase et al.
     1979)
  8. Familiar senile hallucinosis
     (Bergener et al. 1972)
  9. Rare systemic degenerations:
     a) Corticodentatonigral
        degeneration with neuronal
        achromasia
     b) Progressive nuclear palsy
        (Jacob 1969)
     c) Progressive supranuclear palsy
        (Jacob 1969, Albert 1978)
     d) Steele-Richardson-Olszewski
        syndrome (Foerster and
        Regli 1980)
     e) Spinocerebellar degenerations
     f) Unverricht-Lundborg
        myoclonus epilepsy (Norio and
        Koskiniemi 1979)
     g) Progressive multifocal
        leukoencephalopathy
     h) Hallervorden-Spatz' disease
        (Dooling et al. 1974)
II. *Normal pressure hydrocephalus*
   (Jacobs et al. 1978)
III. *Cardiovascular diseases*
   1. Extracranial
      a) Cardiac insufficiency
         (Anonymous 1977)
      b) Myocardial infarction
         (Hontela and Schwartz 1979)
      c) Cardiac rhythm disorders
      d) Extracorporal circulation
         (Meyendorf 1976;
         Götze 1980)
      e) Cardiac arrest (Robinson 1977)
      f) Subacute bacterial endocarditis
         with MID (Wells 1978)
      g) Carotid and vertebral artery
         stenoses

   2. Intracranial
      a) Stenose of cerebral arteries and
         basilar artery
      b) Hypertensive encephalopathy
      c) Thrombangiitis obliterans
         (Scheid 1980)
      d) Arteriovenous malformations,
         kinking (Haase 1971)
      e) Binswanger's syndrome
         (Erbslöh and Kohlmeyer
         1974)

IV. *Blood diseases*
   1. Anemia (Robinson 1977)
   2. Hypercoagulation, polycythemia

V. *Respiratory disorders*
   1. Chronic respiratory insufficiency
      (Hughes 1978)

VI. *Metabolic diseases and avitaminoses*
   1. Diabetes mellitus, hypoglycemia
      (Robinson 1977)
   2. Addison's disease (Katzman and
      Karasu 1975; Roth 1978a)
   3. Cushing's disease (Hughes 1978)
   4. Hypo- and hyperthyroidism,
      myxedema (Robinson 1977;
      Portnoi 1979)
   5. Hypo- and hyperparathyroidism,
      Fahr's disease (Barwich 1976)
   6. Electrolyte imbalance (sodium,
      potassium, calcium) (Jana and
      Romano-Jana 1973; Hughes
      1978)
   8. Lipid storage diseases and
      glycogenoses (Torvik et al. 1974)
   9. Wilson's disease (Foerster and
      Regli 1980)
   10. Nephrotoxic encephalopathy,
      hemodialysis
   11. Hepatotoxic encephalopathy,
      porphyria (Hughes 1978;
      Plum 1978)
   12. Partial malnutrition and
      malabsorption, avitaminoses
      a) B_1 and B_2, mostly in alcoholism
         with Wernicke-Korsakov
         syndrome (Annexton 1978;
         Victor and Baker 1978)
      b) B_{12}, funicular myelosis
         (Wieck 1980a)
      c) Folic acid deficiency
      d) Nicotinic acid deficiency
         (Roth 1978a)

Table 1. (Continued)

VII. *Exogenous intoxications*
  1. Alcoholism (intoxication, delirium)
  2. Other habit-forming agents
    a) Barbiturates
    b) Benzodiazepines
    c) Bromides (RASKIND et al. 1978)
    d) Other sedatives, narcotics
      (HUGHES 1978)
    e) Analgetics
    f) Psychotomimetics
  3. Not habit-forming agents
    a) Corticoids
    b) Anticonvulsants, anti-
      histaminics, antidepressants,
      neuroleptics, digitalis,
      vincristine (HUGHES 1978)
    c) Gases (carbon monoxide)
      (BERGERON and HANUS 1964;
      ROBINSON 1977; BLASS 1980)
    d) Heavy metals (Mn, Pb, Hg, Al)
      (BLASS 1980; FOERSTER and
      REGLI 1980)
    e) Organic compounds (CS_2)
VIII. *Infectious, parainfectious, and*
    immunological diseases
  1. Meningoencephalitis (viral,
    mycotic, tuberculous)
  2. Neurosyphilis, general paralysis
    (BERGERON and HANUS 1964)
  3. Brain abscess
  4. Encephalomyelitis disseminata
  5. Jakob-Creutzfeldt's disease
    (TOSI et al. 1980)
  6. Kuru (HAASE 1971)
  7. Tuberculosis and sarcoidosis
	IX. *Tumorous*
	  1. Brain tumors (BERGERON and
	    HANUS 1964)
	  2. Hodgkin's disease, bronchial
	    carcinoma (ROBINSON 1977;
	    FOERSTER and REGLI 1980)
	X. *Traumatic*
	  1. Cerebral contusion, punch-drunk
	    syndrome (CORSELLIS et al. 1973)
	  2. Brain wounds
	  3. Subdural hematoma
	XI. *Epilepsies, electroconvulsive therapy*
	XII. *Chronic subdural hematoma and*
	    hygroma and subarachnoid bleeding
	XIII. *Psychiatric disorders*
	  1. Endogenous psychoses
	    ("pseudodementia") (WELLS 1979;
	    ROTH 1978a)
	  2. Nonpsychotic disorders
	    a) Reaction to trauma, KZ
	      syndrome, Ganser syndrome
	      ("pseudodementia")
	      (VAN DER HORST 1964)
	    b) Neuroses
	    c) Psychopathy
	    d) Sensory loss, sensory
	      deprivation (ROBINSON 1977)
	    e) Connatal feeble-mindedness
	      (BOWER 1971)

MP (Pick's syndrome) as another presenile dementia is said to occur with a
frequency of about 2% of that of MA (TERRY 1976). Figures are different, since
the distinction of MA and MID in the United States is not as common as in Western Europe (CONSTANTINIDIS et al. 1974). Brain atrophy is accentuated in the frontal lobes and the basal portion of the temporal lobe. Leading in symptomatology
are changes of personality and initiative, affective blunting, moria, indifference,
impairment of reasoning, social responsibility, and moral behavior. Memory, formal intelligence, and orientation are preserved in the initial stage. Aphasic symptoms are not rare and directed toward so-called dynamic aphasia (Luria) superimposed by word-finding difficulties, echo phenomena, reduced fluency, monotony,
and finally mutism. Grasping reflex, oral disinhibition, and rigor appear late in the
course. EEG is often pathological (INGVAR et al. 1978). Nonobligatory neuropathological signs are the Pick cell (argentophilic intraneuronal inclusions) and Hirano

bodies. As the cause of the presumably dominant transmittible disorder, lack of a specific neurotransmitter is suggested.

Parkinson's syndrome (less than 1%) in its final stage can imitate SD but is easily discerned by its preceding neurological symptomatology (BOWEN and DAVISON 1975). Bradyphrenia at second look and with the aid of psychological testing is not to be confused with dementia. Since etiology is manifold, a great number of varieties dominated by rigor, tremor, or akinesia exist.

Jakob-Creutzfeldt's disease (less than 1%) also starts with neurological symptoms of pyramidal, extrapyramidal, cerebellar and nuclear origin; dysarthria, aphasia, myoclonus, visual disorders, and dementia have been observed. Onset during presenium is common, progression rapid, and the course seldom longer than 2 years (ERBSLÖH and KOHLMEYER 1974; TORACK 1978). Typical EEG signs are triphasic sharp-wave complexes; histologically neuronal vacuolization is seen. The disease is thought to be a slow virus infection.

Chorea Huntington (5%) is hereditary and autosomally dominant (BOWEN and DAVISON 1975; TERRY 1976); its typical choreatic hyperkinesias come about through degeneration of the corpus striatum and cerebral fits are no rarity. The so-called choreophrenia comprising personality change, apathy, affective instability, paranoid disturbances, and dementia often leads to suicide. Aphasia is not to be found, while mutism on the other hand not rare. Age of manifestation is clearly presenile (30–45 years) and the course slowly progressive over 12–15 years.

Normal pressure hydrocephalus (6%) is diagnosed more often after the introduction of computer-assisted tomography. Psychopathological features are slight memory disturbances, which are not initial symptoms, and lack of thoughts; focal signs are missing. The differential diagnosis is made neurologically by proof of spastic atactic gait disorders and urine incontinency. Therapy is surgical by ventriculoatrial shunt (SALMON 1969; KATZMAN and KARASU 1975; GOSCH 1976) and successful in 39%–64% of all cases (LAUTER 1980). It is regarded as a primary dysfunction of the formatio reticularis and presents no neocortical changes (JACOBS et al. 1978; TORACK 1978).

Cardiovascular diseases (8%) constitute one of the most important groups for differential diagnosis of SD since they are common, similar, and in 10%–55% of all cases (TOMLINSON et al. 1970; LAUTER 1972; HUGHES 1978; KATZMAN et al. 1978 b; LOEB 1980) combined with primary brain atrophy. Despite the proof that primary brain atrophy is more often the cause of dementing syndromes during senium (51%–90%), many clinicians still favor the assumption of vascular origin (GERHARD 1969; LAUTER 1972; GESCHWIND 1978; STEEL and FELDMAN 1979).

In the case of multiple tiny cerebral infarcts, MID is observed (HACHINSKI et al. 1974; WELLS 1978; LOEB 1980; GOLDENBERG and SAMEC 1981); if one or more of the big extracranial neck arteries is affected, the term "macrovascular" dementia is used, if small intracranial arteries and arterioles are struck, the term "microvascular" dementia.

Depending on the underlying disease, hypertensive, diabetic, hyperuricemic, hyperlipidemic, or immunological vascular changes are met with. Differential diagnosis is made possible through vertigo (vertebrobasilar insufficiency), hemiplegia, and neurological focal signs (carotid insufficiency), headache and nocturnal ex-

Table 2. Clinical differential diagnosis of primary vascular and primary atrophic dementia during senium

Vascular	Atrophic
Abilities to cope with new requirements worsen intermittently and remittently (BLESSED, in ROBERTS 1980). Acute onset, primary personality, social acceptability and insight are preserved better. Affective instability, predominantly depressive, early neurological signs (BIRKETT 1972). Nocturnal exacerbation, marked fluctuations (ANDERSON 1970). Subjective complaints like headache, vertigo, sleep disorders, fatigability (LAUTER 1972). Circumscribed focal signs, pseudo-bulbar palsy; hypertension, coronary heart disease, diabetes, hyperlipidemia not unusual (ROTH 1978). Men affected more often	Abilities to cope with new requirements worsen progressively and steadily (BLESSED, in ROBERTS 1980). SLOW onset, more severe mental deterioration, memory and attention significantly and consistently worse, paranoid symptoms, hallucinations (BIRKETT 1972; PEREZ et al. 1975). Low Hachinski score (HACHINSKI et al. 1975; LADURNER et al. 1981). Highly abnormal EEG without focal signs (INGVAR et al. 1978), no low density lesions in CCT (LADURNER et al. 1981). More frequent during senium than vascular dementia, women affected more often (ROTH 1978a; HACHINSKI 1978)

acerbations (see Table 2). BRAND and GORWITZ (1971) pointed out that prognosis in vascular dementias does not necessarily have to be more favorable than in SD.

Endocrine disorders are represented by thyropathy – myxedema and hyperthyroidism – (less than 1%) and metabolic disorders by liver failure (ammoniacal encephalopathy) (less than 1%). More common are vitamin deficiencies: Lack of vitamin B_1 especially as a consequence of alcoholism, often combined with Wernicke-Korsakov syndrome (6%) and lack of vitamin B_{12} with funicular myelosis (less than 1%). Of increasing importance are chronic intoxications and addiction (3%); of decreasing importance (less than 1%) is general paralysis. Conditions after infectious cerebral diseases were found in less than 1%, space-occupying processes in 5%, chronic subdural hematoma and hygroma and subarachnoid hemorrhage in less than 1%, traumatic lesions and epilepsies in less than 1%, involutional depression in 4%, and other psychiatric disorders in less than 1% in BERGER'S (1979) group. Only in 3% of all the 222 cases could the cause of the dementia not be determined.

Under the term "pseudodementia," heterogenous disorders such as neurotic and psychotic disorders, are thrown together, especially endogenous depression and schizophrenic defects (BIRREN 1959; WELLS 1979; ROTH 1978a). Since the word is also used for exaggeration and simulation of an intellectual deficit and has no true connection with endogenous disorders and SD (LARSSON et al. 1963; TOMLINSON et al. 1970), the ambiguous term should be abandoned (SHRABBER 1980).

F. Pathology and Future Developments

The congophilic angiopathy or amyloid microangiopathy is sometimes found in the brains of demented persons. So far the importance of this observation is difficult to estimate from the neuropathological and clinical point of view. It seems that a unique disease entity is indicated here. Familiar occurrence with cerebellar symptoms, involvement mainly of the occipital lobe, sometimes only of the layers II and IV of the cortex, and the array of amyloid around small vessels with projections to senile plaques, in 25% of the neurofibrillary tangles, are the main reasons in favor of this opinion (Torack 1978, Ulrich et al. 1973).

Senile plaques are mainly observed in the frontal and temporal lobes but also in the cerebellum, brain stem, basal ganglia, and white matter. They are composed of an amyloid core and a surrounding of thickened neurites and destructed organelles. Presently it is assumed that they can either be formed "endogenously," e.g., in analogy to animal experiments by damaging the neurite. An "exogenous" factor also seems to exist in connection with the vascular system. The process possibly begins with an interruption of the flow in dendrites, terminal axons, and synapses. The neurite thickens and is dilated by masses of organelles (Weiss 1961). A neuritic plaque (Wisniewski and Terry 1973), the early form of a senile plaque, originates. Later the amyloid is probably composed of neurofilaments and a mature plaque emerges. In this context some ultrastructural changes of the synapses were explicable. The fibrous astrocytes represent a glious reaction, whereas the microglia could also produce amyloid. Perivascular plaques without neuritic affection suggest another, vascular genesis of senile plaques (Torack 1975, 1978). Tomlinson et al. (1968; Tomlinson 1977) have elucidated the importance of senile plaques. He found, that 14 or more plaques per low-power field are a strong indicator of dementia.

Furthermore the neurofibrillary tangles, bifilar helices of 130-Å filaments (Wisniewski et al. 1976) characterize SDAT. Two ways of development are discussed:

A disturbance in the synthesis of fibrous proteins or of the environmental conditions for their aggregation. An excess production of filaments, answering a distant vulneration of the axon or dendrite (Torack 1978).

Lipofuscin in the neuron increases with age; there has never been any pathogenetical importance to this observation. Especially in senile dementia the pigmentation of neuronal cells represents normal aging. Only in CJD and in Huntington's disease have indications for an involvement of lipofuscin in neuronal degeneration so far been observed (Torack 1969, 1971, 1978; Tellez-Nagel et al. 1973).

The pathogenetical importance of granulovacuolar degeneration, a membrane-bound cytoplasmatic body (Woodard 1962), has also not yet been understood (Scheibel 1979; Torack 1978; Terry 1979). It is found mainly in pyramidal cells of the hippocampus of demented persons. Similarly the bodies described by Hirano et al. (1968) can only be mentioned here.

Scheibel (1978, 1979) emphasizes the importance of the dendritic system, which by its diminution also diminishes the synaptic connectivity of the areas involved. He indicates therefore an eventual loss of processing capabilities despite the known redundancy of neuronal systems. This theory is based on investigations of pyramidal cells in the cortex of senile dements. A deterioration of neuronal plasticity as a pathophysiological substrate of dementia is also postulated by Selkoe and Shelanski (1976), and by Hayflick (1976).

Neurochemical investigations of late have found a marked loss of choline acetyltransferase (CAT), consistent with a loss of presynaptic terminals and cholinergic cell bodies (ROBERTS 1980). The monoaminergic, the acetylcholinergic, and the GABA system are likely to be affected (GOTTFRIES 1980; REISINE et al. 1978). While it is known that there is a significant relationship between the degree of clinical psychic deficiency and the degree of neuropathological alterations (TOMLINSON 1980), a good correlation with levels of cholinergic neurotransmitter enzymes and with the CAT level in the brain could be added to these findings (PERRY et al. 1978, BLESSED 1980; ROBERTS 1980; PERRY and PERRY 1981).

The question of whether the complex AD-SDAT comprises one or several disease entities, could gain additional answers from further epidemiological investigations of already-known populations such as Lundby, Newcastle, or Framingham and from transcultural comparisons. We already have results from Japan (MATSUYAMA and NAKAMURA 1978). Analytical epidemiology can be of great help searching for risk factors, e.g., virus exposition, aluminum, or genetic causes. Chromosome 21 is of special interest because of parallels between AD and Down's syndrome (HESTON 1977). Chromosome 16 being the site of the gene responsible for Haptoglobin Hp^1, which seems to be augmented in AD-SDAT, is also important (STAM and OP DEN VELDE 1978). Indications toward a lack of transmitters, especially cholinergic, rend future neurobiochemical and neuropharmacological investigations rather interesting (MCGEER 1978; DAVIES 1978). The role of aluminum, also, needs further clarification. We need more knowledge about its site and mode of action. Hypotheses about a viral genesis of SDAT (GAJDUSEK and GIBBS 1975), based on animal experiments, so far lack confirmation (JOHNSON 1979). The latest progress in ultrastructural research (TERRY 1979) might promote new results, e.g., on relations between morphological findings and possibly noxious agents such as aluminum, viruses, malnutrition, or on correlations between morphometry and psychopathometry. Immunology also promises further results. There seems to be a correlation between diminution in immunoglobulins and impaired cerebral function (EISDORFER et al. 1978).

G. Treatment

Considering the poor prognosis of senile dementia we must currently confess that there are very few possibilities of influencing the process of neuronal loss. There are more therapeutical approaches in functional brain disturbances than in dementia, for which no accepted treatment exists to date (BAN 1980).

Three reasons for drug therapy in patients with senile dementia have to be mentioned:

First of all the treatment of disturbances in the cardiovascular system, in metabolic conditions, and in endocrinological dysfunctions, as well as in all the multitude of other diseases, which are summarized under the term multimorbidity, can sometimes influence directly the formal etiopathogenesis of senile dementia. Only a few elderly patients have a single complaint or a single disease managed by a single drug; usually several drugs are taken simultaneously.

On the other hand, there is a group of various agents in the treatment of senile dementia which act according to several pathophysiological concepts: nootropic, psychoenergetic, or antihypoxidotic drugs. They are designed to influence CBF and cerebral metabolism. Theoretical concepts are based mainly on vasodilatation, antithrombotic effects, increase of glucose permeation into the neuronal cells, and metabolic stimulation. These various substances – acetylcholine precursors, vincamine, piracetam, centrophenoxin, bencyclan, kallikrein, adamantine, naftidrofuryl, pyritinol, dihydrogenated ergot alkaloids, nicergoline, and vasopressin – (GIURGEA and SALAMA 1978; KUGLER 1975; VENN 1980; CORRODI et al. 1973; GAITZ and HARTFORD 1980; KUGLER et al. 1978; KÜNKEL and WESTPHAL 1970; KUGLER et al. 1975; QUADBECK 1962) are more or less successfully used in vascular and functional brain disease.

Many investigations have indicated a therapeutic efficacy. Unfortunately, ameliorations of dementia syndromes observed so far have only been temporary. Vasoactive drugs might be of some therapeutic value where there is a vascular deficiency. However, these substances and reconstructive arterial surgery appear unlikely to be of much value in the treatment of dementia (ROBERTS 1980). For example, methylxanthinderivatives, naftidrofuryl, vincamine, kallikrein, and papaverine are primarily effective in this way (SATHANANTHAN and GERSHON 1975). Therefore possible impairments of neuronal energy metabolism in the demented brain ought to be considered. A number of drugs have been investigated therapeutically, such as the purported stimulators of cerebral metabolism, e.g., piracetam, dihydrogenated ergot alkaloids, centrophenoxin, and vincamine. However, none of these treatments has so far proved conspicuously successful. Neuroendocrinology in psychoactive drug evaluation in the elderly should be especially considered.

It is evident that most psychotropic substances exert their main effect on behavior through limbic system neurotransmitters, hypothalamic neuropeptides, and endocrine target organ hormones (LIPTO et al. 1978; WURTMAN and RERNSTRON 1976; ORDY et al. 1981). The recently reported significant serum prolactininhibitory effects of hydergine suggest that it may exert major effects on mental dopaminergic activity (CLEMENS and FULLER 1978). Dopamine acts as the major prolactininhibitory factor in the hypothalamus (BÜRKI et al. 1968; MACLEOD 1976).

Finally, the therapeutic possibilities of concomitant syndromes in SD are as manifold as the symptoms themselves. Therapeutic efforts in secondary symptomatic appearances – general psychovegetative disorders, depressive states, paranoid-hallucinatory syndromes, states of psychomotor agitation, sleep disturbances, and neurological symptoms like vertigo, tinnitus, and spasticity – often prove effective and reduce the patient's complaints.

A depressive state caused by senile dementia in our view should first be treated with a benzodiazepine. The antinociceptive effect (WIECK 1980b; BLAHA 1981), especially of the later developed derivatives often calms down tears, excitement, and psychovegetative disturbances and relieves indirectly the depressive mood. If there is no success or the state is severe, one of the new tetracyclic or the other new antidepressant drugs – maprotilin, mianserin, trazodone, nomifensin, viloxazin – may be of additional help. These substances have proved the antidepressant efficacy with less or lacking side effects to cardiovascular and cholinergic systems. Tricyclic antidepressants should be given very cautiously because of their higher rate of side effects (BLAHA 1978; BAN 1980). Paranoid-hallucinatory syndromes and states of excitement require neuroleptic therapy. The indication for high-potency neuroleptics in productive symptoms and low-potency neuroleptics in mere psychomotor agitation can be differentiated. Always the lowest successful dose should be given; butyrophenonderivatives are less complicated by cardiovascular irritations. Sometimes benzodiazepines with more or less sedative properties may prove favorable especially in excited patients. In cases of delirious symptomatology, clomethiazol is effective and well tolerated by older people. But also, depending on the experiences of the physician in charge, neuroleptics or diazepam may be given (BLAHA 1978; STOTSKY 1975). Treatment of sleep disturbances in patients with SD proves quite successful with benzodiazepines and neuroleptics with a sedative and hypnotic component. Chloralhydrat is indicated in isolated difficulties in falling asleep.

With drug treatment in higher-aged groups specific problems have to be considered (SALZMAN et al. 1975; GREENBLATT and SHADER 1981; ISRAILI and WENGER 1981; JELLINGER 1980).

Rarely a patient takes medication exactly the way it is prescribed. The main reason is forgetfulness of the sick elderly patient. A way of improving compliance could be prescription of scheduled drug packages. Another problem is given by the pharmacokinetic changes in the elderly concerning absorption, distribution, metabolism, excretion, altered sensitivity of receptors, and change of the physiological equilibrium of transmitters. Remarkably little information is available on the kinetics of drugs in the elderly, yet adverse drug reactions occur seven times more often in this age group than in persons of the 3rd decade (JARVIK et al. 1981). Absorption is changed by the activity of the intestine, its blood flow, and the physicochemical characteristics. The alteration in distribution is caused by the changes in body composition, in plasma proteins, and in blood flow. Metabolism in elderly is influenced by a decrease of hepatic blood flow, which may decrease drug metabolism (HOLLISTER 1981; GREENBLATT and SHADER 1981) and other factors such as liver enzymes, which diminish by age. Data supporting impaired drug metabolism in the elderly are available for only a few drugs, and many show no impairment (HOLLISTER 1981). Renal function also steadily decreases during life. So drugs with renal excretion should be given cautiously (TOZER 1974). Altered receptor sensitivity is difficult to demonstrate experimentally, but it is a well-recognized clinical phenomenon. Older patients may show toxic confusional states on hypotensive crises following doses of anticholinergic drugs that are well tolerated by younger persons. At any rate the altered susceptibility of the atrophied brain has to be considered (LEHMANN 1972; OCHS 1981). Drugs are only part of the general therapeutic scheme in a multifactorial onset. For instance, sociotherapy in senile dementia is important and should be directed toward accommodation in familiar surroundings, protection against risk of self-damage and least possible restriction (KAUFMANN 1981).

Nowadays a multidisciplinary approach including not only physicians and nurses, but also psychologists and social workers is regarded as the best way to cope with this unfavorable condition (RADEBOLD et al. 1981; OESTERREICH and STETTER 1981; BERGENER 1980).

References

Ackelsberg SB (1944) Vocabulary and mental deterioration in senile dementia. J Abnorm Soc Psychol 39:393–406

Ajuriaguerra J de, Tissot R (1968) Some aspects of psycho-neurologic disintegration in senile dementia. In: Müller C, Ciompi L (eds) Senile dementia. Huber, Bern Stuttgart, pp 69–79

Ajuriaguerra J de, Dias Cordeiro J, Steeb U, Fot K, Tissot R, Richard J (1979) A propos de la désintégration des capacites d'anticipation des déments dégeneratifs du grand âge. Neuropsychologia 7:301–311

Ajuriaguerra J de, Muller M, Tissot R (1960) A propos de quelques problèmes posés par l'apraxie dans les démences. Rev Neurol 102:640–642

Ajuriaguerra J de, Rego A, Tissot R (1963) Le réflexe oral et quelques activités orales dans les syndromes démentiels du grand âge. Encephale 52:189–219

Ajuriaguerra J de, Kluser JP, Velghe J, Tissot R (1965) Praxies idéatoires et permanence de l'objet. Quelques aspects de leur désintégration conjointe dans les syndromes démentiels du grand âge. Psychiat Neurol 150:306–319

Akesson HO (1969) A population study of senile and arteriosclerotic psychoses. Hum Hered 19:546–566

Albert E (1964a) Zur Kenntnis der senilen Demenz. Acta Psychiat Scand 40:287–306

Albert E (1964b) Senile Demenz und Alzheimersche Krankheit als Ausdruck des gleichen Krankheitsgeschehens. Fortschr Neurol Psychiatr 32:625–673

Albert E (1965) Das Bild der Altersdemenz in initialen und fortgeschrittenen Stadien. Internist Prax 5:447–454

Albert E (1968) On the nosology of senile dementia. In: Müller C, Ciompi L (eds) Senile dementia. Huber, Bern Stuttgart, pp 33–34

Albert ML (1978) Subcortical dementia. In: Katzman R, Terry RD, Bick KL (eds) Alzheimer's disease: Senile dementia and related disorders (Aging, vol 7). Raven, New York, pp 173–180

Alexander DA (1972) "Senile Dementia": A changing perspective. Br J Psychiatry 121:207–214

Alexandrowskaja MM (1965) Altersbesonderheiten des Gehirns und damit verbundene Erkrankungen. In: Proceedings 7th international congress of gerontology, Vienna/Austria, June 26–July 2, 1966, Clinical Medicine. Open and special papers, Tom. 3. Wiener Medizinische Akademie, Wien

Allison RS (1962) The senile brain – A clinical study. Arnold, London

Alsen V (1980) Psychopathologie der Defektsyndrome. In: Wieck HH (ed) Somatische Psychosen. Tropon, Köln, pp 52–62

Alsen V (1981) Vaskulär bedingte Wesensänderung und Demenz. Lecture held at the ninth „Fortbildungsveranstaltung in Neurologie und Psychiatrie", April 11th 1981, Erlangen

Alzheimer A (1907) Über eine eigenartige Erkrankung der Hirnrinde. Allg Z Psychiatr 64:146–148

Anderson JP (1970) A study of disturbed behaviour in patients with dementia in two hospital populations. Geront Clin 12:49–64

Angel RW (1977) Understanding and diagnosing senile dementia. Geriatrics 32:47–49

Angst J, Battegay R, Bente D, Berner P, Broeren W, Cornu F, Dick P, Engelmeier MP, Heimann H, Heinrich K, Helmchen H, Hippius H, Pöldinger W, Schidlin P, Schmitt W, Weis P (1969) Das Dokumentationssystem der Arbeitsgemeinschaft für Methodik und Dokumentation in der Psychiatrie (AMP). Arzneim Forsch 19:399–405

Annexton M (1978) Treatable brain diseases in the elderly. JAMA 240:1325–1329

Anonymous (1977) Cardiogenic dementia. Lancet 8001:27–28

Arab A (1960) Unité nosologique entre démence sénile et maladie d'Alzheimer d'après une étude statistique et anatomo-clinique. Sist Nerv 12:189–201

Ban TA (1980) Psychopharmacology for the aged. Karger, Basel München Paris London New York Sydney

Barker MG, Lawson JS (1968) Nominal aphasia in dementia. Br J Psychiatr 114:1351–1356

Barnes RH, Busse EW, Friedman EL (1956) The psychological functioning of aged individuals with normal and abnormal electroencephalograms. II. A study of hospitalized individuals. J Nerv Ment Dis 124:585–593

Barron SA, Jacobs L, Kinkel WR (1976) Changes in size of normal lateral ventricles during aging by comuterized tomography. Neurology 26:1011–1013

Barstein EI (1970) Problems of interrelations between Alzheimer's disease and senile dementia (in Russian). Zh Nevropathol Psikhiatr 70:1242–1246

Barwich D (1976) Symmetrische Stammhirnganglienverkalkungen (Morbus Fahr) und ihr familiäres Vorkommen. Nervenarzt 47:253–257

Bender L (1938) A visual motor Gestalt test and its clinical use. Am Orthopsychiatr Ass Res Monog 3

Benson FD (1979) Neurologic correlates of anomia. In: Whitaker H, Whitaker HA (eds) Studies in neurolinguistics, vol 4. Academic Press, New York San Francisco London, pp 293–326

Benton AL, Spreen O (1972) Handbuch zum Benton-Test. Huber, Bern Stuttgart

Bergener M (1969) Über den Begriff der Demenz - hirnorganisches Syndrom oder psychopathologisches Dogma? Verh Dtsch Ges Inn Med 75:1003–1006

Bergener M (Hrsg) (1978) Mehrdimensionale Psychiatrie. Janssen, Düsseldorf

Bergener M (1980) Alzheimersche Erkrankung – Krankheit sui generis oder psychopathologisches Syndrom? Fortschr Med 98:1001–1007

Bergener M, Jungklaass FK (1970) Genetische Befunde bei Morbus Alzheimer und seniler Demenz. Gerontol Clin 12:71–75

Bergener M, Gerhard L, Husser J (1972) Klinische und morphologische Untersuchungen über eine familiäre Altershalluzinose. Nervenarzt 43:18–33

Berger EY (1980) A system for rating the severity of senility. J Am Geriatr Soc 28:234–236

Berger JP (1979) A propos des démences traitables et du concept d'artériosclérose cérébrale. Rev Med Suisse Romande 99:325–331

Bergeron M, Hanus M (1964) Les états démentiels réversibles. Ann Med Psychol 122:529–553

Bergmann K (1976) The epidemiology of senile dementia. Br J Psychiatry, Spec 9:100–109

Bertelsen E, Wimmer A (1919) Fokalsymptomer ved senil demens. Hospitalstidende 62:421–431

Berzewski H, Selbach H (1970) Neuropsychiatrische Geriatrie: Diagnostik und Therapie. Internist 11:244–250

Birkett DP (1972) The psychiatric differentiation of senility and arteriosclerosis. Br J Psychiatry 120:321–325

Birren JE (1959) Handbook of aging and the individual. University of Chicago Press, Chicago

Blaha L (1978) Behandlungsprobleme in der Gerontopsychiatrie. In: Flügel KA (Hrsg) Neurologische und psychiatrische Therapie. Perimed, Erlangen, pp 397–402

Blaha L (Hrsg) (1981) Psychovegetative Allgemeinstörungen – Diagnose, Therapie und Grundlagen. IMP, Frankfurt

Blass JP (1980) Metabolic dementias. In: Amaducci L, Davison AN, Antuono P (eds) Aging of the brain and dementia. Aging, vol 13. Raven, New York

Blessed G (1980) Clinical aspects of senile dementias. In: Roberts PJ (ed) Biochemistry of dementia. Wiley, Chichester New York Brisbane Toronto, pp 1–14

Blessed G, Tomlinson BE, Roth M (1968) The association between quantitative measures of dementia and of senile change in the grey matter of elderly subjects. Br J Psychiatry 114:797–811

Bleuler E (1915) Die senilen Psychosen. Correspondenz-Blatt für Schweizer Ärzte 45:2–14

Bleuler E (1975) Lehrbuch der Psychiatrie. 13. Auflage. Springer, Berlin Heidelberg New York

Bollerup TR (1975) Prevalence of mental illness among 70 year olds domiciled in nine Copenhagen suburbs. Acta Psychiatr Scand 51:327–340

Bonhoeffer K (1917) Die exogenen Reaktionstypen. Arch Psychiatr 58:58

Bowen DM, Davison AN (1975) Extrapyramidal diseases and dementia. Lancet 7917:1199–1200

Bower HM (1971) The differential diagnosis of dementia. Med J Aust 2:623–626

Brain WR (1977) Brain's diseases of the nervous system. Rev by Walton JN. Oxford University Press, Oxford New York Toronto, 8th ed

Brand FM, Gorwitz K (1971) Relationship of cerebrovascular disease to senile, presenile, and cerebral arteriosclerotic dementia. J Chron Dis 24:569–583

Brody EM, Kleban M, Woldow A, Freeman L (1975) Survival and death in the mentally impaired aged. J Chron Dis 28:389–399

Brückmann J-U (1981) Epidemiologische Aspekte der zerebrovaskulären Insuffizienz. In: Wieck HH, Blaha L (Hrsg) Zerebrovaskuläre Insuffizienz. Perimed, Erlangen, p 13

Brückmann J-U, Blaha L (1980) Zur Problematik der psychopathometrischen Erfassung leichterer Formen der cerebralen Hypoxidose. Vortrag auf dem 9. Internationalen Symposion zur Koordinierung der neurologischen Wissenschaften, Graz 26.–28. Juni 1980

Bürki HR, Asper H, Ruch E, Züger P (1968) Bromocriptine, dihydroergotoxine, methysergide, d-LSD, CF 25–397 and CM 29–712: Effects on the metabolism of the biogenetic amines in the brain of the rat. Psychopharmacology 57:227–237

Burstein SR (1946) Gerontology: A modern science with a long history. Postgrad Med J 22:185–190

Busse EW, Obrist WD (1963) Significance of focal electroencephalographic changes in the elderly. Postgrad Med 34:179–182

Caltagirone C, Gainotti G, Masullo C, Micell G (1970) Validity of some neuropsychological tests in the assessment of mental deterioration. Acta Psychiatr Scand 60:50–56

Cantone G, Orsini A, Grossi D, Michele G de (1978) Verbal and spatial memory span in dementia (An experimental study of 185 subjects). Acta Neurol 33:175–183

Cattell RP (1963) The theory of fluid and crystallized intelligence: A critical experiment. Educ J Psychol 54:1–22

Chase TN, Wexler NS, Barbeau A (1979) Huntington's disease. Advances in neurology, vol 23. Raven, New York

Ciompi L (1972) Allgemeine Psychopathologie des Alters. In: Kisker KP, Meyer J-E, Müller M, Strömgren E (eds) Psychiatrie der Gegenwart – Forschung und Praxis, Bd II/2, Klinische Psychiatrie II. 2. Aufl. Springer, Berlin Heidelberg New York, pp 1001–1036

Ciompi L (1973) Demenz, senile. In: Müller C (ed) Lexikon der Psychiatrie. Springer, Berlin Heidelberg New York, pp 97–98

Ciompi L, Kanowski S (1977) Dokumentationssystem der Arbeitsgemeinschaft für Geronto-Psychiatrie (AGP-System). In: CIPS: Internationale Skalen für Psychiatrie. CIPS, Berlin

Clemens JA, Fuller RW (1978) Chemical manipulation of some aspects of aging. Adv Exp Med Biol 97:187–206

Clouston TS (1884) Clinical lectures on mental disease. Lea & Son, Philadelphia

Coblentz JM, Mattis S, Zingesser LH, Kasoff ES, Wisniewski HM, Katzman R (1973) Presenile dementia. Arch Neurol 29:299–308

Conrad K (1947) Über Struktur- und Gestaltwandel. Dtsch Z Nervenheilk 158:344

Conrad K (1947) Über den Begriff der Vorgestalt und seine Bedeutung für die Hirnpathologie. Nervenarzt 18:289

Constantinidis J (1968) Correlations between the age of onset of dysmnesia and the degree of cerebral degeneration. In: Müller C, Ciompi L (eds) Senile dementia. Huber, Bern Stuttgart, pp 29–33

Constantinidis J (1978) Is Alzheimer's disease a major form of senile dementia? Clinical, anatomical, and genetic data. In: Katzman R, Terry RD, Bick KL (eds) Alzheimer's disease: Senile dementia and related disorders (Aging, vol 7). Raven, New York

Constantinidis J, Garrone G, Tissot R, Ajuriaguerra J de (1965) The familial incidence of Alzheimer's cortical neurofibrillar alterations. Psychiat Neurol 150:235–247

Constantinidis J, Richard J, Tissot R (1974) Pick's disease. Histological and clinical considerations. Eur Neurol 11:208–217

Corrodi H, Fuxe K, Hökfelt T, Lidbrink P, Ungerstedt U (1973) Effect of ergot drugs on central catecholamine neurons: Evidence for a stimulation of central dopamine neurons. J Pharmacol 25:409–412

Corsellis JAN (1962) Mental illness and the aging brain. Maudsley Monograph 9. University Press, Oxford London

Corsellis JAN, Bruton CJ, Freeman-Browne (1973) The aftermath of boxing. Psychol Med 3:270–303

Critchley M (1964) The neurology of psychotic speech. Br J Psychiatr 110:353–364

Dahl G (1972) Reduzierter Wechsler-Intelligenztest (WIP). Hain, Meisenheim

Davies P (1978) Studies on the neurochemistry of central cholinergic systems in Alzheimer's disease: In: Katzman R, Terry RD, Bick KL (eds) Alzheimer's disease: Senile dementia and related disorders. Raven Press, New York, pp 453

Deisenhammer E, Jellinger K (1971) EEG- und morphologische Korrelationen bei organischen Demenzen. Electroenceph clin Neurophysiol 31:529

Demeurisse G, Demol O, Ganty C (1979) Semiological value of the palmo-mental reflex in vascular hemiplegia. Eur Neurol 18:66–72

DeRenzi E, Vignolo LA (1962) The Token Test: A sensitive test to detect receptive disturbances in aphasics. Brain 85:665–678

Diesfeldt HFA (1978) The distinction between long-term and short-term memory in senile dementia: An analysis of free recall and delayed recognition. Neuropsychologia 16:115–119

Dooling EC, Schoene WC, Richardson EP (1974) Hallervorden-Spatz syndrome. Arch Neurol 30:70–83

Eastman M (1978) Senility: The "diagnostic wastebasket." Am Pharm 18:53

Eisdorfer C, Cohen D, Buckley CE III (1978) Serum immunoglobulins and cognition in the impaired elderly. In: Katzman R, Terry D, Bick KL (eds) Alzheimer's disease: Senile dementia and related disorders. Raven Press, New York, p 401

Epstein L, Simon A, Mock R (1964) Clinical neuropathologic correlations in senile and cerebral arteriosclerotic psychoses. In: Hansen PF (eds) Old age with a future. Munksgaard, Kopenhagen, p 272

Erbslöh F, Kohlmeyer K (1974) Diffuse und umschriebene Großhirnatrophien. In: Bodechtel G (ed) Differentialdiagnose neurologischer Krankheitsbilder. Thieme, Stuttgart

Ernst B, Dalby MA, Dalby A (1970a) Luria testing in demented patients. Acta Neurol Scand (Suppl) 46:97–98

Ernst B, Dalby MA, Dalby A (1970b) Aphasic disturbances in presenile dementia. Acta Neurol Scand (Suppl) 46:99–100

Ernst B, Dalby A, Dalby MA (1970c) Gnostic-praxic disturbances in presenile dementia. Acta Neurol Scand (Suppl) 46:101–102

Erzigkeit H (1977) Manual zum Syndrom-Kurztest. Vless, Vaterstetten

Esquirol JED (1827) Esquirol's allgemeine und spezielle Pathologie und Therapie der Seelenstörungen, frei bearb. v. Hille KC. Hartmann, Leipzig

Essen-Möller E (1956) Individual traits and morbidity in a Swedish rural population. Acta Psychiatr Scand 31 (Suppl 100)

Eysenck MD (1945) A study of certain qualitative aspects of problem solving behaviour in senile dementia patients. J Ment Sci 91:337–345

Feigenson JS (1978) Definition of dementia. Stroke 9:523

Feldman P, Cameron DE (1944/45) Speech in senility. Am J Psychiatry 101:64–67

Ferraro A (1967) Senile psychoses. In: Arieti S (ed) American Handbook of psychiatry, vol 2. Kolb, New York

Ferris S, Crook T, Sathananthan G, Gershon S (1976) Reaction time as a diagnostic measure in senility. J Am Geriatr Soc 24:529–533

Fischer O (1910) Die presbyophrene Demenz, deren anatomische Grundlage und klinische Abgrenzung. Z Gesamte Neurol Psychiatr 3:371–471

Fischer O (1912) Ein weiterer Beitrag zur Klinik und Pathologie der presbyophrenen Demenz. Z Gesamte Neurol Psychiatr 12:99–134

Foerster K, Regli F (1980) Zur Ätiologie dementieller Syndrome. Fortschr Neurol Psychiatr 48:207–219

Folstein MF, Folstein SE, McHugh PR (1975) Mini-mental state: A practical method for grading the cognitive state of patients for the clinician. J Psychiatr Res 12:189–198

Fox JH, Topel JL, Huckman MS (1975) Dementia in the elderly – a search for treatable illnesses. J Gerontol 30:557–564

Fürstner (1889) Über die Geistesstörungen des Senium. Arch Psychiatr Nervenkr 20:459–472

Fuld PA (1978) Psychological testing in the differential diagnosis of the dementias. In: Katzman R, Terry RD, Bick KL (eds) Alzheimer's disease: Senile dementia and related disorders (Aging, vol 7). Raven Press, New York, pp 185–193

Fuller S (1911) A study of miliary plaques found in brains of the aged. Am J Ins 68:10–217
Gainotti G, Catagirone C, Masullo C, Miceli G (1980) Patterns of neuropsychologic impairment in various diagnostic groups of dementia. In: Amaducci L, Davison AN, Antuono P (eds) Aging of the brain and dementia. Aging vol 13. Raven, New York
Gaitz CHM, Hartford JT (1980) Ergots in treatment of mental disorders of old age. In: Goldstein M, Calne DB, Liebermann A, Thomer O (eds) Ergot compounds and brain function. Raven Press, New York, pp 349–356
Gajdusek DC, Gibbs CJ (1975) Slow virus infections of the nervous system and the labaratories of slow, latent and temperate virus infections. In: Chase TN, Tower DB (eds): the nervous system, vol 2: The clinical neurosciences. Raven Press, New York
Gedye JL, Exton-Smith AN, Wedgwood J (1972) A method for measuring mental performance in the elderly and its use in a pilot clinical trial of meclofenoxate in organic dementia (preliminary communication). Age Ageing 1:74–80
Gerhard L (1969) Morphologische Befunde zur Differentialdiagnose „Cerebralsklerose" und senile Demenz. In: Seifert G (ed) Alterns- und Aufbrauchkrankheiten des Gehirns. Fischer, Stuttgart, pp 164–174
Gerson IM, John ER, Bartlett F, Koenig V (1976) Average evoged response in the electroencephalographic diagnosis of the normally aging brain: A practical application. Electroencephalogr Clin Neurophysiol 77–91
Geschwind N (1978) Organic problems in the aged: Brain syndromes and alcoholism – discussion. J Geriatr Psychiatry 11:161–166
Giurgea C, Salama M (1978) Nootropic drugs. Prog Neuro-Psychopharmacol 1:235–247
Götze P (1980) Psychopathologie der Herzoperierten. Enke, Stuttgart
Goldenberg G, Samec P (1981) Zur Differentialdiagnose vaskulär bedingter dementieller Syndrome. Nervenarzt 52:405–414
Goldfarb AI (1969) Predicting mortality in the institutionalized aged: A seven year followup. Arch Gen Psychiatry 2:172–176
Gosch HH (1976) Normal pressure hydrocephalus – a treatable cause of dementia. J Fla Med Assoc 63:863–864
Gottfries CG (1980) Amine metabolism in normal ageing and in dementia disorders. In: Roberts PJ (ed) Biochemistry of dementia. Wiley & Sons, Chichester New York Brisbane Toronto, p 213
Greenblatt DJ, Shader RJ (1981) Pharmacokinetics in old age: Principles and problems of assessment. In: Jarvik LF, Greenblatt DJ, Harman D (eds) Clinical pharmacology and the aged patient. Aging vol 16. Raven Press, New York, pp 1–9
Griesinger W (1876) Die Pathologie und Therapie der psychischen Krankheiten. 4. Aufl. Wreden, Braunschweig
Grosch H (1948) Klinisch-hirnpathologische Studien bei der Alzheimerschen und Pickschen Krankheit. Arch Psychiatr Nervenkr 118:568–598
Grossi D, Orsini A, Michele G de (1978) The copying of geometric drawings in dementia. Acta neurol 33:355–360
Gruenberg EM (1961) A mental health survey of older persons. In: Hoch PH, Zubin J (eds) Comparative epidemiology of the mental disorders. Grune and Stratton, New York
Gruenberg EM (1978) Epidemiology. In: Katzman R, Terry RD, Bick KL (eds) Alzheimer's disease: Senile dementia and related disorders. Raven Press, New York, p 323
Grünthal E (1936) Die präsenilen und senilen Erkrankungen des Gehirnes und des Rückenmarkes. In: Bumke O, Foerster O (eds) Handbuch der Neurologie, Bd 11. Traumatische, präsenile und senile Erkrankungen, Zirkulationsstörungen. Springer, Berlin, pp 466–509
Gruhle HW (1956) Verstehende Psychologie, 2. Aufl. Thieme, Stuttgart
Güntz T (1874) Über Dementia senilis. Allg Zeitschr Psychiatr 30:102–109
Gyldensted C, Kosteljanitz M (1975) Measurements of the normal hemispheric sulci with computer tomography: A preliminary study on 44 adults. Neuroradiology 10:147–149
Haase GR (1971) Diseases presenting as dementia. In: Wells CE (ed) Dementia. Blackwell, Oxford, pp 163–208
Hachinski VC (1977) Labioauricular reflex. Lancet Feb 12

Hachinski VC (1978) Cerebral blood flow: Differentiation of Alzheimer's disease from multi-infarct dementia. In: Katzman R, Terry RD, Bick KL (eds) Alzheimer's disease: Senile dementia and related disorders (Aging, vol 7). Raven, New York

Hachinski VC, Lassen NA, Marshall J (1974) Multi-infarct dementia. A cause of mental deterioration in the elderly. Lancet 874:207–210

Hachinski VC, Iliff LD, Zhilka E, duBoulay GHD, McAllister VC, Marshall J, Russell RWR, Symon L (1975) Cerebral blood flow in dementia. Arch Neurol 32:632–637

Hagnell O (1970) Disease expectancy and incidence of mental illness among the aged. Acta Psychiatr Scand 46 (Suppl 219):83–89

Hamster W, Langner W, Mayer K (1980) TÜLUC-Neuropsychologische Untersuchungsreihe. Beltz, Weinheim

Hare M (1978) Clinical check list for diagnosis of dementia. Br Med J 6132:266–267

Hayflick L (1976) Theories of biological aging. In: Scheinberg P (ed) Cerebrovascular diseases. Tenth Princeton Conference, Raven Press, New York

Heilbronner (1900) Über die Beziehungen zwischen Demenz und Aphasie. Arch Psychiatr Nervenkr 33:366–392

Hersch EL, Kral VA, Palmer RB (1978) Clinical value of the London Psychogeriatric Rating Scale. J Am Ger Soc 26:348–354

Hersch EL, Merskey H, Palmer RB (1980) Prediction of discharge from a psychogeriatric unit. Can J Psychiatry 25:234–241

Heston LL (1977) Alzheimer's disease. Trisomy 21, and myeloproliferative disorders: Associations suggesting a genetic diathesis. Science 196:322–332

Hibbard TR, Migliaccio JN, Goldstone S, Lhamon WT (1975) Temporal information processing by young and senior adults and patients with senile dementia. J Gerontol 30:326–330

Hirano A, Dembither HM, Jurland LT, Zimmerman HM (1968) The fine structure of some intraganglionic alterations. J Neuropathol Exp Neurol 27:167–182

Hoff H (1956) Lehrbuch der Psychiatrie. Bd. 1. Schwabe, Basel Stuttgart

Hollister LE (1981) General principles of treating the elderly with drugs. In: Jarvik LF, Greenblatt DJ, Harman D (eds) Clinical pharmacology and the aged patient. Aging vol 16. Raven Press, New York, pp 1–9

Hontela S, Schwartz G (1979) Myocardial infarction in the differential diagnosis of dementias in the elderly. J Am Geriatr Soc 27:104–106

Horenstein S (1971 a) Amnestic, agnosic, apractic, and aphasic features in dementing illness. In: Wells CE (ed) Dementia. Blackwell, Oxford, pp 35–60

Horenstein S (1971 b) The clinical use of psychological testing in dementia. In: Wells CE (ed) Dementia. Blackwell, Oxford, pp 61–80

Horst L van der (1964) Psychiatric deviations in older people. In: Hansen PF (ed) Age with a future. Munksgaard, Kopenhagen, pp 67–73

Hoyer S (1980) Factors influencing cerebral blood flow, CMR-oxygen and CMR-glucose in dementia patients. In: Roberts PJ (ed) Biochemistry of dementia. Wiley, Chichester New York Brisbane Toronto, p 252

Huber G (1962) Typen und Korrelate psychoorganischer Abbau-Syndrome. In: Kranz H (ed) Psychopathologie heute. Thieme, Stuttgart

Huber G (1972) Hirnatrophische Prozesse im mittleren Lebensalter. Münchner Med Wschr 114:429–436

Huber G (1976) Klinik und Psychopathologie der organischen Psychosen. In: Kisker HP, Meyer JE, Müller M, Strömgren E (Hrsg) Psychiatrie der Gegenwart, Bd II, 2. Aufl. Springer, Berlin Heidelberg New York

Huber G (1980) Psychopathologie reversibler Syndrome körperlich begründbarer Psychosen. In: Das ärztliche Gespräch, Bd XXIX Tropon, Köln, p 21

Huckman MS, Fox J, Topel J (1975) The validity of criteria for the evaluation of cerebral atrophy by computed tomography. Radiology 116:85–92

Hughes CP (1978) The differential diagnosis of dementia in the senium. In: Nandy K (ed) Senile dementia: A biomedical approach. Elsevier, p 201–208

Hughes W (1959) Presbyophrenia. Gerontol Clin 1:107–113

Ikeda K, Hori A, Bode G (1980) Progressive dementia with "diffuse Lewy-type inclusions" in cerebral cortex. Arch Psychiatr Nervenkr 228:243–248

Ingvar DH, Brun A, Hagberg B, Gustafson L (1978) Regional cerebral blood flow in the dominant hemisphere in confirmed cases of Alzheimer's disease, Pick's disease, and multi-infarct dementia: Relationship to clinical symptomatology and neuropathological findings. In: Katzman R, Terry RD, Bick KL (eds) Alzheimer's disease: Senile dementia and related disorders (Aging, vol 7). Raven, New York

Irigaray L (1967) Approche psycho-linguistique du langage des déments. Neuropsychologia 5:25–52

Irigaray L (1973) Le langage des déments. Mouton, The Hague

Irigaray L, Dubois J (1966) Les structures linguistiques de la parenté et leurs perturbations dans les cas de démence et de schizophrénie. Cahiers de Lexicologie 8:47–69

Isaacs B, Caird FI (1976) "Brain failure:" A contribution to the terminology of mental abnormality in old age. Age Ageing 5:241–244

Israili ZH, Wenger J (1981) Aging, gastrointestinal disease and response to drugs. In: Jarvik LF, Greenblatt DJ, Harman D (eds) Clinical pharmacology and the aged patient. Aging vol 16. Raven Press, New York, pp 1–9

Jacob H (1969) Psychiatrische Aspekte der Alterns- und Aufbrauchkrankheiten des Gehirns. In: Seifert G (ed) Alterns- und Aufbrauchkrankheiten des Gehirns. Fischer, Stuttgart, pp 21–32

Jacobs L, Kinkel WR, Painter F, Murawski J, Heffner RR (1978) Computerized tomography in dementia with special reference to changes in size of normal ventricles during aging and normal pressure hydrocephalus. In: Katzman R, Terry RD, Bick KL (eds) Alzheimer's disease: Senile dementia and related disorders (Aging, vol 7). Raven, New York

Jakob H (1979) Die Picksche Krankheit. Springer, Berlin Heidelberg New York

Jana DK, Romano-Jana L (1973) Hypernatremic psychosis in the elderly: Case reports. J Am Geriatr Soc 21:473–477

Jarvik LF (1978) Genetic factors and chromosomal aberrations in Alzheimer's disease, senile dementia and related disorders. In: Katzman R, Terry RD, Bick KL (eds) Alzheimer's disease: Senile dementia and related disorders. Raven Press, New York, p 273

Jarvik LF, Greenblatt DJ, Harman D (eds) (1981) Clinical pharmacology and the aged patient. Aging vol 16. Raven Press, New York

Jarvik LF, Blum JE (1971) Cognitive declines as predictors of mortality in twin pairs. A twenty year longitudinal study of aging. In: Palmore E, Jeffers FC (eds) Prediction of life span. D C Heath Co, Lexington, Ky

Jaspers K (1973) Allgemeine Psychopathologie. 9. unveränderte Aufl. Springer, Berlin Heidelberg New York

Jastak JF, Jastak SR (1965) The wide range achievement test. Wilmington, Guidance Associates

Jellinger K (1980) Besonderheiten der Psychopharmakotherapie im Alter. Aktuel Gerontol 10:291–304

Johnson RT (1979) Viral etiology in amentias and dementias. In: Katzman R (ed) Congenital and acquired cognitive disorders Raven Press, New York, p 177

Jones HE, Kaplan OJ (1956) Psychological aspects of mental disorders in later life. In: Kaplan OJ (ed) Mental disorders in later life, 2 nd edn. Standford University Press, Standford, pp 98–156

Jonsson C-O, Mälhammar G, Waldton S (1976) Abnormalities in the orienting response in senile dementia. Acta Psychiatr Scand 54:323–332

Jonsson C-O, Mälhammar G, Waldton S (1977) Reflex elicitation thresholds in senile dementia. Acta Psychiatr Scand 55:81–96

Kahn RL, Goldfarb AI, Pollack M, Peck A (1960) Brief objective measures for the determinations of mental status in the aged. Am J Psychiatr 117:326–328

Kallmann FJ (1956) Genetic aspects of mental disorders in later life. In: Kaplan OJ (ed) Mental disorders in later life. Standford, Standford Univ

Kaplan OJ (1979) Psychological testing of seniles. In: Kaplan OJ (ed) Psychopathology of aging. Academic Press, New York London Toronto Sydney San Francisco, pp 45–77

Kaszniak AW, Fox J, Gandell DL, Garron DC, Huckman MS, Ramsey RG (1978) Predictors of mortality in presenile and senile dementia. Ann Neurol 3:246–252

Kaszniak AW, Garron DC, Fox J (1979) Differential effects of age and cerebral atrophy upon span of immediate recall and paired-associate learning in older patients suspected of dementia. Cortex 15:285–295

Katzman R, Karasu TB (1975) Differential diagnosis of dementia. In: Fields WS (ed) Neurological and sensory disorders in the elderly. Stratton, New York, pp 103–132

Katzman R, Terry RD, Bick KL (1978a) Alzheimer's disease: Senile dementia and related disorders (Aging, vol 7). Raven, New York

Katzman R, Terry RD, Bick KL (1978b) Recommendations of the nosology, epidemology, and etiology and pathophysiology commissions of the Workshop-Conference on Alzheimer's disease – senile dementia and related disorders. In: Katzman R, Terry RD, Bick KL (eds) Alzheimer's disease: senile dementia and related disorders (Aging, vol 7). Raven, New York

Kaufmann R (1981) Care for gerontopsychiatric patients by a multidisciplinary outpatient-station. Z Gerontol 14:40–46

Kay DWK (1970) Senility. Commun Health 2:127–132

Kay DWK (1972) Epidemiological aspects of organic brain disease in the aged. In: Gaitz CM (ed) Aging and the brain. Plenum Press, New York, p 15

Kay DWK, Beamish P, Roth M (1964) Old age mental disorders in Newcastle upon Tyne. Br J Psychiatry 110:146–148

Kay DWK, Bergmann K, Garside RF (1966) Proceedings of the IVth World Congress of Psychiatry Abstr 610, Excerpta Medica Int Congress series, 117. Excerpta Medica Foundation, Amsterdam

Kent S (1977) Classifying and treating organic brain syndromes. Geriatrics 32:87–96

Kimura D (1963) Right temporal lobe damage. Arch Neurol 8:264–271

Kinzel W (1972) Eine Verfahrensweise zur Trennung rückbildungsfähiger und nicht mehr rückbildungsfähiger seelischer Veränderungen körperlich begründbarer Psychosen. Psychiat Clin 5:367–379

Kinzel W (1973) Psychopathometrie des organischen Defektsyndroms. In: Wieck HH (ed) Angewandte Psychopathometrie. Janssen, Düsseldorf, pp 114–137

Kinzel W (1979) Die Notwendigkeit der Unterscheidung von Funktionspsychose und Defektsyndrom. In: Erzigkeit H, Lehrl S, Blaha L, Heerklotz B (eds) Messung und Meßverfahren in der Psychopathologie. Vless, München, pp 119–131

Kinzel W, Galster JV, Erzigkeit H, Lambrecht W (1979) Besteht ein Zusammenhang zwischen dem Schweregrad des psychischen Defektsyndroms nach Hirnkontusion und der Intelligenzleistung? Fortschr Neurol Psychiat 47:67–83

Kleemeier RW (1962) Intellectual change in the senium. In: Proceedings of the Social Statistics Section of the American Statistics Association 290–295

Kolk BA van der (1978) Organic problems in the aged: Brain syndromes and alcoholism – discussion. J Geriatr Psychiatr 11:167–170

Kooi KA, Guvener AM, Tupper CJ, Bagehi BK (1964) Electroencephalographic patterns of the temporal region in normal adults. Neurology 14:1029–1035

Kosaka K, Mehraein P (1979) Dementia-Parkinsonism syndrome with numerous Lewy bodies and senile plaques in cerebral cortex. Arch Psychiatr Nervenkr 226:241–250

Kraepelin E (1910) Psychiatrie. Ein Lehrbuch für Studierende und Ärzte. 8. Aufl, 2. Bd. Klinische Psychiatrie, 1. Teil. Barth, Leipzig, pp 593–632

Kral VA (1972) Somatic therapy in old age. In: Kisker KP, Meyer JE, Müller M (eds) Psychiatrie der Gegenwart – Forschung und Praxis, Band II/2 Klinische Psychiatrie II, 2. Aufl. Springer-Verlag, Berlin Heidelberg New York, pp 1159–1172

Künkel H, Westphal M (1970) Quantitative EEG-analysis of the pyrithioxine action. Pharmakopsychiat 3:41–49

Kugler J (1975) Die Beeinflussung von Vigilanz und Bewußtsein durch Aminoadamantansulfat. Acta Neurol 2:43–51

Kugler J, Schichtl R, Empt J (1975) The influence of kallikrein on the vigilance in the EEG. In: Haberland GL, Rohen JW, Blümel G, Huber P (eds): Kininogenases. Schattauer, Stuttgart New York

Kugler J, Oswald WD, Herzfeld U, Seus R, Pingel J, Welzel D (1978) Langzeittherapie altersbedingter Insuffizienzerscheinungen des Gehirns. Dtsch med Wschr 103:456–462

Ladurner G, Bertha G, Pieringer W, Lytwin H, Lechner H (1981) Klinische Unterscheidungskriterien bei vaskulärer (Multiinfarkt-) und primär degenerativer Demenz (Alzheimer). Nervenarzt 52:401–404

Lang C (1981) Aphasietestung mit psychometrischen Verfahren. Fortschr Neurol Psychiat 49:164–178

Langley GE (1977) Confusion in the elderly. Lancet, Feb 5

Larner S (1977) Encoding in senile dementia and elderly depressives: A preliminary study. Br J Soc Clin Psychol 16:379–390

Larsson T, Sjögren T, Jacobson G (1963) Senile dementia, a clinical sociomedical, and genetic study. Acta Psychiat Scand 39 (Suppl), 1–257

Lauter H (1968) Zur Klinik und Psychopathologie der Alzheimerschen Krankheit. Erhebungen an 203 pathologisch-anatomisch verifizierten Fällen. Psychiat Clin 1:85

Lauter H (1972) Organisch bedingte Alterspsychosen. In: Kisker KP, Meyer J-E, Müller M, Strömgren E (eds) Psychiatrie der Gegenwart – Forschung und Praxis, Band II/2, Klinische Psychiatrie II, 2. Aufl. Springer, Berlin Heidelberg New York, pp 1103–1142

Lauter H (1980) Gerontopsychiatrie – die somatische Dimension. In: Kanowski S (ed) Gerontopsychiatrie. Tropon, Köln, pp 7–54

Lauter H, Meyer JE (1968) Clinical and nosological concepts of senile dementia. In: Müller C, Ciompi L (eds) Senile dementia. Huber, Bern Stuttgart, pp 13–26

Lawson JS, Barker MG (1968) The assessment of nominal dysphasia in dementia: The use of reaction-time measures. Br J Med Psychol 41:411–414

Lehmann HE (1972) Psychopharmacological aspects of geriatric medicine. In: Gaitz CM (ed) Aging and the brain. Advances in behavioral biology, vol 3. Plenum Press, New York London, pp 193–208

Lehrl S (1977) Mehrfachwahl-Wortschatz-Intelligenztest. Manual zum MWT-B. Straube, Erlangen

Lehrl S, Fuchs HH, Lugauer J, Schumacher H, Nusko G (1977) Manual zur Funktionspsychose-Skala-B. Vless, Vaterstetten

Lehrl S, Blaha L, Brückmann J-U (1980) Möglichkeiten zur Differenzierung von Funktionspsychosen und Defektsyndromen mit psychopathometrischen Verfahren. Vortrag auf dem 9. Internationalen Symposion zur Koordinierung der neurologischen Wissenschaften, Graz, 26.–28. Juni 1980

Levert F (1907) Contribution à l'étude des psychoses de l'involution sénile et aliénation mentale. Diss, Paris

Liepmann H (1915) Diseases of the brain. In: Barr CW (ed) Curschmann's textbook on nervous diseases, vol 1. Blakiston, Philadelphia, pp 467–551

Lipto MA, DiMascio A, Killam KF (1978) Psychopharmacology: A generation of progress. Raven Press, New York

Livesly B (1976) In: Action and ageing – Proceedings of Sandoz Symposium held at Basle, p 54

Loeb C (1980) Clinical diagnosis of multiinfarct dementia. In: Amaducci L, Davison AN, Antuono P (eds) Aging of the brain and dementia. Aging vol 13. Raven, New York

Lorr M, McNair DM, Klett CJ, Lasky JJ (1963) Inpatient multidimensional psychiatric scale. Consulting Psychologists Press, Palo Alto

Lungershausen E (1980) Fragen der Abgrenzung zwischen Defekt und reversiblen Syndromen. In: Wieck HH (ed) Somatische Psychosen. Tropon, Köln, pp 92–102

MacLeod RM (1976) Regulation of prolactin seretion. In: Mortini L, Ganong WF (eds) Frontiers in neuroendocrinology, vol 4. Raven Press, New York, pp 169–194

Marchand L, Demay G, Naudascher J (1942) Démence sénile simple, précoce et dégénérescence neurofibrillaire d'Alzheimer. Ann Med Psychol 100:338–341

Marcuse H (1904) Apraktische Symptome bei einem Fall von seniler Demenz. Centralbl f Nervenheilk Psychiat 27:737–751

Matsuyama H, Nakamura S (1978) Senile changes in the brain in the Japanese: Incidence of Alzheimer's neurofibrillary change and senile plaques. In: Katzman R, Terry RD,

Bick KL (eds) Alzheimer's disease: Senile dementia and related disorders. Raven Press, New York, p 287

Mattis S (1976) Dementia rating scale. In: Bellak R, Karasu B (eds) Geriatric psychiatry. Grune & Stratton, New York, pp 108–121

Maudsley H (1868) The physiology and pathology of mind. MacMillan, London

Mayer-Gross W, Slater E, Roth M (1969) Clinical psychiatry. 3rd ed. Bailliere, Tindall and Cassell, London

McDonald C (1969) Clinical heterogeneity in senile dementia. Br J Psychiatr 115:267–271

McGeer EG (1978) Aging and neurotransmitter metabolism in the human brain. In: Katzman R, Terry RD, Bick KL (eds) Alzheimer's disease: Senile dementia and related disorders. Raven Press, New York, p 427

McGhie A (1969) Psychology of attention. In: Vinken PJ, Bruyn GW (eds) Handbook of clinical neurology, vol. 3. Elsevier North Holland Publishing Co. Amsterdam New York p 137

McHugh PR, Folstein MF (1979) Psychopathology of dementia: Implications for neuropathology. In: Katzman R (ed) Congenital and acquired cognitive disorders. Raven Press, New York, p 17-1

McMenemey WH (1968) Present concepts of Alzheimer's disease. In: Bailey OT, Smith DE (eds) Central nervous system. Some experimental models of neurological disease. Williams and Wilkins, Baltimore, pp 201–208

Meese W, Grumme Th (1980) Die Beurteilung hirnatrophischer Prozesse mit Hilfe der Computertomographie. Fortschr Neurol 48:494–509

Meggendörfer F (1925) Über familiengeschichtliche Untersuchungen bei arteriosklerotischer und seniler Demenz. In: Zentralbl Ges Neurol Psychiatr 40:359

Meyendorf R (1976) Hirnembolie und Psychose. J Neurol 213:163–177

Meyer LE, Pudel V, Husziarik-Felgendreher M (1980) Zum Eßverhalten im höheren Lebensalter. Nervenarzt 51:493–497

Mignot H (1950) Problèmes diagnostiques et nosologiques. Compt Rend Séances 2:288–306

Miller E (1974) Dementia as an accelerated ageing of the nervous system: Some psychological and methodological considerations. Age Ageing 3:197–202

Miller E, Lewis P (1977) Recognition memory in elderly patients with depression and dementia: A signal detection analysis. J Abnorm Psychol 86:84–86

Miller M (1977) Abnormal aging: The psychology of senile and presenile dementia. Wiley, New York

Müller C, Ciompi L (1968) Senile dementia – clinical and therapeutic aspects. Huber, Bern Stuttgart

Müller M (1975) Ein einfaches Hilfsmittel (Bildertest) zur Prüfung der mnestischen Funktionen. Nervenarzt 46:467–471

Mulder DW (1976) Organic brain syndromes associated with diseases of unknown cause. In: Freedman AM, Kaplan HI, Sadock BJ (eds) Comprehensive textbook of psychiatry – II, vol 1, 2nd ed. Williams and Wilkins, Baltimore

Mundy-Castle AC, Hurst LA, Beerstecher DM, Pinsloo T (1953) The electroencephalogram in the senile psychoses. Electroencephalogr Clin Neurophysiol 6:245–252

Nandy K (ed) (1978) Senile dementia: A biomedical approach. Elsevier, New York

Nandy K, Sherwin I (eds) (1977) The aging brain and senile dementia. Plenum, New York

Neville HJ, Folstein MF (1979) Performance on three cognitive tasks by patients with dementia, depression or Korsakov's syndrome. Gerontology 25:285–290

Newton RD (1948) The identity of Alzheimer's disease and senile dementia and their relationship to senility. J Ment Sci 94:225–249

Nielsen J (1962) Geronto-psychiatric period-prevalence investigation in a geographically delimited population. Acta Psychiatr Scand 38:307–330

Nielsen J (1968) Chromosomes in senile dementia. Br J Psychiatry 115:303–309

Norio R, Koskiniemi M (1979) Progressive myoclonus epilepsy: Genetic and nosological aspects with special reference to 107 finnish patients. Clin Genet 15:382–398

Obrist WD (1951) The electroencephalogram of normal male subjects over age 75. J Gerontol Suppl to No 3, 2nd. Ant Geriat Cong, September, p 130

Obrist WD (1972) EEG and intellectual function in the aged. Electroencephal. Clin Neurophysiol 33:253

Ochs HR (1981) Arzneimitteldosierung im Alter. Med Welt 32:225

Oesterreich K, Stetter G (1981) Caseworker's intervention during gerontopsychiatric stationary treatment. Z Gerontol 14:69–74

Ordy HM, Brizzeee KR, Bartus RT (1981) Neuropsychopharmacology: Drug modification of memory in relation to aging in human and nonhuman primate brain. In: Jarvik LF, Greenblatt DJ, Harman D (eds) Clinical pharmacology and the aged patient. Aging vol 16. Raven Press, New York, pp 79–102

Orme JE (1957) Non-verbal and verbal performance in normal old age, senile dementia, and elderly depression. J Gerontol 12:408–413

Oswald WD (1980) Das Nürnberger-Alters-Inventar NAI als psychometrische Methode der klinischen Pharmakologie. Vortrag aus dem 7. Rothenburger Gespräch am 6./7.11.1980. Sandoz, Nürnberg

Oswald WD, Roth E (1978) Der Zahlen-Verbindungs-Test ZVT. Verlag für Psychologie, Göttingen

Parker JC Jr (1972) The old age syndrome: Subtle cerebral degeneration and bronchopneumonia. Geriatrics 27:94–102

Paulson GW (1977) The neurological examination in dementia. Contemp Neurol Ser 15:169–188

Pearce J, Miller E (1973) Clinical aspects of dementia. Bailliere Tindall, London

Peck A, Wolloch L, Rodstein M (1978) Mortality of the aged with chronic brain syndrome II. In: Katzman R, Terry RD, Bick KL (eds) Alzheimer's disease: Senile dementia and related disorders. Raven Press, New York, p 299

Peress NS, Kone WX, Aronson SM (1968) Central nervous system findings in a tenth decade autopsy population. In: Wolstenholme GEW, O'Connor MO (eds) Churchill, London, p 473

Perez FI, Gay JR, Taylor RL, Rivera VM (1975) Patterns of memory performance in the neurologically impaired aged. Can J Neurol Sci 2:347–355

Perez FI, Rivera VM, Meyer JS, Gay JRA, Taylor RL, Mathew NT (1975) Analysis of intellectual and cognitive performance in patients with multi-infarct dementia, vertebrobasilar insufficiency with dementia, and Alzheimer's disease. J Neurol Neurosurg Psychiatr 38:533–540

Perez FI, Stump DA, Wray RE, Gay JRA, Bannon MR, Meyer JS (1977) Automated behavioral assessment system: Precise measurement of memory performance in cerebrovascular disease. Stroke 8:140

Perez FI, Gay JRA, Cooke NA (1978) Neuropsychological aspects of Alzheimer's disease and multi-infarct dementia. In: Nandy K (ed) Senile dementia: A biomedical approach. Elsevier, New York, pp 185–199

Perry EK, Tomlinson BE, Blessed G, Bergmann K, Gibson PH, Perry RH (1978) Correlation of cholinergic abnormalities in the senile plaques and mental test scores in senile dementia. Brit Med J 2:1457–1465

Perry EK, Perry RH (1981) Cerebral neurotransmitter and neuropeptide activities in Alzheimer's disease. Proc III rd World Congress Biol. Psychiatry, Stockholm, 28 th June–3 rd July 1981. Elsevier/North Holland Co, New York, to be published

Pfeiffer E (1975) A short portable mental status questionnaire for the assessment of organic brain deficit in elderly patients. J Am Ger Soc 23:433–441

Pfeiffer E (1978) Clinical manifestations of senile dementia. In: Nandy K (ed) Senile dementia: A biomedical approach. Elsevier, New York, pp 171–183

Pick A (1892) Über die Beziehungen der senilen Hirnatrophie zur Aphasie. Prager Medizinische Wochenschrift 17:165–167

Pick A (1906) Über einen weiteren Symptomenkomplex im Rahmen der Dementia senilis, bedingt durch umschriebene stärkere Hirnatrophie (gemischte Apraxie). Monatsschr Psychiatr Neurol 19:97–108

Pick E (1958) Kritische Betrachtungen zur Diagnose „Senile Demenz". In: Doberauer W (ed) Medizinische und soziale Altersprobleme. Wien, pp 217–222

Pilleri G (1961 a) Orale Einstellung nach Art des Klüver-Bucy-Syndroms bei hirnatrophischen Prozessen. Schweiz Arch Neurol Neurochir Psychiatr 87:286–298

Pilleri G (1961 b) Über das chronologische Auftreten von motorischen Schablonen des Oralsinnes, deren ontogenetische Bedeutung und klinisch-anatomische Zusammenhänge bei atrophisierenden Hirnerkrankungen. Schweiz Arch Neurol Psychiatr 88:273–298

Plum F (1978) Metabolic dementias. In: Katzman R, Terry RD, Bick KL (eds) Alzheimer's disease: Senile dementia and related disorders (Aging vol 7). Raven Press, New York

Plutchik R, Conte H, Liverman M, Bakur M, Grossman J, Lehrman N (1976) 040 PLUT, Plutchik geriatric rating scale. In: Guy W (ed) ECDEU Assessment manual for psychopharmacology. National Institute of Mental Health, Rockville

Portnoi VA (1979) Thyrotoxicosis as a mimic of dementia and/or stroke-like syndrome. Postgrad Med 66:219–221

Primrose EJR (1962) Psychological illness – a community study. Maudsley Monograph No 3. Tavistock, London

Quadbeck G (1962) Der Einfluß von Pyrithioxin auf die Blut-Hirnschranke. J Med Exp 7:144

Rabinowicz T (1972) Neuropathologie: In: Kisker KP, Meyer J-E, Müller M, Strömgren E (eds) Psychiatrie der Gegenwart – Forschung und Praxis, Band II/2, Klinische Psychiatrie II, 2. Aufl. Springer, Berlin Heidelberg New York, pp 1059–1076

Radebold H, Bechtler H, Pina I (1981) Therapeutic approach in social work? Impact of social therapy in working with the elderly. Z Gerontol 14:61–67

Raskin N, Ehrenberg R (1956) Senescence, senility, and Alzheimer's disease. Am J Psychiatry 113:133–137

Raskind MA, Kitchell M, Alvarez C (1978) Bromide intoxication in the elderly. J Am Geriatr Soc 26:222–224

Redlich FC, Freedman DX (1976) Theorie und Praxis der Psychiatrie, Band 2. Suhrkamp, Frankfurt am Main

Reisine TD, Yamamura HI, Bird ED, Spokes E, Enna SJ (1978) Pre- and postsynaptic neurochemical alterations in Alzheimer's disease. Brain Res 159:477–481

Reisner TH, Zeiler K, Strobl G (1980) Quantitative Erfassung der Seitenventrikelbreite im CT – Vergleichswerte einer Normalpopulation. Fortschr Neurol Psychiat 48:168–174

Roberts PJ (1980) Summary: Dementia – its biochemistry and prospects for a rational pharmacological approach. In: Roberts PJ (ed) Biochemistry of dementia. J Wiley, Chichester New York Brisbane Toronto, p 263

Robinson RA (1977) Differential diagnosis and assessment in brain failure. Age Ageing (Suppl) 6:42–49

Roth M (1955) The natural history of mental disorder in old age. J Ment Sci 101:289–301

Roth M (1978 a) Diagnosis of senile and related forms of dementia. In: Katzman R, Terry RJ, Bick KL (eds) Alzheimer's disease: Senile dementia and related disorders. Raven Press, New York, p 71

Roth M (1978 b) Epidemiologic studies. In: Katzman R, Terry RD, Bick KL (eds) Alzheimer's disease: Senile dementia and related disorders. Raven Press, New York, p 337

Rothschild D (1937) Pathologic changes in senile psychoses and their psychobiologic significance. Am J Psychiatry 93:757–785

Rothschild D (1941) The clinical differentiation of senile and arteriosclerotic psychoses. Am J Psychiatry 98:324–333

Salmon JH (1969) Senile and presenile dementia. Geriatrics 24:67–72

Salzman C, Shader RI, Harmatz JS (1975) Response of the elderly to psychotropic drugs: Predictable or idiosyncratic? In: Gershon S, Raskin A (eds) Aging, vol 2. Raven Press, New York, pp 259–272

Sathananthan GL, Gershon S (1975) Cerebral vasodilators: A review. In: Gershon S, Raskin A (eds) Aging, vol 2. Raven Press, New York, pp 155–168

Savage RD (1977) Intellect and personality in the aged. In: Smith WL, Kinsbourne M (eds) Aging and dementia. Spectrum Publications, New York

Scheibel AB (1978) Structural aspects of the aging brain: Spine systems and the dendritic arbor. In: Katzman R, Terry RD, Bick KL (eds) Alzheimer's disease: Senile dementia and related disorders. Raven Press, New York, p 353

Scheibel AB (1979) Dendritic changes in senile and presenile dementias. In: Katzman R (ed) Congenital and acquired cognitive disorders. Raven Press, New York, p 107

Scheid W (1962) Die Lehre von den „exogenen Reaktionstypen" vor einem halben Jahrhundert und heute. In: Kranz H (Hrsg) Psychopathologie heute. Thieme, Stuttgart, p 205

Scheid W (1980) Lehrbuch der Neurologie. Thieme, Stuttgart

Scheller H (1965) Über den Begriff der Demenz und unterscheidbare klinische Formen von Demenzen. Nervenarzt 36:1–7

Schneider K (1966) Klinische Psychopathologie. 7. Aufl. Thieme, Stuttgart

Selkoe DJ, Shelanski ML (1976) Neurochemistry of aging. In: Scheinberg P (ed) Cerebrovascular diseases. Tenth Princeton Conference. Raven Press, New York

Shenkin HA, Greenberg J, Bouzarth WF, Gutterman P, Morales JO (1973) Ventricular shunting for relief of senile symptoms. J Am Med Assoc 225:1486–1489

Sheridan FP, Yeager CL, Oliver WA, Simon A (1955) Electroencephalography as a diagnostic and prognostic aid in studying the senescent individual. A preliminary report. J Gerontol 10:53–59

Sishta SK, Troupe A, Marszalek KS, Kremer LM (1974) Huntington's chorea: An electroencephalographic and psychometric study. Electroencephal Clin Neurophysiol 36:387–393

Shibayama H, Hoshino T, Kobayashi H, Iwase S, Takenouchi Y (1978) An autopsy case of atypical senile dementia with atrophy of the temporal lobes – a clinical and histopathological report. Folia Psychiatr Neurol Jpn 32:285–298

Shrabber D (1980) Questioning the concept of pseudodementia. Am J Psychiatr 137:260

Sjögren T, Sjögren HS, Lindgren GH (1952) Morbus Alzheimer and morbus Pick. A genetic, clinical, and pathoanatomical study. Acta Psychiatr Neurol Scand (Suppl 82) p 1

Slater E, Cowie V (1971) The genetics of mental disorders. Oxford University Press, London

Smith WL, Kinsbourne M (eds) (1977) Aging and dementia. Spectrum, New York

Sourander P, Sjögren H (1970) The concept of Alzheimer's disease and its clinical implications. In: Wolstenholme GEW, O'Connor ME (eds) Alzheimer's disease and related conditions. Churchill, London, pp 11–32

Spatz H (1938) Die „systematischen Atrophien". Eine wohlgekennzeichnete Gruppe der Erbkrankheiten des Nervensystems. Arch Psychiatr Nervenkr 108:1–18

Spoerri T (1965) Über Dialogslalie bei Altersdemenz. Akt Fragen Psychiat Neurol 2:175–181

Spreen O (1963) Manual zum MMPI Saarbrücken. Huber, Bern

Stam FC, Op den Velde W (1978) Haptoglobin types in Alzheimer's disease and senile dementia. In: Katzman R, Terry RD, Bick KL (eds) Alzheimer's disease: Senile dementia and related disorders. Raven Press, New York, p 279

Stammler A (1980) Nosologie der Funktionspsychosen. In: Das ärztliche Gespräch, Bd XXIX. Tropon, Köln, p 37

Steel K, Feldman RG (1979) Diagnosing dementia and its treatable causes. Geriatrics 34:79–88

Stengel E (1964a) Speech disorders and mental disorders. In: DeReuck AVS, O'Connor M (eds) Disorders of language. Churchill, London, pp 285–292

Stengel E, (1964b) Psychopathology of dementia. Proc R Soc Med 57:911–914

Sternberg H, Gawrilowa S (1978) Über klinisch-epidemiologische Untersuchungen in der sowjetischen Alterspsychiatrie. Nervenarzt 49:347–353

Steuer J, Bank L, Olsen EJ, Jarvik LF (1980) Depression, physical health and somatic complaints in the elderly: A study of the Zung self-rating depression scale. J Gerontol 35:683–688

Stotsky BA (1975) Psychoactive drugs for geriatric patients with psychiatric disorders. In: Gershon S, Raskin A (eds) Aging, vol 2. Raven Press, New York, pp 229-258

Synek V, Reuben JR, Du Boulay GM (1976) Comparing Evans' index and computerized axial tomography in assessing relationship of ventricular size to brain size. Neurology 26:231–233

Tellez-Nagel I, Kohnson AB, Terry RD (1973) Ultrastructural and histochemical study of cerebral biopsies in Huntington's chorea. Adv Neurol 1:387–398

Terry RD (1976) Dementia – a brief and selective review. Arch Neurol 33:1–4

Terry RD (1979) Ultrastructural changes and quantitative studies. In: Katzman R (ed) Congenital and acquired cognitive disorders. Raven Press, New York, p 99

Tissot R (1968) On the nosological identity of senile dementia and of Alzheimer's disease. In: Müller C, Ciompi L (eds) Senile dementia. Huber, Bern Stuttgart, pp 27–28

Tissot R, Richard J, Duval F, Ajuriaguerra J de (1967) Quelques aspects du langage des démences dégénératives du grand âge. Acta Neurol Psychiatr Belg 67:911–923

Todorov AB, Go RCP, Constantinidis J, Elston RC (1975) Specificity of the clinical diagnosis of dementia. J Neurol Sci 26:81–98

Tomlinson BE (1977) Morphological changes and dementia in old age. In: Smith WL, Kinsbourne M (eds) Aging and dementia. Spectrum, New York, pp 25–86

Tomlinson BE (1980) The structural and quantitative aspects of the dementias. In: Roberts JP (ed) Biochemistry of dementia. Wiley, Chichester New York Brisbane Toronto, p 15

Tomlinson BE, Blessed G, Roth M (1968) Observation on the brains of non-demented old people. J Neurol Sci 7:331–356

Tomlinson BE, Blessed G, Roth M (1970) Observations on the brains of demented old people. J Neurol Sci 2:205–242

Torack RM (1969) Ultrastructural and histochemical studies of cortical biopsies in subacute dementia. Acta Neuropathol 13:43–55

Torack RM (1971) Studies in the pathology of dementia. In: Wells C (ed) Dementia, the failing brain. F A Davis, Philadelphia

Torack RM (1975) Congophilic angiopathy complicated by surgery and massive haemorrhage. Am J Pathol 81:349–366

Torack RM (1978) The pathologic physiology of dementia. Springer, Berlin Heidelberg New York

Torvik A, Dietrichson P, Svaar H, Hudgson P (1974) Myopathy with tremor and dementia: A metabolic disorder? Case report with postmortem study. J Neurol Sci 21:181–190

Tosi C, Regli F, Wenk J (1980) Die Creutzfeldt-Jakobsche Krankheit. Fortschr Neurol Psychiat 48:353–384

Tozer TN (1974) Nomogram for modification of dosage regimens in patients with chronic renal functional impairment. J Pharmacokinet Biopharm 2:13–28

Trueblood CK (1935) The deterioration of language in senility. Psychol Bull 32:735

Ulrich G, Taghavy A, Schmidt H (1973) Zur Nosologie und Ätiologie der kongophilen Angiopathie. Z Neurol 206:39–59

Uyematsu S (1923) On the pathology of senile psychosis. The differential diagnostic significance of Redlich-Fischer's miliary plaques. J Nerv Ment Dis 57:1–25, 131–156, 243–260

Varsamis J, Zuchowski MS, Maini KK (1972) Survival rates and causes of death in elderly psychiatric patients: A six year follow-up study. Can Psychiatr Assoc J 17

Venn RD (1980) Review of clinical studies with ergots in gerontology. In: Goldstein M, Calne DB, Lieberman A, Thomer MO (eds) Ergot compounds and brain function. Raven Press, New York, pp 363–376

Victor M, Banker BQ (1978) Alcohol and dementia. In: Katzman R, Terry RD, Bick KL (eds) Alzheimer's disease: Senile dementia and related disorders (Aging, vol 7). Raven, New York, p 151

Waldton S (1974) Clinical observations of impaired cranial nerve function in senile dementia. Acta Psychiatr Scand 50:539–547

Wallace M (1971) Speech therapy with geriatric aphasia patients. In: Kastenbaum R (ed) New thoughts on old age. Springer, New York, pp 161–178

Wang HS (1978) Prognosis in dementia and related disorders in the aged. In: Katzman R, Terry RD, Bick KL (eds) Alzheimer's disease: Senile dementia and related disorders. Raven Press, New York, p 309

Wechsler D (1956) Die Messung der Intelligenz Erwachsener. Huber, Bern

Wechsler AF (1977) Presenile dementia presenting as aphasia. J Neurol Neurosurg Psychiatry 40:303–305

Weigl E, Goldstein K, Scheerer M (1945) Color form sorting test. Psychological Corporation

Weinstein E, Kahn R (1955) The denial of illnes. Charles C Thomas, Springfield, Ill.

Weiß E (1968) Die reine senile Demenz – eine Spätmanifestation der Alzheimerschen Krankheit? Diss. München

Weiss P (1961) The concept of perpetual neuronal growth and proximo-distal substance convection. In: Kety SS, Elkes J (eds) Regional neurochemistry. Pergamon Press, New York, pp 220–242

Weitbrecht HJ (1962) Zur Frage der Demenz. In: Kranz H (Hrsg) Psychopathologie heute. Thieme, Stuttgart, pp 221–233

Wells CE (1971) The symptoms and behavioral manifestations of dementia. In: Wells CE (ed) Dementia. Blackwell, Oxford, pp 1–11

Wells CE (1977) Dementia: Definition and description. Contemp Neurol Ser 15:1–14

Wells CE (1978) Role of stroke in dementia. Stroke 9:1–3

Wells CE (1979) Pseudodementia. Am J Psychiatry 136:895–900

Wever R (1975) Die Bedeutung der circadianen Periodik für den alternden Menschen. Verh Dtsch Ges Pathol 59:160–180

Wieck HH (1956) Zur Klinik der sogenannten symptomatischen Psychosen. Dtsch Med Wochenschr 81:1345–1349

Wieck HH (1962) Zur Analyse der Syndromgenese bei körperlich begründbaren Psychosen. In: Kranz H (Hrsg) Psychopathologie heute. Thieme, Stuttgart, p 212

Wieck HH (Hrsg) (1972) Klinische Psychopathometrie. Byk Gulden, Konstanz

Wieck HH (1973) Zur Psychopatometrie. In: Wieck H (ed) Angewandte Psychopathometrie. Janssen, Düsseldorf, pp 1–23

Wieck HH (1978) Lehrbuch der Psychiatrie. 2. Aufl. Schattauer, Stuttgart New York

Wieck HH (1980a) Merkmale der Funktionspsychose. In: Wieck HH (ed) Somatische Psychosen. Tropon, Köln, pp 12–20

Wieck HH (1980b) Diagnostik und therapeutische Situationen in der Sprechstunde. Schriftenreihe Bay Landesärztekammer 51:162–174

Wille (1873) Die Psychosen des Greisenalters. Allg Z Psychiat Psychisch-gerichtl Med 30:269–294

Wisniewski HM, Terry RD (1973) Reexamination of the pathogenesis of the senile plaque. In: Zimmerman HM (ed) Progress in neuropathology, vol 2. Grune and Stratton, New York, pp 1–26

Wisniewski HM, Narang HK, Terry RD (1976) Neurofibrillary tangles of paired helical filaments. J Neurol Sci 27:173–189

Wolstenholme GEW, O'Connor M (eds) (1970) Alzheimer's disease and related conditions. Churchill, London

Woodard JS (1962) Clinicopathologic significance of granulovacuolar degeneration in Alzheimer's disease. J Neuropathol Exp Neurol 21:85–91

Wurtman RJ, Rernstron JD (1976) Neuroendocrine affects on psychotropic drugs. In: Uschin E (ed) Hormons, behaviour and psychopathology. Raven Press, New York, pp 145–152

Yamaura H, Ito M, Kubota K, Matsuzawa T (1980) Brain atrophy during aging: A quantitative study with computed tomography. J Gerontol 35:492–498

Zangwill OL (1964) Psychopathology of dementia. Proc R Soc Med 57:914–917

Zerbin-Rüdin E (1972) Genetische Aspekte der Erkrankungen des höheren Lebensalters. In: Kisker KP, Meyer J-E, Müller M, Strömgren E (Hrsg) Psychiatrie der Gegenwart. Bd II/2, 2. Aufl, pp 1037–1058

Zutt J (1964) Was lehren uns die Demenzzustände über die menschliche Intelligenz. Nervenarzt 35:1–5

Alzheimer's Disease and its Clinical Implications

A. Brun

A. Definition of Alzheimer's Disease and Scope of Chapter

Alzheimer's disease (AD) may be defined clinicopathologically as a progressive presenile dementing organic brain disease, starting insidiously between 40 and 65 years of age. The dominant psychiatric symptoms are amnesia, apraxia, agnosia, and aphasia, the most prominent pathoanatomical correlate of which is cerebral atrophy with striking histological changes such as senile plaques and neurofibrillary degeneration.

Alois Alzheimer in a lecture in 1906 first presented the disease that was to bear his name and later published a more complete account (1907, 1911). It is striking how he was able to identify from a limited material most of its major features including the clinical picture. Thus he reported a bilaterally symmetrical cerebral atrophy that was most pronounced in the temporal and parietal lobes, less marked in the frontal lobes but spared the central areas. This pattern he found also to be parallelled by the distribution of senile plaques and neurofibrillary tangles, which latter structure he discovered. He also described other changes such as degeneration mainly of the superficial cortical layers, various forms of neuronal alterations and spongy degeneration. Since then many of these findings seem, however, to have been forgotten or neglected.

Alzheimer regarded the disease as separate from senile dementia. The question whether senile dementia of the Alzheimer type (SDAT) (dementia senilis alzheimerisata) and AD are separate diseases or not is still debated. Attempts or suggestions to separate the diseases have been made on structural and topographic (Shefer 1977; Sourander and Sjögren 1970; Scheibel 1979b), clinical (Roth 1971, Sjögren et al. 1952) or genetic (Larsson et al. 1963) grounds. The evidence has been regarded by others (Terry 1978a; Constantinidis 1978) as unconvincing. An epidemiological approach is recommended by Grufferman (1978). The delineation from ageing is equally unclear. Bowen et al. (1979), however, arrives at the conclusion that with its selective loss of cholinergic neurons AD is a primary degenerative nerve-cell disorder and not just simple premature ageing. Furthermore, aged brains do not always show senile plaques and tangles and in SDAT tangles may be missing.

By definition, AD and SDAT are presently mainly separated by age of onset, and also intensity of the degenerative process, differing thus rather on quantitative than on qualitative grounds. The three "conditions" AD, SDAT, and ageing may be regarded as facets of the same process (Constantinidis 1978) or AD and SDAT as the same disease regardless of age of onset (Neumann and Cohn 1978).

Among cases designated as AD there are some which do not conform to the majority with regard to main features and which are therefore set aside as atypical and treated separately. The main presentation to follow here concerns the great bulk of cases with AD conforming to the definition given above but not SDAT, which is treated in Chap. 8 in this volume, although structural and many clinical features are alike.

Our concept stems from experiences in a collaborative study on AD involving psychiatrists (L. GUSTAFSON), neuropsychologists (J. RISBERG and B. HAGBERG), neurophysiologists (D. H. INGVAR), and neuropathologists (A. BRUN) at the University of Lund in Sweden. AD and SDAT have been the subject of many extensive and elegant clinicopathological presentations through the years. During the last 10–15 years new techniques and new branches of basic medical science have tremendously expanded our knowledge in this and neighbouring fields. This has resulted in a vast literature, difficult to cover, ranging from e.g. bio- and histochemical, ultrastructural, virological, immunological, and cytogenetic research to neurophysiological, e.g. electroencephalographic and isotope-guided blood flow studies. This has led to important new findings and elucidation of many older problems. With reverence and reference to the older literature it will therefore be covered less thoroughly than recent writings.

B. Frequency and Sociomedical Importance

AD is the most common of all organic presenile dementias. The real prevalence or incidence is, however, difficult to define since most figures refer to AD and SDAT together. Studies including cases of dementia above 65 (TOMLINSON, cit TERRY 1978a) and 55 (JELLINGER 1976) years of age agree on a figure of about 50% for dementias caused by Alzheimer lesions, while, e.g. Pick's disease accounts for little more than 2%. SJÖGREN et al. (1952) calculated a morbidity risk of 0.1% for Pick's disease and presenile AD together, meaning 75 new cases per year in Sweden, viz. mostly examples of presenile AD. The frequency of AD in a geriatric patient material, well documented both clinically and histopathologically, was a high as 5.6% (SJÖGREN and SOURANDER 1962). Most studies concern relatively small groups or communities, but a large scale investigation may be more enlightening such as that presently under way in Finland (PALO et al. 1979).

Exact figures are thus difficult to obtain for the presenile AD under discussion. However, with the approximate figures available and a disease duration of a few to 15 or even 20 years, with a considerably shortened life span, it is obvious that AD is a great social problem and a heavy burden to medical institutions. This statement is even more valid if SDAT is included in a unitarian concept of the disease.

C. The Clinical Picture of Alzheimer's Disease

I. Clinical Characteristics and Course of the Disease

As early as 1907, when ALOIS ALZHEIMER in his lecture „Über eine eigenartige Erkrankung der Hirnrinde" first described what he considered a new disease entity, several of the core characteristics of Alzheimer's disease were reported. Alzheimer described a progressive mental deterioration starting in a 51-year-old woman. She developed loss of memory, disorientation as to time and place, severe language disturbances, perseveration and apraxia. The patient also manifested anxiety, paranoid delusions and auditory hallucinations. The neurological investigation was normal. The patient died after 4½ years of disease, mutistic, incontinent, and bedridden. Alzheimer and other investigators have added new information from studies on Alzheimer's disease and thereby subsequently modified and developed the clinical description (PERUSINI 1909; STERTZ 1922; SJÖGREN et al. 1952; SIM and SUSSMAN 1962; LAUTER 1968, 1970; SOURANDER and SJÖGREN 1970; BRUN and GUSTAFSON 1976, 1978).

Presenile AD, which will be described here, starts by definition between 40 and 65 years of age. Few cases with the clinical and pathological characteristics of AD have so far been reported before the age of 40 (except in cases of Down's syndrome) (ROTHSCHILD 1934; SJÖGREN et al. 1952; McMENEMY 1963).

The duration of the disease is given with some uncertainty since its onset is always difficult to define. SJÖGREN (1950), in his material of 20 deceased cases, found a mean duration of the disease of 8.5 years (range 5–16 years) and in a presentation of 18 post-mortem verified cases from 1952 (SJÖGREN et al. 1952) reported 7.1 years. LAUTER (1968), in his extensive material of 203 verified cases of AD, found a mean duration at death of 5.8 years (range 1–20 years) and BRUN and GUSTAFSON (1976) a mean duration of 8.9 ± 2.1 years in 7 cases.

Few systematic studies exist of the premorbid personality and psychopathological characteristics during the preclinical stage of Alzheimer's disease. LAUTER (1968) found no specific pathological premorbid traits while SIM and SUSSMAN (1962) observed premorbid obsessional and anxiety features in 8 of 22 verified cases of AD. In general, however, patients developing AD have been reported previously to be normal and socially well adapted.

The clinical picture and the course of AD can best be described using the classical three stages of the disease (SJÖGREN 1950; SJÖGREN et al. 1952; JERVIS 1956; LAUTER 1968).

In most cases of AD the intellectual impairment starts and develops insidiously. A more acute onset has been described but most of these cases seem to be atypical from the clinical and neuropathological point of view (e.g. HOLLANDER and STRICH 1970). In several cases there has been reported somatic or psychological events in close connection with the onset of AD (SIM and SUSSMAN 1962; LAUTER 1968). The significance of somatic disorders such as infections, skull trauma, subarachnoid haemorrhage or emotional stress, such as berievement, have been discussed. The first stage of AD lasts 1–3 years. The consistent clinical finding during this stage is memory failure, affecting learning and recent events but also to some extent the remote past. The memory dysfunction involves verbal as well as spatial material. It has often been pointed out that patients with AD manifest some spatial disorientation already at an early stage though perhaps only intermittently. Language disturbances are often observed by the patient himself. Nominal expressive aphasia is most easy to recognize but also receptive aphasia might appear in stage 1.

Non-specific but still obvious changes of behaviour are observed during stage 1. The patient becomes less active and efficient, emotionally shallow and unconcerned about what used to interest him. The patient often complains of anxious and depressed feelings, tiredness and other unspecific symptoms such as headache and dizziness. Fainting spells and attacks of vertigo are sometimes reported but their relationship to AD are unclear. The attacks might be seen as participating factors in the development of the disease or as events secondary to the underlying pathological process (BRUN and GUSTAFSON 1976). Suspiciousness, jealousy, and sometimes even paranoid psychosis are observed during AD. Often the paranoid delusions are less well organized and such reactions may disappear spontaneously.

In general, patients with AD do not appear prematurely old or mentally deteriorated in the first stage. The patients may, however, suffer severely and plead for assistance or medical help referring to diffuse somatic complaints. Habitual personality traits are preserved and remain so even at an advanced stage of AD. The patient's ambition is to retain a facade of ,normal' behaviour, and all possible resources are used by the patient to conceal the cognitive impairment and to protect the patient from catastrophic reactions. Questions are answered with general phrases or guesses or short confabulations may be used to conceal embarrassment. Fanciful confabulation is sometimes observed. The patient's general passivity is sometimes concealed by an aimless restlessness which might be misunderstood as hyperactivity.

As pointed out by several authors (STERTZ 1922; SJÖGREN et al. 1952; SOURANDER and SJÖGREN 1970; PEARCE 1974), a change of muscular tension may be observed early in the course of AD. The akinetic-hypertonic character of this feature might be revealed by neurological investigation or seen as a disturbed rhythmicity, especially evident when the patient is walking. This symptom is often misinterpreted as Parkinson's disease.

The second stage of Alzheimer's disease is dominated by the classical A-A-A syndrome, aphasia, apraxia, and agnosia. Stage 2 has a duration of 1–3 years. During this stage, the memory dysfunction increases severely, affecting also memory of remote events. Confabulation, if present, is mostly restricted and not of the productive, fanciful type. The expressive and receptive aphasias greatly restrict the verbal communication. The speech becomes uncertain, paraphrasic, perseverating, sometimes voluble, and completely incomprehensible. A peculiar clonic type of stammering, logoclonia, has been related to AD, as well as echolalia. Dysarthria is common as well as dyslexia and dysgraphia. In spite of these language disturbances, it is possible to achieve emotional, non-verbal social contact with most patients.

During the second stage, the mental deterioration causes severe apraxia, spatial disorientation, and agnosia. The visual agnosia affects recognition of faces, sometimes even the patient's own (mirror sign). At this stage the patient lacks insight, appears euphoric or rather unconcerned about his disabilities. Restless, stereotype movements are common but anxiety or depressive reactions are less frequent.

In the second stage, neurological investigation reveals no or only slight sensory impairment including visual and hearing capacities. Simple motor functions are also retained and only inconstant neurological defects are reported, such as paresis of the facial nerve (SJÖGREN et al. 1952; BRUN and GUSTAFSON 1976).

Paroxysmal motor phenomena, such as epileptic seizures and myoclonic twitchings, become more frequent in the second stage of AD. SOURANDER and

SJÖGREN (1970) reported epilepsy in 75% of 68 verified AD cases. Minor spells described as dropfits or hypokinetic fits (SJÖGREN et al. 1952) were observed in 64% and generalized epileptic seizures in 44% of the cases. Grand mal was most common in the terminal stage. SOURANDER and SJÖGREN (1970) pointed out that masticatory seizures related to temporal lobe damage, were observed in 45% of the patients. LAUTER (1968, 1970) reported seizures in 16% of 203 AD cases. Grand mal was recorded in 9%, syncope in 3%, and non-specific seizures in another 3% of this material. He found a strong relationship between frequency of epileptic seizures, the patient's age and onset of AD. Seizures were observed in 37.5% when the onset of AD was before 49 years, in 22% between 50 and 59 years and in 8.8% when the onset was between 60 and 69 years of age. This finding indicates the age dependency of certain symptoms in AD, which have also been shown in presenile dementia in general (GUSTAFSON 1975). Myoclonic twitchings appear in the earliest descriptions of AD (PERUSINI 1909). Myoclonic twitchings may even appear already at an early stage but are manifested mostly at an advanced stage of AD. Frequencies varying from 10% (TARISKA 1970) to 80% (SOURANDER and SJÖGREN 1970) have been presented. A high frequency, however, refers to the terminal stage of AD. When myoclonia appears early in AD the differentiation from Jacob-Creutzfeldt's disease is difficult (JACOB 1970; BRUN and GUSTAFSON 1976; FADEN and TOWNSEND 1976).

During the third and terminal stage of AD most patients become increasingly passive, vegetative, incontinent, and incapacitated. The patients are largely bedridden with stiff, rigid extremities, and an expressionless facies. Epileptic seizures and myoclonic phenomena are common. The myoclonic jerkings involve small groups of muscles, a limb, all or part of the face or the whole body. The jerkings are often elicited by touching the body, which may lead to strong mass discharges. The patients also have spells of crying or shrieking (SJÖGREN et al. 1952), sometimes recurring at regular intervals.

A syndrome similar to the Klüver-Bucy syndrome (KLÜVER and BUCY 1938, 1939) has been reported in AD, especially during its terminal stage (PILLERI 1966; SOURANDER and SJÖGREN 1970; BRUN and GUSTAFSON 1976). The syndrome consists of visual agnosia, hyperorality, hypermetamorphosis, loss of emotions and sometimes hypersexuality and bulimia. Sometimes emotional deterioration changes to aggressiveness. The Klüver-Bucy syndrome has been correlated with temporal lobe lesions but the importance of other brain structures has also been pointed out (PILLERI 1966). The hypersexuality and bulimia have been related to frontal lobe involvement in the terminal stage of AD (JELGERSMA 1964; BRUN and GUSTAFSON 1976, 1978).

II. Psychometric Assessment

The cognitive dysfunction in AD has been evaluated using psychometric tests at different stages of the disease. Some authors (SIM 1979; PEREZ et al. 1975) have disputed the efficiency of psychometric tests for early recognition of AD and for differential diagnosis. However, a proper use of psychometry and standardized observations have been shown most helpful both for differentiating presenility from normal ageing (HAGBERG and INGVAR 1976) as well as for promoting a better differentiation especially between early stages of the various forms of presenile dementia (HAGBERG 1978a, b, 1980a, c).

In general the results emphasize the gnostic character of the intellectual dysfunction in AD. This is shown as a general reduction of the capacity for handling symbols and abstractions in a logical-inductive way. This deficiency is generally found in some forms in most of the psychometric tasks offered to the patient. Two aspects of this cognitive defect are especially apparent: an incapacity to form abstractions (understand symbols) and to process symbols and abstractions in a logical fashion. The results indicate that the processing capacity is most vulnerable and gives way in the early stages of AD. It should also be stressed that AD less often starts out as a selective memory deficit but has a gnostic dysfunction already at an early stage (HAGBERG 1978b). When this is the case, the diagnosis of multi-infarct dementia seems more likely. AD cases compared to patients with hydrocephalic dementia or normal pressure hydrocephalus (ADAMS et al. 1965; GRANVILLE-GROSSMAN 1971) have a test profile that differs significantly from that of hydrocephalic dementia, which more often seems to be characterized by the presence of constructional apraxia (GUSTAFSON and HAGBERG 1978). When psychometric tests are used for a differential diagnosis between AD and dementia of the Pick type, not only quantitative but also qualitative differences must be considered. These differential behaviour characteristics refer foremost to reactions upon and attitudes towards the test situation (HAGBERG 1978a, 1980b). In dementia a correlation between the degree of cognitive reduction as measured by psychometric tests and the degree of EEG abnormality also exists (JOHANNESSON et al. 1979) as well as with rCBF and structural abnormalities (HAGBERG and INGVAR 1976; HAGBERG 1978b; GUSTAFSON et al. 1978).

III. EEG Findings

HANS BERGER in 1931 reported a pathological EEG in a case of Alzheimer's disease later confirmed histologically. In general the proportion of abnormal EEGs in patients with verified AD approaches 100% (GREEN et al. 1952; LETEMENDIA and PAMPIGLIONE 1958; SWAIN 1959; GORDON and SIM 1967; NEVIN 1967; JOHANNESSON et al. 1977). In most cases a diffuse, irregular slowing was found and in later stages a complete disorganization of the EEG pattern. A longitudinal EEG study of AD cases, verified post-mortem, showed progressive worsening of the abnormalities in most cases (JOHANNESSON et al. 1977). The first EEG was pathological in all AD cases while a normal or essentially normal EEG was often recorded early in Pick's disease. In addition to the general slowing of EEG, bifrontal episodic delta was recorded in four of seven AD cases but also in two of five Pick cases. This EEG characteristic seems to be connected to brain stem changes. Thus EEG is most useful for the differential diagnosis of Alzheimer's disease and Pick's disease. An abnormal EEG in presenile dementia favours the diagnosis of AD while a normal EEG makes the diagnosis of Pick's disease more likely (JOHANNESSON et al. 1977; SIM and SUSSMAN 1962; CHRISTIAN 1968). The relationship between EEG and rCBF was analysed by JOHANNESSON et al. (1977).

IV. Regional Cerebral Blood Flow

Since cerebral blood flow is treated in Chap. 1, only some problems pertaining to AD will be briefly accounted for. The cerebral blood flow and oxygen metabolism is markedly reduced in senile and presenile dementia including Alzheimer's and Pick's diseases (FREYHAN et al. 1951; LASSEN et al. 1957; MUNCK and LASSEN 1957; INGVAR and GUSTAFSON 1970; OBRIST et al. 1970; GUSTAFSON and RISBERG 1979; and others). Development of the rCBF techniques based on extracranial recording of local clearance rates of the gamma-emitting, inert and diffusible tracer ^{133}Xenon has made it possible to study focal circulatory disturbances in Alzheimer's disease and other dementing disorders. In the first studies the unilateral intra-arterial injection technique was used (INGVAR and LASSEN 1961) while later investigations have been based on the non-traumatic ^{133}Xe-inhalation method, which allows bilateral and repeated measurements (OBRIST et al. 1975; RISBERG et al. 1975). In GUSTAFSON et al. (1977) and BRUN et al. (1975) a comparison was made between the distribution of degeneration of the cortex and areas of focal decrease of the rCBF. In AD the most marked atrophy and the lowest flow values were seen in postcentral, mainly parietotemporal regions, while frontal and frontotemporal flow changes were seen in Pick's disease. Using the ^{133}Xenon inhalation technique, GUSTAFSON and RISBERG (1979) could confirm the earlier findings, including a small number of patients with a diagnosis verified at autopsy.

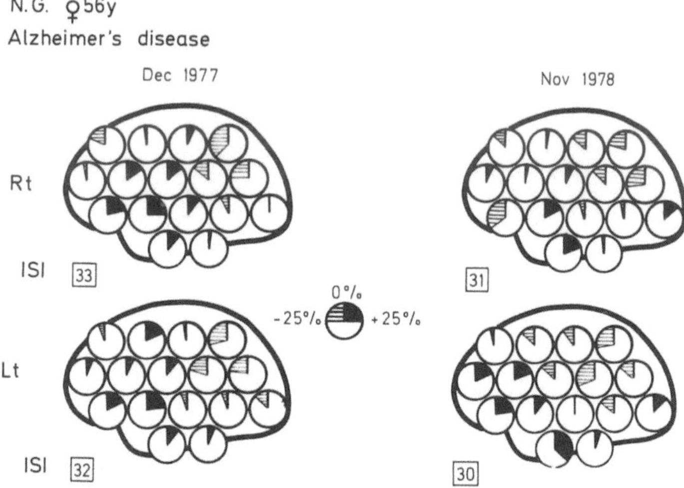

Fig. 1. Regional cerebral blood flow in a case of progressing AD. A woman aged 56 years with heredity for organic dementia, who, at the time of the first investigation (December 1977), presented a 4-year history of progressing dementia with amnesia, dyscalculia, spatial disorientation and apraxia. She displayed symptoms of dysphasia but enjoyed a superficial and friendly conservation. The personality seemed fairly well preserved. Mean hemispheric flow is shown in *boxes. Clock symbols* show deviations from hemispheric mean. The rCBF showed a subnormal flow level with focal decreases in parietal and parieto-occipital regions. At the time of the second investigation (November 1978), the symptoms of dementia showed a marked progression with agrafia, agnosia, (jargon) aphasia and total apraxia. The rCBF results showed a slightly lower mean level with more marked focal flow decreases in parietotemporal regions

In a group of 22 patients diagnosed as Alzheimer's disease based on clinical features, the earliest cases had a normal rCBF level with a tentative focal low decrease in postcentral regions. With further progress of the disease the hemispheric flow was significantly reduced compared to age-matched patients with depressions, who had a normal rCBF. In 19 of the AD cases there were focal flow decreases of at least 20% below the hemispheric mean in postcentral regions, predominantly in the parietal area but usually with sparing of most of the frontal area. A typical case is illustrated in Fig. 1. In more advanced cases, temporal and also frontal regions showed low flow values with less subnormal values seen in the Rolandic and occipital regions.

D. The Neuropathological Picture of Alzheimer's Disease

I. Gross Findings

The brain may be entirely unremarkable in mild or early cases with little or no weight loss and no gross atrophy at all. In more advanced cases the brain weight is usually reduced to about 1,000 g, but often 800–900 g or even less is recorded (SOURANDER and SJÖGREN 1970). The brain weight for normal 40–60 year old men is about 1,350 g and women 1,250 g (ARENDT 1972; BRAUNMÜHL 1957).

In these more advanced stages of the disease there is commonly noticeable gross atrophy. The cortical atrophy is usually not circumscribed though in some cases it has been of a Pick-like appearance, viz. of a more lobular, demarcated character (TARISKA 1970). The cortical atrophy thus is usually referred to as diffuse and bilaterally symmetrical, though with an accent on the frontal lobes (JERVIS 1971; CORSELLIS 1976a; BRAUNMÜHL 1957). In later years it has, however, been repeatedly stressed also that preponderantly temporal, especially medial basal limbic structures are involved (SOURANDER and SJÖGREN 1970; CORSELLIS 1970; HOOPER and VOGEL 1976; BRION 1966; TOMLINSON and HENDERSON 1976; MEHRAEIN and ROTHEMUND 1976). BRION (1966) points out an accentuation in the parietal lobe.

Notably spared according to many authors, however, are the occipital lobes and the basal gyri except for the medial temporal limbic areas. In our own experience not only the medial temporal lobe but also its basal and inferior lateral areas are severely atrophic (Fig. 2a, b) together with adjoining portions of the parietal, postcentral areas, whereas the frontal lobe is less involved in the average case. In between, the central gyri stand out well preserved (Fig. 3b). On the medial aspect of the hemisphere the cingulate gyrus in its posterior portion (area 23 of Brodmann) often appears shrunken but the pericalcarine cortex and anterior cingulate gyrus (area 24) are well preserved (BRUN and GUSTAFSON 1976, 1978). As often pointed out there is, however, a discrepancy between gross and microscopic degree of involvement, which is why topographic mapping of the degeneration has to include a microscopical study.

The ventricular system is generally widened and the callosal body narrowed. Basal ganglia are in most cases grossly well preserved while the substantia nigra is somewhat pale. The mamillary bodies usually appear normal. The brain stem, and cerebellum in the average case is unremarkable or shows a slight atrophy, while the spinal cord is normal.

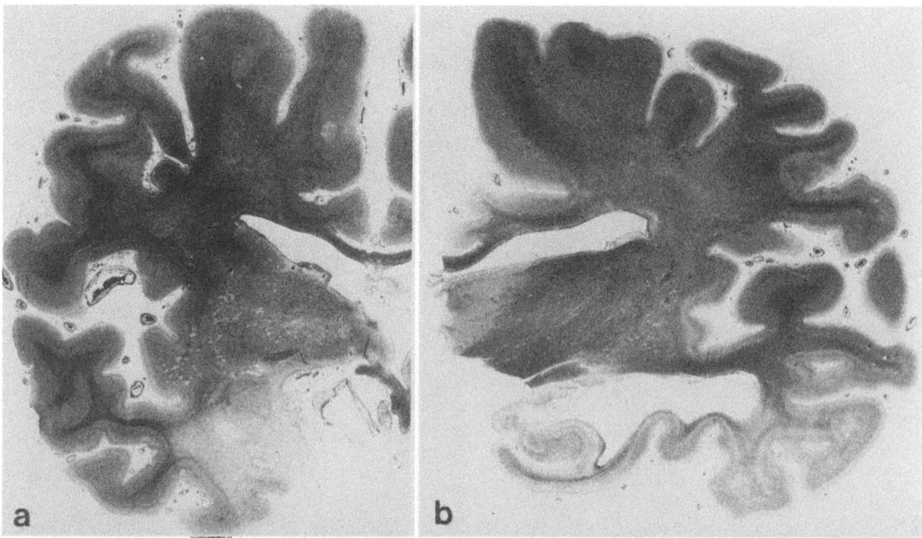

Fig. 2. a Alzheimer's disease. Frontal section through anterior temporal lobe with severe degeneration of the amygdaloid nucleus and adjoining basal temporal cortex but with relative sparing of other areas including anterior part of middle and superior temporal gyrus (temporal pole area). Compare **a** with **b**, a section posterior to **a**, and Fig. 3 a, a normal section through the anterior temporal lobe. Hematoxylin and eosin, × 1.5, reduced to 65%. **b** Alzheimer's disease. Frontal section through midtemporal area showing pronounced collapse of basal parts of temporal lobe with atrophy of cortex and partial degeneration of white matter in hippocampal, inferior and middle temporal gyrus but with sparing of superior temporal gyrus. Note also atrophy of posterior part of cingulate gyrus but preservation of adjoining motor and sensory cortex on the convexity. Hematoxylin and eosin, × 2, reduced to 65%

The meninges, particularly the frontal, are sometimes thickened. The cerebral vessels in the great majority of cases often show mild or no arteriosclerotic changes, in only a few percent with occlusive atherosclerosis and then with a clinical picture showing an admixture of cerebrovascular disease.

Similar findings have also been reported in SDAT and normal ageing: namely, an atrophy of the medial temporal limbic structures, frontal, and parietal lobes with some sparing of the calcarine and sensory-motor areas (ARENDT 1972).

II. Microscopical Findings

The most well-known microscopical alterations in AD are the neurofibrillary changes (NF) in the perikaryon of neurons, and senile or neuritic plaques (SP). These were the fundamental changes reported initially 1906 by ALZHEIMER and have since been the subject of a vast literature. However, elucidation of their nature and detailed composition had to await the use of the electron microscope, and biochemical and subcellular fractionation methods. These changes have in common that they are best shown by silver impregnation methods and also react positively to amyloid-staining procedures and thioflavine fluorescence methods. Furthermore the basic structure of NF, the paired helical filament (PHF), is also found in SP, possibly transported there from the nerve cell body (TERRY 1978 b).

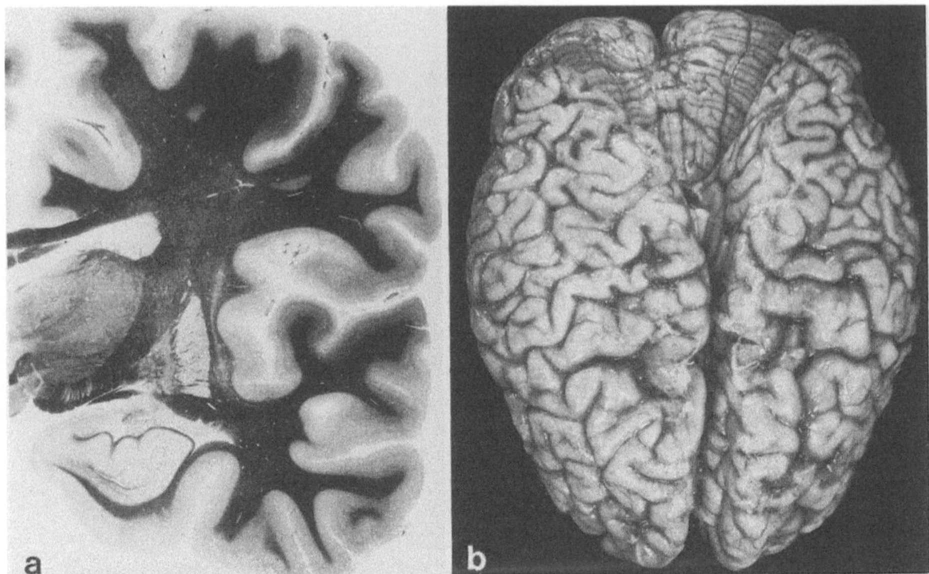

Fig. 3. a Normal case with pseudodementia without morphological or blood flow changes, for comparison with Figs 2a, b. Note preserved, not collapsed temporal structures. Luxol fast blue, × 1.3, reduced to 65%. **b** Top view of brain from a case of Alzheimer's disease. Note postcentral parietal lobe atrophy with shortening of hemispheres, which do not cover cerebellum, but with preservation of central and also frontal gyri

1. Senile (Neuritic) Plaques

The SP are concentrated in grey matter, mostly the cortex, sometimes with some spill over into the adjoining white substance. SP are usually rounded with a diameter of 5–200 µm (TOMLINSON 1977) and involve the synaptic apparatus of the neuron rather than the cell body. The classical plaque consists of a central argyrophilic core of amyloid, surrounded by a halo and a ring of granules and rods, made up of axon terminals and preterminals and in the periphery some astrocytes and microglial cells (Fig. 4a). The axonal terminals and preterminals are distended by abnormal mitochondria, dense bodies, lipid granules and PHF. Consequently the plaque is not only argyrophilic to a large extent but also PAS and Congo-red positive and contains an excess of acid phosphatase demonstrable by, e.g. the Gomori method (FRIEDE 1965), a method which is rapid and reliable for the demonstration of SP.

Numerous subtypes of plaques have been described and arranged in a sequential order according to their supposed stepwise development. Here only the extremes will be mentioned. An early or primitive plaque has been described as a condensation of the ground substance often in connection with amyloid components (DIVRY 1927) though from ultrastructural studies the earliest change is now known to be degenerative changes in a few neurites, later supplemented with amyloid (TERRY et al. 1964; KIDD 1964; WISNIEWSKI and TERRY 1973a, b) in increasing amounts, and reactive glial cells to form the classical plaque. In the end the neurites

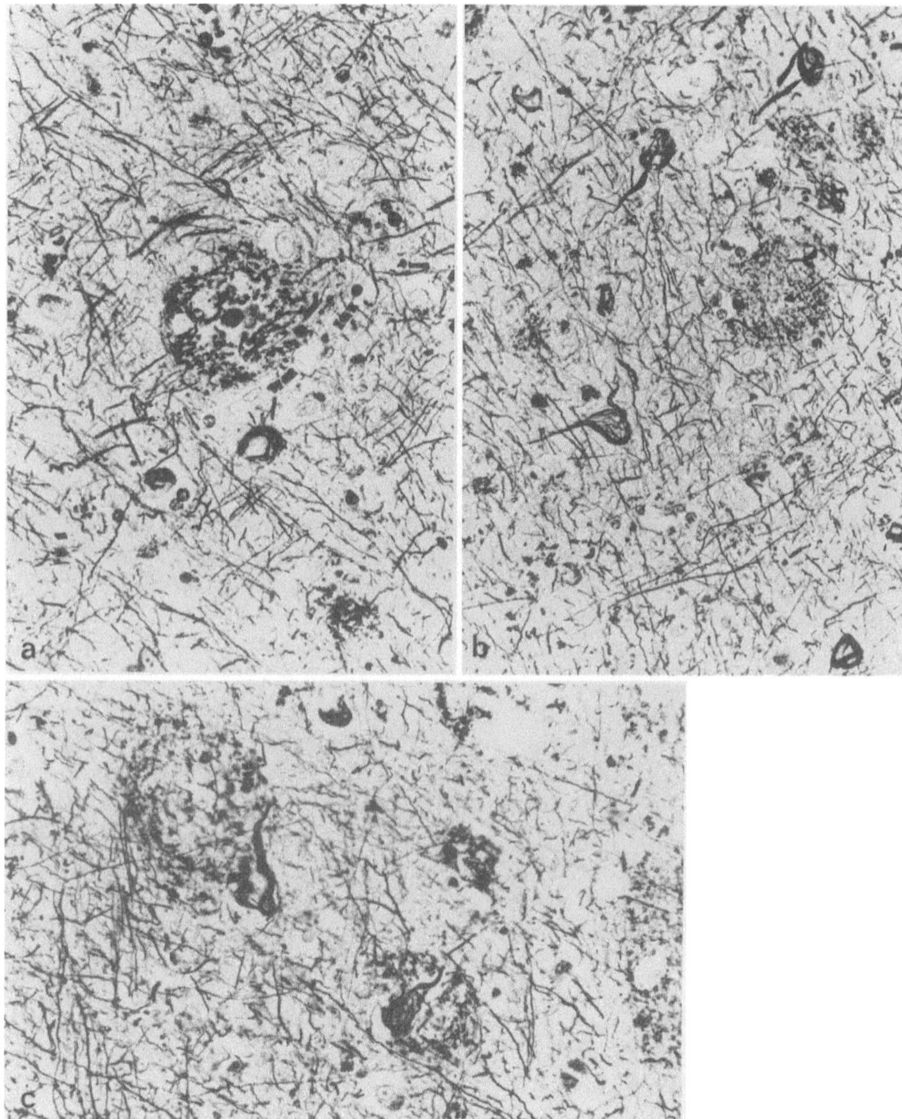

Fig. 4a–c. Senile (neuritic) plaques (SP) and neurofibrillary degeneration (NF). Naoumenko, × 63. **a** SP in the centre of picture with dense central core surrounded by "empty" halo and a corona of rods and granules. Below is a NF. **b** Various forms of NF around three SP, which tend to coalesce. **c** NF within and at the periphery of SP

decrease and disappear, and an amyloid mass may remain, bordered by some glial cells, representing a "burnt out," old plaque (TERRY and WISNIEWSKI 1970).

A number of additional types have been described, though basically they are all variations on the same theme (BRAUNMÜHL 1957; HABERLAND 1969; JERVIS 1971).

A certain proportion of SP develop in connection with amyloid infiltration of intracortical arterioles and capillary vessels, the dyshoric angiopathy of Morel and Wildi (1952). Here the amyloid extends out into surrounding brain tissue, but it is not always associated with perivascular plaque formation (Terry and Wisniewski 1970). Even if in some animals the SP are chiefly perivascular (Wisniewski et al. 1973, 1970), the relationship is not consistent enough to support a vascular theory of origin of SP. Other theories center around the neuron, glial cell or the role of neurotoxic antigen–antibody complexes with amyloid formation (Wisniewski 1979), as reviewed by Torack (1978).

2. Neurofibrillary Degeneration

Alzheimer's neurofibrillary degeneration (NF) constitutes the second most extensively studied alteration in AD. It consists light microscopically of argyrophilic fibrils, often assembled in loops, torch-like formations or globose forms in the neuronal perikaryon (Fig. 4 b). There it displaces the cell organelles, which together with the nucleus, tend to disintegrate, leaving in the end an isolated NF lying seemingly free in the neuropil. They take up Congo red and become birefringent, though they are not believed to be composed of amyloid (Wisniewski and Terry 1976). They may be found within or next to a SP (Fig. 4 c).

Not until more than half a century after their recognition was their true nature unveiled in the electron microscope. Terry (1963) designated them twisted tubules and Kidd (1963) suggested a bifilar helix, a shape later confirmed by Wisniewski et al. (1976). They thus consist of a single or usually a pair of 10-nm-wide pathological filaments, helically wound with twists every (65-)80 nm (Wisniewski and Soifer 1979). Named therefore paired helical filaments (PHF) they vary in width between 10 and 22 nm. They are assembled in bundles in the perikaryon creating an NF (Fig. 5 a, b). Their derivation has aroused much speculation. Chemical and immunological studies suggest that the PHF is composed of a protein similar to β-tubulin of normal neuronal tubules, which thus may be involved in the origin of PHF and consequently also in the pathogenesis of AD (Grundke-Iqbal et al. 1979). This composition is supported also by immunofluorescencent studies by Ishii et al. (1979). PHF characterize NF in humans but not in animals with experimentally induced or spontaneously occurring NF, where they consist of single straight filaments. PHF are found both in the neuronal perikaryon and its processes including the axon and its terminals and dendritic terminals involved in the formation of SP. This and the fact that the SP and NF usually appear together in AD and that PHF occupy many of the changed neurites in SP (Terry and Wisniewski 1970) serves to unify them as interrelated parts of the same lesion affecting soma and synaptic region of the neurons. They may appear in large numbers but their functional importance is unclear (Torack 1978) a problem discussed by Crapper (1976). (See also Chap. 3.)

3. Dendritic Changes

Alterations in the synaptic ultrastructure, such as abnormal mitochondria, multilamellar dense bodies and fibrillar and tubulovesicular material have been found

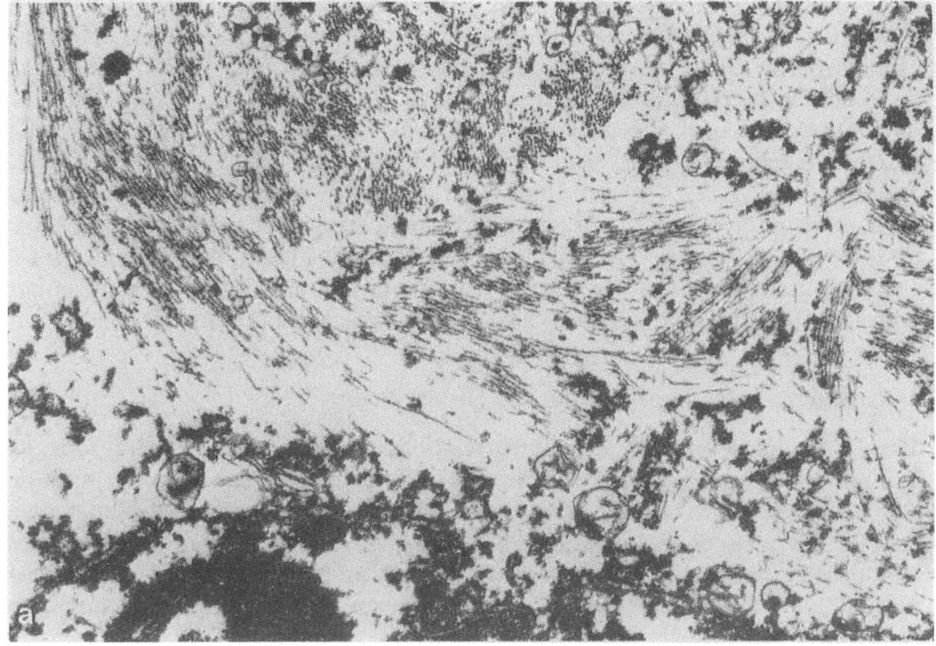

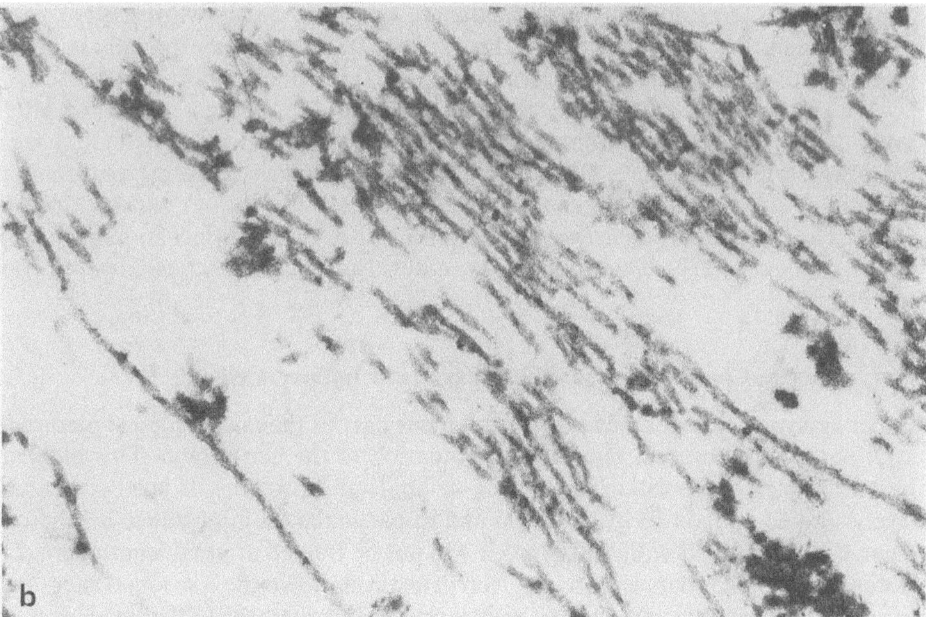

Fig. 5a, b. Electron microscopical picture of NF. **a** NF, consisting of bundles of paired helical filaments (PHF) sweeping past the nucleus *(bottom left)* of a neuron. × 17,100. **b** Part of **a** at higher magnification, showing the double helical character of the PHF with "twists" at regular intervals. × 76,800

in or around SP (Gonatas and Moss 1975; Gonatas and Gambetti 1970). The dendritic tree also suffers a reduction of its extent including the density of spines as indicated by ultrastructural studies (Wisniewski and Terry 1973 a) and by Golgi technique investigations (Mehraein et al. 1975; Scheibel 1979 a; Feldman 1976). In this process of degeneration, neurons may also exhibit signs of irregular dendritic regeneration, possibly restricted to familial AD (Scheibel 1979 b). Buell and Coleman (1979), however, found that normally dendrites of at least one class of neurons in the hippocampal gyrus continue to grow while in SDAT they fail to do so or even retrogress. These synaptic and dendritic alterations involve a considerable proportion of neurons with a deafferentation, most likely of great importance for their function and thus also for the clinical picture of AD.

4. Granulovacuolar Degeneration and Hirano Bodies

These two changes, which are mainly restricted to the medial temporal lobe, are less intense than those reported above. Granulovacuolar degeneration, first described by Simchowitz (1911), consists of neuronal cytoplasmic membrane bound vesicles 3–5 μm in diameter, which are "empty" save for a central 1-μm-wide electron-dense granule, which is argyrophilic (Terry and Wisniewski 1972). Their nature and derivation is not clear. They are almost entirely restricted to the hippocampus and adjoining cortex where they may involve up to 50% of neurons, mainly in the posterior half of the hippocampus, where their distribution largely parallels that of NF (Ball and Lo 1977). Heavily affected neurons show a reduced RNA content and alteration in shape indicative of neuronal death (Mann 1978).

Although thus limited in extent this form of degeneration, especially in cooperation with other neuronal lesions, may be of functional importance.

Hirano bodies described by Hirano et al. (1966) are the least impressive alteration in AD. These are eosinophilic rods, roughly 15 μm wide and 30 μm long with a paracrystalline structure, situated mainly extracellularly, close to neurons but sometimes also found within glial, and neuronal cells (Schochet and McCormic 1972). They occur particularly in the Sommer sector of the hippocampus (Gibson and Tomlinson 1977). Their derivation, nature, and importance is, however, not clear.

5. Lipofuscin, Chronic Neuronal Shrinkage, and Inflated Cells

Other neuronal changes make up a prominent part of the microscopical picture in AD, above all lipofuscin pigment accumulation in the perikaryon. This pigment has a complex composition, consisting of lipids and proteins. It has been extensively studied and yet its exact origin and in particular its importance is far from clear. Since it is dealt with in Chap. 5 it will not be treated at great length here. Lipofuscin pigment is deposited as electron dense granules in the lysosomal vacuome, assembled in cytoplasmic masses rich in acid phosphatase. Different classes of neurons display different tendencies to accumulate the pigment. Thus cells of the inferior olive and lateral geniculate body show large amounts early on, whereas Purkinje cells of the cerebellar cortex are virtually free from lipofuscin. Though Mann and Sinclair (1978) found no increase of lipofuscin in SDAT, other consider cortical neurons, especially the larger neurons of lamina III and V, to become increasingly and heavily involved in AD.

The importance of this change has been interpreted differently, from a harmless feature or even the expression of a protective mechanism (storing away of useless or harmful waste products) to an injurious process, consuming organelle space and manufactured neuronal enzymes, interfering with neuronal metabolism, transport mechanisms, and membrane functions, or more likely blocking of the normal functions of the lysosomal vacuome (WISNIEWSKI and TERRY 1973a; BRUN and BRUNK 1974; BRUNK and BRUN 1972; MANN and YATES 1979; BOWEN et al. 1973; HOCHSCHILD 1971). The neurons so changed show a reduced amount of RNA, resulting in a paler-staining cytoplasm.

Other neurons may be pale and appear empty without pigment accumulation but sometimes with an argyrophilic inclusion, obtaining a rounded shape, so-called inflated cells (BRAUNMÜHL 1957).

In this context an additional form of neuronal change may be mentioned, namely chronic neuronal shrinkage or sclerosis (Nissl) (BRAUNMÜHL 1957). The nerve cells have the appearance of a dark neuron, elongated, and darkly staining with loss of organelles. These neurons are often found in AD, especially in lamina III and V in increasing numbers corresponding to increasing severity of the cortical degeneration (Fig. 6a, b). This may however, at least in part, be an artefact as pointed out by CAMMERMEYER (1961).

6. Glial Alterations

Glial changes are seen in more advanced degeneration of the cortex. Microglial proliferation is readily noted in the molecular layer of the cortex (Fig. 6c). It is not known whether the original astrocytic population remains unaltered or decreases, though BOWEN et al. (1979) noted a decrease in glial cells by age. Reactive astrocytes, however, increase in number at all depths of the cortex but most prominently in its superficial layers (BRAUNMÜHL 1957), where they form dense aggregations or nests similar to SP in shape and size but different in other respects (Fig. 7a, c, d). These nests spread through the depth of the cortex with increasing severity of degeneration (BRUN and ENGLUND 1981). Glial conglomerates similar to these nests are mentioned by TARISKA (1970). Glial cells or fibrils form a dense layer along the vessels and ventricular linings as well as the cortical surface as seen also in ageing (ARENDT 1972).

7. Spongiosis

Spongy degeneration or spongiosis of the cortex is a feature only rarely mentioned in recent literature (ALZHEIMER 1907; TARISKA 1970). It was included by BRAUNMÜHL (1957) in his extensive review of the pathology of AD together with a discussion on its pathogenesis. The sponginess represents a loosening of the neuropil due to the presence of minute vacuoles often with a laminar distribution. The spongiosis first appears in laminae I–II, descending through the cortex with increasing severity of the degeneration (BRUN and ENGLUND 1981). It is non-specific and of the same appearance as that seen in other conditions, many of which have been surveyed by COLMANT (1968) (Fig. 7b).

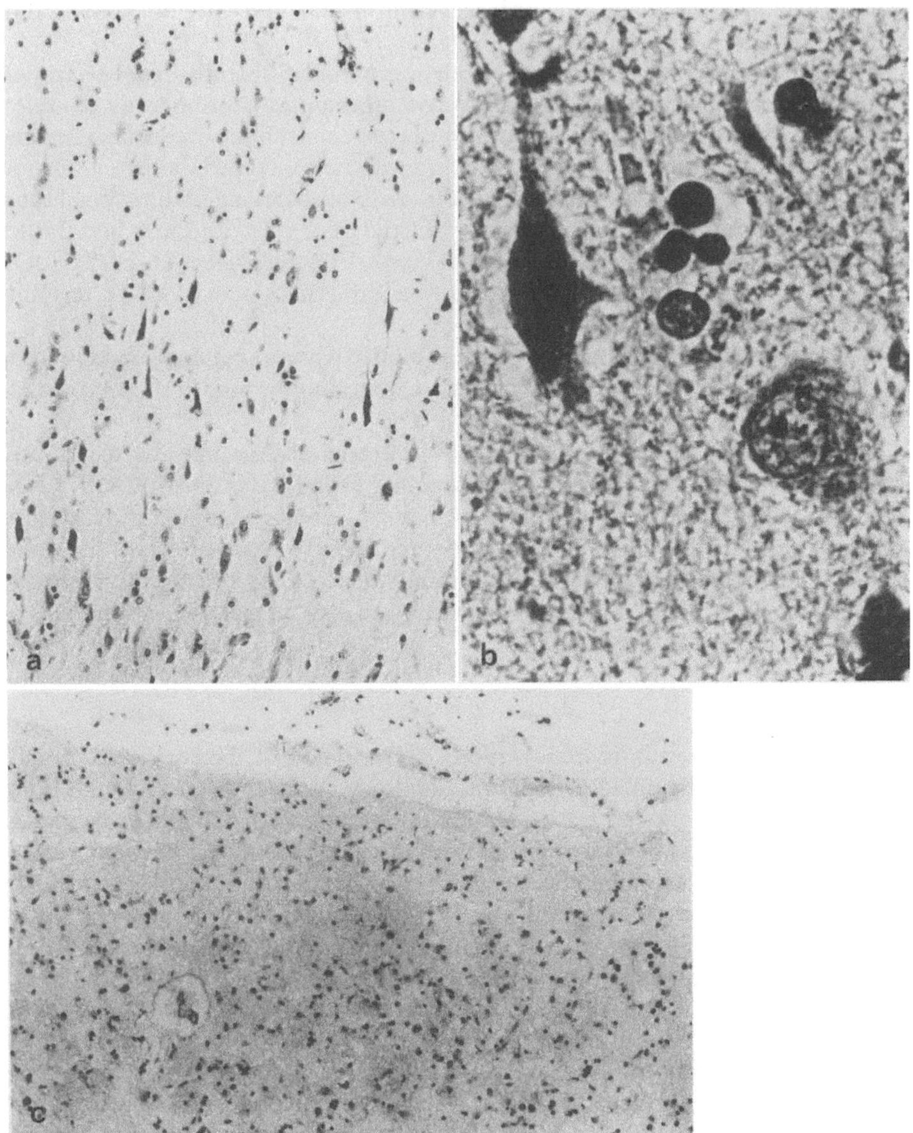

Fig. 6 a–c. Neuronal shrinkage (sclerosis) and gliosis. Cresyl violet. **a** Cerebral cortex with "dark" slender neurons in lamina III among preserved neurons. ×150. **b** Dark cortical neuron with partial obliteration of internal structures and loss of contact with surrounding neuropil. Compare preserved neighbouring neuron. ×690. **c** Superficial layers of cerebral cortex with gliosis, especially obvious in lamina I. ×100

8. Neuronal Loss

The question of accelerated loss of neurons in AD is a matter of controversy.

Cortical neuronal loss in ageing was documented in several papers by BRODY (1955, 1970, 1976) but a loss in excess of that has not been found in SDAT by TER-

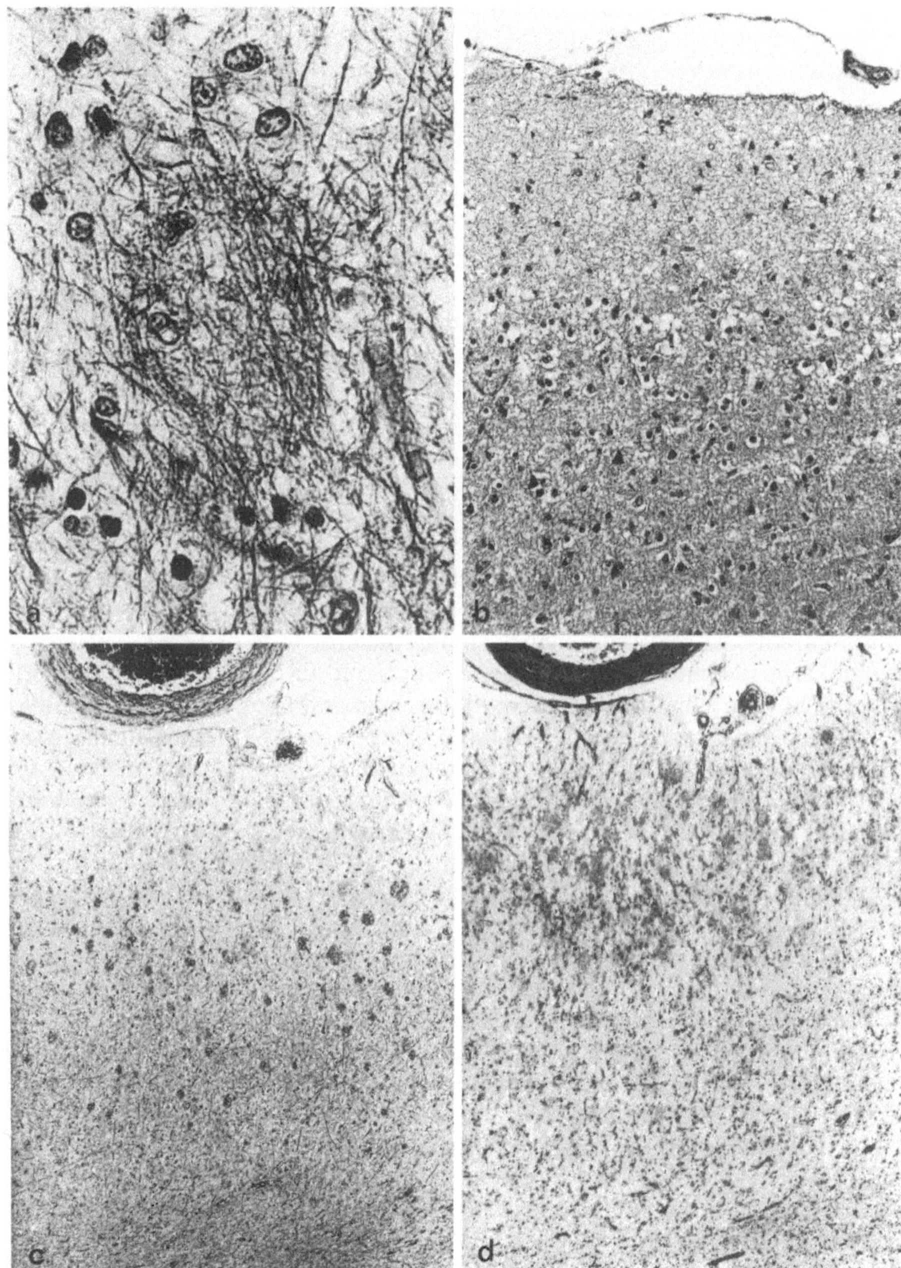

Fig. 7. a Cerebral cortex with glial nest consisting of a meshwork of glial fibrils and surrounded by glial (astrocytic) nuclei. Note abscence of central core or other characteristics of a SP. Holzer's stain, × 275. **b** Cerebral cortex with slight (grade I) degeneration. Note spongy degeneration concentrated in lamina II. Hematoxylin and eosin, × 150. **c** Cerebral cortex with SP mainly in laminae III–IV. Same area as in **d**, for comparison. Naoumenko, × 45. **d** Cerebral cortex with many glial nests in laminae I–II. Same area as **c** for comparison of location of SP versus glial nests. Holzer's stain, × 45

RY et al. (1977; TERRY 1978c, 1979) and TOMLINSON and HENDERSON (1976), and DEKOSKY and BASS (1980) and the cortical thickness was reported as unchanged.

BOWEN, however, found with biochemical methods a temporal lobe neuronal loss in SDAT expressed as 57%–70% reduction in neuronal markers (BOWEN et al. 1976; BOWEN 1979). In AD others have found a severe decrease of neurons, e.g. in the hippocampus or its subicular part (BALL 1977; SHEFER 1972, 1977) and COLON (1973) noted an overall 57% loss of cortical neurons, with a distribution different from that in ageing, and in addition a reduction in cortical thickness. Also SHEFER (1972) noted a neuronal loss from the neocortex. There are also reports, based more on impression than quantitation, which are in agreement with the latter opinion and state that neuronal loss and shrinkage occur. In view of the profound and extensive neuronal lesions in AD it would be surprising not to find a neuronal decrement if AD and SDAT are closely related. Ageing and SDAT may, however, be different from AD on this point with additional amplification of the difference in terms of a tendency to regional accentuation of the degenerative process in AD. Our results of cell counting have shown a marked loss of neurons and a concomitant shrinkage of the cortical thickness in AD. Thus in advanced cases some areas such as the posterior cingulate gyrus and superior and inferior parietal lobules loose as much as 60%–80% of their neurons, whereas in the motor and sensory area and anterior cingulate gyrus the loss is only around 30%. In between falls the temporal lobe with average figures comparable to those of BOWEN, whereas the frontal lobe is somewhat less damaged (BRUN and ENGLUND 1981). There is thus a regionally varying loss of neurons to be compared later with rCBF alterations.

Within the cortex, JERVIS (1971) and CORSELLIS (1969) found a neuronal loss in the outer three layers of the cortex, more than in its inner layers in AD in agreement with ALZHEIMER's own findings. The opposite opinion has been expressed by others (COLON 1973) while layers II and IV have been pointed out by BRODY (1976, 1978).

The neuronal loss, SP, NF, gliosis, dark neurons, spongiosis, and other parameters result in a blurring of the cortical cytoarchitecture (Fig. 8c) and an atrophy increasing with the severity of the degenerative process. On the basis of these parameters a rough grading of the severity of the neocortical degeneration was done for a correlation with clinical parameters (BRUN and GUSTAFSON 1976, 1978). This grading was further analysed and supplemented with neuronal countings and measurements of the cortical shrinkage (BRUN and ENGLUND 1981). Four grades, 1–4, of advancement of the degeneration were defined beyond a basic stage, 0, with only SP and NF (Fig. 8a–c). These grades correlated well with brain weight reduction, neuronal loss, and cortical shrinkage, as well as rCBF changes and symptoms as discussed later in connection with correlations between the clinical and pathological picture.

9. Regional Variations

A lobe or even gyrus is rarely uniformly involved in this "diffuse encephalopathy." Smaller adjoining compartments of the cortex show a variation in severity of the various parameters constituting the degeneration, especially in not too far advanced cases. A well-known example of this is the great abundance of SP in the

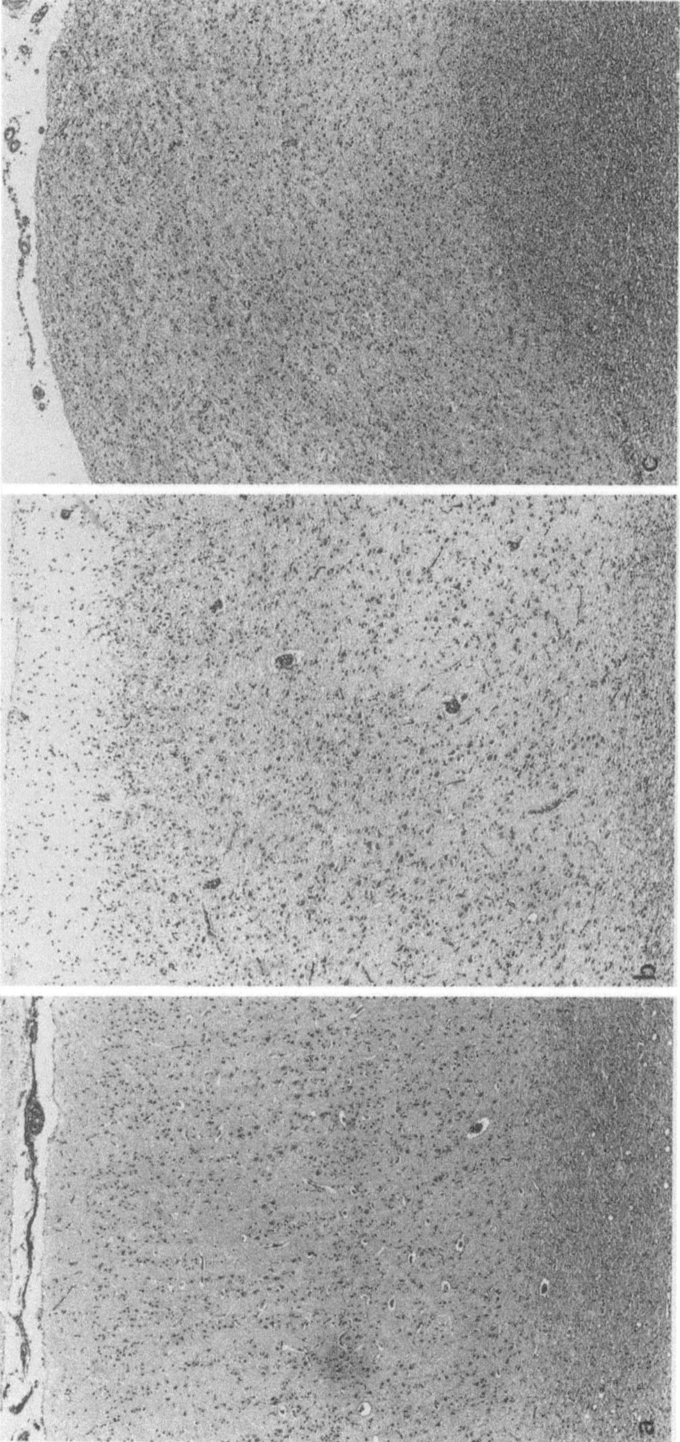

Fig. 8a–c. Varying serverity of cortical degeneration. Hematoxylin and eosin, × 40. **a** No discernible degeneration (SP and NF present but not shown with the staining used); grade 0. **b** Anterior cingulate gyrus. Slight degeneration with gliosis, slight spongiosis and less distinct lamination than in **a**; grade I. **c** Posterior cingulate gyrus. Severe degeneration with intense gliosis, shrinkage of cortex and blurring of lamination, grade 4. From the same case and same cingulate gyrus as **b**

depth of sulci compared to the adjoining bank or crown of the gyrus and also their preference for superficial compared to deeper cortical layers. These small scale variations may not be traceable in terms of symptoms or rCBF changes.

There are, however, consistent variations between larger brain regions, though mostly described on the basis of studies on SDAT.

SP and NF in general vary concomitantly. JAMADA and MEHRAEIN (1968) found the highest counts in the amygdala compared to other limbic and some non-limbic areas. Others have also stressed the limbic involvement though again mostly in SDAT. Thus HOOPER and VOGEL (1976), in a study including quantitation of NF, SP, and granulovacuolar degeneration, reported a preponderance of limbic degeneration, especially in the amygdala and hippocampus with entorhinal cortex, less in the mamillary bodies. Similarly CORSELLIS (1970) found the amygdaloid nucleus, particularly its medial half, to bear the brunt of the disease in AD. Only mild changes were found in the mamillary bodies (CORSELLIS 1970; JAMADA and MEHRAEIN 1968).

Within the hippocampus the posterior portion was much more affected in AD with cell loss and NF (BALL 1977) and in the hippocampal cortex the same author (BALL 1978) mapped out the varying density of NF and granulovacuolar degeneration in different regions.

In SDAT KEMPER (1978) also recorded the distribution of NF within the hippocampus, arriving at striking regional variations with an accent on the subicular cortex and adjoining first portion of the pyramidal hippocampal band, areas which may be cardinal zones for the production of the clinical symptoms of dementia. SOURANDER and SJÖGREN (1970) also stressed a medial temporal limbic involvement with numerous tangles in these structures and even in the temporal neocortex and somewhat less in the frontal and especially the occipital cortex.

MANDYBUR (1975) found least NF in prefrontal portions of the hemispheres. The central sensory motor area was the least involved according to JAMADA and MEHRAEIN (1968). It may be pointed out here that there are regional variations also in ageing, with more severe atrophy reported to occur in the temporofrontal areas whereas the calcarine and motor areas appear resistant (ARENDT 1972).

In very advanced degeneration the SP become less prominent or even tend to disappear (BRUN and ENGLUND 1981) (Fig. 9a–c). A preservation in AD of the superior temporal gyrus, especially the auditory area with clearly less neuronal drop out, SP, and NF compared to adjoining areas, was noted by MUTRUX (1947). In SDAT these changes were less pronounced than in AD, a point of differentiation between the two diseases.

The distribution with preponderance in, e.g. the amygdala even in early and mild cases, points to these structures and possibly also the hippocampal formation as the starting area with later and less intense involvement of other areas. Regional variations are of importance for the clinical picture and rCBF variations and thereby for diagnostic considerations.

It is difficult to pin down a lesion pattern in AD on the basis of a compilation of opinions put forward in the literature due to the admixture of SDAT, which brings with it a contamination of pure ageing phenomena. Some opinions may also be based on the gross picture, which can give an erroneous impression of degeneration or lack thereof. Taking these factors into account and on the basis of our own

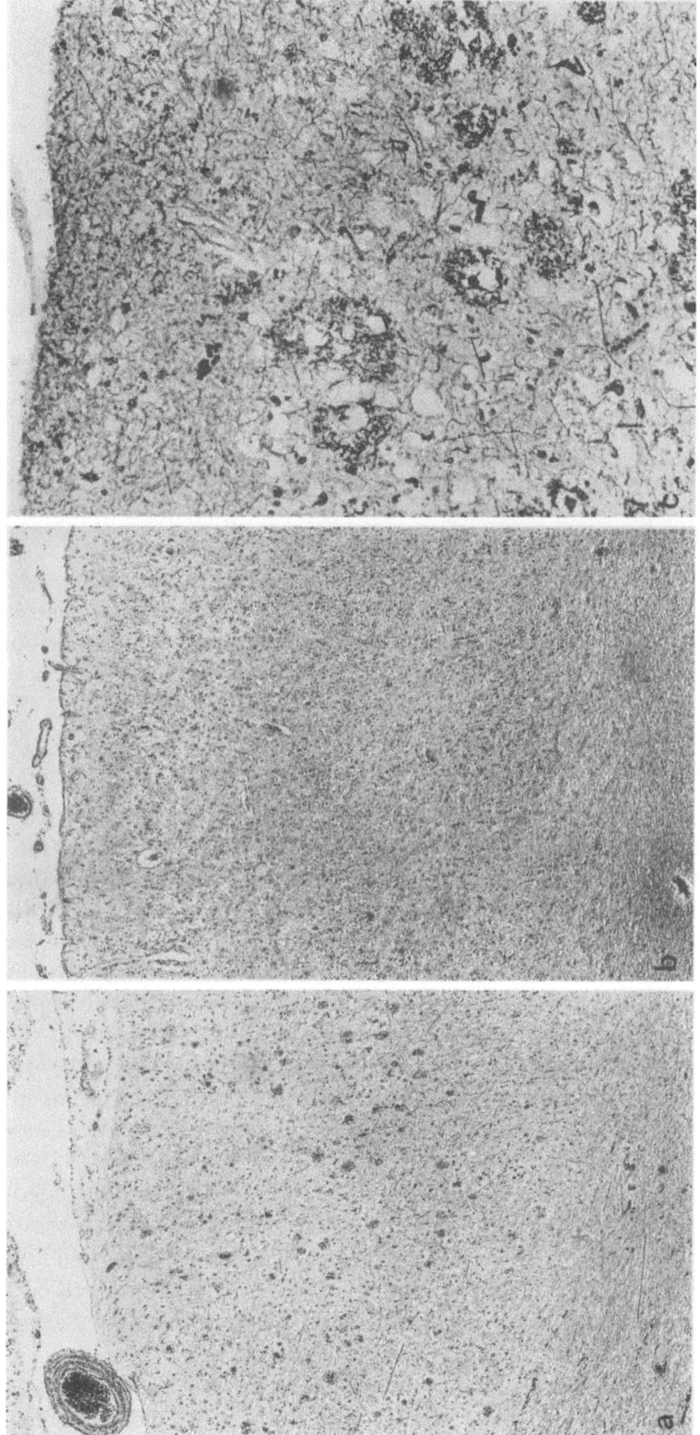

Fig. 9 a–c. Disintegration of SP. Naoumenko. **a** Cerebral cortex. Moderately severe degeneration and many SP, ×37. **b** Cerebral cortex with severe degeneration and only few remaining SP (bottom of sulcus, usually rich in SP), ×50 **c** Cerebral cortex with moderately severe to severe degeneration in same case as **b**. SP disintegrating with spongy degeneration and disappearance of abnormal neurites, ×63

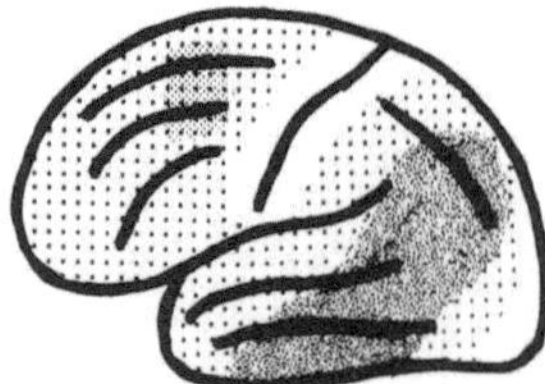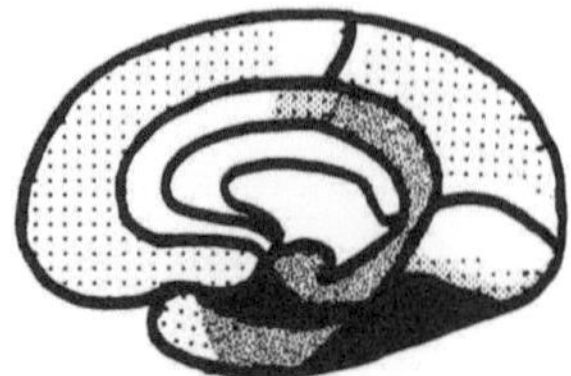

Fig. 10. Schematic picture of typical case of rather advanced AD, showing the distribution of cortical degeneration. The darker the shade the more severe the degeneration. The delineation of areas with different severity of degeneration is less sharp than shown in figure. Subject to a certain individual variation in distribution, the regional accentuations largely follow the pattern shown in the figure of the lateral and medial aspect of the cerebral hemisphere and as detailed in the text

experience we have arrived at the following pattern, which also finds support in clinical parameters. The main and earliest changes are found in the limbic grey, predominantly the amygdaloid nucleus, the hippocampus and, possibly somewhat later, in the posterior cingulate gyrus. Then follow changes in the neocortex, especially in the postcentral portion of the parietal lobe and particularly in the superior parietal lobule and basolateral temporal areas. When very severe the disease also involves the frontal lobes more heavily, still with a relative sparing of the sensorimotor and calcarine areas, the anterior cingulate gyrus and often parts of the superior temporal gyrus (Fig. 2a, b and 10).

10. Changes in Non-cortical Including Limbic Areas

At sites other than cortical and limbic areas there are also changes, according to Braunmühl (1957) in his large workup on SDAT and AD. Thus the white matter suffers a reduction in volume with some pallor of myelin staining and astrocytic gliosis but with little deposition of breakdown products. As a consequence the ventricles are widened. The striate body, pallidum, and thalamus show some atrophy with loss of neurons and lipofuscinosis, but NF and SP only to a limited extent. Here a relationship between cortical areas of accentuated involvement and subcortical nuclear degeneration may exist. Also the substantia nigra in AD is mildly or less involved than in the older patients with SDAT. Pearce (1974) on the other hand reports on the common occurrence of Parkinson symptoms in AD, though the diagnosis in these cases was not verified histopathologically. Large numbers of Lewy bodies in the substantia nigra were found in a case of AD (Rosenblum and Ghatak 1979), though lacking Parkinson symptoms. The pons, medulla, and cerebellum are by some regarded as atrophied though less than the telencephalon (Tomlinson 1977, 1979). Corsellis (1976b) found a Purkinje cell loss and an 18% difference in total cerebellar volume between dements of unspecified type and normals of the same age. The situation is often different in atypical and familial cases where, e.g. SP occur in the cerebellum (Braunmühl 1957).

It is our impression that in sporadic AD the cerebellum, pons, and medulla largely escape the Alzheimer type of degeneration, showing only few SP and NF in agreement with Mandybur (1975). The Purkinje cells thus never show NF and little, if any, lipofuscin. Yet these cells become reduced in number in ageing and to some extent also in AD. This then may be a secondary loss rather than a primary effect of the AD, e.g. due to the common epileptic seizures of the later stages of AD or secondary to fallout of other neuronal groups. This may be true also for other nuclei of the brain stem, though some have been reported to have a stable cell population (KONIGSMARK and MURPHY 1972). The spinal cord likewise shows little or no primary involvement but may suffer secondarily when long tracts degenerate due to cerebral neuronal fallout. YAMADA (1978) noted no NF in spinal cord neurons in AD but some in SDAT, together with lipofuscin increase.

11. Vascular Changes

Congophilic angiopathy (CA) has for a long time been known to occur in both ageing and SDAT and AD, though some regard it as unusual. Familial and sporadic forms of CA appear to be primary microangiopathies distinct from AD in several ways (TORACK 1978), though some features may be shared by the amyloid angiopathy in AD, such as involvement of the same calibre of vessels and also a related perivascular plaque formation. One of the pioneers in this field was SCHOLZ (1938) and also DIVRY, who wrote a series of papers on amyloid in SP and vessels. His concept was summarized by VAN BOGAERT (1970), who stated that cerebral amyloid angiopathy is most frequently found in AD, a conclusion also arrived at by SCHWARTZ (1968).

MANDYBUR (1975) in material to a large extent composed of AD of the type under consideration here, found CA in 13 of 15 cases. In agreement with this we have found CA to be very common in AD (BRUN and CAMERON 1981) and entirely missing in only few cases. It is usually of a regionally varying extent and severity, though there are reports on a more consistent regional accentuation (SCHOLZ 1938). It involves both meningeal and intracerebral, especially cortical vessels. The amyloid is deposited under the endothelium and in the media, sometimes extending through the adventitia out into the surrounding brain tissue. Here it is not always associated with plaque formation (TERRY and WISNIEWSKI 1970).

The amyloid shows a clearly segmental distribution in the meningeal and often also the intracerebral vessels, the involved segments often being expanded in a bead-like manner (BRUN and CAMERON 1981).

CA has been implicated as a cause of cerebral haemorrhage or small infarcts in cases reported as hereditary cerebral haemorrhage (GUDMUNDSSON et al. 1972), senile dementia, hypertensives or atypical AD (OKAZAKI et al. 1979; LEE and STEMMERMAN 1978; MANDYBUR and BATES 1978; SCHMITT and BARZ 1978). JELLINGER (1977) in a survey of the problem found it to be a rare cause of haemorrhage. To our knowledge it is distinctly rare in the presenile AD under consideration here. Not a single instance of either haemorrhage or infarction occurred in our large material of AD where CA is of common occurrence. Using thioflavine fluorescence SCHWARTZ (1968) found amyloid in the heart, pancreas, and also aorta, not only in ageing and senile dementia but also in AD. We are of the opinion, however, that in presenile AD the cerebromeningeal CA appears to be selective with little or no amyloid deposition at extracranial sites. This also agrees with findings of others, e.g. PANTELAKIS (1954) as well as HOLLANDER and STRICH (1970) in atypical AD.

Arteriosclerosis of the meningeal or basal vessels is not a prominent feature of AD (SOURANDER and SJÖGREN 1970; SJÖGREN et al. 1965). Intracerebral capillary vessels often show a non-amyloid change (MANCARDI et al. 1980), a thickening of the basal membrane clearly in excess of what is seen in controls. It is, however, not specific for AD since the same change is found in several other dementing cerebral disorders. The cerebral vessels in addition show the hyaline thickening and fibrosis seen in ageing (GELLERSTEDT 1933), thus also a non-specific change, as well as more severe degeneration similar to hypertensive angiopathy. Such vascular changes may play a part in the pathogenesis of the encephalopathy in AD (SJÖGREN et al. 1965), but is probably of greater relevance in SDAT with its more frequent white matter sclerosis.

E. Atypical Alzheimer's Disease

If AD is defined as a presenile disorder with the clinical character, course and histopathological picture quantitatively and topographically described above, then there are a number of cases which for one reason or other fall outside that frame and which should be designated according to deviating, dominating features, or called atypical.

The age of onset may be considerably lower than 40–65 years of age, particularly in familial cases. This is exemplified by the father and three children who all between 31 and 34 years of age developed AD, according to LOEWENBERG and WAGGONER (1934, cit. BRAUNMÜHL 1957), or the juvenile case with Alzheimer changes reported by LÖKKEN and CYVIN (1954).

The clinical picture may be ‚typical' of AD but the histopathology lacks some or all features of AD. Thus in some cases there have been NF but no SP (RASKIN and EHRENBERG 1956, CORSELLIS 1976a). Other cases have neither SP nor NF, though a clinical diagnosis of AD was regarded as firmly established (BRAUNMÜHL 1957). It is, however, conceivable that cerebral changes other than those of AD could, e.g. with limbic and temporoparietal distribution produce symptoms like those of AD.

The opposite situation, SP, and NF without the clinical picture of AD or SDAT is not a rare occurrence in patients succumbing from other causes, e.g. patients with Down's syndrome dying in their thirties or forties due to leukemia or heart malformation.

The latter combination of Alzheimer lesions and Down's syndrome was sporadically mentioned prior to JERVIS' (1948) paper on the subject, followed by, e.g. OLSON and SHAW (1969). A survey of such cases from the literature is presented by WHALLEY and BUCKTON (1979). This association is almost universal. Clinically some report a non-characteristic brain-ageing syndrome (HIRABAYASHI et al. 1979) while others also find, except for mental retardation, a reduced abstract reasoning in slightly retarded cases (STICKLAND 1954) and a reduced short-term memory above 43 years of age (DALTON et al. 1974). Such features were also reported by WISNIEWSKI et al. (1978). In a retrospective and prospective study (BRUN et al. 1978b), there were signs of dementia with onset between the ages 47 and 63, often combined with the onset of epilepsy. Symptoms included increasing incapacity to manage daily living activities, memory disturbances and also spatial disorientation. Myoclonic phenomena and insecure gait were also found. rCBF and EEG abnormalities were of the same kind as in sporadic presenile AD. In younger cases there were the same though less intense brain changes, slowly increasing from around age 20. The neuropathology was identical to that of sporadic AD in its full extent including electron microscopical features, as found by others (ELLIS 1974; SCHOCHET et al. 1973; OHARA 1972; HABERLAND 1969).

There are thus enough clinical and especially pathoanatomical similarities between sporadic AD and the presenile dementing disorder in Down's syndrome to include it as a subgroup of AD.

There are also cases on record which, in addition to SP, NF, and other changes met with in AD, show numerous Lewy-type inclusions in the neocortical neurons (YAGISHITA et al. 1980).

CA with dementia and histopathological changes of AD may be termed an atypical form or separate disease since not only symptoms but even distribution of changes is often at variance with that of AD (TORACK 1978). It occurs as a sporadic or familial disease with amyloid microangiopathy and perivascular plaques, originally called *drüsige Entartung* (SCHOLZ 1938) and dyshoric angiopathy (MOREL and WILDI 1952). The onset of dementia may be acute and NF may be missing (HOLLANDER and STRICH 1970). The amyloidosis is, however, as in ordinary AD, restricted to the brain.

A further divergent feature may be the circumscription of the atrophy in certain restricted areas. In our experience the focal atrophies are just accentuations of the general process with no abrupt transitions towards better preserved parenchyma, and sharp limits should arouse suspicion of Pick's disease or a vascular etiology. Combinations of Pick's disease and AD or a severe frontotemporal atrophy in AD are also known to occur (cit. CORSELLIS 1976 a). AD may also concur with Jacob-Creutzfeldt's disease (GACHES et al. 1977).

Cases of this type often show features clearly departing from ordinary AD. Thus in the series reported by TARISKA (1970) there was a circumscribed type of atrophy with "knife blade" atrophy. In addition the distribution of NF and SP was unusual, seen especially in the brain stem while there were no SP in some cases. On the other hand the sponginess and plaque-like gliosis reported in the cortex is a regular feature of ordinary AD in our experience.

At the far end of this spectrum there are a number of conditions which have little or nothing to do with AD but in which one finds one or more of the prominent histopathological changes of AD. Thus NF and SP in varying proportions and even granulovacuolar degeneration have been recorded in various structures, often the central grey nuclei and brain stem in a large number of diverse diseases such as "normal pressure hydrocephalus," certain inborn errors of metabolism, Parkinsonism-dementia complex of Guam, kuru, amyotrophic lateral sclerosis syndrome of Guam, progressive multifocal leucoencephalopathy, encephalitis lethargica, subacute sclerosing panencephalitis, postencephalitic Parkinsonism, and progressive supranuclear palsy. In most of these the NF is of the same PHF type as in AD except in progressive supranuclear palsy where they are found to be straight filaments (WISNIEWSKI and SOIFER 1979). Also the posttraumatic dementia after single or repeated trauma shows the changes seen in AD including CA, NF, and

SP and with much the same distribution as in AD, though in some examples with few or no SP.

These examples underscore the non-specificity of the individual pathological traits of AD.

F. Correlation Between Clinical and Pathological Features

The functional impairment has been related to the tissue changes. Thus the concentration of SP and to a lesser extent NF in the cortex have been found to correlate with degree of dementia (CORSELLIS 1962; ROTH et al. 1967; TOMLINSON et al. 1970). Beyond a mean count of about 10 SP per low-power field the intellectual capacity was impaired. This amount constitutes a threshold level. Above that level, BLESSED and TOMLINSON (1965) found a decline of test scores for the mental performance. This relationship exists only until the degeneration is severe. This would fit in with a decrease in plaque density in the severest degree of degeneration (Fig. 9 b).

The plaque count also correlates with a decrease in CAT activity but not with γ-aminobutyric acid changes (PERRY et al. 1978), the latter system thus being less closely associated with AD than the cholinergic.

A plaque count of an area may be significant and related to the dementia in a diffuse disease like AD where regional accentuations in a constant pattern are implicit and responsible for much of the symptomatology. This also means that the same count may not be related to the degree of dementia in other diseases or varieties of AD with a different pattern of regional accentuations and other lesions as often met with in atypical, e.g. familial cases. This may explain some of the situations where a correlation is lacking.

There are also other pitfalls inherent in the use of SP as a correlate, not only those connected with regional accentuations of the degenerative process, and the tendency of SP to decrease in more advanced stages, as mentioned above, but also a well-known variability in the outcome of silver impregnations mostly used for their demonstration, and the considerable morphological variation of SP, e.g. a diameter varying between 5 and 200 μm!

The relationship between SP and dementia may reflect a destruction of synaptic structures. This as well as the loss of dendrites and their spines may make early dementia and other symptoms an effect of a deafferentation of the neurons. Neuronal loss is the next level of morphological expression of the degeneration. Our own results show a relationship between decrease in neuronal cell counts in AD (relative to age-matched controls) and severity of the disease expressed as length of history and severity of clinical picture in general.

The pattern of accentuated neuronal loss also corresponds very well with the topographic pattern of lesions summarized in Fig. 10. This means that neuronal loss may relate directly to rCBF or symptom patterns especially in more advanced stages of AD. In early stages a synaptic decrement may be the only and less easily documented structural correlate.

The distribution of lesions shows important correlations to symptoms in AD with early presenile onset under consideration here. This tallies with LAUTER's finding (1968, 1970) that the earlier the onset the more pronounced the focalization of the symptom pattern becomes.

A correlation exists between the early and progressive memory failure and the early and severe degeneration of the medial, temporal limbic structures, underlined by so many neuropathologists.

When productive confabulation of the fantastic type is found in AD as well as in Pick's disease it possibly indicates lesions in the hypothalamic diencephalic structures, the prefrontal cortex or the anterior cingulum (ULE 1958; BRIERLY 1961; MEHRAEIN and ROTHEMUND 1976; PETERS 1967; BRUN and GUSTAFSON 1978). Also the epileptic phenomena in AD might be related to a severe degeneration of the temporal limbic structures including the amygdaloid nucleus. Subcortical lesions, as indicated by EEG (INGVAR and GUSTAFSON 1970; JOHANNESSON et al. 1977, 1979) might also be of importance for epileptic seizures. It also seems justified to relate the typical symptom constellation of aphasia, agnosia, spatial desorientation, and apraxia to the consistent involvement of the association cortex of the temporoparieto-occipital region of the brain (MUTRUX 1947; BRION 1966; SJÖGREN 1950; BRUN and GUSTAFSON 1976). This focalized symptom pattern dominates the second stage of AD and is also to some extent to be found as early as stage 1. The early manifestation of these symptoms indicates the significance of temporoparieto-occipital lesions for the mental deterioration in AD as well as in dementia in general (GUSTAFSON and RISBERG 1974; INGVAR et al. 1975; BRUN and GUSTAFSON 1976).

Moreover, the widespread involvement of the temporal lobe might be related to the Klüver-Bucy-like syndrome observed in AD. The syndrome is, however, only partial and indicates the importance of other brain structures for the symptom pattern (PILLERI 1966; BRUN and GUSTAFSON 1976). The relative lack of hypersexuality and bulimia is possibly due to less marked frontal lobe involvement in presenile AD as discussed by BRUN and GUSTAFSON (1976, 1978).

The emotional and personality changes in AD may relate to the involvement of limbic structures. Even at an advanced stage most AD cases appear amiable and cautious, capable of a non-verbal emotional contact. These characteristics might be related to the relative sparing of the frontal lobe cortex and especially of the anterior cingulate gyrus. When euphoria and disinhibition are present it possibly indicates a more pronounced frontal degeneration. These findings are in contrast with the pronounced personality alterations appearing early and dominating the clinical picture of Pick's disease, where prefrontal, anterior temporal and anterior cingulate cortex degeneration is more important.

As long as an adequate neurological examination can be performed, no or only slight sensory, sight and hearing impairment is noted in AD, and simple motor functions are retained. This correlates well with the sparing of the sensorimotor and calcarine areas and with the relative preservation of the superior temporal gyrus. However, motor disturbances of an akinetic-hypertronic character, unsteady gait or a "supranuclear type of extrapyramidal disorder" (PEARCE 1974) may be present. This seems to be related to the basal ganglia or cerebellar alterations which are encountered in some cases (BRUN and GUSTAFSON 1976), rather than to motor or prefrontal cortical lesions.

The relationship between ratings of symptoms of dementia and the rCBF results was studied by GUSTAFSON and RISBERG (1974). Significant correlations were found, the most important being a coupling between postcentral decrease of flow

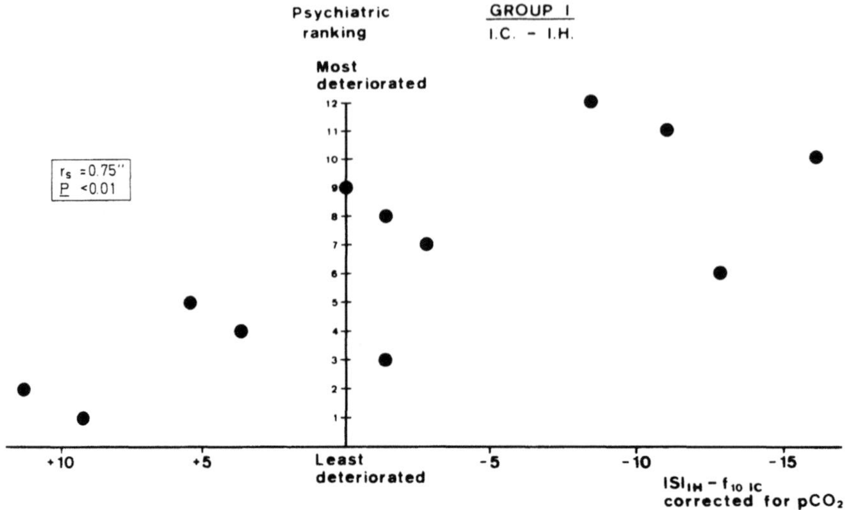

Fig. 11. Progress of dementia related to changes of mean rCBF. Correlation diagram between ranking of the degree of mental deterioration over a 5–6 year period in 12 patients with presenile dementia and changes of left hemisphere mean CBF. The first rCBF examination was made by the ^{133}Xe intra-arterial injection technique (f_{10}, height over area flow) and the second by the ^{133}Xe inhalation method (ISI). A highly significant correlation (rank) is found

and severity of symptoms such as amnesia, apraxia, confusion, agraphia, and alexia. More productive psychiatric symptoms such as paranoia, delusions, and depressions were coupled to more preserved flow conditions. Similar close relationships between scores on psychometric tests and the rCBF results have been reported by HAGBERG (1978a) and HAGBERG and INGVAR (1976).

Yearly examinations make it possible to relate changes of the clinical picture to changes in rCBF (Figs. 1 and 11). Figure 11 illustrates such a relationship regarding average CBF in a group of 12 patients (mixed group of AD and multi-infarct dementia) comparing change of flow level to degree of mental deterioration during a 5–6 year period of disease (RISBERG 1980a). A highly significant correlation of 0.75 was found, implying that a fast progression of dementia was accompanied by a rapid decrease in mean CBF. In cases of progressing AD an early more focal flow decrease in postcentral regions was recognized in the first examination while a more widespread and severe flow decrease was seen in later re-examinations (Fig. 1). It should be added that further significant information is obtained if the rCBF measurements are made during mental activation. INGVAR et al. (1975) showed a reduced amplitude of the flow response to mental activation as well as abnormal patterns of flow changes in some cases. These findings have been confirmed in series, studied by the inhalation technique (RISBERG 1980b).

G. Differential Diagnosis of Alzheimer's Disease

The differentiation of AD from other presenile dementias is difficult especially at an early stage. In dementia of the Pick type, the brain disease predominantly involves frontal and anteriotemporal regions. The clinical picture is from the onset dominated by emotional and personality deterioration and less by cognitive dysfunction (ONARI and SPATZ 1926; SCHNEIDER 1927; SJÖGREN et al. 1952; MANSVELT 1954; ESCOUROLLE 1958; ROBERTSON et al. 1958; SIM and SUSSMAN 1962). Loss of insight, disinhibition in behaviour and emotional bluntness are common and appear early, in contrast with the emotional amiability and relatively preserved personality traits in Alzheimer's disease even at an advanced stage. Memory function is less affected at an early stage as are practical abilities and spatial orientation. Confabulation of a fanciful, productive type may dominate. There is often after a period of disinhibited overactivity a change to apathy and stereotypy in behaviour. This change also involves language and mimical functions. Verbal spontaneity decreases, often ending in a mutistic state. Mimical movements disappear, sometimes ending in complete amimia. The combination of pallilalia, ecolalia, mutism, and amimia, the PEMA syndrome (GUIRAUD 1956), is considered pathognomonic of Pick's disease (ESCOUROLLE 1958). Other clinical features that might differentiate between AD and Pick's disease are epileptic seizures and myoclonia, which are more common in AD. The increased muscle tension and small-stepped gait, which are common in an advanced stage of AD, are rarely seen in Pick's disease. Moreover hyperalgesia is often reported in early and middle stages of Pick's disease (ROBERTSON et al. 1958).

EEG gives important information for the differentiation of AD and Pick's disease. In Alzheimer's disease EEG is always pathological while in Pick's disease it is considered normal at an early stage and may remain so for several years. For further information on this subject see the section on EEG findings in this chapter. The differentiation between AD and Pick's disease using psychometric tests is described in the section on psychometric assessment in this chapter.

The most common differential diagnostic problem involves AD and dementia due to cerebrovascular disorders also known as multi-infarct dementia (HACHINSKI et al. 1974). Various diagnostic procedures have been developed for this purpose, e.g. ischemic score (HACHINSKI et al. 1975), and for differentiating AD, Pick's disease, and cerebrovascular dementia (GUSTAFSON and NILSSON 1981). In cerebrovascular dementia the onset is more abrupt and the course often shows marked fluctuations with stepwise deterioration.

Confusional episodes, preservation of personality, and depressive reactions are more common in cerebrovascular dementia as are hypertension, strokes, atherosclerosis, and focal neurological symptoms and signs. Psychometric tests, EEG, rCBF, and computerized tomography can give clues important to the differential diagnosis.

The differentiation of AD from Jacob-Creutzfeldt's disease is usually easy due to the rapid course and the type of neurological defect in Jacob-Creutzfeldt's disease. However, when myoclonic twitchings and extrapyramidal signs appear early in the course of AD the differentiation might be difficult.

Differentiations between AD and hydrocephalic dementia may be important with respect to therapeutic shunting. The possibility of differentiation on psychiatric and psychometric grounds has been discussed by GUSTAFSON and HAGBERG (1978). The typical patient with hydrocephalic dementia shows a Korsakoff-like syndrome, gait disturbance and urinary incontinence, but not aphasia, agnosia,

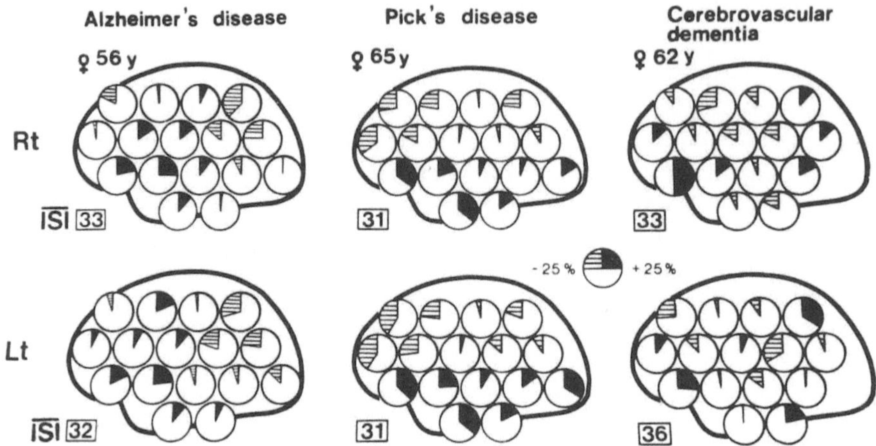

Fig. 12. Typical cases of AD, Pick's disease and multi-infarct dementia. Diagnoses confirmed at autopsy. Mean hemispheric flows shown in the *boxes*. Regional flows are indicated as *clock symbols* showing percent deviation from hemispheric mean

and apraxia to the same extent as AD cases. In AD, however, the increase in muscle tension and a small-stepped gait might sometimes resemble the gait disturbance of hydrocephalic dementia. In AD the urinary incontinence begins later in the course of the disease.

Regional cerebral blood flow measurements will in many cases add significant and sometimes decisive information for the differential diagnosis of organic dementia. In the early cases of AD the first pathological sign in rCBF is a focal flow diminution in postcentral, especially parietal regions. The abnormality commonly involves both hemispheres to an equal extent. The mean hemispheric flow level is in the lower normal range in these early cases, but will fall to subnormal levels during the progress of the disease. In moderately severe AD the focal flow pathology will be more marked involving major postcentral, except occipital, areas, and sometimes also temporal regions (a typical case is illustrated in Fig. 12). In the late and terminal stages of AD the flow level is markedly subnormal (sometimes down by 60%) with pronounced flow decreases now also in frontal regions and thus with a global distribution.

In Pick's disease the typical sign is sometimes a very marked flow decrease in frontal and frontotemporal regions with better preserved perfusion in other parts of the hemispheres. In some cases a mixture of decreased and elevated flows might be seen in frontal and frontotemporal regions. A typical picture is shown in Fig. 13. The flow changes are symmetrically distributed in the hemispheres. The flow level is generally reduced but shows larger variations than in AD with occasionally rather high values in fairly advanced cases.

Early cases of cerebrovascular dementia commonly have a normal CBF level and regional pattern and are difficult to differentiate from normal healthy control subjects with regard to rCBF. In later stages the typical indication is a spotty and asymmetrical rCBF pattern (a typical case is shown in Fig. 13) in marked contrast to the symmetrical flow changes seen in AD and Pick's disease.

A global decrease of the rCBF without focal flow changes is seen in many cases of suspected brain stem infarcts but is also seen in many other, e.g. toxic conditions. The results thus indicate that a differential diagnosis of organic dementia is possible with the bilateral ^{133}Xe-inhalation method, the degenerative dementias being more easily recognizable than the cerebrovascular ones. rCBF can also be used for a differential diagnosis between AD and pseudodementia (GUSTAFSON and RISBERG 1979).

H. Aetiology and Pathogenesis

I. Immunological, Toxic, Viral, and Hereditary Factors

The aetiology of AD is unknown. This is not surprising for a disease in which the separate structural components are non-specific or non-pathognomonic and in which up until now the early or preclinical stages of development of the disease have been beyond the reach of scientific exploration. Nevertheless a number of new hypotheses exist, which are presently under scrutiny and deserve a short review.

The possibility of immunological or auto-immune factors was suggested originally by the presence of amyloid both in vessel walls (CA) and in the central core of SP, and lately by the immunodeficiencies in Down's syndrome. Further evidence has been added, such as the finding of immunoglobulins in the central (amyloid) core of the SP. Others have found this amyloid to be closer to apud amyloid (POWERS and SPICER 1977). The exact derivation of this and the vascular amyloid is unclear though several possibilities exist (GLENNER 1978). In the SP a possible macrophage-mediated production of amyloid from local proteins may be a likely alternative, though circulating systemic factors such as immunoglobulins or SAA proteins may also be the source. The amyloid may also be a viral derivative as seen in other diseases caused by a virus or virus-like micro-organism, e.g. kuru; scrapie and Jacob-Creutzfeldt's disease, where amyloid is also found in SP. In CA the amyloidogenic source would most likely be a serum factor though the peculiar segmental deposition requires supplementary explanations not yet available.

Further, neuron-specific antibodies (NANDY 1978) have been found to increase in the serum of the aged and particularly in AD. This is of great interest with respect to neuronal loss in AD. The stimulus may be a NF protein, shown by SCHLAEPFER and LYNCH (1976) to be antigenic. The neurotubular proteins presumed to be precursors of the NF (GRUNDKE-IQBAL et al. 1979) should then be in a central position in the etiopathogenesis of AD.

A prerequisite may be an incompetence of the blood-brain barrier and presumably also of the immune apparatus such as an inability of T cells to respond properly to cell mitogens with a protein synthesis (BEHAN and BEHAN 1979) or a B-cell dyscrasia related to the former (for further information on immunological aspects see Chap. 7). As with many other factors a genetic predisposition may play an important or supplementary role.

The theory of a toxic environmental agent has also been entertained. Lead has been shown to produce in the rabbit, though not in the humans, encephalopathy with NF. The metal most often and most vividly proposed as an aetiological agent is aluminum. The aluminum is bound to neuronal nuclear chromatin in AD (DE

BONI et al. 1974), a feature of importance with respect to cellular functions such as information transfer. As with many other substances it has been shown experimentally to produce NF (KLATZO et al. 1965), though not of the PHF type seen in AD (WISNIEWSKI and SOIFER 1979), and of a different distribution. Aluminum also produced NF-like changes, again not of the PHF type, in cultured human neurons (CRAPPER et al. 1978). The validity of the latter finding, however, is not clear. Aluminum has also been found in increased amounts in the cortex in AD, both the sporadic form and in Down's syndrome with AD (CRAPPER et al. 1978). McDERMOTT et al. (1979) did not find aluminum increase in SDAT in excess of that in age-matched controls. TRAPP et al. (1978) reported the same finding in SDAT but a 1.4-fold increase in AD. A condition in which clearly raised levels of non-nuclear aluminum have been documented by several authors (e.g. ALFREY et al. 1976; McDERMOTT et al. 1978) is dialysis dementia, though NF and SP have not been reported. BRUN and DICTOR (1981), however, found SP and NF in the cortex of five out of seven dialysed patients, of which four had developed dementia. SP were more frequent than NF and the distribution was different from that usually seen in AD. All cases belonged to the presenile age group.

Even if aluminum is more closely related to NF than SP, an effect on SP would not be entirely unexpected since SP contain PHF in the distended neurites. DUCKETT and GALLE (1976) furthermore found aluminum increase in SP, and also in lysosomes using electron microprobe technique (GALLE et al. 1980).

Speculation has been aroused as to the mechanism involved in the production of PHF. One possibility is that altered protein metabolism occurs in response to nuclear deposition of aluminum or more directly through interference with the assembly of microtubules, the constituent proteins of which may be essential to the production of NF.

The aluminum debate was summarized by HENIG (1980), Parenthetically it was added that fluoridation of water may prevent aluminum from being absorbed since fluoride competes with aluminum for absorption. This measure is not therapeutic but preventive and of interest for aetiological considerations. In view of the conflicting results of quantitation studies, however, no conclusions can at present be drawn with respect to the aetiological role of aluminum, which could even be secondarily absorbed by the nervous system deteriorating from other causes.

Other metals studied include iron, the amount of which is not increased in the cortex but possibly redistributed, resulting in an increase of stainable iron (HALLGREN and SOURANDER 1960).

The possibility of a slow virus aetiology both of the conventional (EDMOND 1979) and unconventional type as in, e.g. Jacob-Creutzfeldt's disease has also been proposed, on the basis of e.g. the concurrence of Jacob-Creutzfeldt's disease and AD (GACHES et al. 1977). Jacob-Creutzfeldt's disease is characterized by neuronal loss and spongiform encephalopathy, both present also in AD though of somewhat different character and seen also in scrapie. Also suggestive of a viral theory is the appearance of complete SP as in AD, neurite thickening and amyloid depositions in experimental scrapie (WISNIEWSKI et al. 1975) and the appearance of NF in subacute spongiform panencephalitis and progressive multifocal leucoencephalopathy (HADFIELD et al. 1974; MANDYBUR et al. 1977), examples of unconventional and conventional virus diseases respectively.

Cultured fetal human neurons, exposed to extracts, including cell-free preparations, from a deceased case of AD, developed PHF in many of the neuronal processes (DE BONI and CRAPPER 1978). This could be due to metabolic products or a viral agent, the latter alternative being favoured by the authors. A viral mechanism is possible (WISNIEWSKI 1978) with regard to the microtubule involvement in virus replication (DALES 1975). Tubulin does not make neurotubules but forms PHF with viral protein.

Attempts have also been made to induce AD in experimental animals by transmission from human cases. Two such familial cases resulted in a spongiform encephalopathy in the animal brain though without SP or NF, and the disease proved to be serially transmissible (GIBBS and GAJDUSEK 1978; REWCASTLE et al. 1978). However, material from sporadic cases did not result in an experimental disease. This may be a difference between familial and sporadic AD in addition to those pointed out above.

If reduced immunocompetence is required, then the above-mentioned decrease in this function with advancing age, particularly in SDAT, may again become important. In this context it is of interest that AD may be associated with histocompatibility antigens, e.g. HLA-BW 15 as discussed by RENVOIZE et al. (1979) or HLA-A 2, suggesting a role for immune response genes (BEHAN and BEHAN 1979) though WHALLEY and BUCKTON (1979) and WHALLEY et al. (1979, 1980) found no such association with AD.

Genetic factors have been touched upon in connection with aetiological or precipitating factors. The association between AD and Down's syndrome, which has an extra chromosome 21, has led to a search for chromosomal abnormalities in AD, in particular pertaining to chromosome 21, which by TAN et al. (1973) was proposed to harbour the gene for antiviral protein. This brings up again the possibility of a viral cause. Chromosomal abberrations in AD have also been reported (NIELSEN 1968; BERGENER and JUNGKLAASS 1970) but were not verified by others (MARK and BRUN 1973; BRUN et al. 1978a; SULKAVA et al. 1979) using Giemsa banding technique and sister chromatid exchange studies. In ageing patients, however, GALLOWAY and BUCKTON (1978) found a loss of chromosome 21 in peripheral blood lymphocytes. WHALLEY and BUCKTON (1979) argue that such an abnormality of the immune surveillance cell system can not be excluded in AD until a large proportion of cells have been studied. If present, such a defect would allow a conventional virus to contribute to the development of the neuropathological changes, especially in the senile group.

WARD et al. (1979) reported aneuploidy in both sporadic and especially familial cases of presenile AD and to some extent in groups of siblings of affected patients. The question was asked whether this change might herald the onset of the disease.

Further indications of a genetic factor are the increased risks for first degree relatives of AD patients to develop the disease and the increased morbidity risk for Down's syndrome and haematological malignancies (HESTON and MASTRI 1977). Furthermore the female relative of an AD patient is much more likely to have a Down's child than a male relative, this occurring in nearly 2% of female relatives of AD patients (HESTON 1979).

There are a limited number of population studies, the results of which are difficult to interpret since in some, AD and SDAT and even Pick's disease are not treated separately, nor is more than a proportion of cases histologically verified. According to some investigators (Pratt 1970; Zerbin-Rüdin 1967), 10%–15% of cases with AD have a positive heredity, while thus the majority is of the sporadic type. The true familial cases often deviate from the great bulk of sporadic cases by showing a dominant genetic pattern and, in addition, differ with respect to many clinical and histopathological features as noted above.

For the sporadic cases the possibility of multifactorial inheritance was pointed out (Sjögren et al. 1952), though an exact determination of the mode of inheritance could not be made. Further careful studies by Larsson et al. (1963) and Constantinides et al. (1962) disagree on the occurrence of AD among first degree relatives. Pratt (1970) in his review on the matter concludes that a polygenic inheritance with a shared predisposition both to AD and SDAT is more likely than a single autosomal dominant gene.

Against this background we feel, however, that it would be premature to nominate the most likely aetiological agent or agents or a sequence of pathogenetic events. The aetiological alternatives, viral, immunological, and toxic environmental agents may interact to produce the disease (Crapper and De Boni 1978), and may also interact with hereditary factors.

II. Transmitters

Newer research results include the finding of a disturbance of transmitter substances and functions.

Catecholamine disturbances and substitution therapy with L-dopa and dopamine agonists have been reported in AD and SDAT by, e.g. the Gottfries group (Adolfsson et al. 1978, 1979), with increase of monoamine oxidase activity and reduced levels of dopamine and norepinephrine though without direct correlation to dementia. The main interest has lately shifted from catecholamines, GABA, and peptides towards cholinergic mechanisms, though Reisine et al. (1978, 1980) point out the importance of the other systems and their dependence on the cholinergic system. Both in monkeys and humans the short-term memory is less dependent on dopamineergic than cholinergic systems (Bartus 1978), which have a specific relationship to memory and other cognitive functions (Drachman 1977). There are some conflicting or hard to interprete results but it now appears safe to conclude that on the presynaptic side cholinacetyltransferase (CAT) is reduced in AD (Davies and Maloney 1976), a reduction that is selective and possibly a key change in AD (Bowen et al. 1979), separating AD from ageing. It may be an early indicator of synaptic failure preceeding the disappearance of the neuron and the appearance of regional blood flow changes. There seems also to be a reduction in acetylcholine esterase (AChE) though this would be less specific (Davies and Maloney 1976). The reduction in CAT also correlates with the neuropathology. Thus Bowen (1979) found that whole temporal lobe assessment revealed no loss of CAT in non-demented controls but a significant loss in AD. This is interesting in view of the regional accentuation of the atrophy in the temporal lobe in AD. The atrophy is, however, not uniformly distributed in the temporal cortex but spares some neocortical areas such as the temporal pole and superior temporal gyrus with a corresponding preservation of neurons. The atrophy is much more pronounced than in SDAT and especially in ageing. It seems reasonable to assume that exclusion of these less affected areas would have further amplified the difference between AD and controls in the biochemical study.

A CAT reduction was also found by PERRY et al. (1977, 1978) to occur in the parietal lobe. This is another area of accentuated degeneration with prominent cell loss according to our experience. DAVIES (1978, 1979) found a loss of choline acetylase to be greater than 87% in hippocampus, amygdala, midtemporal gyrus, and parietal cortex, 79%–83% in the frontal cortex and insignificant in, e.g. occipital and central gyri. The pattern revealed by loss of cholinergic substances thus shown by BOWEN, PERRY and DAVIES above agrees well with the pattern of accentuated degeneration (BRUN and GUSTAFSON 1976, 1978) and distribution of neuronal cell loss and degree of severity of the degeneration in AD (BRUN and ENGLUND 1981). Unfortunately, figures for the cingulate gyrus are not specified as to anterior or posterior part, which are dramatically different with respect to severity of degeneration. The low figures for the hippocampus correspond well with several observations on the extent and severity of lesions including cell loss here (BALL 1977; KEMPER 1978; SHEFER 1977). It still remains to be clarified whether CAT reduction is primary or secondary, whether it is due to loss of synaptic structures or chemical synthesis alone and also whether acetylcholine is reduced (BOWEN 1979). The answer to such questions will be decisive for future therapeutic attempts. Neurotransmitters are more fully treated in Chap. 6.

I. Treatment with Transmitter Substances

In the decline of the synaptic apparatus described, part of it may long remain intact, in particular on the postsynaptic side. Muscarinic acetylcholine receptor binding capacity was found by DAVIES and VERTH (1978) to be preserved, something that can be taken to indicate a compensatory increase in these receptors by the surviving neurons. Preservation of such neuronal structures and functions would be a prerequisite for meaningful treatment. The knowledge that enhanced cholinergic activity facilitates cognitive functions and the discovery of a failure of mainly, but not exclusively cholinergic transmitters in AD has prompted attempts to substitute or preserve the transmitters in analogy with therapeutics in Parkinsons disease. Therapeutic pilot studies have been made with, e.g. choline in moderately advanced cases of AD or rather SDAT with no definite clinical improvement (ETIENNE et al. 1978 a). Some clinical benefit was noted when lecithin was given at early stages of the disease (ETIENNE et al. 1978 b). Others have not shown an effect, which may be due either to insensitivity of the test instrument or of the patient, having too far advanced structural changes to respond to treatment (RENVOIZE and JERRAM 1979). Other as yet mostly theoretical alternatives, such as selectively centrally active anticholinesterase, remain to be tested. Before that or any other therapeutic measure can be tested, other problems have to be solved, above all that of an early and reliable diagnosis of AD.

J. Early Diagnosis of Alzheimer's Disease

Early recognition of AD has for a long time been of mainly academic interest. A more relevant objective has now been added, viz. the possibility of symptomatic treatment as outlined above. An early diagnosis is important considering the irreparable tissue damage with loss of irreplacable structures including neurons in later stages of AD.

Biopsy has been evaluated (SMITH et al. 1966) and is by some regarded as not justified. With reference to the pattern of regional accentuation of the disease process the best site would be the parietal superior lobule both from a practical point of view and with regard to its early and prominent involvement. Intraregional variations influence the size of the biopsy specimen needed for a safe diagnosis.

The computerized tomography scan has been employed for diagnostic purposes and for a correlation with degree of dementia. It is the opinion of several writers that this method has little positive help to offer (e.g. RAMANI et al. 1979; Fox et al. 1979) but may exclude other causes of dementia such as infarctions, haemorrhages, and tumours. This is important especially in early stages (DONALDSON 1979) when there may be little weight loss, gross atrophy or ventricular widening in spite of a clear-cut dementia. The problems of early diagnosis were debated at a colloquium in Edinburgh (GLEN and WHALLEY 1979). Criteria for an early diagnosis have been outlined by, e.g. GLEN and CHRISTIE (1979 and SIM (1979).

The early diagnosis of AD has to rest upon the exclusion of other causes, above all Pick's disease, Jacob-Creutzfeldt's disease, cerebrovascular disease, normal pressure hydrocephalus, and inorganic dementias but also alcoholism, head injury, anaemias including pernicious anaemia and other metabolic or deficiency states. The positive diagnostic criteria of AD have been outlined in the clinical workup of the disease. As pointed out there, an early diagnosis, based on the symptomatology alone is hardly practicable at present but may be supported by psychometric tests, EEG and rCBF (JOHANNESSON et al. 1977; GUSTAFSON 1979). Diagnostic criteria must, however, be tested against neuropathological data until the criteria for the various methods for an early diagnosis are well worked out.

K. Concluding Remarks

The fact that all the histopathological changes in AD and SDAT are identical and are furthermore also seen in many other conditions makes these changes rather unspecific and may also indicate a varied aetiology. The same might apply to the symptomatology, which would rather be based on the structures involved than on the nature of the underlying tissue process. Consequently these factors are of limited value as evidence for identity between AD and SDAT.

The main differences between these two diseases relate to age of onset, course and intensity of the disease process, differences which are again rather vague. According to our experience however, SDAT differs from AD with respect to a distinctly higher rate of not only infarctions but also white matter "degeneration," a demyelination possibly related to intracerebral vascular sclerosis. The question of identity or not between the two diseases can thus presently not be settled convincingly. For the time being it would therefore be an advantage to state the type of disease under discussion or keep the diseases apart in scientific reports simply by setting the age limit at 65 years of age. This would help avoid confusion, e.g. as to prevalence or cell loss and enable the reader to evaluate similarities or differences. It is reasonable to assume, however, that research results pertaining to the PHF in particular might apply to both conditions, since they belong to the two main lesions, the NF and SP, of both AD and SDAT. They can be induced experimentally in vivo and in vitro and can be logically associated with several of the aetiological and pathogenetic possibilities.

Alzheimer's disease is a diffuse mainly cortical disorder but with regional accentuations, appearing chronologically and topographically in a fairly consistent pattern. Chronology, topography, and intensity of the regional accentuations are reflected in the course and intensity of symptoms and rCBF changes. These accentuations thus seem to characterize the disease.

Before the changes reach the level of intensity that produces symptoms, they may have run through a long period of build up, possibly as protracted as in Down's syndrome, where the lesions may develop during 25–30 years or more before symptoms set in. During such a "preclinic" period these changes may create an erroneous impression of a particular "premorbid personality."

Considering the short period of survival sometimes reported and an average survival of 5–7 years this latter phase of the disease appears to be one of accelerated progression. Against this background AD may be regarded as an extremely protracted disease with a slow preclinical and a fast clinical phase.

In spite of the considerable recent research achievements much remains to be done, in particular with regard to aetiology and pathogenesis and also epidemiology and even purely diagnostic especially early diagnostic criteria. A preclinical period would presumably be of greater interest from the aetiological and pathogenetic point of view than even the earliest definable period of clinical symptoms.

An early diagnosis is also of importance with respect to therapeutic, e.g. symptomatic, transmitter-related or curative, attempts since any response is dependent upon structural integrity, and little would be gained by halting the disease in a severely incapacitated phase. Furthermore, the possibility of regeneration of synaptic structures at an early stage cannot be excluded. The magnitude of the problem from a medical and social point of view and the promises afforded by recent research work certainly make this field of investigation one of the most worthwhile and important.

List of Abbreviations

AD: Alzheimer's disease; CA: Congophilic angiopathy; CAT: Choline acetyltransferase; EEG: Electroencephalogram; NF: Neurofibrillary degeneration; PHF: Paired helical filaments; rCBF: Regional cerebral blood flow; SDAT: Senile dementia of Alzheimer's type; SP: Senile plaue

Acknowledgements: Thanks are in particular due to L. Gustafson, D. Ingvar, J. Risberg, and B. Hagberg for contributions and collaboration on clinical, cerebral blood flow and psychometric aspects. The excellent histotechnical, photographic, and secretarial assistance of K. Sturesson, E. Andersson, and G. Behm, P. Posselwhite, and C. Nilsson, K. Carlsson, and G. Kungberg is gratefully acknowledged.

References

Adams RD, Fisher CM, Hakin S, Ojemann RG, Sweet WH (1965) Symptomatic occult hydrocephalus with „normal" cerebrospinal fluid pressure. New Engl J Med 3:117–126

Adolfsson R, Gottfries CG, Oreland L, Roos BB, Winblad B (1978) Reduced levels of catecholamines in the brain and increased activity of monoamine oxidase in platelets in Alzheimer's disease: Therapeutic implications. In: Katzman A, Terry RD, Bick KL (eds) Alzheimer's disease: Senile dementia and relates disorders (Ageing vol 7). Raven Press, New York, p 441

Adolfsson R, Forsell Å, Gottfries CG, Kajsajuntti C (1979) Substitution therapy with *l*-dopa and dopamine agonist in dementia disorders of Alzheimer type. In: Orimo H, Shimada K, Iriki M, Maeda O (eds) Recent advances in gerontology. Excerpta Medica, Amsterdam, p 173

Alfrey AC, LeGendre GR, Kaehny WD (1976) The dialysis encephalopathy syndrome. Possible aluminum intoxication. New Engl J Med 294:184–188

Alzheimer A (1906) Lecture, 37 Versammlung Südwestdtsch Irrenärzte, Tübingen Nov 1906, noted by title only; published 1907

Alzheimer A (1907) Über eine eigenartige Erkrankung der Hirnrinde. Verh psychiatr Vereine: Verein südwestdeutscher Irrenärzte. Allg Z Psychiatr 64:141–148

Alzheimer A (1911) Über eigenartige Krankheitsfälle des späteren Alters. Z. Ges Neurol Psychiat 356–385

Arendt A (1972) Altern des Zentralnervensystems. In: Holle G (ed) Handbuch der allgemeinen Pathologie, B IV/4. Springer, Berlin Heidelberg New York, p 490

Ball MJ (1977) Neuronal loss, neurofibrillary tangles and granulovacuolar degeneration in the hippocampus with ageing and dementia. A quantitative study. Acta Neuropathol (Berl) 37:111–118

Ball MJ (1978) Topographic distribution of neurofibrillary tangles and granulovacuolar degeneration in hippocampal cortex of aging and demented patients. A quantitative study. Acta Neuropathol (Berl) 42:73–80

Ball MJ, Lo P (1977) Granulovacuolar degeneration in the ageing brain and in dementia. J Neuropath Exp Neurol 36:474–487

Bartus RT (1978) Short-term memory in the rhesus monkey: Effects of depamine blockade via acute haloperiodol administration. Pharmacol Biochem Behav 9(3):353–357

Behan PO, Behan NMH (1979) Possible immunological factors in Alzheimer's disease. In: Glen AIM, Whalley LJ (eds) Alzheimer's disease. Early recognition of potentially reversible deficits. Churchill Livingstone, Edinburgh London New York, p 33

Bergener M, Jungklaass FK (1970) Genetische Befunde bei Morbus Alzheimer und seniler Demenz. Geront Clin 12:71–75

Berger H (1931) Über das Elektroencephalogramm des Menschen. Fünfte Mitteilung. Arch Psychiat Nervenkrankh 98:231–254

Blessed G, Tomlinson BE (1965) Senile plaques and intellectual deterioration in old age. In: Psychiatric disorders of the aged. Geigy (UK) Ltd, Basle, pp 310–321

van Bogaert L (1970) Cerebral amyloid angiopathy and Alzheimer's disease. In: Wolstenholme and O'Connor M (eds) Alzheimer's disease and related conditions. Churchill, London, p 95

Bowen DM (1979) Neurochemical findings in Alzheimer's disease. In: Glenn AIM, Whalley LJ (eds) Alzheimer's disease. Early recognition of potentially reversible deficits. Churchill Livingstone, Edinburgh London New York, p 17

Bowen DM, Smith CB, Davison AN (1973) Molecular changes in senile dementia. Brain 96:849–856

Bowen DM, Smith CB, White P, Davison AN (1976) Senile dementia and related abiotrophies: Biochemical studies on histologically evaluated human postmortem specimens. In: Terry RD, Gershon S (eds) Neurobiology of Aging. Raven Press, New York, p 361

Bowen DM, Spillane JA, Curzon G, Meier-Ruge W, White P, Goodhardt MJ, Iwangoff P, Davison AN (1979) Accelerated ageing or selective neuronal loss as an important cause of dementia? Lancet 1; 8106:11–14

Braunmühl A (1957) Alterserkrankungen des Zentralnervensystems. Senile Involution. Senile Demenz. Alzheimersche Krankheit. In: Lubarsch O, Henke F, Rössle R (eds) Handbuch der speziellen pathologischen Anatomie und Histologie. Band XIII/1. Springer, Berling Göttingen Heidelberg, p 337

Brierly JB (1961) Clinico-pathological correlations in amnesia. Gerontol Clin 3:97–109

Brion S (1966) Démences par atrophie cérébrale primitive. Le concours médical 15-I-88-3, Dossier EPU no 31:313–324

Brody H (1955) Organization of the cerebral cortex III. A study of ageing in the human cerebral cortex. J Comp Neurol 102:511–556

Brody H (1970) Structural changes in the aging nervous system. Interdiscipl Topics Gerontol 7:9–21

Brody H (1976) An examination of cerebral cortex and brainstem aging. In: Terry RD, Gershon S (eds) Neurobiology of Aging. Raven Press, New York, p 177

Brody H (1978) Cell counts in cerebral cortex and brain stem. In: Katzman R, Terry RD, Bick KL (eds) Alzheimer's disease. Senile dementia and related disorders (Aging vol 7). Raven Press, New York, p 345

Brun A, Brunk U (1974) Lysosomal alterations related to age. In: Viidik A (ed) Proc 4 th Europ Sympos on basic res in Geront. Scand J Clin Lab Invest Suppl 141:18–19

Brun A, Cameron R (to be published 1981) The appearance of cerebrovascular amyloidosis in Alzheimer's disease and Down's syndrome

Brun A, Dictor M (1981) Senile plaques and tangles in dialysis dementia. Acta path microbiol Scand 89:193–198

Brun A, Englund E (1981) The pattern of degeneration in Alzheimer's disease. Neuronal loss and histopathological grading. Histopathology 5:549–564

Brun A, Gustafson L (1976) Distribution of cerebral degeneration in Alzheimer's disease. A clinico-pathological study. Arch Psychiat Nervenkr 223:15–33

Brun A, Gustafson L (1978) Limbic lobe involvement in presenile dementia. Arch Psychiat Nervenkr 226:79–93

Brun A, Gustafson L, Ingvar DH (1975) Neuropathological findings related to neuropsychiatric symptoms and regional cerebral blood flow in presenile dementia. VII th Int Congress of Neuropathology. Excerpta Medica, Amsterdam, p 101

Brun A, Gustafson L, Mitelman F (1978 a) Normal chromosome banding pattern in Alzheimer's disease. Gerontology 24:369–372

Brun A, Gustafson L, Risberg J (1978 b) The development of Alzheimer's encephalopathy and its clinical expression. J Neurpath exp Neurol 37, 5, p 595

Brunk U, Brun A (1972) The effect of aging on lysosomal permeability in nerve cells of the central nervous system. An enzyme histochemical study in rat. Histochemie 30:315–324

Buell SJ, Coleman PD (1979) Dendritic growth in the aged human brain and failure to grow in senile dementia. Science 206:854–856

Cammermeyer J (1961) The importance of avoiding "dark" neurons in experimental neuropathology. Acta Neuropath (Berlin) 1:245–270

Christian W (1968) Elektroencephalographie. Lehrbuch und Atlas. Georg Thieme, Stuttgart

Colmant HJ (1968) Spongiöse Dystrophien. Verh d Dtsch Ges f Path 52 Tagung 1968. G Fischer Verlag, Stuttgart, p 126–152

Colon EJ (1973) The cerebral cortex in presenil dementia. A quantitative analysis. Acta Neuropathol (Berl) 23:281–290

Constantinidis J (1978) Is Alzheimer's disease a major form of senile dementia? Clinical, anatomical and genetic data. In: Katzman R, Terry RD, Bick KL (eds) Alzheimer's disease: Senile dementia and related disorders (Aging vol 7). Raven Press, New York, p 15

Constantinidis J, Garrone D, deAjuriaquerra J, (1962) L-hérédité de démenes de l'âge avance. L'Encépale 4:301–344

Corsellis JAN (1962) Mental illness and the ageing brain. Oxford University Press, London

Corsellis JAN (1969) The pathology of dementia. Br J Hosp Med 1969:695–702

Corsellis JAN (1970) The limbic areas in Alzheimer's disease and in other conditions associated with dementia. In: Wolstenholme GBW, O'Connor M (eds) Alzheimer's disease and related disorders. A CIBA Foundation Symposium, Churchill, London, p 37

Corsellis JAN (1976a) Ageing and the dementias. In: Blackwood W, Corsellis JAN (eds) Greenfield's Neuropathology, 3rd ed. Edward Arnold publishers Ltd, London, p 796

Corsellis JAN (1976b) Some observations on the Purkinje cell population and on brain volume in human aging. In: Terry RD, Gershon S (eds) Neurobiology of aging. Raven Press, New York, p 205

Crapper DR (1976) Functional consequenses of neurofibrillary degeneration. In: Terry RD, Gershon S (eds) Neurobiology of Aging. Raven Press, New York, p 405

Crapper DR, Karlik S, De Boni U (1978) Aluminum and other metals in senile (Alzheimer) dementia. In: Katzman R, Terry RD, Bick KL (eds) Alzheimer's disease: Senile dementia and related disorders (Aging vol 7). Raven Press, New York, p 471

Crapper DR, De Boni U (1978) Brain aging and Alzheimer's disease. Can Psychiat Assoc J 4:229–233

Dales S (1975) Involvement of the microtubule in replication cycles of animal viruses. Ann NY Acad Sci 253:440–444

Dalton AJ, Crapper DR, Schlotter GR (1974) Alzheimer's disease in Down's syndrome: Visual retention deficits. Cortex 10:366–377

Davies P (1978) Studies on the neurochemistry of central colinergic systems in Alzheimer's disease. In: Katzman R, Terry RD, Bick KL (eds) Alzheimer's disease: Senile dementia and related disorders (Aging vol 7). Raven Press, New York, p 453

Davies P (1979) Biochemical changes in Alzheimer's disease-senile dementia: Neurotransmitters in senile dementia of the Alzheimer's type. In: Katzman R (ed) Congenital and aquired cognitive disorders. Raven Press, New York, p 153

Davies P, Maloney AJF (1976) Selective loss of central cholinergic neurons in Alzheimer's disease. Lancet II:1403

Davies P, Verth AH (1978) Regional distribution of muscarinic acetylcholine receptor in normal and Alzheimer's-type dementia brains. Brain Res 138:385–392

DeBoni U, Crapper DR (1978) Paired helical filaments of the Alzheimer type in cultured neurones. Nature 271:566–568

DeBoni U, Scott JM, Crapper DR (1974) Intracellular aluminum binding: A histochemical study. Histochemistry 40:31–37

DeKosky ST, Bass NH (1980) Effects of aging and senile dementia on the microchemical pathology of human cerebral cortex. In: Amaducci L, Davison AN, Antuono P (eds) Aging of the brain and dementia (Aging vol 13). Raven Press, New York

Divry P (1927) Etude histochimique des plaques séniles. J Belge Neurol 27:643–657

Donaldson AA (1979) CT scan in Alzheimer pre-senile dementia. In: Glen AIM, Whalley LJ (eds) Alzheimer's disease: Early recognition of potentially reversible deficits. Raven Press, New York, p 97

Drachman DA (1977) Memory and cognitive function in man: Does the cholinergic system have a specific role? Neurology 27:783–790

Duckett S, Galle P (1976) Mise en évidence de l'aluminium dans le plaques séniles de la maladie d'Alzheimer: Etude a la microsonde de Castaign. C R Acad Sci (0) Paris 282:393–395

Edmond E (1979) Conventional viruses in slow infection of the central nervous system. In: Glen AIM, Whalley LJ (eds) Alzheimer's disease: Early recognition of potentially reversible deficits. Churchill Livingstone, Edinburgh London New York, p 46

Ellis WG (1974) Presenile dementia in Down's syndrome. Ultrastructural identity with Alzheimer's disease. Neurology 24, no 2:101–106

Escourolle R (1958) La maladie de Pick. Etude critique d'ensemble et synthese anatomo-clinique. Imprimerie R Foulon, Paris

Etienne P, Gauthier S, Johnson G, Collier B, Mendis T, Dastoor D, Cole M, Muller HF (1978a) Clinical effects of choline in Alzheimer's disease. Lancet I:508–509

Etienne P, Gauthier S, Dastoor D, Collier B, Ratner J (1978b) Lecithin in Alzheimer's disease. Lancet II:1206

Faden AI, Townsend JJ (1976) Myoclonus in Alzheimer disease. A confusing sing. Arch Neurol 33:278

Feldman ML (1976) Aging changes in the morphology of cortical dendrites. In: Terry RD, Gershon S (eds) Neurobiology of aging. Raven Press, New York, p 211

Fox JA, Kaszniak AW, Huckman M (1979) Computerized tomography scanning not very helpful in dementia. New Engl J Med 300/8:437

Freyhan FA, Woodford RB, Kety SS (1951) Cerebral blood flow and metabolism in psychoses of senility. J Nerv Ment Dis 113:449–456

Friede RL (1965) Enzyme histochemical studies of senile plaques. J Neuropath Exp Neurol 24:477–491

Gaches J, Supino-Viterbo V, Foucin JF (1977) Association de maladies d'Alzheimer et de Creutzfeldt-Jakob. Acta Neurol Belg 77:202–212

Galle F, Berry J-P, Duckett S (1980) Electron microprobe ultrastructural localization of aluminum in rat brain. Acta Neuropathol (Berlin) 49:245–247

Galloway SM, Buckton RE (1978) Aneuploidy and ageing: Chromosome studies on a random sample of the population using G-banding. Cytogenet Cell Genet 20:78–95

Gellerstedt N (1933) Zur Kenntnis der Hirnveränderungen bei der normalen Altersinvolution. Diss Uppsala Läk-fören Förh 38:191

Gibbs CJ, Gajdusek DC (1978) Subacute spongiform virus encephalopathies. The transmissible virus dementias. In: Katzman R, Terry RD, Bick KL (eds) Alzheimer's disease: Senile dementia and related disorders (Aging vol 7). Raven Press, New York, p 559

Gibson PH, Tomlinson BE (1977) Numbers of hirano bodies in the hippocampus of normal and demented people with Alzheimer's disease. J Neurol Sci 33:199–206

Glen AIM, Christie IE (1979) Early diagnosis of Alzheimer's disease: working definitions for clinical and laboratory criteria. In: Glen AIM, Whalley LJ (eds) Alzheimer's disease. Early recognition of potentially reversible deficits. Churchill Livingstone, Edinburgh London New York, p 122

Glen AIM, Whalley LJ (1979) Alzheimer's disease. Early recognition of potentially reversible deficits. Churchill Livingstone, Edinburgh London New York

Glenner GG (1978) Current knowledge of amyloid deposits as applied to senile plaques and congophilic angiopathy. In: Katzman R, Terry RD, Bick KL (eds) Alzheimer's disease and related disorders (Aging vol 7). Raven Press, New York, p 493

Gonatas NK, Gambetti P (1970) The pathology of the synapse in Alzheimer's disease. In: Wolstenholme GEW, O'Connor M (eds) Alzheimer's disease and related conditions. A CIBA Foundation Symposium Bd 6. Churchill, London, p 169

Gonatas NK, Moss A (1975) Pathologic axons and synapses in human neuropsychiatric disorders. Human Pathology 6:5:571–582

Gordon EB, Sim M (1967) The EEG in presenile dementia. J Neurol Neurosurg Psychiat 30:285–291

Granville-Grossman K (1971) Hydrocephalic dementia. In: Recent advances in clinical psychiatry. Churchill, London, p 246

Green MA, Stevenson LD, Fonseca JE, Wortis SB (1952) Cerebral biopsy in patients with presenile dementia. Dis Nerv Syst 13:303–307

Grufferman S (1978) Alzheimer's disease and senile dementia: one disease or two? In: Katzman R, Terry RD, Bick KL (eds) Alzheimer's disease: Senile dementia and related disorders (Aging vol 7). Raven Press, New York, p 35

Grundke-Iqbal I, Wisniewski HM, Johnson AB, Terry RD, Iqbal K (1979) Evidence that Alzheimer neurofibrillary tangles originate from neurotubules. Lancet I:578–579

Gudmundsson G, Hallgrímsson J, Jónasson TA, Bjarnason O (1972) Hereditary cerebral haemorrhage with amyloidosis. Brain 95:387–404

Guiraud P (1956) Psychiatrie clinique. Le Françcois, Paris, p 533–550

Gustafson L (1975) Psychiatric symptoms in dementia with onset in the presenile period. Acta Psychiat Scand suppl 257, p 9

Gustafson L (1979) Regional cerebral blood flow in Alzheimer's disease – differential diagnosis, the possibility of early recognition and evaluation of treatment. In: Glen AIM, Whalley LJ (eds) Alzheimer's disease. Early recognition of potentially reversible deficits. Churchill Livingstone, Edinburgh London New York, p 102

Gustafson L, Hagberg B (1978) Recovery in hydrocephalic dementia after shunt operation. J Neurol Neurosurg Psychiat vol 41, no 10:940–947

Gustafson L, Nilsson L (1981) Differential diagnosis of presenile dementia on clicinal grounds. Acta Psych Scand (accepted)

Gustafson L, Risberg J (1974) Regional cerebral blood flow related to psychiatric symptoms in dementia with onset in the presenile period. Acta Psychiat Scand 50:516–538

Gustafson L, Risberg J (1979) Regional cerebral blood flow measured by the 133-Xe inhalation technique in differential diagnosis of dementia. Acta Neurol Scand 60, suppl 72:546–547

Gustafson L, Brun A, Ingvar DH (1977) Presenile dementia: Clinical symptoms, pathoanatomical findings and cerebral blood flow. In: Meyer JS, Lechner H, Reivich M (eds) Cerebral vascular disease. Proceedings of the 8 th International Salzburg Conference. Excerpta Medica, Amsterdam, p 5

Gustafson L, Hagberg B, Ingvar DH (1978) Speech disturbances in presenile dementia related to local blood flow abnormalities in the brain. Brain Language 5:103–118

Haberland C (1969) Travauz originaux. Alzheimer's disease in Down's syndrome. Clinical-neuropathological observations. Acta Neurol Belg 69:369–380

Hachinski VC, Lassen NA, Marshall J (1974) Multi-infarct dementia, a cause of mental deterioration in the elderly. Lancet II:207–210

Hachinski VC, Iliff LD, Zilhka E, duBoulay GH, McAllister VL, Marshall J, Ross Russell RW, Symon L (1975) Cerebral blood flow in dementia. Arch Neurol 32:632–637

Hadfield MG, Martinez AH, Gilmartin AC (1974) Progressive multifocal leukoencephalopathy with paramyxovirus-like structures, Hirano bodies and neurofibrillary tangles. Acta Neuropathol (Berl) 27:277–288

Hagberg B (1978 a) Defects of immediate memory related to the cerebral blood flow distribution. Brain Language 5:366–377

Hagberg B (1978 b) Cognitive impairment and personality change in relation to brain dysfunction. Thesis. Studiae Psychol et pedag. Series altera 44. Liber, CWK Gleerup, Lund

Hagberg B (1980 a) Psychometry and regional cerebral blood flow (rCBF) measurements. An evaluation of central concepts in the dynamic localization theory of behaviour determination. Psychological research, in Luria Memorial Issue, vol 41 (2–3)

Hagberg B (1980 b) Cognitive impairment and test taking attitudes in organic dementia. A comparison between diffuse pre- and postcentral lesions. Psychol Bull, Lund University, Lund, Sweden

Hagberg B (1980 c) Bedömning av tidiga demenstillstånd (Evaluation of dementia with early onset). In: Kongressrapport från 4: e nord kongr i Gerontologi, Oslo 28–30 maj 1979. Universitetsförlaget, Oslo, Norway

Hagberg B, Ingvar DH (1976) Cognitive reduction in presenile dementia related to regional abnormalities of the cerebral blood flow. J Psychiatr 128:209–222

Hallgren B, Sourander P (1960) The non-haemin iron in the cerebral cortex in Alzheimer's disease. J Neurochem 5:307–310

Henig AM (1980) Aluminum neurotoxicity studied. Gerontologists emphasize the aging brain. Bio Sci 30:61–63

Heston LL (1979) Alzheimer's disease and senile dementia: Genetic relationships to Down's syndrome and hematologic cancer. In: Katzman R (ed) Congenital and aquired cognitive disorders. Raven Press, New York, p 167

Heston LL, Mastri AR (1977) The genetics of Alzheimer's disease. Arch Gen Psychiatry 34:976–981

Hirabayashi K, Ikeda K, Shimokawa K, Orthner H (1979) Vorzeitiges Gehirnaltern bei Down-Syndrom. Folia Psychiatr Neurol Japon 33:1:81–95

Hirano A, Malamud N, Elizan TS, Kurland LT (1966) Amyotrophic lateral sclerosis and Parkinsonism-dementia complex on Guam. Arch Neurol 15:35–51

Hochschild R (1971) Lysosomes, membranes and aging. Exp Geront 6:153–166

Hollander D, Strich SJ (1970) Atypical Alzheimer's disease with congophilic angiopathy presenting with dementia of acute onset. In: Wolstenholme GE, O'Connor M (eds). Alzheimer's disease and related conditions. A CIBA Foundation Symposium, Churchill Ltd, London, p 105

Hooper MV, Vogel S (1976) The limbic system in Alzheimer's disease. A neuropathologic investigation. Am J Pathol 85:1–20

Ingvar DH, Gustafson L (1970) Regional cerebral blood flow,in organic dementia with early onset. In: Juul-Jensen P (ed) Proceedings of the 19th Congress of Scandinavian Neurologists. Acta Neurol Scand suppl 43, vol 46. Munksgaard, Copenhagen, p 42

Ingvar DH, Lassen NA (1961) Quantitative determination of regional cerebral blood flow in man. Lancet I:806–807

Ingvar DH, Risberg J, Schwartz MS (1975) Evidence of subnormal function of association cortex in presenile dementia. Neurology 25:964–974

Ishii T, Haga S, Tokutake S (1979) Presence of neurofilament protein in Alzheimer's neurofibrillary tangles (ANT). An immunofluorescent study. Acta Neuropathol 48:105–112

Jacob H (1970) Muscular twitchings in Alzheimer's disease. In: Wolstenholme GE, O'Connor M (eds) Alzheimer's disease and related conditions. A CIBA Foundation Symposium, Churchill LTD, London, p 75

Jamada M, Mehraein P (1968) Verteilungsmuster der senilen Veränderungen im Gehirn. Die Beteiligung des limbischen Systems bei hirnatrophischen Prozessen des Seniums und bei Morbus Alzheimer. Arch Psychiatr Ges Neurol 211:308–324

Jelgersma HC (1964) Ein Fall von juveniler hereditärer Demenz vom Alzheimer Typ mit Parkinsonismus und Klüver-Bucy-Syndrom. Arch Psychiatr Z Ges Neurol 205:262–266

Jellinger K (1976) Neuropathological aspects of dementias resulting from abnormal blood and cerebrospinal fluid dynamics. Acta Neurol Belg 76:83–102

Jellinger K (1977) Cerebrovascular amyloidosis with cerebral hemorrhage. J Neurol 214:195–206

Jervis GA (1948) Early senile dementia in mongoloid idiocy. Am J Psychiatr 105:102–106

Jervis GA (1956) The presenile dementias. In: Kaplan OJ (ed) Mental disorders in later life, 2nd ed. Stanford University Press, Stanford, Calif, p 262

Jervis GA (1971) Alzheimer's disease. In: Minckler J (ed) Pathology of the nervous system, vol 2. McGraw Hill Co, New York, p 1385

Johannesson G, Brun A, Gustafson L, Ingvar DH (1977) EEG in presenile dementia related to cerebral blood flow and autopsy findings. Acta Neurol Scand 56:89–103

Johannesson G, Hagberg B, Gustafson L, Ingvar DH (1979) EEG and cognitive impairment in presenile dementia. Acta Neurol Scand 59:225–240

Kemper TL (1978) Senile dementia: A focal disease in the temporal lobe. In: Nandy K (ed) Senile dementia: A biomedical approach. Developments in neuroscience, vol 3. Elsevier/North Holland Biomedical Press, New York Amsterdam, p 105

Kidd M (1963) Paired helical filaments in electron microscopy of Alzheimer's disease. Nature 197:192–193

Kidd M (1964) Alzheimer's disease – an electronmicroscopical study. Brain 87:307–320

Klatzo I, Wisniewski H, Streicher E (1965) Experimental production of neurofibrillary degeneration. J Neuropathol Exp Neurol 24:187–199

Klüver H, Bucy PC (1938) An analysis of certain effects of bilateral temporal lobectomy in the rhesus monkey with special reference to "psychic blindness". J Psychol 5:33–54

Klüver H, Bucy P (1939) Preliminary analysis of functions of the temporal lobes in monkeys. Arch Neurol Psychiat 6, 42:979–1000

Konigsmark BW, Murphy EA (1972) Volume of the ventral cochlear nucleus in man – its relationship to neuronal population and age. J Neuropathol Exp Neurol 31:304–316

Larsson T, Sjögren T, Jacobson G (1963) Senile dementia, a clinical, sociomedical and genetic study. Acta Psych Scand 39 (suppl 167):1–257

Lassen NA, Munck O, Tottey ER (1957) Mental function and cerebral oxygen consumption in organic dementia. Arch Neurol Psych 77:126–133

Lauter H (1968) Zur Klinik und Psychopathologie der Alzheimerschen Krankheit. Psychiat Clin 1:85–108

Lauter H (1970) Über Spätformen der Alzheimerschen Krankheit und ihre Beziehung zur senilen Demenz. Psychiat Clin 3:169–189

Lee Sh-Sh, Stemmermann GN (1978) Congophilic angiopathy and cerebral hemorrhage. Arch Pathol Lab Med 102:317–321

Letemendia F, Pampiglione (1958) Clinical and electroencephalographic observations in Alzheimer's disease. J Neurol Neurosurg Psychiat 21:167–172

Lökken A, Cyvin K (1954) A case of clinical juvenile amaeurotic idiocy with the histological picture of Alzheimer's disease. J Neurol Neurosurg Psychiat 17:211–215

Mancardi GL, Perdelli F, Rivano C, Leonardi A, Bugiani O (1980) Thickening of the basement membrane of cortical capillaries in Alzheimer's disease. Acta Neuropathol (Berl) 49:79–83

Mandybur TI (1975) The incidence of cerebral amyloid angiopathy in Alzheimer's disease. Neurology 25:120–126

Mandybur TI, Bates SRD (1978) Fatal massive intracerebral hemorrhage complicating cerebral amyloid angiopathy. Arch Neurol 35:246–248

Mandybur TI, Nagpaul AS, Pappas S (1977) Alzheimer neurofibrillary change in subacute sclerosing panencephalitis. Ann Neurol 1:103–107

Mann DMA (1978) Granulovacuolar degeneration in pyramidal cells of the hippocampus. Acta Neuropath (Berl) 42:149–151

Mann DMA, Sinclair KGA (1978) The quantitative assessment of lipofuscin pigment, cytoplasmic RNA and nucleolar volume in senile dementia. Neuropathol Appl Neurobiol 4:129–135

Mann DMA, Yates PO (1979) The effects of ageing on the pigmented nerve cells of the human locus caeruleus and substantia nigra. Acta Neuropathol (Berl) 47:93–97

Mansvelt J (1954) Pick's disease. A syndrome of lobar cerebral atrophy; its clinical-anatomical and histopathological types. Thesis. Enschede, Utrecht

Mark J, Brun A (1973) Chromosomal deviations in Alzheimer's disease compared to those in senescence and senile dementia. Gerontol Clin 15:253–258

McDermott JR, Smith AI, Ward MN, Parkinson S, Kerr DNS (1978) Brain-aluminium concentration in dialysis encephalopathy. Lancet 1:901–903

McDermott JR, Smith AI, Iqbal K, Wisniewski HM (1979) Brain aluminum in aging and Alzheimer disease. Neurology 29:809–814

McMenemy WH (1963) The dementias and the progressive disease of the basal ganglia. In: Blackwood W, McMenemy WH, Mayer A, Norman RM, Russell DS (eds) Greenfield's neuropathology, 2nd ed. Edward Arnold, London, p 520

Mehraein P, Rothemund E (1976) Neuromorphologische Grundlagen des amnestischen Syndrom. Arch Psychiat Nervenkr 222:153–176

Mehraein P, Yamada M, Tarnowska-Dziduszko E (1975) Quantitative study on dendrites and dendritic spines in Alzheimer's disease and senile dementia. In: Kreutzberg GW (ed) Advances in neurology, 12. Raven Press, New York, p 453

Morel F, Wildi E (1952) General and cellular pathochemistry of senile and presenile alterations of the brain. Proc 1st Int Cong Neuropathol 2:347–374

Munck O, Lassen NA (1957) Bilateral cerebral blood flow and O_2 consumption in man by use of krypton 85. Circ Res 5:163–168

Mutrux S (1947) Diagnostic différentiel histologique de la maladie d'Alzheimer et de la démence sénile. Pathophobie de la zone de projection corticale. Mrschr Psychiat Neurol 113:100–117

Nandy K (1978) Brain-reactive antibodies in aging and senile dementia. In: Katzman R, Terry RD, Bick KL (eds) Alzheimer's disease: Senile dementia and related disorders (Aging vol 7). Raven Press, New York, p 503

Neuman M, Cohn R (1978) Epidemiological approach to questions of identity of Alzheimer's and senile brain disease. A proposal. In: Katzman R, Terry RD, Bick KL (eds) Alzheimer's disease: Senile dementia and related disorders (Aging vol 7). Raven Press, New York, p 27

Nevin S (1967) On some aspects of cerebral degeneration in later life. Proc R Soc Med 60:517–526

Nielsen J (1968) Chromosomes in senile dementia. Br J Psychiat 114:303–309

Obrist WD, Chivian E, Cronqvist S, Ingvar DH (1970) Regional cerebral blood flow in senile and presenile dementia. Neurology 20:315–322

Obrist WD, Thompson HK, Wang HW, Wilkinson WE (1975) Regional blood flow estimated by 133-Xenon inhalation. Stroke 6:245–256

Ohara PT (1972) Electron microscopical study of the brain in Down's syndrome. Brain 95:681–684

Okazaki H, Reagan TJ, Campbell RJ (1979) Clinicopathological studies of primary cerebral amyloid angiopathy. Mayo Clin Proc 54:22–31

Olson MI, Shaw C-M (1969) Presenile dementia and Alzheimer's disease in mongolism. Brain 92:147–156

Onari K, Spatz H (1926) Anatomische Beiträge zur Lehre von der Pickschen umschriebenen Großhirnrinden-Atrophie („Picksche Krankheit"). Z Ges Neurol Psychiat, pp 470–511

Palo S, Sulkava R, Wikström J, Pukonen A-R (1979) An approach to the epidemiology of dementia in general population. In: Glen AIM, Whalley LJ (eds) Alzheimer's disease. Early recognition of potentially reversible deficits. Churchill Livingstone, Edinburgh London New York, p 86

Pantelakis S (1954) Un type particulier d'angiopathie sénile du systéme nerveux central: l'angiopathie congophile. Topographie et fréquence. Monatsschr Psychiat Neurol 128:219–256

Pearce J (1974) The extrapyramidal disorder of Alzheimer's disease. Eur Neurol 12:94–103

Perez FI, Rivera VM, Meyer JS, Gay JRA, Taylor RL, Mathew NT (1975) Analysis of intellectual and cognitive performances in patients with multi-infarct dementia, vertebrobasilar insufficiency with dementia and Alzheimer's disease. J Neurol Neurosurg Psychiat 38:533–540

Perry EK, Perry RH, Blessed G, Tomlinson BE (1977) Necropsy evidence of central cholinergic deficits in senile dementia. Lancet 1:189

Perry EK, Tomlinson BE, Blessed G, Bergmann, Gibson, Perry RH (1978) Correlation of cholinergic abnormalities with senile plaques and mental test scores in senile dementia. Br Med J 2:1457–1459

Perusini G (1909) Über klinisch und histologisch eigenartige psychische Erkrankungen des späteren Lebensalters. Histologische und histopathologische Arbeiten über die Großhirnrinde. In: Nissl F (ed) Nissl-Alzheimers Arbeiten 3. Fischer, Jena, p 297

Peters G (1967) Neuropathologie und Psychiatrie. In: Kisker KP, Meyer JE, Müller C, Stromgren E (eds) Psychiatrie der Gegenwart, Band 1/1, Teil A. Springer, Berlin Heidelberg New York, p 286

Pilleri G (1966) The Klüver-Bucy sundrome in man. A clinicoanatomical contribution to the function of the medial temporal lobe structures. Psychiat Neurol, Basel 152:65–103

Powers JM, Spicer SS (1977) Histochemical similarity of senile plaque amyloid to apudamyloid. Virchows Arch (Pathol Anat) 376:107–115

Pratt RTC (1970) The genetics of Alzheimer's disease. In: Wolstenholme GEW, O'Connor U (eds) CIBA Foundation Symposium. Churchill Livingstone, Edinburgh London New York, p 137

Ramani SV, Loewenson RB, Gold L (1979) Computerized tomographic scanning and the diagnosis of dementia. New Engl J Med 300:23

Reisine TD, Yamamura HI, Bird ED, Spokes E, Enna SJ (1978) Pre- and postsynaptic neurochemical alterations in Alzheimer's disease. Brain Res 159:477–481

Reisine TD, Pedigs VW, Meiners B, Iqbal K, Yamamura HI (1980) Alzheimer's disease; studies on neurochemical alterations in the brain. In: Amaducci L, Davison AN, Antuono P (eds) Aging of the brain and dementia (Aging vol 13). Raven Press, New York

Renvoize EB, Jerram T (1979) Choline in Alzheimer's disease. New Engl J Med 301:330

Renvoize EB, Hambling MH, Pepper MD, Rajah SM (1979) Possible association of Alzheimer's disease with HLA-BW 15 and cytomegalovirus infection. Lancet 1:1238

Rewcastle NB, Gibbs CJ, Gajdusek DC (1978) Transmission of familial Alzheimer's disease to primates. Proc VIII th Intern Cong of Neuropath 295:679

Risberg J (1980a) Regional cerebral blood flow measurements by 133 Xe-inhalation: Methodology and applications in neuropsychology and psychiatry. Brain Language 9:9–34

Risberg J (1980b) Non-invasive measurements of CBF during brain work in chronic cerebrovascular disease. In: Gallad D (ed) Cerebrovascular disease: Drugs and methods. Proceedings of the symposium on "Experimental and clinical methodologies for the study of acute and chronic cerebrovascular diseases. Clinical applications to vasoactive drug studies. Pergamon Press, Paris, p 24

Risberg J, Ali Z, Wilson EM, Willis EL, Halsey JH (1975) Regional cerebral blood flow by 133 Xenon inhalation. Preliminary evaluation of an initial slope index in patients with unstable flow compartments. Stroke 6:142–148

Robertson EE, leRoux AVS, Brown JH (1958) The clinical differentiation of Pick's disease. J Ment Sci 104:1000–1024

Rosenblum WI, Ghatak NR (1979) Lewy bodies in the presence of Alzheimer's disease. Arch Neurol 36:170–171

Roth M (1971) Classification of and aetiology in mental disorders of old age: some recent developments. In: Kay DWK, Wack A (eds) Recent developments in psychogeriatrics. Brit J Psych Spec publ no 6. Headley Brothers Ltd, Ashford Kent, p 1

Roth M, Tomlinson BE, Blessed G (1967) The relationship between quantitative measures of dementia and of degenerative changes in the cerebral grey matter of elderly subjects. Proc R Soc Med 60:14–18

Rotschild D (1934) Alzheimer's disease. A clinicopathologic study of five cases. Am J Psychiat 91:485–575

Scheibel AB (1979a) The hippocampus: organizational patterns in health and senescence. Mech Ageing Develop 9:89

Scheibel AB (1979b) Dendritic changes in senile and presenile dementias. In: Katzman R (ed) Congenital and aquired cognitive disorders. Raven Press, New York, p 107

Schlaepfer WW, Lynch RG (1976) Immunofluorescent studies of neurofilaments in the peripheral and central nervous system of rats and humans (abstr). J Neuropathol Exp Neurol 35:345

Schmitt HP, Barz J (1978) Cerebral massive hemorrhage in congophilic angiopathy and its medicolegal significance. Forens Sci Intern 12:187–201

Schneider C (1927) Über Picksche Krankheit. Monatschr Psychiat Neurol 65:230–275

Schochet Jr SS, McCormic WF (1972) Ultrastructure of Hirano bodies. Acta Neuropath (Berl) 21:50–60

Schochet Jr SS, Lampert PW, McCormick WF (1973) Neurofibrillary tangles in patients with Down's syndrome: A light and electron microscopic study. Acta Neuropath (Berl) 23:342–346

Scholz W (1938) Studien zur Pathologie der Hirngefäße. II: Die drüssige Entartung der Hirnarterien und Kapillaren. Z Neurol Psychiat 162:694–715

Schwartz Ph (1968) New patho-anatomic observations on amyloidosis in the aged. Fluorescence microscopic investigations. In: Madama I (ed) Amyloidosis. Excerpta Medica, Amsterdam, p 403

Shefer VF (1972) Absolute number of neurons and thickness of the cerebral cortex during aging, senile and vascular dementia, and Pick's and Alzheimer's diseases. Zhurnal Nevropathol Psikhiatr, Korsak 72:1024–1029

Shefer VF (1977) Hippocampal pathology as a possible factor in the pathogenesis of senile dementias. Neurosci Behav Physiol 8(3):236–239

Sim M (1979) Early diagnosis of Alzheimer's disease. In: Glen AIM, Whalley LJ (eds) Alzheimer's disease. Early recognition of potentially reversible deficits. Churchill Livingstone, Edinburgh London New York, p 78

Sim M, Sussman I (1962) Alzheimer's disease: its natural history and differential diagnosis. J Nerv Ment Dis 135:489–499

Simchowitcz T (1911) Histopathologische Studien über die senile Demenz. In: Nissl F, Alzheimer A (eds) Histologie und histopathologische Arbeiten über Großhirnrinde. Fischer, Jena, p 267

Sjögren H (1950) Twenty-four cases of Alzheimer's disease. A clinical analysis. Acta Med Scand, suppl 246:225–233

Sjögren H, Sourander P (1962) Histopathological studies in Alzheimer's disease. Proc 4th Int Congr Neuropath, vol III. Thieme, Stuttgart, p 319

Sjögren H, Sourander P, Svennerholm L (1965) Clinical, histological and chemical studies on presenile and senile neuropsychiatric diseases. Proc V th Int Congr Neuropathol. Exc Med Int Congr ser no 100, p 555–559

Sjögren T, Sjögren H, Lindgren ÅGH (1952) Morbus Alzheimer and morbus Pick. A genetic, clinical and pathoanatomical study. Acta Psychiat Scand suppl 82:1:1–52

Smith WTh, Turner E, Sim M (1966) Cerebral biopsy in the investigation of presenile dementia. Br J Psychiat 112:127–133

Sourander P, Sjögren H (1970) The concept of Alzheimer's disease and its clinical implications. In: Wolstenholme GEW, O'Connor M (eds) Alzheimer's disease and related conditions. A CIBA Foundation Symposium. Churchill, London, p 11

Stertz S (1922) Zur Frage der Alzheimerschen Krankheit. Allg Zeitschr Psych 336

Stickland CA (1954) Two Mongols of unusually high mental status. Br J Med Psychol 27:80–83

Sulkava R, Rossi L, Knuutila S (1979) No elevated sister chromatid exchange in Alzheimer's disease. Acta Neurol Scand 59:156–159

Swain JM (1959) Electroencephalographic abnormalities in presenile atrophy. Neurology 9:722–727

Tan YH, Tischfield J, Ruddle FH (1973) The linkage of genes for the human interferon-induced antiviral protein and indolphenoloxidase-B traits to chromosomes G-21. J Exp Med 137:317–330

Tariska I (1970) Circumscribed cerebral atrophy in Alzheimer's disease: A pathological study. In: Wolstenholme GE, O'Connor M (eds) Alzheimer's disease and related conditions. A CIBA Foundation symposium. Churchill Ltd, London, p 51

Terry RD (1963) The fine structure of neurofibrillary tangles in Alzheimer's disease. J Neuropath Exp Neurol 22:629–634

Terry RD (1978a) Aging, senile dementia and Alzheimer's disease. In: Katzman R, Terry RD, Bick KL (eds) Alzheimer's disease: Senile dementia and related disorders. Raven Press, New York, p 11

Terry RD (1978b) Ultrastructural alterations in senile dementia. In: Katzman R, Terry RD, Bick KL (eds) Alzheimer's disease: Senile dementia and related disorders (Aging vol 7). Raven Press, New York, p 375

Terry RD (1978c) Senile dementia. Fed Proc 37:2837–2840

Terry RD (1979) Morphological changes in Alzheimer's disease – Senile dementia: Ultrastructural changes and quantitative studies. In: Katzman R (ed) Congenital and aquired cognitive disorders. Raven Press, New York, p 99

Terry RD, Wisniewski H (1970) The ultrastructure of the neurofibrillary tangle and the senile plaque. In: Wolstenholme GEW, O'Connor M (eds) Alzheimer's disease and related conditions. CIBA Foundation Symposium, Churchill, London, p 145

Terry RD, Wisniewski H (1972) The ultrastructure of senile dementia and of experimental analoge. In: Gaitz CM (ed) Aging and the brain. Plenum Publ Corp, New York, p 123

Terry RD, Gonatas NK, Weiss M (1964) Ultrastructural studies in Alzheimer's presenile dementia. Am J Path 44:269–281

Terry RD, Fitzgerald C, Peck A, Millner J, Farmer P (1977) Cortical cell counts in senile dementia. J Neuropathol Exp Neurol 36:633

Tomlinson BE (1977) The pathology of dementia. In: Wells K (ed) Contemporary neurology series. FA Davis Co, Philadelphia, p 113–153

Tomlinson BE (1979) The ageing brain. In: Smith WT, Cavanagh JB (eds) Recent advances in neuropathology. Churchill Livingstone, New York, p 129

Tomlinson BE, Henderson G (1976) Some quantitative cerebral findings in normal and demented old people. In: Terry RD, Gerson S (eds) Neurobilogy of aging. Raven Press, New York, p 183

Tomlinson BE, Blessed G, Roth M (1970) Observations on the brains of demented old people. J Neurol Sci 11:205–242

Torack RM (1978) The pathologic physiology of dementia. With indications for diagnosis and treatment. In: Hippius H, Janzarik W, Müller C (eds) Monographien aus dem Gesamtgebiete der Psychiatrie, Psychiatry Series. Springer, Berlin Heidelberg New York, p 1

Trapp GA, Miner GD, Zimmerman RL, Mastri AR, Heston LL (1978) Aluminum levels in brain in Alzheimer's disease. Biol Psychiatry vol 13 no 6:709–717

Ule G (1958) Pathologisch-anatomische Befunde bei Korsakow-Psychosen und ihre Bedeutung für die Lokalisationslehre in der Psychiatrie. Ärztl Wochenschr 13:6–13

Ward BE, Cook RH, Robinson A, Austin JH (1979) Increased aneuploidy in Alzheimer's disease. Am J Med Genet 3:137–144

Whalley LJ, Buckton KE (1979) Genetic factors in Alzheimer's disease. In: Glen AIM, Whalley LJ (eds) Alzheimer's disease. Early recognition of potentially reversible deficits. Churchill Livingstone, Edinburgh London New York, p 36

Whalley LJ, Urbaniak SJ, Darg C, Peutherer JF, Christie E (1980) Histocompatibility antigens and antibodies to viral and other antigens in Alzheimer pre-senile dementia. Acta Psychiat Scand 61:1–7

Wisniewski HM (1978) Possible viral etiology of neurofibrillary changes and neuritic plaques. In: Katzman R, Terry RD, Bick KL (eds) Alzheimer's disease: Senile dementia and related disorders (Aging vol 7). Raven Press, New York, p 555

Wisniewski HM (1979) Neurofibrillary and synaptic pathology in senile dementia of the Alzheimer's type (SDAT). In: Glen AIM, Whalley LJ (eds) Alzheimer's disease. Early recognition of potentially reversible deficits. Churchill Livingstone, Edinburgh London New York, p 7

Wisniewski HM, Soifer D (1979) Neurofibrillary pathology: current status and research perspectives. Mechanisms of Ageing and Development 9:119–142

Wisniewski HM, Terry RD (1973a) Morphology of the aging brain, human and animal. In: Ford DH (ed) Progress in brain research, vol 40. Neurobiological aspects of Maturation and Aging, p 167

Wisniewski HM, Terry RD (1973b) Reexamination of the pathogenesis of the senile plaque. In: Zimmermann HM (ed) Progress in neuropath vol II. Grune Stratton, New York, pp 1–26

Wisniewski HM, Terry RD (1976) Neuropathology of the aging brain. In: Terry RD, Gershon S (eds) Neurobiology of aging. Raven Press, New York, p 265

Wisniewski HM, Johnson AB, Raine CS, Kay WS, Terry RD (1970) Senile plaques and cerebral amyloidosis in aged dogs. Lab Invest 23:287–296

Wisniewski HM, Ghetti B, Terry RD (1973) Neuritic (senile) plaques and filamentous changes in aged rhesus monkeys. J Neuropathol Exp Neurol 32:566–584

Wisniewski HM, Bruce ME, Fraser H (1975) Infectious etiology of neurotic (senile) plaques in mice. Science 190:1108–1110

Wisniewski HM, Narang HK, Terry RD (1976) Neurofibrillary tangles of paired helical filaments. J Neurol Sci 27:173–181

Wisniewski K, Howe J, Williams DG, Wisniewski HM (1978) Precocious aging and dementia in patients with Down's syndrome. Biol Psychiatry 13

Yagishita S, Itoh Y, Amano N, Nakano T (1980) Atypical senile dementia with widespread Lewy type inclusion in the cerebral cortex. Acta Neuropathol (Berl) 49:187–191

Yamada M (1978) On the distribution of senile changes in the spinal cord. Folia Psychiat Neurol Jpn 32:249–251

Zerbin-Rüdin E (1967) Hirnatrophische Prozesse. In: Becker PE (ed) Humangenetik vol V/2. Thieme, Stuttgart, p 84

Stroke

K.A. Flügel

A. Introductory Remarks on Physiology and Pathophysiology

I. Cerebral Blood Flow and Disorders

The normal amount of cerebral blood flow (CBF) lies around 750–1,000 ml/min or, related to brain weight, 50–55 ml/100 g per minute. These data refer to the global blood flow of the brain whereas there are considerable differences in regional cerebral blood flow between various brain areas. The relationship between gray and white matter is approximately 4:1.

Continuous blood flow is necessary to provide the brain with oxygen and glucose. The consumption of oxygen is 500–600 ml/min and that of glucose 75–100 mg/min.

Because of the relatively high consumption of oxygen, the brain is dependent on continuous blood flow. This demand is accomplished by means of special regulatory mechanisms of cerebral blood flow. In spite of the variations of systemic blood pressure and cardiac output, global cerebral blood flow is kept constant by these mechanisms, which are termed *"autoregulation."* However, depending on the actual functional state, regional blood flow varies considerably.

The cerebral blood flow results from the relationship of effective blood pressure to cerebral vascular resistance. Blood pressure is influenced by cardiac performance and the distribution of the blood volume including arterial flow toward and venous flow from the brain. Vascular resistance, on the other hand, is determined by the diameter of the vessels and by vessel content, i.e., rheologic factors.

Autoregulation is effected mainly by reflectory changes of vessel caliber, which are probably performed through constriction and dilatation of the arteries.

1. Cerebral Blood Flow and Blood Pressure

Investigating the relationship between blood pressure and the magnitude of cerebral blood flow, two ranges can be distinguished. There is a lower range up to about 70 mm Hg, in which with rising blood pressure there is an increase of blood flow. Then the profile of blood flow values stays constant over a blood pressure range from 60–70 mm Hg upward. This steadiness is the effect of autoregulation, whereby adaptive regulation of vascular resistance is causative. These mechanisms are, however, not indefinitly effective. With very high blood pressure values the autoregulation fails to work. Moreover, in patients with fixed hypertonia the critical threshold for autoregulatory adaptation is shifted, so that when blood pressure is decreased ischemia may occur at far higher pressures than usual.

Autoregulation prevents the brain from getting more oxygen offered than it needs. In brain lesions, especially ischemic lesions, autoregulation can be impaired. Thus a surplus of oxygen supply of infarcted brain tissue may occur in spite of normal blood pressure with or without intracerebral steal. This phenomenon has been described as *luxury perfusion* (LASSEN 1966).

Whether the cardiac output itself influences cerebral blood flow or whether this happens via an increase of arterial blood pressure has been discussed in cases in which cardiac output was increased by implantation of electronic pacemaker.

2. Cerebral Blood Flow and the Influence of Carbon Dioxide Tension and Blood pH

There is a significant relationship between the pCO_2 of the arterial blood and cerebral blood flow, which can be expressed in a characteristic response curve. Low pCO_2 values of 15–20 mm Hg are accompanied by an equally low blood flow of about half normal, followed by a rather steep increase of blood flow with rising pCO_2 in the range 20–70 mm Hg. Then in the upper range of 70–80 mm Hg and above the cerebral blood flow is maximally raised but remains on a constant level, presumably due to extreme vasodilatation.

The relationship between $paCO_2$ and cerebral blood flow is influenced by blood pressure. The curve presenting this relationship becomes less steep when arterial blood pressure decreases. In low values around 50 mm Hg this relationship completely disappears.

Contradictory results have been obtained in experiments on the influence of pH of arterial blood upon cerebral blood flow. The same is true of the extracellular pH and of the difference of intra- and extracellular pH.

3. Cerebral Blood Flow and the Influence of Oxygen and Glucose

Acute hypoxia leads to an elevation of blood flow in the brain, as can be seen in experiments with inhalation of gas mixtures of various oxygen content. With normal pCO_2 an increase of CBF occurs only when the arterial pO_2 is less than 60 mm Hg. In hypercapnia the rate of CBF increase is higher. It has been shown that the relationship is more evident for the oxygen tension of venous blood (pvO_2) so that this may be the parameter relevant for changing cerebral blood flow. A rise under normal conditions will begin at a venous oxygen tension of 25–28 mm Hg. When a critical threshold of venous oxygen tension of 70 mm Hg is reached, clinical signs of severe hypoxia occur, the most important being disorders of consciousness. Brain edema results from failure of the blood-brain barrier. The situation is different when there is a chronic hypoxia.

There is obviously no dependency of cerebral blood flow on the glucose blood level or glucose consumption of brain tissue; at least there is no compensatory rise of CBF in glucose deficit.

4. Cerebral Blood Flow and Nervous Influences

Findings on influences of stimulation of sympathetic or parasympathetic nerves on the cerebral blood flow are inconsistent. The role of nervous influences on cerebral blood flow in normal and abnormal situations is not yet precisely known. It seems as if the actual initial situation influences the nervous reactions in experimental situations decisively.

The nervous elements possibly concerned with regulation of cerebral blood flow via vascular innervation and vasomotor control are sympathetic fibers arising from cervical ganglia, parasympathetic fibers partly running in the superficial petrosal nerve, and others. Following stimulation of sympathetic fibers, a constriction of pial vessels has been described (BETZ 1972b, survey). This constriction would lead to decrease of cerebral blood flow, although this is not proven in man.

Stimulation of the dilatatory parasympathetic fibers may increase cerebral blood flow. Neurogenic dilatation following ischemia is supposed to come also from fibers not accompanying the pial vessels but arising directly from the gray matter lying underneath.

There is supposed to be an interaction between vegetative vasomotor control mechanisms and autoregulation i.e., the pCO_2 response. In animal experiments the responses to blood pressure and to pCO_2 changes were shown to be different in sympathectomy, stimulation of sympathetic nerve fibers, and normals. Controversial effects were described after transsection and stimulation of the vagus nerve.

II. Energetic Brain Metabolism and Its Disorders

The human brain needs about 17 cal/100 g per minute. For the total adult brain this would amount to around 250 cal/min, which is approximately 20% of the energy need of the whole organism at rest. In relation to brain weight (2% of the body weight) the cerebral enery need is about ten times as high as that of other organs.

The energy is necessary for different purposes: for the preservation of brain structure, various metabolic processes, and for the maintenance and restitution of electric excitability. Energy-consuming processes include, for example, those maintaining balance of electrolytes which cause the resting potential of the cells and synthesis of proteins.

Energy for brain functions is physiologically provided by the aerobic (oxidative) reduction of glucose. One mole of glucose delivers 38 mol energy-producing ATP. About 92% of glucose is reduced in the aerobic and only about 8% in the anaerobic way. Anaerobic glycolysis is much less effective in producing ATP and would not be sufficient for the energy demands of the brain.

The consumption or cerebral metabolic rate of glucose (CMR gluc.) can be calculated by the product of cerebral blood flow and arteriovenous difference of glucose concentration (a–v D gluc.) to lie between 5 and 5.5 mg/100 g per minute. The uptake of glucose into the brain tissue is influenced by a carrier function between blood and brain.

Oxidation of glucose is performed in two ways. It can run via glycolysis and the Krebs cycle (according to Embden-Meyerhof) and via a hexose monophosphate shunt.

Storage of glucose in brain cells is only very poor. It would merely suffice for a few minutes if there was no supply and if the rate of oxidation remained equal.

The effects of hypoglycemia on brain functions is of great practical importance. The term hypoglycemia is applied if blood glucose level sinks below 50 mg-%. Up to this level the glucose uptake remains fairly constant and fluctuations of glucose level in the physiological range practically do not influence glucose uptake of the brain. In hypoglycemia below 40–50 mg-%, disorders of cerebral functions occur but even in low levels of about 20 mg-% their intensity varies from one case to another. Glucose uptake decreases in hypoglycemia but not to the same extent as the glucose blood level. Clinical symptoms following severe hypoglycemia are disorders of consciousness, seizures, and neurological deficits including focal disorders, such as hemiparesis, aphasia, or others.

Other substrates besides glucose are believed to be used in the case of glucose deficit, for instance, amino acids and phosphatides. Amino acids can be directed into the Krebs cycle via the GABA shunt and thus be called upon for energetic needs in emergency situations.

The glucose uptake in the brain is not a matter of pure diffusion. Increased blood glucose level does not cause an increase of glucose uptake, except when glucose is infused together with insulin (GOTTSTEIN et al. 1970).

In the case of chronic glucose deficit or very slow decrease of glucose input, keto bodies can take part in energetic metabolism.

Oxygen consumption [cerebral metabolic rate of oxygen (CMR O_2)] is fairly constant during rest. This concerns the total amount for the whole brain, although there are regional differences depending upon the active or resting state. According to some experimental data, regional oxygen consumption of the cortex may vary between 8 and 12 ml/100 g per minute. It is decreased in barbiturate narcosis. An increase is found in states of activity of the brain region investigated and in experimental stimulations. Thus oxygen consumption rises in attention, mental tasks, emotional stress, and during seizure activity, in which maximal increase occurs. In hypothermia a decrease of oxygen consumption is found as in various pathologic states of diffuse brain disorder (metabolic coma, acute intoxications, dementia).

The oxidative process necessary for energy gain in the tissue is performed in the mitochondria. Inside the mitochondria are respiratory enzymes, especially cytochromoxydase, the sites of which oxygen reactions take place at. Corresponding to differences of oxygen consumption in different brain regions regional differences of enzyme concentrations have also been found.

Oxygen transport from the capillaries to the mitochondria is performed mainly by diffusion. According to the classic model of Krogh, the capillaries supply cylindric areas in such a way that in the case of insufficient perfusion the venous end first becomes hypoxic. The model was modified by Diemer and by Lübbers and Grunewald. As a consequence of oxygen diffusion, distribution curves of oxygen tension in tissue can be measured. In mitochondria oxygen tension can be as low as 1 mm Hg without disorder of oxidation, but in hypoxia the histogram of oxygen tensions shows an increase of low values. A decrease of venous oxygen tension below a critical value of 20 mm Hg leads to diminution of cerebral oxygen consumption.

III. Special Features in Old Age

Cerebral blood flow differs, depending on age. Above the age of 50 years mean cerebral blood flow begins to decrease. In healthy aged, however, cerebral blood flow may be the same as in younger adults. The difference of mean values, therefore, seems to be due to a relatively high percentage of arteriosclerosis in the older people investigated.

The same profile of the age curve is found for oxygen consumption and for glucose uptake of the brain. There is a nearly parallel course of all three variables.

Differences of cerebral blood flow were found between healthy old people, persons with mild cerebral ("pseudoneurasthenic") disorders and old people with marked mental deterioration (GOTTSTEIN 1965). The decrease of oxygen consumption in old age is also explained with the frequency of arteriosclerotic vascular changes and with the decrease of brain weight following loss of nerve cells.

B. Morphologic Findings in Stroke and Underlying Disorders

I. Cerebral Infarction

The morphologic substrata of the clinical event "stroke" (or apoplexy) are cerebral infarction (or encephalomalacy) and intracerebral hemorrhage. Infarcts can occur as the consequence of a vascular obturation or without obturation. In the latter case there may be a proximal stenosis and infarction can also be caused by hemodynamic insufficiency or failure of collateral circulation. Frequently more than one factor work together to cause acute localized ischemia.

In transient ischemia causing reversible clinical disorders, morphological changes are not found, at least with conventional histological methods.

Infarctions can be distinguished according to their *topography* (ZÜLCH 1971) into (a) infarcts in borderline areas of different regions of arterial supply, (b) infarcts in the terminal area of arterial supply, and (c) infarcts in the center of an area supplied by the artery. Borderline infarctions are mainly situated at the convexity in a borderline zone of the middle and anterior cerebral artery (frontotemporal cortex) or between the middle and posterior cerebral arteries. Further areas frequently concerned are the occipital cortex and the cerebellum. In the genesis of these borderline infarcts mostly diffuse cerebrovascular or hemodynamic changes are involved. Infarcts of the terminal region often concern the middle and anterior cerebral arteries, corresponding to the caudatum and the centrum semiovale. Infarcts within the area of arterial blood supply can have the character of total infarction (affecting the whole territory supplied) or they can include only parts, for instance, the central part of the territory.

Sometimes very small (minimal) infarctions occur, for example, including the Broca area of the frontal lobe, causing selective expressive aphasia. Incomplete infarctions of the regions supplied by the vertebral and basilar arteries and their branches may cause a number of different clinical syndromes as little differences of localization can change the symptomatology markedly.

There are *different stages* of ischemic brain lesions (CERVÓS-NAVARRO 1980). One type is described as elective necrosis of parenchyma or anoxic (ischemic) necrosis of ganglion cells and in association there may be glial reaction of varying extent. In "total necrosis" there is not only anoxic lesion of the ganglion cells but also breakdown of glial metabolism and even of vascular and connective tissue. In total necrosis also, different phases can be distinguished. First there is necrosis characterized by the fact that nuclei will not be stained and the necrotic tissue becomes edematous and softened. In the second phase, which can last over weeks to months, one finds colliquation and resorption of necrotic material. The third phase is that of the formation of scars (or pseudocysts). In the case of multiple small cortical glial scars the cortical surface appears bumpy and this finding has led to the term *"granular atrophy."* Small foci of the myelon have a spongious character. Large infarcts will be transformed into cysts in which ependyma remains preserved.

Hemorrhagic infarcts exhibit a secondary diapedic bleeding and must not be mistaken for intracerebral hemorrhage or for hemorrhagic infarction in venous cerebral thrombosis. Hemorrhagic infarcts usually affect terminal parts of the region supplied by an artery and are mostly limited to the gray matter, whereas intracerebral hemorrhage may transgress the area of supply of one single artery. As to the pathogenesis of hemorrhagic infarcts, secondary bleeding into the ischemic necrotic lesion may be caused by increase of hemodynamic blood pressure in the venous compartment to such an extent that capillaries in the necrotic area become retrogradely filled with blood. Because of the capillary lesion, hemorrhage into the necrotic tissue will result. Experimental hemorrhagic infarcts were produced by embolization, additional venous compression, stasis, and recirculation after temporary arterial occlusion.

II. Diffuse Ischemic Lesions

In *global ischemia*, which in most cases is preceded by heart arrest and reanimation, different morphologic changes dependent on the duration of cerebral hypoxia are found. They can be generalized and usually predominantly affect the borderline zones of cerebral and cerebellar cortex, frequently also the hippocampal and thalamic areas. Patterns of ischemic encephalopathy are influenced by brain edema and effects of mass shifting and compression. Histologic changes range from elective laminar necrosis to total necrosis of the cerebral cortex. Early changes are ischemic cell alterations (tigrolysis, shrinking, vacuolization) and they are followed by cell necrosis, excrescence of microglia, and degeneration of myelin sheath in the deep medullary substance. A mechanism involved in causing irreversible damage is the so-called no-reflow-phenomenon, which results from compression of vascular lumen.

In cerebrovascular disease *multifocal* ischemic lesions with the histologic changes of infarction are more important than global affection. Small multiple microinfarcts with prevalence in the basal ganglia and pons constitute *"status lacunaris."* The clinical symptoms correlated with these findings are disseminated neurologic disorders of a chronic and progressive kind.

Another type of generalized cerebrovascular lesion is found as a sequela of severe long-lasting hypertension. Multiple and symmetric small perivascular lesions forming the morphologic pattern of *"status cribrosus"* and the diffuse degeneration of medullar substance and cysts characteristic of *Binswanger's encephalopathy* are explained as complications of hypertension and arteriosclerosis. The term "hypertensive encephalopathy" is clinically and morphologically not clearly defined.

III. Intracerebral Hypertensive Hemorrhage

There are several possible causes of intracerebral hemorrhage. Most frequent and especially predominant in old age is hypertensive hemorrhage. Usually there is a history of severe hypertension and cerebral or general arteriosclerosis. About three-quarters of hypertensive bleedings are situated in the basal ganglia, especially the putamen. They originate from ruptures of the lenticulostriate arteries and can primarily affect lateral, intermediate, or medial parts of the basal ganglia and also the thalamus and internal capsule. Other sites of predilection are the pons, the thalamus, and rarely the cerebellar hemispheres. Hemorrhages of the basal ganglia often penetrate into the ventricular system. The sequelae of intracerebral hematoma for the brain are determined by direct destructive lesions and compression of the hematoma as a space-occupying process.

In the course of time following hemorrhagic apoplexy the blood will be cleared away and finally a cystic cave or a narrow gap with brownish or yellowish color will remain. This change of color may be the only feature permitting differentiation between the end stage of an infarct or that of a hemorrhage.

Hypertension causes the alterations of the arterial wall (hyalinosis) as well as the actual rupture when it happens during an acute hypertensive crisis. Other causes of hemorrhage will be mentioned later in this article. They may concern other vascular diseases (next chapter) or pathologic disorders of blood vessel content, for instance, hemorrhagic diathesis and anticoagulant treatment.

IV. Diseases of Cerebral Blood Vessels Leading to Stroke

1. Arteriosclerosis

Arteriosclerosis is the most frequent disease underlying ischemic and hemorrhagic stroke. Although in the individual cases there are differences of incidence and severity of arteriosclerosis between the arteries of different regions, i.e., coronaries, peripheral arteries, and cerebral arteries, arteriosclerosis is fundamentally a general disease of the arterial vascular system. Nevertheless there may be cases of selective affection of cerebral vessels. Mostly, however, and especially in old age, arteriosclerosis concerns cerebral as well as other arteries. Cerebral arteries usually become involved later than the coronaries and aorta.

The general morphologic findings and epidemiologic data are valid for the vascular disease irrespective of the organs affected. Arteriosclerosis is localized predominantly at the intima of the arterial wall. The process is of a multifocal character and has a predilection to certain parts of the arterial system. At the extracranial parts of the carotids the internal carotid is most frequently affected at the level of the carotid sinus near the bifurcation and at the syphon. The segment between the sinus and syphon is only rarely involved. At the vertebral artery there is predilection of arteriosclerosis near the origin of the subclavian artery and here the plaques often have their origin.

At these extracranial places the process leads to ulcerations, stenosis, and finally complete obturation.

The basal cerebral arteries are usually affected later in the course of arteriosclerosis and to a lesser extent than the internal carotid artery. Arteries with wide lumina are more strongly involved than those with narrow lumina. Typical sites of predilection are the initial part of the middle cerebral artery and regions with curves in the course of the anterior, middle, and posterior cerebral arteries. The arteries of cerebral convexity may show arteriosclerotic changes in cases with or without involvement of basal arteries. They are relatively rare in comparison to other localizations. Of the intracerebral arteries the small vessels supplying the basal ganglia are mainly involved.

As to the pathogenetic mechanisms causing arteriosclerosis, the decisive initial mechanism is not yet known. There has been a lot of discussion about various theories. Mechanisms claimed to be a primary lesion are subintimal edema, deposition of lipids, fibroelastic plaques of the intima, and mechanic lesions like shearing.

Theories concerning the etiology of arteriosclerosis include those of primary abnormalities of lipid metabolisms, inflammation, and hemodynamic-mechanical causation. Because of the multitude of etiologic and pathogenetic concepts and the lack of a single theory explaining all findings, a multifactorial constellation of pathogenesis is generally assumed.

Risk factors of arteriosclerosis are advanced on the basis of epidemiologic studies. Old age is highly correlated with the incidence of arteriosclerosis. This is true for all manifestations including cerebral arteriosclerosis. Nevertheless, even very aged persons in the 9 th decade need not be affected.

Between 3% and 11% of autopsied patients of this age in a general hospital exhibited no cerebral arteriosclerosis (ULE and KOLKHANN 1972, survey). These findings and the occurrence of arteriosclerosis in younger persons indicate that age is not an essential condition for the development of arteriosclerosis. Hypertension undoubtedly promotes arteriosclerosis and this also seems to be true for obesity and diabetes mellitus. The role of genetic factors is uncertain. There are geographical differences, the reasons of which are not clear. A possible role of nutritional influences is discussed. The significance of cigarette smoking is not entirely clear for cerebral arteriosclerosis in contrast to myocardial infarct and peripheral arteriosclerosis. This also refers to the problem of silent stress.

2. Hypertensive Cerebrovascular Disease

Apart from the role of hypertension in the genesis of arteriosclerosis there are vascular alterations of another type associated with long-lasting and severe hypertension. They concern mainly the arterioles and may be independent from arteriosclerosis. Typical features are hypertrophy of the media, hyalinosis, miliary aneurysms, and hemorrhage.

3. Congophilic Angiopathy (Cerebrovascular Amyloidosis)

This rare type of angiopathy previously described as "dysoric angiopathy" and "senile necrosis of vessel wall" occurs predominantly in old age. It is a disease of the intracerebral and meningeal arterioles with a predilection in the occipital lobes. There is metachromatic mass deposition in the tunica media and it can be stained with Congo red.

Senile plaques are constant findings. In congophilic angiopathy too, etiology is not yet certain. An unspecific toxic or inflammatory reaction was discussed together with a local disorder of polysaccharide metabolism. Familiar occurrence,of clinical disorders combined with congophilic angiopathy was reported (GUDMUNDSSON et al. 1972). Relatively frequent sequelae are intracerebral hemorrhages (ULRICH et al. 1973; TORACK 1975; JELLINGER 1977; SCHMITT et al. 1978). There is also often a brain atrophy of mild or moderate degree.

4. Inflammatory Diseases of Brain Vessels

Angiitis may represent primary vascular disease or a secondary affection in connection with meningoencephalitis. In the cases of primary angiitis etiology is frequently one of immunologic pathology. The position of cerebrovascular *thrombangitis obliterans* is controversial. Two forms had been differentiated: one with irregular multifocal localization and a second type with regular affection of distal parts of intracerebral arteries. The first type manifests itself with multiple infarcts and the second type with a diffuse granular cortical atrophy.

Panarteriitis nodosa is a generalized angiitis and the incidence of cerebrovascular affection is estimated to lie between 10%–80%. Distinct predilections at the brain arteries are not found. The intensity of proliferations at the intima and granulomatous alterations is variable. Sequelae at the brain parenchyma are ischemic lesions, focal areas of demyelinization, infarctions, and hemorrhages (FLÜGEL et al. 1980b).

Together with *lupus erythematodes, sclerodermia,* and *dermatomyositis,* periarteriitis nodosa is classified as so-called collagen disease.

Giant cell arteritis (Horton's arteritis) mostly manifests itself at the extracerebral cranial arteries (not merely at the temporal artery), the ophthalmic artery and the aortic arch, but occasionally also at the intracranial arterial system. Giant cell arteritis is a disease of old age and is met most frequently in the 7th and 8th decades. It will only extremely seldomly represent the cause of stroke (HUGHES and BROWNELL 1966; BURGER et al. 1977; RUSSI et al. 1980; WEISS et al. 1980). Central hemorrhage may in occasional instances occur as a late complication of *Wegener's granulomatosis.*

Young females are seized with Takayasu's disease, a special form of aortic arch syndrome with inflammatory etiology. There may be similarities to luetic aortitis. The disease has practically no significance for old age.

5. Other Vascular Diseases

Traumatic lesions of cerebral and extracerebral vessels may give rise to thrombotic obstruction and thus to the clinical picture of stroke. The trauma itself may be remarkably mild when there is preexisting arteriosclerosis. This is especially true for the extracranial internal carotid artery and neck trauma. The lesions involved are dissections of the intima and media, and intramural hematomas may result. The problem of late hemorrhagic apoplexy after cranial trauma and the possible role of traumatic aneurysm is regarded as very controversial.

Obliterative alterations of blood vessels and secondary lesions of brain tissue have been postulated to occur as sequelae of radiotherapy.

A rare nonarteriosclerotic type of angiopathy is *fibromuscular dysplasia* (or hyperplasia) with a yet unknown etiology. Morphologic and angiographic characteristics are pathognomonic. The internal carotid artery is often affected. Female patients of younger or middle adult age prevail. The disease can lead to stenosis or obturation of the affected artery with consecutive brain infarct.

Similar consequences are observed in Ehlers-Danlos syndrome, a rare congenital disease of connective tissue.

6. Anomalies and Dysplasias of Cerebral Blood Vessels

Anomalies (aplasia, hypoplasia, anomalies of origin, and others) of cranial arteries have generally no direct effect on cerebral function, but they may modify the consequences of additional vascular disease. Arterial dysplasias not infrequently cause intracerebral hemorrhage and also ischemic stroke. The most important forms of malformations are *angiomas* and *aneurysms*. Hemorrhages from angiomas are more likely to occur in angioma cavernosum than in angioma capillare ectaticum. Another type of angioma, namely, angioma capillare et venosum calcificans (Sturge-Weber syndrome) leads to atrophic changes, focal nutritional disorders, and frequently convulsions with consecutive lesions. The *arteriovenous angiomas* (angioma arteriovenosum aneurysmaticum) cause arteriovenous shunt (fistula) and malnutrition leading to atrophy. These angiomas can also rupture and bring about intracerebral hemorrhage.

Aneurysms of the basal cerebral arteries are important sources of intracerebral hemorrhage, which are regularly combined with subarachnoid bleedings. Another complication is the occurrence of spasms of the intracerebral arteries, which can cause ischemic infarcts or diffuse ischemic lesions. It seems as though the incidence of ischemic infarcts is increased with antifibrinolytic treatment, which itself lowers the risk of relapsing hemorrhage. Late complications of spasms after proliferative subarachnoid hemorrhages and necrotic lesions of the arteries have been observed.

C. Clinical Manifestations of Stroke

I. Symptoms of Stroke Affecting the Carotid System

1. General Remarks

The term stroke marks the apoplectic occurrence of a neurologic deficit caused by cerebrovascular disorder. Primarily, it describes a purely clinical event which can be brought about by different mechanisms including thrombosis, embolism, and hemorrhage. In many cases stroke is associated with unilateral palsy and therefore stroke and hemiplegia are sometimes spoken of synonymously, although this symptom is present only in a part of cases. Symptoms depend upon the region of the brain affected by the disorder of circulation. On the other hand the course of time of manifest symptoms is closely related to the underlying pathogenetic mechanisms. The symptoms described in the following chapters according to the affected artery can principally be reversible and transient, or permanently persisting.

2. Internal Carotid Artery

Of all cranial arteries the internal carotid artery most frequently shows arteriosclerotic changes with stenosis or occlusion. Sites of predilection are the area of bifurcation and less frequently the syphon. Other causes than arteriosclerosis play a subordinate role.

Cases labeled "asymptomatic" are those in which stenosis or even occlusion is present without any corresponding neurologic symptoms. There is frequently a bruit to be heard in the area of carotid bifurcation when the neck region is auscultated. The special problems of asymtomatic cases concerning ways of prophylaxis will be discussed later.

In manifest cases characteristic symptoms are: hemiparesis and/or sensory disorders on the contralateral side, pronounced at or even limited to the face and upper extremity (brachiofacial hemiparesis) and when the dominant (mostly left) hemisphere is affected, aphasia (dysphasia) of a motor, sensory or mixed type. The symptoms are more or less identical to those of a lesion in the area supplied by the middle cerebral artery. Horner's syndrome or initial disorders of vision caused by ischemia in the area of the ophthalmic artery indicate that the obturation is situated in the carotid artery.

Further possible symptoms are epileptiform seizures, generalized, or Jacksonian. Optical atrophy is rare. In the case of abnormal vascular topography, for instance, if both anterior arteries and one posterior cerebral artery originate from the internal carotid artery, then homonymous hemianopsia and psychopathologic disorders will be present. In completed stroke these symptoms may persist but they can also be transient and last only a very short time. The fact that occlusion of internal carotid artery may remain without clinical symptoms in asymptomatic cases is explained by the collateral circulation via the communicating anterior artery and the vertebrobasilar system and also via the external carotid artery, i.e., the collaterals of ophthalmic artery.

3. Common Carotid Artery

When a stenosis or occlusion is located in the common carotid artery, a rare event, no carotid pulse will be felt on the affected side. Asymptomatic unilateral occlusion is not infrequent. In this case there is collateral supply with retrograde circulation of the external carotid artery, leading blood from the vertebral artery via occipital arterial anostomosis and from the external carotid artery of the opposite side and other sources. Even asymptomatic bilateral occlusion of the common carotid arteries may occur in rare instances.

In cases of brain infarction resulting from common carotid artery occlusion, marked edema covering the whole hemisphere may be seen in computerized tomography, corresponding to severe neurologic deficit on the contralateral side.

4. Aortic Arch

Obliterating disease of the aortic arch and the large vessels originating there is mainly of arteritic origin and as it affects younger adults more frequently than old people it is of minor interest to gerontologists. In Japan Takayasu syndrome or pulseless disease was first observed. The aortic arch syndrome has, in respect to the low blod pressure in craniocervical vessels, been attributed as a kind of reverse to stenosis of isthmus aortae. Occlusion of common carotid artery (uni- or bilateral) and subclavian steal syndrome are parts of the manifestations of aortic arch syndrome together with ophthalmic symptoms and ischemic signs of the face and upper extremities.

5. Anterior Cerebral Artery

Obliterations of the anterior cerebral artery are seen only less than 10% as frequently as those of the middle cerebral artery. If the communicating anterior artery leading blood from the opposite side is involved, a paresis of the contralateral lower extremity results. Primitive motor phenomena like grasping and oral automatisms can also be present, as well as apraxia of ideomotor type. Infarcts in both frontal lobes in the case of bilateral occlusion are followed by marked psychopathologic disturbances mainly affecting drive and producing a stuporous and akinetic syndrome. They may be associated with spastic paraparesis of both legs.

If the artery is occluded before the communicating anterior artery leaves, a syndrome results which cannot be definitely differentiated from internal carotid or medial cerebral artery occlusion on clinical grounds. One finds brachiofacial hemiparesis as the ischemia affects the anterior part of the internal capsule.

6. Middle Cerebral Artery

Of all intracranial arteries, the middle cerebral artery is most often involved. This is true for thrombotic disorders as well as for embolism. Symptoms depend on the location of the obstruction. Proximal thromboses have more severe consequences than occlusion of distal artery branches. They cause ischemia of the dorsal part of the internal capsule and of the basal ganglia. Occlusion of single distal branches can at best occur without persistent deficit. In lesions of the dominant hemisphere, complete aphasia will be combined with hemiplegia and disorders of epicritic sensory perception. Ischemia in the area of anterior parietal artery causes a disorder of postural sensitivity and stereoagnosia in the contralateral hand. Dorsal parietal lesion is associated with hemianopsia, akalkulia, finger agnosia, disturbances of body image, and a sensory aphasia if the dominant hemisphere is damaged and anosognosia if the lesion is of the nondominant hemisphere. A mild hemiparesis sometimes only affecting the face and dysarthria is found in ischemia of anterior branches.

7. Anterior Choroid Artery

This artery arises from the internal carotid artery near the posterior communicating artery and supplies parts of the temporal lobe, the occipital part of the internal capsule, tractus opticus, and lateral geniculate body. Isolated occlusion is very rare and may be asymptomatic but hemiplegia, hemihypalgesia, and homonymous hemianopsia to the opposite side are reported.

8. Posterior Communicating Artery and Posterior Cerebral Artery

The posterior communicating artery forms an anastomosing artery between the carotid and vertebrobasilar part of the circulus arteriosus. The posterior cerebral artery itself may originate in the internal carotid artery (between 5% and 30%) but usually this is the terminal artery of the basilar artery. Posterior comunicating and posterior cerebral arteries belong embryologically to the carotid system but in respect to hemodynamics must be regarded as a part of the basilar system. Therefore, clinical symptoms are described in the next section.

II. Symptoms of Strokes Affecting the Vertebrobasilar System

Occlusion and stenoses in the vertebral artery and basilar artery and ischemia in brain areas supplied by these arteries and their branches cause a variety of clinical syndromes depending on the place and size of the ischemic lesion.

The classic brain stem syndromes of mesencephalon, pons, and medulla oblongata are observed only in a part of cases and in others there are variations. Most of the classic syndromes are characterized by a combination of ipsilateral cranial nerve disorders and contralateral hemiparesis or sensory deficit. Relatively often Wallenberg's syndrome can be seen.

The syndromes of transitory ischemic attacks (TIAs) in the vertebrobasilar system usually are even more variable and ambiguous. Vertigo, dizziness, blurred vision, and diplopia can be caused by different disorders apart from those of cerebrovascular origin. Also the so-called drop attacks, a relapsing sudden loss of muscle control and muscle tone in the legs with falling down and only lasting for a few seconds, are not pathognomonic. On the other hand, this symptom is a very important sign of vertebrobasilar ischemia and apparently it is also often misinterpreted.

When occurring only transiently, cranial nerve disorders – evoked by transitory ischemia of brain stem structures – are difficult to recognize on the strength of anamnestic data when the attack has passed by.

Persistent syndromes of disorder may follow the classic brain stem syndromes as mentioned before or show some aberrations. A relatively frequent type is Wallenberg's syndrome or the syndrome of posterior inferior cerebellar artery, supplying the dorsolateral part of medulla oblongata. The syndrome cannot only occur on the base of an occlusion of the posterior inferior cerebellar artery (which is an end artery) but often in more proximally situated occlusion or stenosis of a vertebral artery.

A very severe pattern of disorders is seen in total basilar artery occlusion leading to an infarction of the ventral pons and clinically characterized by "locked-in" syndrome with tetraplegia and cranial nerve palsies leading to de-efferentiation in spite of unclouded consciousness. The locked-in syndrome can be incomplete with some motor functions preserved.

Ischemia in a region of posterior cerebral artery is seen in cerebral arteriosclerosis of these vessels or basilar artery but also in embolism. Areas of supply are the visual cortex and visual tract, parts of the thalamus, and rostral brain stem. The most prominent symptom is disorder of visual field in the form of homonymous hemianopsia or quadrantanopsia.

Because of the topographic situation both posterior cerebral arteries are often involved, leading to cortical (bilateral) blindness, which can be combined with anosognosia in respect to the visual deficit (Anton's syndrome). In these cases amaurosis is present in spite of normal light reaction of the pupils. In unilateral infarction of the posterior cerebral artery, one finds besides hemianopsia a contralateral hypalgesia and loss of proprioception and transient and mild hemiparesis. As a late sequela spontaneous pains and hyperpathia of the contralateral extremities may be observed.

There is some evidence to assume that the syndrome of *transient global amnesia* (TGA) is caused by acute transitory ischemia in portions of the medial temporal lobe supplied by arterial branches from the vertebrobasilar system. Older persons are affected frequently and in many cases signs of cerebrovascular disease are evident (FRANK 1981, survey). We observed the onset of an attack of TGA in one patient immediately after selective catheter arteriography of a vertebral artery. The opposite artery had been hypoplastic in this case. It has been discussed that in cases of TGA the affected brain areas concerned with short-term memory are supplied by arteries originating from only one communicating posterior cerebral artery (GANNER 1974).

TGA is characterized by a failure of recent memory with apoplectic onset, lasting for some hours and followed by amnesia for the time of the attack. It is, however, not proven that TGA really is a cerebrovascular local symptom. A combination with other vertebrobasilar symptoms is not usual and remittent occurrence seems to be exceptional.

III. Symptoms in Diffuse Cerebrovascular Disorders

In bilateral, multifocal, and diffusely localized cerebrovascular disorders, psychopathologic symptoms used to be predominant features. The symptoms are generally included in the term organic brain syndrome. The psychopathologic phenomena themselves are unspecific with regard to the etiology of brain dysfunction, i.e., whether ischemic, neoplastic, degenerative, or otherwise. However, the course of disease, its acuity, and dynamics would influence symptomatology. Still more important is the degree of severity of impairment and this corresponds with the severity of underlying cerebral dysfunction. Another important question to determine is whether the disorders are reversible or whether they are persisting deficits caused by irreversible loss of brain tissue.

Organic brain syndrome has been classified into syndromes with global cognitive impairment (delirium, subacute amnestic-confusional state, dementia), syndromes with selective psychological deficit (amnestic syndrome and others), and "symptomatic functional syndromes" showing similarity to endogenous psychoses.

In subacute or chronic cerebral diseases, like most instances of diffuse cerebrovascular disorders, psychological deficits appear as alterations of personality.

Multifocal neurologic symptoms, including the extrapyramidal system, can be combined with psychopathologic disturbances. These combinations of symptoms can be present both in degenerative cerebral atrophy and in cerebrovascular disease. In the differential diagnosis of multifocal and diffuse cerebrovascular disorders, Jakob-Creutzfeldt's disease (spongiform encephalopathy), a slow virus infection of the brain, must also be considered.

Fluctuations of severity and intercurrent appearance of acute symptoms can indicate ischemic etiology of organic brain syndrome *(multiinfarct dementia)* and help to differentiate it from progressive degenerative brain atrophy.

There is increasing evidence that in the dementias of middle and late life cerebral vascular disease is not the major cause but that these processes in most cases must be ascribed to Alzheimer's disease, which itself is not etiopathogenetically linked with cerebrovascular disorders. In only about 8% of dementias does arteriosclerosis seem to be responsible (WELLS 1978).

D. Clinical Stages of Stroke

Four stages of stroke are distinguished on the grounds of clinical conditions.

Stage I means the stenoses or occlusions of a cerebral or extracranial artery without neurologic symptoms and signs (asymptomatic stage). Stage II is that of transient ischemic attacks (TIAs). With stage III a condition is described in which neurologic deficits develop acutely but stepwise. This stage is also called stroke in evolution or progressive stroke. In stage IV, completed stroke, neurologic symptoms are manifest and have occurred in an apoplectic manner. In the further course there can be protracted recovery or the deficit may fully persist.

I. Asymptomatic Stenosis or Occlusion (Stage I, "Asymptomatic Bruit")

This stage of arteriosclerotic disease has gained practical interest as to the question of surgical preventive procedures. Stenosis or occlusion of one or both extracranial carotid arteries can in the asymptomatic stage be discovered by chance or after carefully directed diagnosis. Most frequently asymptomatic stenosis is diagnosed on the grounds of a carotid bruit searched for because of known peripheral or coronary arteriosclerotic disease.

The typical bruit caused by carotid stenosis is localized in the middle of the carotid artery and diminished toward the thoracic outlet. The bruit is most evident in stenosis of 50% and more but may disappear when stenosis is more than 85%. In about 80% of cases audible bruit is correlated with a stenosis of internal carotid artery. However, only about 60% of all stenoses are combined with a bruit. In the differential diagnosis one must consider bruits that are propagated, stenosis of external carotid artery, incipient murmurs, kinking, and other possible causes. Doppler sonography is a useful tool in the diagnosis of asymptomatic stenosis of higher degree and occlusion.

The diagnosis of an asymptomatic stenosis raises the question which consequences will have to be drawn (Fields 1978). The procedures are of an entirely prophylactic character as there is actually no need for therapy. The justification to prophylaxis results from the fact that asymptomatic stenosis may at any time become symptomatic. Transient ischemic attacks can follow the asymptomatic stage but completed stroke can also develop acutely without preceding attacks. The acute manifestation can be caused by thrombotic occlusion of the previously stenotic artery. On the other hand, even asymptomatic occlusion can suddenly become symptomatic because of acute failure of collateral circulation or other conditions.

Considerations about prophylaxis can be of immediate interest in different situations. A bruit can, for instance, be recognized in a patient who exhibits symptoms that indicated a lesion of the opposite side and in whom bilateral carotid alterations are found, one being asymptomatic. Another situation would be a patient who is about to be operated on for thoracic, peripheral, or renal arteriosclerotic disease and in whom uni- or bilateral stenosis (bruit) is found by directed investigation. Finally, diagnosis can be made on the grounds of routine examination in clinically healthy persons, diabetic or hypertonic patients, or others.

Under the assumption that these vascular alterations are prestroke lesions, ideas about possible prevention have been propagated. The indication for surgery in these cases is a relative one. Patients who have risk factors as to the operation itself will generally be excluded. If such risk factors are not present, the surgical treatment of asymptomatic carotid stenosis in patients about to undergo major arterial reconstructive operations on other organs is able to reduce the frequency of intra- or postoperative stroke.

In the group of healthy persons with asymptomatic stenosis diagnosed by chance, the risk of complications of operation and preoperative angiography must be set off against the probability of spontaneous stroke. In most cases nonsurgical methods of prophylaxis, i.e., antiplatelet adherent agents, but not anticoagulants, will be preferred.

Until now no randomized prospective study of surgically and nonsurgically matched groups has been completed and most investigators agree that such a study is urgently needed to decide the proper way of proceeding.

II. Transient Ischemic Attacks (Stage II)

Transient ischemic attack (TIA) is regarded to be the most important warning symptom of impeding stroke. TIA is defined as temporary focal cerebral dysfunction which lasts for only short time between a few minutes and maximally 24 h and which is fully reversible without any resting disorders. The attack is always of vascular origin. The focal dysfunction can concern the carotid or vertebrobasilar system. The number of attacks and the frequency of their occurrence is very variable. The more frequent they are, the more probable is the transition into completed stroke. Altogether, roughly a third of the patients with TIAs will suffer from stroke within 1 year's time.

TIAs in the carotid system are most frequently associated with stenosis of the internal carotid artery at the bifurcation; less common are lesions at the syphon. As extracranial carotid stenosis is suitable for vascular surgery and because of the high risk of completed stroke in untreated TIAs, this stage is of utmost importance in respect to diagnostic and therapeutic or prophylactic procedures.

The pathogenetic mechanisms underlying TIA in the carotid system is either transitory hemodynamic insufficiency, or platelet-fibrin emboli or atheromatous (cholesterol) emboli arising from arteriosclerotic ulcerated plaques in the carotid artery. In these cases the degree of stenosis is not of major significance.

The diagnosis of TIA is based on clinical symptoms, whereas the recognition of the causative lesion requires special investigation. In most cases clinical signs are no longer present when the patients come to medical examination. The decision on whether TIA or other transient disorders has occurred must rely on the patient's statements. Essential criteria that must be established are the type of transient neurologic deficits, details of their incidence and cessation, their duration and possible concomitant phenomena (e.g., unilateral headache in migraine accompagnée), relapsing occurrence with identical symptoms, and others. The diagnosis is less difficult to make when clinical signs are still present when the physician sees the patient. If investigation can be done during an attack of amaurosis fugax, it may be possible to observe cholesterol or platelet-fibrin emboli directly in the retinal arterioles.

The common symptoms of carotid and vertebrobasilar attacks are specified in Sect. C. In summary, they are for the carotid artery and branches: amaurosis fugax, i.e., monocular blindness or monocular blurring of previously normal vision, aphasia, contralateral paresis of the arm or leg or both, contralateral sensory disturbances (numbness), and unilateral facial weakness. Symptoms of vertebrobasilar attacks are vertigo, bilateral visual blurring, diplopia, ataxia, drop spells, and rarely bilateral weakness or numbness in the face and extremities.

Differential diagnosis of TIAs in the carotid system include: acute and brief confusional states, focal epileptic seizures, migrainous attacks, and syncopal episodes. These disorders can in many cases be ruled out on the grounds of anamnestic and purely clinical data.

In the differential diagnosis of vertebrobasilar attacks distinction is more difficult as the symptoms are less characteristic. Recurrent attacks of vertigo are also found in Menière's syndrome, but this is more frequent in younger persons than in the aged. Moreover, "dizziness" is a very ambiguous complaint and must be differentiated from true vertigo. Diplopia can occur in many different disorders ranging from cerebral pathology to myasthenia gravis. Episodic ataxia must be distinguished from toxic states caused by alcohol or drug intake. Similar difficulties are to be encountered in the interpretation of drop attacks.

Transient ischemic attacks are defined on the basis of clinical phenomena, which include short duration and complete recovery. Studies of computerized tomography (CT) in patients with TIA have, however, frequently shown signs of persisting parenchymatous lesions without corresponding neurologic deficit. Even in asymptomatic patients CT sometimes reveals small areas of hypodensity indicating previous ischemic lesions. These experiences show that the clinical regression is not identical with morphologic integrity.

TIA is not a disease entity. The definition and classification as stage II of stroke is arbitrary in still another respect. Ischemia can be transient and fully reversible but can take a longer time than 24 h. Therefore, regardless of its duration reversible neurologic deficit can be distinguished from completed stroke with only partial or no recovery at all. However, for the time being TIAs are still defined, as it were, with the limitation of 24 h and strokes with recovery taking more than this limit are classified as prolonged reversible ischemic neurologic deficit (PRIND) or as prolonged TIAs but properly ascribed to stage II.

Outside the attacks signs of neurologic deficit are not to be found but there may be a carotid bruit depending on the degree of stenosis. However, the absence of a bruit does not rule out stenosis and, on the other hand, bruits may have an origin different from carotid stenosis.

Transient vertebrobasilar attacks are of a minor practical importance compared with those of the carotid system. Both a reduction of blood flow and embolism can also obviously occur in the posterior circulation. The significance of localized obliteration is not comparable with that of the carotids, for usually the arteriosclerotic plaquing is more diffuse. Also in stenosis of the subclavian artery and the subclavian vertebral junction, vascular surgery is in most cases not as efficient as in carotid stenosis. If TIAs of the vertebrobasilar system are diagnosed, the treatment of choice will generally be the use of antiplatelet drugs.

III. Stroke in Evolution (Stage III)

This stage is really a special variant of completed stroke with regard to its development. Neurologic deficit does not manifest itself at once in full strength but it develops with a stepwise progression over a period of hours or a few days. The progression may be more or less continuous or going on with attacks frequently following one another and producing an increasing deficit. The pathogenetic mechanism seems in most cases to be the propagation of a thrombus in the carotid or basilar arteries. Accordingly, the clinical symptoms advance under the physician's eyes without being influenced by the therapy usually performed in acute stroke. Therefore, some clinicians propagate an active strategy using anticoagulant or even fibrinolytic therapy at the start of progressive stroke. These procedures require an immediate diagnosis. Differential diagnosis must consider lesions with very rapid space occupation including intracranial hemorrhages and cerebral venous thrombosis.

IV. Completed Stroke (Stage IV)

Stage IV of stroke or completed stroke means cerebral infarction. Clinical symptoms develop rapidly over minutes and there may be some further progression in the first hours. Apoplexies with succeeding complete recovery but taking longer time than classical TIAs are regarded as a special kind of reversible ischemia distinct from completed stroke with permanent deficit. However, if the recovery takes a long time (for instance, some weeks) the stroke will generally be regarded as stage IV or completed stroke.

The typical symptoms of completed stroke depend on the affected areas of brain and have been described earlier.

In most cases of completed stroke with sudden onset, neither etiology nor prognosis can be recognized with security. Computerized tomography (CT) has shown that previous views on differentiation between ischemia and hemorrhage on the basis of clinical symptoms cannot be relied on, especially in the case of smaller hemorrhages and extensive infarction. Emboli of cardiac origin have some typical features which, however, are not sufficiently specific to prove embolic etiology. The features are: sudden onset of focal deficit up to a maximum in a few minutes, focal or generalized seizures, some degree of hemorrhage (erythrocytes) in the CBF, hemorrhagic infarction (CT), frequently multiple lesions, and preference of the left hemisphere.

In the case of nonembolic thrombotic vascular occlusion different vascular diseases or lesions must be considered concerning etiology, but in old people arteriosclerosis is most common.

The treatment must depend upon the question whether stroke is caused by infarction or hemorrhage and in the case of infarction whether it is of thrombotic or embolic origin.

As far as the prognosis is concerned, this can also not be definitely decided in the initial stage. Even in the case of maximal hemiplegia, recovery cannot be predicted or ruled out, even if there is no tendency to be seen during the first days.

A maximum of neurologic deficit is found mostly within the first 48–72 h. Progressive deterioration with fatal outcome may occur on the basis of an extensive brain edema. Start of recovery is usually observed within 2–4 weeks from the onset and in most cases recovery is achieved after 12 weeks.

Further improvement cannot be expected when 6 or 9 months have passed since the apoplexy.

E. Pathogenetic Mechanisms of Stroke

I. Vascular Stenosis and Thrombotic Occlusions

1. Basic Diseases

Arteriosclerosis is by far the most important vascular disease leading to stroke, especially in old age. As stated in Sect. B.IV.1 arteriosclerotic plaquing shows certain places of predilection in the carotid system whereas it is more diffusely spread in the vertebrobasilar system. Poststenotic ischemia occurs acutely if the mechanisms which help in compensating the increased vascular resistance fail to work. Moreover, stenosis can suddenly reach such a degree that poststenotic circulation becomes insufficient. These mechanisms can manifest themselves under the clinical syndrome of transient attack, progressive stroke, or acute completed stroke. Thrombotic obstruction will lead to progressive stroke or a completed stroke with apoplectic onset.

Nonarteriosclerotic vascular diseases occurring in old age and possibly causing neurologic deficit are congophilic angiopathy (cerebral amyloidosis) and related angiopathies, described as dysoric or senile angiopathy. Congophilic angiopathy is often combined with hypertension and intracerebral hemorrhage.

Inflammatory angiopathies may form the cause of thrombotic or hemorrhagic complications also in old age, although they are more frequent in younger patients. Vasculitis belonging to the group of collagen diseases are periarteritis nodosa and generalized lupus erythematodes. Extremely rare are cerebral dysfunctions in cranial giant cell arteriitis, which is found nearly exclusively in old age. Affected are in most cases extracranial arteries, mainly the superficial temporal artery, occipital arteries, and ophthalmic artery. In exceptional cases, however, also cerebral arteries can be involved.

2. Additional Factors

In addition to the increase of vascular resistance caused by arteriosclerotic obliteration, some other factors take part in the development of stroke. *Acute hypotonia* can be involved and this can happen spontaneously or can be induced by antihypertensive treatment. *Acute cardiac arrhythmia* may not only bring about embolism but also may be an additional factor in producing poststenotic ischemia. Although the medical lowering of blood sugar is an important and useful measure for improving one risk factor of cerebrovascular disease, the induced *hypoglycemia* can provoke symptoms of stroke, for instance, when oral antidiabetics or insulin is given in an overdosage and in the case of preexisting vascular disease. These accidents are more likely to happen in older patients.

Apart from the insufficiency of cerebral blood flow in poststenotic and postthrombotic brain areas, another mechanism of acute neurologic dysfunction is to be considered, namely, *microembolisms* of fibrin platelets or cholesterol particles from ulcerating plaques in an artery, especially the internal carotid artery. Whether this pathogenetic mechanism of stroke is perhaps overestimated is under discussion.

Another way that ischemia or infarction can develop is by *steal-syndromes*. Vascular occlusion leads to a reverse direction of blood flow in order to compensate for the obstructive lesion and this is realized at the expense of another brain area. Steal phenomena can also be produced by incorrect treatment of acute cerebrovascular disorders.

Spasms play no role in the genesis of spontaneous stroke but they are a common feature in direct lesions of vessels and in subarachnoid hemorrhage. In the latter, factors originating from the blood in the subarachnoid space are made responsible for vasoconstriction. These spasms can be very marked and spread and they not infrequently cause infarction in one or more brain regions. Although subarachnoid hemorrhage is more frequently found in middle-aged persons it can also occur in old age.

Traumatic lesions of arteries occasionally lead to thrombotic stroke. Younger persons are affected in connection with head or neck trauma, which can appear relatively harmless and a similar situation can also arise in older persons. Cervical manipulation has repeatedly been the cause of vertebrobasilar stroke and in some cases older patients were involved. Arteriosclerosis may be a predisposing factor in such cases.

II. Embolism

It is important to differentiate between the situations brought about by stenosis or thrombosis and by embolism of cardiac origin. The diagnosis of cardiac embolization is based either on the proof of cardiac disorder associated with stroke or on certain characteristics of the history and findings. In old people cerebrovascular arteriosclerosis much more frequently causes stroke than embolism, whereas in younger people the relationship is different.

Therefore, embolism of cardiac origin is more a problem of stroke in early and middle life, but, of course, it can also occur in older age.

Cerebral emboli can be caused by rheumatic heart disease with mitral or aortic valvular disease with and without atrial fibrillation. Heart disease is often indicated by murmur.

Prostetic aortal and mitral valves may be the source of embolization of platelet-fibrin clots. Following myocardial infarction cerebral embolism can occur arising from a thrombus due to ischemic lesion of endocardium and subsequent nidation of thrombosis. There can be an interval of some months between myocardial infarction and cerebral embolism. Other possible sources of cerebral embolism with cardiac origin are congenital vitium cordis, myopathies of the heart muscle, prolapse of the mitral valve and atrial myxoma – both occurring more frequently in younger than in old people – congestive heart failure, and marantic, nonbacterial endocarditis, which may be associated with malignant neoplasma.

Apart from the signs of cardiac disease other criteria indicating cerebral embolism are the finding of multiple embolic infarctions, especially if there is disseminated location, and the finding of a hemorrhagic infarction. In respect to clinical symptomatology focal or generalized epileptiform seizures are more frequent with embolic than with other causes of cerebral infarction. Neurologic deficit usually occurs suddenly and becomes maximal in the course of minutes. Unless there is generalized seizure activity, consciousness remains unclouded.

Infected emboli arise from acute or subacute bacterial endocarditis, which develops on the base of a lesion of heart valves, prosthetic valves, and congenital cardiac defects. In addition to a neurologic deficit one can find symptoms resembling meningitis, such as nuchal rigidity, psychopathologic disorders (acute brain syndrome), and general symptoms of infection. Embolization in other organs may or may not be recognizable from clinical symptoms.

Important clinical signs of cardiac origin are arrhythmia and episodes of atrial fibrillation, anamnestic data of myocardial infarction, and abnormal heart sounds. Intermittent arrhythmia is diagnosed with long-term continuous electrocardiographic monitoring. Intracardiac thrombus, tumor, and valve disease can be recognized with echocardiography.

The main ways of preventing embolism are anticoagulant therapy and surgical elimination of the source of embolization. For both alternatives, old age means a limitation as the risk of bleeding complications in anticoagulation and the risk of intra- and postoperative complications increase with age.

III. Hemorrhages

Spontaneous intracerebral hemorrhage is a frequent complication of arteriosclerosis and severe hypertension, sometimes occurring in connection with hypertensive crisis. Hypertensive hemorrhage is caused by the rupture of a cerebral arterial vessel. Neurologic deficit and destruction of brain tissue is not limited to the area of one definite artery. Clinical symptoms are dependent on the localization and size of the hematoma. Large bleedings cause the destruction of great parts of a brain hemisphere and mass shifting. In these situations consciousness will be grossly deteriorated. Small hemorrhages, on the other hand, can be associated with pure neurologic deficit and cannot be differentiated from ischemic stroke on the grounds of clinical signs alone. Diagnosis is settled by CT. Sites of predilection are mentioned in Sect. B.III. Apart from the site and size of the hemorrhage and surrounding edema, symptoms and prognosis also depend on age, the state of general brain function, and additional disorders.

Hemorrhages in the posterior fossa and intraventricular bleedings are liable to cause obstruction of CSF flow, resulting in hydrocephalus and raised intracranial pressure and demanding surgical CSF drainage.

Other vascular diseases causing cerebral hemorrhage are various types of angiitis and amyloid (congophilic) angiopathy. A possible cause of intracerebral hemorrhage of great practical importance is anticoagulant treatment. Together with subdural hematoma and sub- and epidural spinal hematomas, intracerebral hemorrhage is one of the most frequent and most serious complications of the long-lasting treatment with coumadin. Arteriosclerosis, hypertension, and old age promote this complication. Apparently it is not dependent on the reason of anticoagulation. Other therapy apart from coumadin influencing hemostasis may occasionally cause intracerebral hemorrhage, as for instance, fibrinolytic substances. Moreover, there may be underlying hemorrhagic diathesis on the ground of hematologic disease or severe hepatic dysfunction.

A very important cause of spontaneous hemorrhage is the rupture of a cerebral aneurysma or angioma. Bleedings of aneurysmatic origin mostly concern the subarachnoid space, causing the typical symptoms, but in about a third of all cases a subarachnoid hemorrhage is associated with an intracerebral hematoma. Rupture of aneurysma is not uncommon in old aged persons. Intracerebral hemorrhage is to be distinguished from a hemorrhagic infarction, and this differentiation is generally possible with the aid of CT.

IV. Rheologic Causes

Alterations of blood condition with increased viscosity can be the cause of thrombotic ischemia either as an additional factor to arterial wall disease or as an isolated disorder.

The best-known disorder of this kind is *polycythemia* which both in its primary and secondary variant can cause cerebrovascular disease (MILLIKAN et al. 1960). Increase of blood viscosity begins with a hematocrit of more than 55%. Abnormal platelet function can be a further pathogenetic factor in polycythemia vera and in secondary polycythemia there may be hypoxemia in addition.

States of *hypercoagulability* and *hyperviscosity* are brought about by various disorders and different types of coagulopathy. There can be increased rate of coagulation, diminution of factors that inhibit coagulation, increase of activities inhibiting fibrinolysis, or decrease of fibrinolytic activity. Disorders of coagulation have been reported in patients with arterial vascular diseases and with cardiac and cerebral infarction. Special interest is attributed to the problem of platelet aggregation on the vessel wall.

An increase of thrombotic brain infarctions has been reported as a complication of antifibrinolytic therapy in subarachnoid hemorrhage.

In hemoglobinopathies like sickle cell anemia and in some other disorders of blood proteins and cells, stroke may occur as a consequence of thrombosis.

F. Diagnostic Technical Procedures

I. Cerebral Angiography

Cerebral angiography, nowadays generally performed with catheter technique, is the only method of directly demonstrating extra- and intracranial blood vessels. Stenoses and occlusions, irregularities of vascular caliber, and spasms and malformations like aneurysma and angioma are therefore diagnosed angiographically. Moreover, serial angiography provides information on collateral circulation, velocity of blood flow, and modes of venous drainage.

The changes in the nervous parenchyma, i.e., outside the vessel itself, is not directly shown in the angiogram and can be best indicated by shifting and other indirect signs. The parenchymatous alterations can be displayed by CT and brain scanning.

Angiography can thus give certain information and the possibilities and limitations of this method must be known when it is indicated. One must take into account that cerebral angiography is not without risks and that complications consisting of seizures, neurologic deficit, or general symptoms of allergic reaction occur in between 0.7% and 2%, even fatal outcome in a small proportion of cases (SCHIEFER 1972b, survey). Therefore, the risks and benefits of angiographic diagnoses must be carefully considered. The question of possible therapeutic consequences is decisive, and here age must again be taken into account as a factor that restricts the indications for surgical treatment.

Complications due to puncture and injection can be largely reduced by catheter technique and selective angiography. Old age favors the incidence of permanent complications (PATTERSON et al. 1964), whereas the overall frequency is not dependent on age. However, cardiovascular diseases are a strongly predisposing factor and these disorders occur predominantly in older patients.

II. Measurements of Cerebral Blood Flow

Quantitative and regional cerebral blood flow (CBF) is measured on the basis of determining the clearance of radioactive substances. For practical diagnostic purposes ^{133}Xenon has proven to be a suitable substance.

The traditional method of Kety and Schmidt can only give a mean value of the global cerebral blood flow, whereas local differences are not indicated.

The intracarotid injection method (INGVAR et al. 1965) has the disadvantage of being an invasive procedure. In this respect progress was achieved with the establishment of the ^{133}Xenon inhalation method of determining regional cerebral blood flow (OBRIST et al. 1975; MEYER et al. 1978). Investigations with this technique have shown that in normal individuals with advancing age, blood flow in the gray matter declines progressively. A differentiation of CBF into gray and white matter and of extracranial structures is possible using a 2 or 3 compartmented analysis proposed by OBRIST et al. Values were found to agree well with those of the intracarotid injection technique.

Following cerebral infarction, flow values are reduced but in ischemia with recovery, increased flow in circumscribed areas indicates relative hyperemia (luxury perfusion). In the acute phase of infarction there may be regional reduction of blood flow not only in the area of infarction but also in other regions such as the corresponding area of the opposite hemisphere. Severe reduction of mean blood flow (below 23 ml/100 g/min) in the area of ischemia following stroke generally indicates a pure prognosis for functional recovery. Regional CBF changes can be found in subarachnoid hemorrhage due to ischemia caused by spasms. Following bypass and reconstructive surgery, CBF measurements can prove the effectiveness of the procedure. In spite of the various indications, measurements of CBF are not yet available as a routine method in most departments but are restricted to some specialized departments, although with the improvement of noninvasive technique, increased and more widespread application can be expected.

III. Computerized Tomography

Computerized tomography (CT) shows to some extent the alterations that are produced by circulatory disorders in the brain tissue. The morphologic alterations of the blood vessels themselves are not visible except for large malformations like angioma or aneurysma.

The great importance of CT diagnosis in the initial stage of stroke is the possibility of differentiating between hemorrhage and ischemia, and this is possible immediately after the apoplexy on account of increased density of fresh blood. The ischemic lesion is not immediately visible but takes about 20–40 h until lowered density can be seen. For direct differentiation CT is a unique diagnostic tool. In the acute stage hemorrhagic infarction can also be demonstrated and in general it can be distinguished from primary hemorrhage.

Both hyperdensity of hematoma and hypodensity of infarcted tissue change in the course of time, leaving a scar expressing itself in the zone of lowered density, which can be very discrete. In this late stage, whether intracerebral hemorrhage or infarction has preceded cannot be recognized.

Apart from the differential diagnosis of stroke disorders which may simulate stroke can also be ruled out, such as primary or metastatic brain tumor, venous thrombosis, traumatic lesions, and others.

The fact that CT changes can be found following TIAs shows that tissue damage not always goes parallel with clinically recognizable disorders of function. In some parts of the brain small ischemic lesions can apparently even pass without clinical symptoms, at least none that are realized by the patient and his environment.

IV. Electroencephalography

The information given by electroencephalography (EEG) in stroke is predominantly indirect and nonspecific. Ischemic stroke and hemorrhage cause localized abnormalities of bioelectric activity. Alterations of background (basic) activity can indicate the state of general brain function and are correlated with consciousness and disorders. In brain stem lesions discrepancies between the state of consciousness and EEG can be found.

Unlike CT, angiography, brain scanning, and other methods, the EEG reflects cerebral function at the time of investigation. A great advantage is that recordings can be repeated unobjectionably. Investigations in the course of illness can give prognostic information (VAN DER DRIFT et al. 1972, 1973).

A differential diagnosis between causes of stroke and cerebrovascular disease and other disorders is not possible on the basis of EEG except for some rare situations, such as acute or subacute encephalitis. Diffuse cerebrovascular disorders will manifest themselves in diffuse slow wave activity, which, however, is also not specifically different from other pathologic conditions.

Special significance is attributed to the EEG for the diagnosis of epileptic syndromes. Embolic or thrombotic stroke can produce a focus of epileptic activity and in these cases EEG is the most suitable method for recognition and control of therapeutic effectiveness.

V. Doppler Sonography

Doppler ultrasonics has proven a useful method for evaluating the state of extracranial carotid arteries and especially of carotid bifurcation.

Directional Doppler sonography of the supratrochlear artery, a branch of the ophthalmic artery anastomosing with the external carotid artery indicates occlusion of the internal carotid artery when blood flow takes a reverse direction, i.e., from external to internal carotid artery. Antidromic blood flow occurs in complete obstruction and in very severe stenosis. Direct investigation of the carotid arteries at the neck allows differentiation between common, external, and internal carotid arteries in most cases. Stenoses can be recognized on account of increased current flow and turbulence and in the poststenotic part pulse amplitude is decreased. In complete occlusion above it, no pulse signal can be recorded. Similar findings can be obtained in stenoses and occlusions of the internal and external carotid artery.

Findings are much less reliable in vertebral artery investigations. The rate of correct ultrasonic diagnosis depends on the special skill and experience of the investigator.

In severe stenoses and occlusion this is correctly established by directional Doppler sonography in 80%–90% of cases. VON REUTERN et al. (1979) found positive findings with direct sonography of the carotids in all cases with angiographically verified severe stenosis of the internal carotid artery. Stenoses were distinguished from occlusions in more than 95% of cases.

A modification of direct carotid sonography has been developed using continuous-wave Doppler-shift ultrasound (SPENCER et al. 1974) and spectral analysis for imaging the carotid bifurcation (LEWIS et al. 1978).

Negative results of sonography are likely to be received in stenoses of less than 50% of vessel lumen. As small ulcerating stenoses can cause TIAs by way of embolism, angiography has to be performed in cases of TIA, even if Doppler sonography is normal.

VI. Brain Scanning

Until the introduction of CT, conventional brain scanning was the most important noninvasive method of revealing structural changes of the brain parenchyma. Abnormal findings rest on localized disorders of the blood-brain barrier, leading to abnormal enhancement of radioactive marked isotope, as for instance, Te^{133m} as pertechnatate.

A characteristic feature of infarction is the change of enhancement in the course of time. During the first 5 days there is generally no positive finding but between the 2nd and 3rd week increased activity occurs and disappears after the 4th or 6th week. Hematomas in general keep the enhancement a little longer but a definite differentiation is not possible. The time-dependent changes enable cerebrovascular lesion to be distinguished from brain tumor.

Scintigraphy is now considerably less important since the establishment of CT, which gives much more direct information.

An extension that conventional brain scanning has experienced is the developement of *radioangiography* or *dynamic brain scanning*, in which, following intravenous injection, a serial scanning is performed with a gamma camera and different phases of blood flow are analyzed. Pathologic vascularization and unilateral retardation of perfusion can thus be seen.

VII. Other Noninvasive Methods

Some other methods can give partial information on cerebral circulation and are used as screening procedures before angiography.

Thermography can indicate localized differences of skin temperature which may be caused by different blood flow. Decrease of skin temperature in the medial supraorbit region of one side may be caused by severe stenosis or occlusion of the internal carotid artery. Altogether, thermography is far less instructive than Doppler sonography.

Ophthalmodynamography is one of the oldest of these methods. Systolic and diastolic blood pressure of the ophthalmic artery and the volume of pulsations are measured on both sides, applying external pressure on both eyes. Side differences can indicate unilateral stenosis or occlusion of the carotid artery. This method, too, is insecure and vague. In the case of bilateral stenoses (or occlusion), which is not very rare, no side differences and thus no signs will be received.

Rheoencephalography is also an almost traditional method. Findings are influenced by many different factors, making the method only of very little use.

G. Prevention, Treatment, and Prognosis

I. Prevention

1. Treatment and Prevention of Risk Factors

A first step of preventing cerebrovascular disease is the prophylaxis and therapy of risk factors, which are involved in the etiopathogenesis of stroke. These include the factors that are looked upon as favoring the development of arteriosclerosis. Factors that induce or favor cardiovascular disease like obesity and lack of physical activity can also be regarded as risk factors for cerebrovascular pathology.

As *hypertension* plays an important role in most kinds of stroke, early and sufficient treatment of hypertension can help prevent arteriosclerotic thrombosis and hypertensive hemorrhage. A reduction of the incidence of cerebrovascular disease in the United States has been referred to an intensified treatment of this risk factor (SOLTERO et al. 1978).

Similarly early and adequate treatment of diabetes mellitus will be able to prevent diabetic angiopathy and stroke in many patients. This may also be true for disorders of lipid metabolism.

2. Medical Prevention

a) Anticoagulant Treatment

Thrombosis is the most important mechanism leading to cerebral infarction and embolism. Antithrombotic therapy therefore means an ingenious approach of prophylaxis and it can theoretically be indicated in cases of disturbed hemostasis (hypercoagibility), in patients with obliterating and ulcerating vascular disease, and in cases with cardiac disorders with the tendency of cerebral embolism.

There has been a lot of investigation and discussion about the application of antithrombotic treatment and its objections.

Two main ways of therapy are available:
1. Anticoagulant agents including oral anticoagulants and heparin
2. Substances interfering with platelet aggregation and not influencing the factors of hemostasis.

The *oral anticoagulants*, as for instance, warfarin, inhibit the synthesis of coagulation factors II, VII, IX, and X in the liver and the action of vitamin K. Depression of clotting factor activity after warfarin sets in only some time after the start of therapy and the restoration of coagulation to normal after withdrawal is reached with some delay.

Heparin, on the other hand, does not cause deficiencies of coagulation factors, but it interferes with the process of coagulation in a different respect. Activation of factor IX as well as IXa, Xa, and thrombin is inhibited and by the inhibition of thrombin factor XIII cannot be activated. The propagation of thrombosis is interrupted. Heparin can only be given intravenously or subcutaneously and is therefore not suited for a long-term prophylaxis.

The use of oral anticoagulants is mainly limited by the risk of hemorrhagic complications and among these especially intracerebral and subdural hematoma.

The decision whether anticoagulants should be given must be taken for each individual case.

Contraindications include previous hemorrhages of the CNS and peptic ulcer, hepatic, and renal dysfunctions, hypertension (blood pressure above 160/90 mm Hg), and hemorrhagic diathesis of any kind. Moreover, trustworthy cooperation with the patient and his family (patient compliance) and careful control of diagnostic tests of hemostasis must be guaranteed.

The risk of complication is increased if the treatment is performed for more than 12 months. Therefore, limitation of the application to some months is advisable.

In patients with TIA the indications are controversial and depend on the individual situation. The prevention of subsequent stroke is not sure enough to justify the risk of bleeding. Also in ischemic progressive stroke the risk of hemorrhagic infarction is great; on the other hand, in this situation one has to try all possible measures to influence the otherwise progressive lesion. There is no sense in giving anticoagulant treatment in completed stroke. An important indication can be embolism of cardiac origin as in these cases younger persons without hypertension often are affected.

b) Platelet-Inhibiting Agents

Under platelet antagonists or platelet-inhibiting agents, one understands drugs which can quantitatively alter certain platelet properties, such as aggregation, adhesion, and retention and inhibit thrombus formation induced by platelets. Furthermore, they can prolong survival of platelets in states of pathologic or experimentally induced decrease of survival as can be the case in increased activation.

The most prominent agent of this group is *acetylsalicylic acid (ASA)*. Platelet aggregation is partly inhibited by the means of interference with the prostaglandin and thromboxane A 2 synthesis. Platelet survival is not definitely affected. Acetylsalicylic acid is administered in therapeutic doses of 1–1,5 g daily and usually means a long-term therapy. Prophylaxis in patients with TIA has proven useful in various studies (FIELDS et al. 1977; BARNETT et al. 1978; FIELDS et al. 1978). Some authors propagate a short-term initial treatment with anticoagulants for a few months and thereafter antiplatelet therapy (OLSSON et al. 1980). FIELDS found a significant reduction of TIA under ASA compared with placebo but no difference of the lethality, which is mostly determined by cardiovascular disorders (FIELDS et al. 1977, 1978).

The Canadian cooperative study revealed a sex difference of prophylactic effect, as there was a significant antithrombotic effect of ASA in men but not in female patients. This difference was not found by OLSSON et al. (1980), who described an equally significant antithrombotic effect of long-term anticoagulant and antiplatelet treatment. Bleeding complications are rare under ASA. Other side effects mainly concern the gastrointestinal tract.

Some other antiinflammatory drugs show antithrombotic efficacy to some extent, which, however, is not proven for the prophylaxis of stroke.

Sulfinpyrazone affects platelet adhesiveness in vitro and platelet survival, but bleeding time, release reaction, and collagen-induced platelet aggregation are not influenced. The substance is introduced as a uricosuric agent for the treatment of gout.

Dipyridamole used as a coronary vasodilator was found to have antithrombotic effects by decreasing platelet adhesion and aggregation, probably via potentiation of endogenous prostacyclin (MONCADA and KORBUT 1978). A prophylactic effectiveness against cerebral infarction was not proven in patients with reversible cerebrovascular disorders. The combined application of acetylsalicylic acid and dipyridamole and of ASA and sulfinpyrazone is widespread. The effectiveness is, according to the Canadian report, equivalent to that of ASA alone.

The indication for antiplatelet agents is given in many cases of reversible ischemic strokes including typical TIA if surgical treatment is for any reason not possible and in cases that have undergone reconstructive operation of the carotid artery or bypass operation.

3. Surgical Prevention

a) Reconstructive Surgery

Thirty years ago the first reconstruction of carotid artery in its extracranial part was performed. In the meantime carotid surgery is a routine procedure indicated in many situations. Operative mortality depends on the clinical situation (stage of stroke), general physical condition, and the skill and experience of the surgeon. In special centers mortality of operation performed in patients with TIA (stage II) lies between 0.7% and 1%, morbidity (neurologic deficit after operation) around 1%, and transient deficits a little more frequent than permanent disorders. In an asymptomatic stage of carotid stenosis mortality is cited to be far less than 1% and morbidity between 0% and 3%. In stage III (stroke in evolution) the risks of operative therapy are very great, mortality lying over 20%. Some authors refuse to perform vascular surgery in this stage. In completed stroke operation is, if at all, not executed in the acute stage but some weeks to months after apoplexy. Mortality ranges between 3% and 8% (WYLIE et al. 1970; THOMPSON et al. 1970, 1976; FLEMING et al. 1977; RAITHEL 1977, 1978).

Carotid reconstruction can be indicated in obliterations leading to poststenotic insufficiency of blood flow. This is the case when stenoses amount to more than 50% of the vessel lumen. Also in stenosis of lesser severity, operation can be indicated as in these cases ulcerative plaques may be the origin of intermittent embolism. Both situations can manifest themselves as TIA and this clinical situation is generally regarded as the most important indication for carotid reconstruction.

Not infrequently stenoses are bilateral and in this case operation is performed with an interval of 1–2 weeks on both sides. In purely ulcerative plaque without marked stenosis prophylaxis of stroke can at first be attempted with antiplatelet medication (or anticoagulants) and if TIAs continue, surgery can be performed subsequently.

Carotid kinking will be the reason for surgery only if combined with stenosis or if it causes intermittent neurologic deficit.

Complications may arise from remittent thrombosis, embolism, and intracerebral hemorrhage (CAPLAN et al. 1978). Further risks are local hemorrhagic complications and peripheral nerve lesions at the neck.

In most cases of stenoses at the bifurcation and internal carotid artery, endarterectomy is sufficient. Stenoses at the proximal portion of the common carotid artery, the truncus branchiocephalicus, and the subclavian artery are mostly corrected with an extrathoracal bypass. Stenoses of the vertebral arteries are generally not suitable for surgical treatment. Besides, the lesions in vertebrobasilar insufficiency are usually more diffusely localized. In some cases with a combination of vertebrobasilar symptoms and carotid stenosis, carotid reconstruction can improve or even remove the neurologic symptoms.

b) Extraintracranial Arterial Anastomosis

In vascular disorders that are not accessible to extracranial vascular reconstruction, such as intracranial stenoses and occlusions, complete extracranial occlusion, or extended obliterations of the internal carotids, improvement of arterial blood supply can be achieved by means of operative bypass between the superficial temporal artery (originating from external carotid artery) and the medial cerebral artery in the form of end-to-side anastomosis (Gratzel et al. 1976). With this method a condition is produced, which on principle is a physiologic process of adaptation, i.e., the formation of collaterals between external and internal carotid systems.

Clinical situations or stages of stroke in which extra-intracranial arterial bypass can be indicated include TIAs, prolonged reversible neurologic deficit, and completed stroke (eventually developed as stroke in evolution), but stages III and IV not in the initial phase. The underlying pathogenetic situations at the vascular system are crucial for the indication. They are diagnosed with angiogram and CT. Measurement of regional cerebral blood flow can be useful for determining perfusion in the affected region pre- and postoperatively (Fenske et al. 1980). The pathologic situations are: stenosis of internal carotid artery in the area of the syphon, extracranial occlusion of internal carotid artery in the region of bifurcation, and occlusion of medial cerebral artery (and its branches). In cases with extracranial stenosis of the internal carotid artery on one side and occlusion on the other, Koos (1980) recommends performing endarterectomy on the stenotic side first and bypass on the side of occlusion some time afterwards, if this is necessary.

Reserve is advisable concerning indication in stenoses of medial cerebral artery in younger persons as these are not infrequently reversible, and in occlusions of the syphon with persistent neurologic deficit.

There is no indication for operation in stroke with severe neurologic deficit without tendency toward restitution, stroke in the acute phase, and if combined with other diseases which exclude operability altogether, and in generalized severe cerebrovascular disease with multiple obliterations. Old age per se is no contraindication. Of the patients treated by Koos, 18% were over 60 years.

After the operation with functioning bypass, its full effect on perfusion is seen only after a few months. Improvement was found in 72% of cases with moderate neurologic deficit and in 44% of cases of severe deficit, whereas the incidence of unchanged findings was 19% in the cases with moderate deficit and 50% in the patients with severe deficit (Koos 1980).

II. Treatment

1. Management of Stroke in the Initial Stage

In acute stroke a differentiation between ischemic lesion and hemorrhage is necessary for adequate treatment. In the acute phase of ischemic stroke, therapy aims at the following effects: improvement and normalization of perfusion in the affected region, limitation of the extent of infarction, and prevention of secondary lesions. Ultimate morbidity is to be decreased as far as possible and acute illness shortened and relieved.

General treatment of the acute stage includes management of respiratory function, prophylaxis against aspiration, clearing the airway of secretions, prevention of bronchopneumonia and other infections, control of urinary excretion, balancing of fluid and electrolytes, and prophylaxis against venous thrombosis of the extremities. Special problems are met in unconscious or severely obnubilated patients.

In order to normalize cerebral blood flow, therapy must provide for improvement of heart function, normal blood pressure, rheologic properties of the blood, and abolition of brain edema.

Cardiac therapy is not only necessary in cerebral embolism of cardiac origin but also in other causes of stroke, which in most cases are accompanied with hypertension and arteriosclerosis and often lead to cardiac insufficiency in the initial period. In old patients suffering from stroke, cardiac therapy is of major importance. Cardiac output should be kept on an optimal level. Digitalis glycosides are administered in an individual fashion. Arrhythmia is to be treated adequately, by the implantation of a pacemaker if necessary.

Blood pressure must be held on a level as near to normal as possible. There may initially be low pressure or hypertension and sometimes blood pressure strongly fluctuates. Medical decrease of pressure must be performed carefully as hypotension would favor cerebral ischemia. It is, on the other hand, necessary to treat hypertension as physiologic autoregulation of CBF is impaired in acute ischemia and high blood pressure may cause secondary hemorrhage. There is usually no need to lower blood pressure if it is moderately elevated in the first days after stroke in a previously normotensive patient, as hypertension can be a regulatory mechanism in order to improve CBF. A transient elevation of catecholamines in the plasma during the initial stage of stroke has been reported by KOMATSUMOTO et al. (1980). In patients with long-lasting hypertension, values should not be decreased to below 160–180 mm Hg.

Improvement of *rheologic blood properties* can influence blood perfusion and this is attempted with various substances. Hemodilution, decreased viscosity, and platelet adhesiveness with the consequence of increased CBF can be achieved by infusion of low molecular weight dextran (GILROY et al. 1969; GOTTSTEIN et al. 1976). As in some cases anaphylactic reactions after dextran may occur and exceptionally may be lethal (RICHTER et al. 1980), Dextran should not be infused without premedication. Some clinicians renounce dextran altogether for this reason.

Brain edema is counteracted with glucocorticoids, diuretics, and hyperosmolar solutions. Although the efficacy of corticosteroids against ischemic edema is not definitely proven, steroid therapy (dexamethasone) is generally performed in acute stroke (PATTEN et al. 1972; NORRIS 1976). Recommended dosages differ. The value of glycerol, which is also frequently used, is controversial. Mannitol is often given in combination with dextran. Among the diuretics furosemide mainly is used but in most cases it is also combined with other agents such as dexamethasone.

Application of vasodilatory drugs in the initial phase is not recommended because of the risk of provoking steal phenomena as vasodilators will act on peripheral vessels and CBF may be decreased via drop of blood pressure. Vasodilators may be used in a later stage of cerebrovascular disease.

Symptomatic treatment is indicated if seizures occur in the course of stroke, and also concerning pain, sleep disorders, depression, or other psychopathologic troubles. Special treatment is indicated in inflammatory vascular disease causing stroke, polycythemia, subarachnoid hemorrhage with ischemia on the base of spasms, and in other conditions. Intracerebral hemorrhage will demand the general measures described. The management of brain edema is of primary importance. Space occupation may demand for surgical relief (shunt or removal of hematoma). Indications for the operative removal of the hematoma are dependent on consciousnes, size and localization of the hemorrhage, and the patient's general condition.

In all stroke patients naturally proper nursing and physical training are of crucial importance for prognosis.

2. Rehabilitation

Rehabilitation *sensu strictiori* is of minor importance in gerontology. If the term is used in this context it does not refer to working capability but to a maximum of independence in everyday life.

Rehabilitation begins in the acute phase, as many possible complications arising at that time influence prognosis persistently. Lack of correct placement of paretic extremities will lead to painful contractures and Sudeck syndrome and can delay or even prevent restoration of function. Decubitus and infections also obstruct the process of recovery.

In completed stroke with permanent neurologic deficit, differentiated physical training aims at an optimal compensation of impaired functions and this happens with special regard to practical everyday performances like dressing, taking meals, realizing defecation, and so on. The patient's mental state influences the capability of rehabilitation and so do preexistent and independent diseases. Dysphasia offers special problems of training.

III. Prognosis

In TIA the risk of turning over into completed stroke is high and therefore surgical or medical prevention must be performed if possible. Both ways of prophylaxis improve the prognosis as to the incidence of further cerebrovascular accidents. The probability of completed stroke is greater in typical TIAs – especially with frequent occurrence – than in prolonged reversible ischemic neurologic deficit (PRIND).

The prognosis of completed stroke with persistent symptoms depends among other things on the size and site of the infarction, the patient's age, and concomitant disorders.

Large infarctions with severe and long-lasting impairment of consciousness generally have a poorer prognosis than cases without these features. Old age also impairs the prognosis. Mortality of patients beyond 80 years is about twice as high as that of patients between 51 and 80 years (FEIGENSON et al. 1977a, b). Coronary arteriosclerosis and hypertension are factors that negatively influence prognosis. FEIGENSON et al. found that concerning outcome and length of stay at the stroke rehabilitation unit the following factors had negative prognostic influence: severe weakness at admission, long interval between onset and admission, presence of perceptual or cognitive dysfunction, homonymous hemianopsia and multiple neurologic deficits as well as slow recovery and poor motivation. No influence was found for dysphasia, hemisensory deficit, age (up to 80 years and more) and the presence of diabetes and hypertension.

Patients who survive 2–5 years after stroke in approximately 40%–60% of cases are independent of external care and aids and 10%–20% of cases remain in a state that requires constant nursing and medical care (MARX 1977).

References

Abu-Zeid HAH, Choi NW, Maini KK et al. (1977) Relative role of factors associated with cerebral infarction and cerebral hemorrhage. Stroke 8:106–112

Acheson J, Danta G, Hutchinson EC (1969) Controlled trial of dipyridamole in cerebrovascular disease. Br Med J 1:614–615

Alberti E (1978) Antikoagulantien-Behandlung in der Neurologie. In: Flügel KA (Hrsg) Neurologische und psychiatrische Therapie. Perimed, Erlangen

Anderson DC, Cranford RE (1979) Corticosteroids in ischemic stroke. Stroke 10:68–71

Barnett HJM and the Canadian Cooperative Study Group (1978) A randomized trial of aspirin and sulfinpyrazone in threatened stroke. New Engl J Med 299:53–59

Barolin GS (1980) Die zerebrale Apoplexie. Enke, Stuttgart

Barolin GS, Scherzer E, Schnaberth G (1975) Die zerebrovaskulär bedingten Anfälle. Huber, Bern

Barolin GS, Hodkewitsch E, Saurugg D (1980) Die Rehabilitation beim Zerebralinsult. In: Barolin H (Hrsg) Die zerebrale Apoplexie. Enke, Stuttgart, pp 180–201

Bauer RB, Tellez H (1973) Dexamenthasone as treatment in cerebrovascular disease. Stroke 4:547–555

Betz E (1972a) Pharmakologie des Gehirnkreislaufs. In: Gänshirt H (Hrsg) Der Hirnkreislauf. Thieme, Stuttgart

Betz E (1972b) Cerebral blood flow: its measurement and regulation. Physiol Rev 52:595–630

Birkett DP(1972) The psychiatric differentiation of senility and arteriosclerosis. Br J Psychiat 120:321–325

Blauenstein UW, Halsey JH, Wilson EM, Wills EL, Risberg J (1977) [133]Xenon inhalation method. Analysis of reproducibility: some of its physiological implications. Stroke 8:92–102

Böger J (1974) Rehabilitation zerebraler Durchblutungsstörungen und ihrer Folgen. Z Präklin Geriatr 5:95–100

Brinker RA, Lundiss DJ, Croley RF (1968) Detection of carotid artery bifurcation stenosis by Doppler ultrasound. J Neurosurg 29:143–148

Burger PC, Burch JG, Vogel FS (1977) Granulomatous angiitis. An unusual etiology of stroke. Stroke 8:29–35

Càmpbell JK, Houser OW, Stevens JC et al. (1978) Computerized tomography and radionuclide imaging in the evaluation of ischemic stroke. Radiology 126:695–702

Canadian Cooperative Study Group (1978) A randomized trial of aspirin and sulfinpyrazone in threatened stroke. New Engl J Med 299:53–59

Caplan LR (1979) Occlusion of the vertebral or basilar artery. Follow-up analysis of some patients with benign outcome. Stroke 10:277–782

Caplan LR, Skillman J, Ojemann R, Fields WS (1978) Intracerebral hemorrhage following carotid endarterectomy: a hypertensive complication? Stroke 9:450–457

Carter AB (1972) Clinical aspects of cerebral infarction. In: Vinken PJ, Bruyn GW (eds) Handbook of clinical neurology. North Holland Publ Co, Amsterdam

Cervós-Navarro J (1980) Gefäßerkrankungen und Durchblutungsstörungen des Gehirns. In: Spezielle pathologische Anatomie. Bd 13/I. Pathologie des Nervensystems I. Springer, Berlin Heidelberg New York, pp 1–510

David TE, Humphries AW, Young IR et al. (1973) A correlation of neck bruits and arteriosclerotic carotid arteries. Arch Surg 107:729

Dawber TR, Wolf PA, Colton Th, Nickerson CJ (1977) Risk factors: comparison of the biological data in myocardial and brain infarctions. In: Zülch KJ, Kaufmann W, Hossman K-A, Hossman V (eds) Brain and heart infarct. Springer, Berlin Heidelberg New York, pp 226–250

DeWeese JA, Rob DG, Satran R et al. (1973) Results of carotid endarterectomy for transient ischemic attacks five years later. Arch Surg 178:258–264

Dorndorf W (1975) Schlaganfälle. Thieme, Stuttgart

Dorndorf W, Gänshirt H (1972) Klinik der arteriellen zerebralen Gefäßverschlüsse. In: Gänshirt H (Hrsg) Der Hirnkreislauf. Thieme, Stuttgart

Drift van der JHA, Kok NUD (1972) The EEG in Cerebro-Vascular Disorders in relations to pathology. In: Handbook of electroencephalography and clinical neurophysiology, vol 14 A–12. Elsevier, Amsterdam

Drift van der JHA, Kok NUD (1973) EEG prognosis in cerebrovascular disease. In: Meyer JS, Lechner H, Heinrich M, Eichhorn O (eds) Cerebral vascular disease. Proceedings of the VI International Symposium of Salzburg 1972. Thieme, Stuttgart, pp 127–135

Dyken ML (1978) Clinical studies of cerebral ischemia and antiplatelet drugs. In: Breddin K, Dorndorf W, Loew D, Marx R (eds) Acetylsalicylic acid in cerebral ischemia and coronary heart disease. Schattauer, Stuttgart New York, pp 79–84

Easton JD, Sherman DG (1977) Stroke and mortality rate in carotid endarterectomy. 228 consecutive operations. Stroke 8:565–568

Easton JD, Sherman DG (1980) Management of cerebral embolism of cardiac origin. Stroke 11:433–442

Estler C-J (1978) Zur Behandlung zerebraler Durchblutungsstörungen verwendete Arzneimittel. Pharmakologische Übersicht. In: Flügel KA (Hrsg) Neurologische und psychiatrische Therapie. Perimed, Erlangen

Feigenson JS, McDowell FH, Meese P, McCartly ML, Greenberg SD (1977a) Factors influencing outcome and length of stay in a stroke rehabilitation unit. Part 1. Stroke 8:651–656

Feigenson JS, McCartly ML, Greenberg SD, Feigenson WS (1977b) Factors influencing outcome and length of stay in a stroke rehabilitation unit. Part 2. Stroke 8:657–662

Fenske A, Meinig G, Schürman K (1980) Die regionale und globale Hirndurchblutung bei zerebraler Ischämie sowie nach EC/IC Anastomosierung. In: Reisner H, Schnaberth G (Hrsg) Fortschritte der technischen Medizin in der neurologischen Diagnostik und Therapie. Wien, pp 145–148

Fields WS (1978) The asymptomatic carotid bruit-operate or not? Stroke 9:269–271

Fields WS, Lemak NA, Frankowski RF, Hardy RJ (1977) Controlled trial of aspirin in cerebral ischemia. Part I. Stroke 8:301–316

Fields WS, Lemak NA, Frankowski RF, Hardy RJ (1978) Controlled trial of aspirin in cerebral ischemia. Part II. Stroke 9:309–317

Fleming JFR, Griesdale DE, Schutz H et al. (1977) Carotid endarterectomy: Changing morbidity and mortality. Stroke 8:14

Flügel KA (1974) Die zerebralen Durchblutungsstörungen. Klinik, Ätiopathogenese, Diagnostik. In: Wieck HH (Hrsg) Zerebrale und periphere Durchblutungsstörungen. Aesopus, München Lugano, pp 93–138

Flügel KA (1975) Transitorische globale Amnesie – ein paroxysmales amnestisches Syndrom. Fortsch Neurol Psychiat 42:471–485

Flügel KA (1980a) Prophylaxe und Therapie des Schlaganfalls. Fortschr Med 98:773–778

Flügel KA, Fuchs HH (1980b) Intrazerebrale Blutungen bei entzündlichen Gefäßerkrankungen. In: Reisner H, Schnaberth G (Hrsg) Fortschritte der technischen Medizin in der neurologischen Diagnostik und Therapie. Wien, pp 671–677

Flügel KA, Fuchs HH (to be published) Intrazerebrale Blutungen im höheren Lebensalter. Akt Gerontol 1982

Frank G (1981) Amnestische Episoden. Springer, Berlin Heidelberg New York

Freeman J, Ingvar DH (1968) Elimination by hypoxia of cerebral blood flow autoregulation and EEG relationship. Exp Brain Res 5:61–71

Furlan AJ, Whisnant JP, Baker HL (1980) Long-term prognosis after carotid artery occlusion. Neurology 30:986–988

Gänshirt H (Hrsg) (1972) Der Hirnkreislauf. Physiologie, Pathologie, Klinik. Thieme, Stuttgart

Gänshirt H (1977) Indikationen für gefäßchirurgische Eingriffe. In: Wieck HH (Hrsg) Zerebrovaskuläre Insuffizienz. Perimed, Erlangen, pp 149–156

Ganner H (1974) Ictus amnesticus. Ärztl Prax 26:1872–1876

Genton E, Barnett HJM, Fields WS, Gent M, Hoak JC (1977) Cerebral ischemia: the role of thrombosis and of antithrombotic therapy. Study group on antithrombotic therapy. Stroke 8:150–175

Gerhard L, Bergener M, Homayun S (1972) Angiopathie bei Alzheimerscher Krankheit. Z Neurol 201:43–61

Gilroy J, Burnhart MI, Meyer JS (1969) Treatment of acute stroke with Dextran Forty. JAMA 210:292–298

Goran A, Moore G (1980) Value of non-invasive cerebrovascular laboratory in diagnosis of extracranial carotid artery disease. Stroke 11:325–328

Gottstein U (1965) Physiologie und Pathophysiologie des Hirnkreislaufs. Med Welt I:715

Gottstein U (1974) Behandlung der zerebralen Mangeldurchblutung. Internist 15:575

Gottstein U (1977) Pathogenese und Risikofaktoren der zerebralen Ischämie. Akt Neurol 4:65–76

Gottstein U, Held K, Büttner H et al. (1970) Continuous monitoring of arterial and cerebral venous glucose differences in human subjects during intravenous infusion of glucose and insulin. In: Meyer JS, Lechner H, Eichhorn O (eds) Research on cerebral circulation. Thomas, Springfield

Gottstein U, Sedlmeyer I, Heuß A (1976) Behandlung der akuten zerebralen Mangeldurchblutung mit niedermolekularem Dextran. Dtsch med Wochenschr 101:223–227

Gratzel O, Schmiedek P, Spetzler RF, Marguth F (1976) Clinical experience with extra-intracranial arterial anastomosis in 65 cases. J Neurosurg 44:313–324

Grobe Th (1980) Zur Häufigkeit psychischer Auffälligkeiten bei Karotisstenosen. Krankenhausarzt 53:117–119

Grobe Th (1981) Diagnostik und Behandlungsmöglichkeiten extrakranieller Verschlußprozesse der Arteria carotis. Fortschr Neurol Psychiat 49:335–367

Gudmundsson G, Hallgrimsson J, Jónasson TA, Bjarnason O (1972) Hereditary cerebral hemorrhage with amyloidosis. Brain 95:387–404

Hachinsky VC, Lassen NA, Marshall J (1974) Multi-infarct dementia. Lancet 2:207–210

Halsey JH, O'Brien M, Strong ER (1980) Amelioration of cerebral ischemia by prior treatment of hypertension. Stroke 11:235–240

Harrer G (1974) Die Therapie der akuten zerebrovaskulären Dekompensation im Alter. Geriatrie 1:20–24

Harrison MJG (1978) Evidence for thromboembolism as a cause of transient cerebral ischemia. In: Breddin K, Dorndorf W, Loew D, Marx R (eds) Acetylsalicylic acid in cerebral ischemic and coronary heart disease. Schattauer, Stuttgart New York, pp 75–77

Hartmann A (1978) Der Schlaganfall. Therapie in der Akutphase. In: Flügel KA (Hrsg) Neurologische und psychiatrische Therapie. Perimed, Erlangen, pp 170–180

Heiss WD, Reisner T, Herles H, Bruck J (1974) Störungen der regionalen Hirndurchblutung bei vaskulär bedingten passageren neurologischen Ausfällen. Wien Klin Wochenschr 86:614

Held K, Gottstein U (1972) Pathogenese und Therapie cerebraler Zirkulationsstörungen. Z Gerontol 5:324

Herrschaft H (1975) Die regionale Gehirndurchblutung. Springer, Berlin Heidelberg New York

Heyden S, Heiss G, Heyman A, Tyroler AH, Hames CH, Patzschke U, Manegold C (1980) Cardiovascular mortality in transient ischemic attacks. Stroke 11:252–255

Huber P (1979) Zerebrale Angiographie für Klinik und Praxis (Krayenbühl/Yasargil) 3. Aufl. Thieme, Stuttgart

Hughes JT, Brownell B (1966) Granulomatous giant-celled angiitis in the central nervous system. Neurology 16:293

Ingvar DH, Cronquist S, Ekberg R et al. (1965) Normal values of regional cerebral blood flow in man, including flow and weight estimates of grey and white matter. Acta Physiol Scand 41 (Suppl 14):72–78

Jellinger K (1977) Cerebrovascular amyloidosis with cerebral hemorrhage. J Neurol 214:195–206

Jones HR, Millikan CH, Sandok BA (1980) Temporal profile (clinical course) of acute vertebrobasilar system cerebral infarction. Stroke 11:173–177

Kannel WB (1971) Current status of the epidemiology of brain infarction associated with occlusive arterial disease. Stroke 2:295–318

Kannel WB, Dawber T, Cohen M et al. (1965) Vascular diseases of the brain-epidemiologic aspects: the Framingham study. Am J Publ Health 55:1355–1366

Katzman R, Clasen R, Klatzo I, Meyer JS et al. (1977) Report of Joint Committee for stroke resources. IV. Brain edema in stroke. Stroke 8:512–540

Komatsumoto S, Gotoh F, Shimazu K et al. (1980) Autonomic nervous activity in stroke. In: Betz E, Grote J, Heuser D, Wüllenweber R (eds) Pathophysiology and pharmacotherapy of cerebrovascular disorders. Witzstrock, Baden-Baden Köln New York, pp 217–220

Koos W (1980) Die Behandlung zerebrovaskulärer Insulte mittels des extra- und intrakraniellen arteriellen Bypass. In: Barolin G (Hrsg) Die zerebrale Apoplexie. Enke, Stuttgart, pp 153–165

Ladurner G, Sager SD (1980) Die klinische Wertigkeit der Computertomographie bei zerebrovaskulären Erkrankungen. In: Reisner H, Schnaberth G (Hrsg) Fortschritte der technischen Medizin in der neurologischen Diagnostik und Therapie. Wien, pp 59–65

Lassen NA (1966) The luxury perfusion syndrome and its possible relation to acute metabolic acidosis localised within the brain. Lancet 2:1113–1115

Lassen NA, Ingvar DV (1963) Regional cerebral blood flow measurement in man. Arch Neurol 9:615–622

Lechner H, Ott E (1978) Zerebrovaskuläre Insuffizienz. Pharmakotherapie. In: Flügel KA (Hrsg) Neurologische und psychiatrische Therapie. Perimed, Erlangen

Lechner H, Ladurner G, Ott E (Hrsg) (1979) Die zerebralen transitorisch-ischämischen Attacken. Huber, Bern Stuttgart Wien

Lewis RR, Beasley MG, Hyams DE, Gasling RG (1978) Imaging the carotid bifurcation using continuous-wave Doppler-shift ultrasound and spectral analysis. Stroke 9:465–471

Lubic LG, Plakovitz HP (1979) Stroke. Discussion in patient management. Huber, Bern

Lübbers DW (1972) Physiologie des Gehirnkreislaufs. In: Gänshirt H (Hrsg) Der Gehirnkreislauf. Thieme, Stuttgart, pp 3214–3260

Mandybur TI (1975) The incidence of cerebral amyloid angiopathy in Alzheimer's disease. Neurology 25:120–126

Marsden CD, Harrison MJG (1972) Outcome of investigation of patients with presenile dementia. Br Med J 2:249–252

Marx P (1977) Die Gefäßerkrankungen von Hirn und Rückenmark. Fischer, Stuttgart New York

Matthew NT, Meyer JS, Rivera VM et al. (1972) Double blind evaluation of glycerol therapy in acute cerebral infarction. Lancet 2:1327–1329

McDowell FH, Millikan CH (1980) Summary of the 12th conference on cerebrovascular disease. Stroke 11:442–451

McDowell FH, Millikan CH, Goldstein M (1980) Treatment of impending stroke. Stroke 11:1–3

Mchedlishvili G (1980) Physiological mechanisms controlling cerebral blood flow. Stroke 11:240–248

Meyer JS (1978) Improved method for noninvasive measurement of regional cerebral blood flow by ^{133}Xenon inhalation. Part II. Stroke 9:205–210

Meyer JS, Ishihara N, Deshmukh VD, Naritomi H, Sakai F, Hsu M-C, Pollack P (1978) Improved method for noninvasive measurement of regional cerebral blood flow by ^{133}Xenon inhalation. Part I. Stroke 9:195–205

Millikan CH (1971) Reassessment of anticoagulant therapy in various types of occlusive cerebrovascular disease. Stroke 2:201–208

Millikan CH, McDowell FH (1978) Treatment of transient ischemic attacks. Stroke 9:299–308

Millikan CH, Siekert RG, Whisnant JP (1960) Intermittent carotid and vertebrobasilar insufficiency associated with polycythemia. Neurology 10:188–196

Moncada S, Korbut R (1978) Dipyridamole and other phosphodiesterase inhibitors act as antithrombotic agents by potentiating endogenous prostacyclin. Lancet 1:1286–1289

Müller HR (1972) Diagnosis of internal carotid artery occlusion by directional Doppler sonography of the ophthalmic artery. Neurology 22:816–823

Nelson RF, Pullicing P, Kendall BE, Marschall J (1980) Computed tomography in patients presenting with lacunar syndromes. Stroke 11:256–261

Norris JW (1976) Steroid therapy in acute cerebral infarction. Arch Neurol 33:69–71

O'Brien MD (1977) Vascular disease and dementia in the elderly. In: Smith WL, Kinsbourne M (eds) Aging and dementia. Spectrum Publ, New York, pp 77–90

Obrist WD, Thompson HK Jr, King H et al. (1967) Determination of regional cerebral blood flow by inhalation of ^{131}Xenon. Circ Res 20:124–135

Obrist WD, Thompson HK Jr, Wang HS et al. (1975) Regional cerebral blood flow estimated by ^{131}Xenon inhalation. Stroke 6:245–256

Olsson J-E, Brechter C, Bäcklund H, Krook H, Müller R, Nitelius E, Olsson O, Tornberg A (1980) Anticoagulant vs anti-platelet therapy as prophylactic against cerebral infarction in transient ischemic attacks. Stroke 11:1–4

Ostendorf P (1979) Therapie mit Antikoagulantien und Thrombozytenaggregationshemmern bei extrakraniellen Gefäßstenosen und Gefäßverschlüssen. Internist 20:539–546

Patten BM, Mendel J, Bruun G et al. (1972) Double blind study of the effects of dexamethasone on acute stroke. Neurology 22:377–383

Patterson RH, Goodell H, Dunning HS (1964) Complications of carotid arteriography. Arch Neurol (Chic) 10:513–520

Pilgeram LO, Chee AN, von dem Bussche G (1973) Evidence for abnormalities in clotting and thrombolysis as a risk factor for stroke. Stroke 4:643–657

Prosenz P, Heiss WD, Tschabitscher H (1974) The value of regional blood flow measurements compared to angiography in the assessment of obstructive neck vessel disease. Stroke 5:19–31

Quandt J (1969) Die zerebralen Durchblutungsstörungen des Erwachsenenalters. Schattauer, Stuttgart

Raithel D (Hrsg) (1977) Zerebrale Insuffizienz durch extrakranielle Gefäßverschlüsse. Perimed, Erlangen

Raithel D (1978) Gefäßchirurgische Therapie bei zerebralen Durchblutungsstörungen. In: Flügel KA (Hrsg) Neurologische und psychiatrische Therapie. Perimed, Erlangen, pp 197–202

Regli F (1971) Die flüchtigen ischämischen zerebralen Attacken. Dtsch med Wschr 13:525–530

Reisner H (1977) Therapeutische Probleme beim frischen cerebralen Insult. Therapiewoche 27:1167–1173

Reivich M (1972) Regional cerebral blood flow in physiologic and pathophysiologic states. Progr Brain Res 35:191–228

Reuther R, Dorndorf W (1978) Aspirin in patients with cerebral ischemia and normal angiograms or non-surgical lesions: the results of a double-blind trial. In: Breddin K, Dorndorf W, Loew D, Marx R (eds) Acetylsalicylic acid in cerebral ischemia and coronary heart disease. Schattauer, Stuttgart New York, pp 97–106

Richter W, Seemann C, Hedin H, Ring J, Messmer K (1980) Dextranunverträglichkeit. Immunologische, tierexperimentelle und klinische Studie. Med Welt 10:2–12

Russi E, Aebi M, Kraus-Ruppert R, Mumenthaler M (1980) Riesenzellarteriitis mit intrakranieller Lokalisation. In: Reisner K, Schnaberth G (Hrsg) Fortschritte der techn. Medizin in der neurologischen Diagnostik und Therapie. Wien, pp 655–659

Sandok BA, Furlan AJ, Whisnant JP, Sundt TM (1978) Guidelines for the management of transient ischemic attacks. Mayo Clin Proc 53:665–674

Santambrogio S, Marfiotti R, Sardella et al. (1978) Is there a real treatment of stroke? Clinical and statistical comparison of different treatments in 300 patients. Stroke 9:130–132

Scheid W (1953) Die Zirkulationsstörungen des Gehirns und seiner Häute. In: v. Bergmann G, Frey W, Schwiegk H (Hrsg) Handbuch der inneren Medizin. Springer, Berlin Göttingen Heidelberg

Schiefer W (1972a) Zwischenfälle bei der Hirngefäßdarstellung. In: Gänshirt H (Hrsg) Der Hirnkreislauf, Physiologie, Pathologie, Klinik. Thieme, Stuttgart

Schiefer W (1972b) Klinik der intrazerebralen Massenblutungen und spontanen Hämatome. In: Gänshirt H (Hrsg) Der Hirnkreislauf. Thieme, Stuttgart

Schmitt HP, Barz J (1978) Cerebral massive hemorrhage in congophilic angiopathy and its medicolegal significance. Forens Sci Internat 12:187–201

Soltero J, Lin K, Cooper R, Stamler J, Garside D (1978) Trends in mortality from cerebrovascular disease in the United Stated, 1960 to 1975. Stroke 9:549–555

Soyka D (1972) Prozesse der extrakraniellen Strombahn als Ursache von Hirndurchblutungsstörungen. Fortschr Neurol Pschiat 40:229–269

Spencer MP, Reid JM, Davis EE et al. (1974) Cervical carotid imaging with a continuous-wave Doppler flowmeter. Stroke 5:145–154

Sydney L, McDowell F (1970) Age: its significance in nonembolic cerebral infarction. Stroke 1:449–453

Thompson JE, Talkington CM (1976) Surgical progress in carotid endarterectomy. Ann Surg 184:1

Thompson JE, Austin DJ, Patman RD (1970) Carotid endarterectomy for cerebrovascular insufficiency: long-term results in 592 patients followed up to thirteen years. Ann Surg 172:663

Thompson JE, Pathman RD, Persson AV (1976) Management of asymptomatic carotid bruits. Ann Surg 42:77–80

Tomlinson BE, Blessed G, Roth M (1970) Observations on the brains of demented old people. J Neurol Sci 11:205–242

Toole JF, Patel AN (1980) Zerebrovaskuläre Störungen. Springer, Berlin Heidelberg New York

Toole JF, Yuson CP, Janeway R et al. (1978) Transient ischemic attacks: a prospective study of 225 patients. Neurology 28:746–753

Torack RM (1975) Congophilic angiopathy complicated by surgery and massive hemorrhage. Amer J Pathol 81:349–366

Troost BT (1980) Dizziness and vertigo in vertebrobasilar disease. Stroke 11:301–303, 413–415

Ule G, Kolkmann F-W (1972) Pathologische Anatomie des Hirngefäßsystems. In: Gänshirt H (Hrsg) Der Hirnkreislauf. Thieme, Stuttgart

Ulrich G, Taghavy A, Schmidt H (1973) Zur Nosologie und Ätiologie der kongophilen Angiopathie (Gefäßform der zerebralen Amyloidose). Z Neurol 206:39–59

von Arnim D (1978) Physikalische Therapie und Rehabilitation des Schlaganfalles. In: Flügel KA (Hrsg) Neurologische und psychiatrische Therapie. Perimed, Erlangen

von Reutern GM, Büdingen HJ, Hennerici M, Freund HJ (1979) Doppler-sonographische Diagnostik von Stenosen und Verschlüssen. In: Lechner H, Ladurner G, Ott E (Hrsg) Die zerebralen transitorisch-ischämischen Attacken. Huber, Bern Stuttgart Wien, pp 200–210

Waltz AG, Sundt TM (1968) Influence of systemic blood pressure on blood flow and microcirculation of ischemic cerebral cortex: a failure of autoregulation. Progr Brain Res 30:107–112

Weaver RG, Howard G, McKinney WM, Ball MR, Jones AM, Toole JF (1980) Comparison of Doppler ultrasonography with arteriography of the carotid artery bifurcation. Stroke 11:402–404

Weiss R, Jellinger K, Sunder-Plassmann E (1980) ZNS-Beteiligung bei granulomatöser Riesenzell-Angiitis. In: Reisner H, Schnaberth G (Hrsg) Fortschritte der technischen Medizin in der neurologischen Diagnostik und Therapie. Wien, pp 661–664

Wells CE (1978) Role of stroke in dementia. Editorial. Stroke 9:1–3

West H, Burton R, Roon AJ, Malone JM et al. (1979) Comparative risk of operation and expectant management for carotid artery disease. Stroke 10:117–121

Whisnant JP (1976) A population study of stroke and TIA: Rochester Minnesota. In: Gillingham FJ, Mawdsley C, Williams AF (eds) Stroke. Churchill Livingstone New York, pp 21–39

Whisnant JP, Cartlidge NEF, Elveback LP (1978) Carotid and vertebral-basilar transient ischemic attacks: Effect of anticoagulants, hypertension and cardiac disorders on survival and stroke occurence. A population study. Ann Neurol 3:107–115

Wieck HH (Hrsg) (1977) Zerebrovaskuläre Insuffizienz. Konservative Therapie in der Praxis. Perimed, Erlangen

Wylie EJ, Ehrenfeld WK (1970) Extracranial occlusive cerebrovascular disease. Diagnosis and management. Saunders, Philadelphia

Yarnell P, Earnst M, Kelly G, Sanders B (1978) Disappearing carotid defects. Stroke 9:258–262

Ziegler DK, Hassanein R (1973) Prognosis in patients with transient ischemic attacks. Stroke 4:666–673

Zülch KJ (1961) Die Pathogenese von Massenblutung und Erweichung unter besonderer Berücksichtigung klinischer Gesichtspunkte. Acta Neurochir (Wien) Suppl VII:51

Zülch KJ (1971) Cerebral circulation and stroke. Springer, Berlin

Zülch KJ (1977) Clinical ischemia: brain infarcts. In: Zülch KJ, Kaufmann W, Hossmann K-A, Hossmann V (eds) Brain and heart infarct. Springer, Berlin Heidelberg New York, pp 288–254

Vertebrobasilar Syndrome

M. S. J. Pathy

A. Introduction

The prevalence of the vertebrobasilar syndrome in later life reflects the age-related multifactorial determinants of this condition.

Davenmuehle et al. (1961) found clinical evidence of arteriosclerosis in 27% of community volunteers over the age of 60. Obrist et al. (1963) noted a close correlation between the EEG pattern and investigatory evidence of cardiovascular or cerebrovascular arteriosclerosis in elderly asymptomatic volunteers. In critically evaluated studies of cerebral blood flow, Geraud et al. (1969) and O'Brien and Mallet (1970) presented evidence of early cerebrovascular disease in a proportion of elderly subjects. Autopsy studies clearly confirm the increasing prevalence and degree of atherosclerosis in the aorta and cerebral vessels after the 6th decade (Sadoshima et al. 1973). The incidence of strokes increases markedly with age (Kurtzke 1976).

The prevalence rates of transient ischaemic attacks (TIAs) without subsequent established strokes increase from approximately 1% in the decade 65–74 to almost 2% in those aged 75 and over (Whisnant et al. 1973). The established stroke rate with TIAs in either the carotid or the vertebrobasilar system increases with age (Matsumato et al. 1973). Serious cardiac dysrhythmias occur with increasing frequency in later life. Yates (1976) considered that a quarter of patients with TIAs belong to the group of patients with episodic failure of cardiac output. Difficulty arises over the clinical term TIA, which covers brief strokes of heterogenous causation.

During normal ageing, the water content of cartilage slightly decreases and the proteoglycan content slightly increases (Maroudas and Venn 1977). The fibres of the annulus fibrosis of the intervertebral discs become thickened (Hirsch et al. 1953) with occasional areas of mucoid degeneration and calcifation (Boemke 1951). With increasing age, clefts and cavities develop with subsequent fibrous scarring (Hirsch et al. 1953). The nucleus pulposus also shows considerable age-related change. It becomes progressively more acellular with increasing reduction of the mucoid gel and subsequent fibrous replacement. Weightman (1975) and Kempson (1975) have demonstrated a significant reduction of biomaterial wear properties of articular cartilage as a function of ageing. The combination of these cervical disc changes and osteoarthrosis of the cervical diarthrodial joints increase the vulnerability of the vertebral arteries to compression as they traverse the vertebral canal, with possible vertebrobasilar ischaemia.

Ostberg (1973) found evidence of arteritis in 1.7% of routine autopsy cases. Histological findings suggested that at least 2% of elderly subjects may have been affected by the giant-cell arteritis-polymyalgia rheumatica complex. DIXON et al. (1966) noted that the giant-cell arteritis-polymyalgia rheumatic complex usually occurs in persons over the age of 60.

The vertebral arteries arise from the first part of the subclavian arteries in 91% of cases (DASELER and ANSON 1959), but occasionally from the aorta or carotid arteries. The vertebral arteries transverse the foramina of the upper six cervical vertebrae. Within the vertebral canal they are closely related on their anteromedial aspect to the neurocentral joints of Luschka and on their posterior aspect to the apophyseal joints; they lie immediately anterior to the emerging cervical nerve roots. On leaving the axis for the atlas, the vertebral artery passes around and under the lateral mass of the atlas and enters the skull below the lower border of the posterior atlanto-occipital membrane and foramen magnum. The vertebral arteries commonly unite at the level of the lower border of the pons to form the basilar artery. MECKEL (1828) noted both a variation in the diameter of the two vertebral arteries and in the precise level of the formation of the basilar artery. Variability in size of the vertebral arteries is common and might range from minor calibre differences to atresia of one artery and the presence of a large dominant vessel on the other side (HUTCHINSON and YATES 1956). Absence of union of the two vertebral arteries, either due to occlusion or from developmental anomaly is not uncommon. In this event the basilar artery is the continuation of one vessel with the other vertebral artery largely supplying the cerebellum.

The vertebrobasilar syndrome may result from any condition which compromises the blood flow in the vertebrobasilar territory sufficiently to produce significant ischaemia of brain stem, cerebellum, occipital lobe or temporal lobe. One or a combination of any of these areas of the nervous system may be affected. The presence of an adequate collateral circulation may obviate the effect of an occlusive lesion as was clearly demonstrated by WILLIS in 1720. BRAIN (1957) considered that the function of the circle of Willis is to equilibrate the distribution of blood to all parts of the brain whatever the position of the head in relation to the trunk may be. TOOLE and TUCKER (1960) and HARDESTY et al. (1962) support this thesis. In addition to this normal function, the circle of Willis acts as a major site of collateral circulation in the event of obstruction in the carotid and vertebral artery territory. The potential of the circle of Willis to circumvent the consequences of occlusion in the carotid or vertebrobasilar system is dependent on the absence of significant intraluminal calibre reduction of its component vessels, either from congenital or pathological causes. VAN DER EEKEN and ADAMS (1953) and GILLIAN (1959) discuss the role of leptomeningeal anastomoses in modifying the ischaemic impact of occlusions distal to the circle of Willis. LOEB and MEYER (1965) reviewed the anastomotic channels between the vertebrobasilar and carotid circulations and FIELDS et al. (1965) discussed the extensive potential collateral systems that might moderate the effect of occlusive arterial disease involving the brain.

B. Determinants of the Vertebrobasilar Syndrome

The vertebrobasilar blood supply of the brain stem, cerebellum, and occipital lobes may be jeopardised by a wide variety of haemodynamic or mechanical factors.

NARITOMI et al. (1979) have drawn attention to the importance of disordered autoregulation in the pathogenesis of symptoms of long-standing vertebrobasilar insufficiency. DE KLEYN (1939) clearly showed that obstruction of blood flow in the contralateral-vertebral artery may occur following rotation and extension of the head. Patients with evidence of severe cervical atherosclerosis may develop transient neurological symptoms, mainly dysarthria, and nystagmus following combined rotation and extension of the neck (BIEMOND 1951). HUTCHINSON and YATES (1956) showed at autopsy that the vertebral arteries could be markedly distorted by osteophytic outgrowths and they concluded that transient vertebrobasilar ischaemia could well have occurred in life following rotation of the head. The vertebral arteries may be compressed due to subluxation and deformation of the cervical apophyseal joints (KOVACS 1955). The consequences of stenosis or occlusion of the vertebral artery may range from symptomless or insignificant to catastrophic, depending on the integrity and calibre of the opposite vertebral artery, the adequacy of the cardiac output, the systemic blood pressure and on a functional collateral circulation. The clinical phenomena associated with the vertebrobasilar syndrome may be manifested by recurrent momentary neurological symptoms from brief external obstruction of the vertebral artery in its course along the vertebral canal; transient neurological deficits due to platelet or thrombotic emboli; or more substantial and lasting neurological features due to infarction of any part of the nervous system whose blood supply is derived from the vertebrobasilar system.

The relationship between stenosis of the vertebral arteries to the occurrence of infarction remains a topic of dispute. HUTCHINSON and YATES (1956) in a systematic autopsy examination of 100 subjects who had had clinical evidence of cerebrovascular disease, found stenosis greater than 50% in 46 cases of infarction. Subsequent studies by SCHWARTZ and MITCHELL (1961), WHISNANT et al. (1961), and McGEE et al. (1962) produced broadly similar results and indicated that severe atherosclerosis was commonly present in the vertebral arteries of people with and without cerebrovascular lesions. FISHER et al. (1965), BATTACHARJI (1965), MITCHELL and SCHWARTZ (1965), and BATTACHARJI et al. (1967) found that approximately a quarter of cases over the age of 35 years had evidence of severe vertebral artery stenosis, based on unselected autopsy series. The predominant site of vertebral artery stenosis has been variously located at the point of origin of the vertebral artery from the subclavian artery (MARTIN et al. 1960; SCHWARTZ and MITCHELL 1961; WHISNANT et al. 1961; BAUER et al. 1962), in the vertebral artery in the vertebral canal (HUTCHINSON and YATES 1956; McGEE et al. 1962) or the ostium of the artery (FISHER et al. 1965; BATTARCHARJI et al. 1967). FISHER et al. (1965) considered that brain infarction commonly followed intracranial vertebral artery occlusion, but did not occur when the cervical segment of the vertebral artery was occluded. Later FISHER (1970) recorded patients presenting with symptoms of recurrent transient brain stem ischaemia associated with bilateral occlusion of the first part of the vertebral arteries.

CASTAIGNE et al. (1973) found that 50% of cases of vertebral artery thrombosis were associated with infarction in the territory of blood supply of the vertebrobasilar artery. Though stenosis of the extracranial cervical arteries is common, other factors such as thrombosis or emboli from atherosclerotic plaques, acute haemodynamic states causing sudden hypotension or hypertensive crises may be necessary to precipitate infarction. The influence of stenosis or occlusion of the extracranial and/or cerebral arteries in the pathogenesis of infarction in the boundary zones between major cerebral arteries, has been considered by Romanul and Abramowicz (1964) and by Romanul (1970, 1976). They pointed out that the site of infarction following occlusion of the vertebral arteries was unpredictable and inconstant due to variability in the vertebrobasilar arterial tree and in the calibre of the posterior communicating arteries. The variability in the site and extent of atherosclerotic changes in the basilar artery is often critical. Castaigne et al. (1973) dealt with both vertebral and basilar occlusions in a study of 44 patients with postmortem data. "In 35 of the 44 patients the demonstrable cause of the arterial occlusion was atherosclerosis, in four patients cardiac embolism was responsible and in five the occlusion was classified as undetermined."

Of 31 patients with primary occlusive thrombosis there were 40 occlusions, 95% of which were in or near pre-existing stenosis and 95% of the stenoses were classified as "tight." They pointed out that only 9% of vertebral and/or basilar occlusions resulted from cardiac emboli as against 22% in the carotid arteries. Antegrade thrombosis was noted to progress occasionally along the vertebral artery to the junction of the two vertebral vessels. Retrograde spread of thrombosis from the basilar artery may obstruct the vertebral artery, but more commonly, antegrade spread from the vertebral artery involves the basilar artery. Kubik and Adams (1946) found that occlusion of the basilar artery occurred from an embolus in 39% of their 18 cases, but Castaigne reported that basilar artery occlusion resulted from atherosclerotic thrombosis in 94.4% of 18 cases. Loeb and Meyer (1965) summarised the clinicopathological findings of 64 cases of basilar artery thrombosis in a literature survey. They noted that "the ischaemic lesion was regional in 34.4%, usually in the pons (28.1%), rarely in the occipital lobe (3.1%) and extremely rarely in the medulla or in the cerebellum. In 61% there were scattered infarcts and rarely (4.6%) there were combined softenings".

Posterior cerebral artery occlusion may be due to either thrombosis or an embolus, but where infarction occurs in the territory of the posterior cerebral artery, Castaigne and his colleagues found that all cases in their study were due to an embolism.

It is no longer tenable to use some of the past eponymic names allegedly associated with precise segmental syndromes following infarction within the territory of the vertebrobasilar blood supply. However, in a more general way it is meaningful to identify focal infarction of brain stem, occipital lobe, cerebellum or temporal lobe or lesions involving two or more of these areas or lesions involving both the carotid and vertebral-basilar systems. As noted earlier the role of stenosis of the extracranial arteries in the pathogenesis of infarction has been overstated in the past. Gross vertebral artery stenosis may certainly be a major component of the complex amalgam of factors that may lead to under-perfusion of the hind-brain sufficient to precipitate infarction. It may more significantly be a source of recurrent emboli. Jörgensen and Torvik (1966) considered the majority of infarcts to be caused by thrombo-emboli. Stenosis of the cerebral arteries is more identifiably associated with thrombotic infarction (Kameyama and Okinaka 1963).

I. Cervical Spondylosis

With advancing age the progressive desiccation of the mucopolysaccharide gel (PÜSCHEL 1930) and diminution of the mucopolysaccharide protein complex (TAYLOR 1953) of the nucleus pulposus encourages disc degeneration and subsequent degenerative changes. Loss of height in the cervical spine from multiple disc degeneration leads to the vertebral arteries, which are only loosely attached to the transverse foramina, becoming tortuous, and kinked.

Radiological evidence of cervical disc degeneration is common after the age of 65. PALLIS et al. (1954) found significant radiological changes in 75% of persons aged 65 and over and LAWRENCE et al. (1963) found evidence of disc degeneration in 87% of males and 74% of females in the age group 65–74 years. FRYKHOLM (1951) classified disc protrusions into four main types based on the predominate site of disc change. An annular lateral disc protrusion comes from the uncinate part of the disc and may compress the vertebral artery. Disc degeneration gives rise to secondary osteophytosis around the margins of the vertebral bodies which may displace the vertebral arteries. Depending on the magnitude of the spondylotic bosses, the vertebral arteries may be displaced laterally or even posteriorly (PALLIS et al. 1954).

The neurocentral and apophyseal joints are diarthrodial joints and are susceptible to osteoarthrosis. As previously noted these joints are in close relationship to the vertebral artery. Osteophytes may cause angulation or compression of the closely related vertebral artery, particularly on head rotation. SHEEHAN et al. (1960) undertook a detailed angiographic study in 46 patients with cerebrovascular symptoms due to cervical spondylosis. Percutaneous retrograde subclavian vertebral angiography was initially employed, but in the later part of the study this was changed to transbrachial vertebral artèriography, which was considered to be a less hazardous technique. In 26 patients with symptoms due to spondylosis, vertebral artery displacement was demonstrated in all cases. The vertebral arteries were exceedingly tortuous in the presence of severe spondylosis. The fifth and sixth and fourth and fifth intervertebral spaces were the most common sites of arterial displacement. Sheehan and her colleagues noted that severe vertebral artery compression due to osteophytes may be converted to complete obstruction by rotating the head. Angiographic retrograde filling of the basilar artery and its branches may occur from transient complete vertebral arterial osteophytic obstruction (VAN DER ZWAN 1954). Some patients with cervical osteoarthritic spurs may have associated constricting peri-arterial fibrosis which plays a role in the pathogenesis of symptoms (P'ASZTOR 1978).

The clinical sequelae of vertebral artery obstruction in cervical spondylosis is influenced by the calibre of the opposite vertebral artery. During continuous ambulatory ECG tape monitoring in patients with repeated transient ischaemic attacks and evidence of symptomatic cervical spondylosis, we have been impressed by the alleviation of repeated syncopal or dizzy attacks by either controlling the dysrhythmia or by preventing recurrent transitory vertebral artery occlusion by immobilising the neck in a well-fitting cervical collar. We noted a similar correlation between postural hypotension and cardiac dysrhythmia in the development of symptoms; the treatment of either factor may give symptomatic relief. A single operative factor may not impair cerebral perfusion to a sufficient degree to induce symptoms.

II. The Subclavian Steal Syndrome

The subclavian steal syndrome (TOOLE 1964) is also termed the subclavian artery obstruction syndrome (CONTORNI 1960) or the brachial-basilar insufficiency syndrome (NORTH et al. 1962). Atheromatous lesions develop at any point throughout the subclavian arteries. Atherosclerotic occlusive disease may involve the innominate, right subclavian or right or left common arteries, usually at or in the vicinity of their origins. Multiple lesions are not uncommon. However, isolated occlusions occur five times more commonly in the left subclavian artery than in any of the other vessels (DE BAKEY and CRAWFORD 1969). Atheromatous stenosis of the subclavian artery proximal to the origin of the vertebral artery, which is severe enough to reduce the pressure beyond the stenosis, may cause blood to flow down the vertebral artery into the subclavian artery instead of caudally along the vertebral artery. The reversed flow allows the vertebral artery to act as a significant collateral to the deprived upper limb. A steal syndrome may occasionally occur on the right when the stenosis is in the innominate artery. The physiopathogenesis of the subclavian steal syndrome was convincingly established by the experimental work of REIVICH et al. (1961) on dogs using an electromagnetic flow metre. In man, the major collateral role of the vertebral artery was simply demonstrated by reducing retrograde vertebral blood flow during cuff-induced ischaemia of the arm (MAGAARD and EKESTROM 1975). Postischaemic hyperaemia of the affected upper limb magnifies the retrograde vertebral flow.

III. Other Causes of the Vertebrobasilar Syndrome

Intermittent symptoms of vertebrobasilar insufficiency may be a manifestation of atlanto-axial subluxation in rheumatoid arthritis (JONES and KAUFMAN 1976) or more rarely tumour emboli (DE REUCK et al. 1979). MARSHALL et al. (1978) have suggested that the frequency of vertebrobasilar spasm as a sequelae of head injury has been overlooked in the past.

IV. Giant-Cell Arteritis

In a review of deaths from giant-cell arteritis, CARDELL and HANLEY (1961) considered that cerebrovascular accidents were responsible for the fatal outcome in half the reported cases. Vertebral or, less commonly carotid artery occlusion is the predominant cause of brain infarction from giant-cell arteritis. The vertebral or basilar arteries may be involved in polyarteritis nodosa, but lesions are usually small and multiple and rarely associated with infarction. Syphilis may be the aetiological factor in thrombosis at any point in the vertebrobasilar system and HENDIN et al. (1973) report occlusion of the basilar artery due to tuberculous meningitis. Vertebral artery occlusion by cervical hour-glass neurofibroma has been described by GEISSINGER et al. (1971).

V. Transient Vertebrobasiliar Ischaemic Attacks: Aetiology

1. Haemodynamic Crises

This hypothesis was introduced by DENNY-BROWN (1951) to emphasise the dependence of collateral circulations on systemic blood pressure in the presence of arteriosclerotic narrowing in the caroticovertebrobasilar system. A temporary generalised fall in cerebral perfusion might result in a transient ischaemic event localised to the region of the collateral blood supply or to watershed areas of anastomoses of distal branches of major territorial arteries. If hypotension persists, focal infarction may occur. KENDALL and MARSHALL (1963) studied the effect of lowering the blood pressure in patients with transient ischaemic attacks, but were unable to produce focal before generalised ischaemia. In an unpublished study of a group of elderly patients with postural hypotension and intermittent dysrhythmia recorded by 24-h ambulatory ECG monitoring, we found that treatment of either the arrhythmia or the postural hypotension would abolish the frequent brief TIAs.

2. Embolic Mechanisms

ZUCKER (1947), FISHER (1954), and DENNY-BROWN (1960) produced evidence that embolic phenomena play a causal role in TIA. Subsequent work has underlined the pre-eminence of thrombo-embolism. FISHER (1959) and ROSS-RUSSELL (1961, 1963) were able to demonstrate micro-emboli traversing the retinal vessels, which at autopsy have been shown to variously consist of platelet aggregation (McBRIEN et al. 1963), cholesterol esters (HOLLENHORST 1961; DAVID et al. 1963) or lipid (COGAN et al. 1964). Emboli from infective endocarditis, non-bacterial thrombolic endocarditis, cardiac aneurysm or a postmyocardial infarction akinetic ventricular segment may give rise to transient ischaemic attacks, though more persistent neurological deficits are likely from emboli from these cardiac sites.

Vertebral artery compression by spondylotic spurs due to cervical spondylosis may induce TIAs (SHEEHAN et al. 1960), particularly in association with rotation of the cervical spine (TOOLE 1964).

The neurological manifestations of polycythaemia vera are many and TIA's are among the more common features (MILLIKAN et al. 1960; SILVERSTEIN et al. 1962). MODAN and MODAN (1968) have suggested that transient CNS ischaemia may be associated with benign erythrocytosis. Hyperviscosity due to multiple myeloma or macroglobulinaemia may also be associated with TIAs.

TIAs may occur in the presence of severe anaemia and subside once the anaemia is corrected (SIEKERT et al. 1960). Transient cardiac arrhythmias may give rise to characteristic features of vertebrobasilar ischaemic attacks, presumably due to a fall in cerebral perfusion subsequent to a fall in left ventricular output in the presence of vertebrobasilar arterial disease or compression. Sudden hypertensive crises have been recorded as precipitating TIAs (KENDALL and MARSHALL 1963; MARSHALL 1968; WHISNANT 1974; VARNETT 1976; KEITH 1977).

Dissecting aneurysms due to cystic medial necrosis or due to trauma may involve the vertebral arteries producing transient ischaemic episodes (LHERMITTE 1966; ROSS-RUSSEL 1976).

VI. Clinical Features of the Vertebrobasilar Syndrome

The clinical presentation of disorders of the vertebrobasilar system may be characterised not only by a group of symptoms or signs at a point in time, but often by repetitive constellations of symptoms occurring over days, weeks, months or longer periods. The association of visual disorders due to occipital lobe dysfunction with brain stem symptoms can only be due to vascular insufficiency involving the vertebrobasilar distribution. The variable involvement of brain stem, occipital lobes and part of a temporal lobe, determines the wide spectrum of clinical presentation. The grouping of symptoms is almost kaleidoscopic, but visual phenomena occur in two-thirds (WILLIAMS 1969) to 83% (IVANOV and MATEV 1973) of patients. Visual hallucinations of spots before the eyes are common; more elaborate hallucinations are uncommon. However, visual hallucinations may be associated with formalised auditory hallucinations from temporal lobe ischaemia due to hypoperfusion of the anterior temporal branch of the posterior cerebral artery, which is derived from the termination of the basilar artery. Other visual features include blurring of vision, visual field defects, teichopsia, diplopia or uncommonly hemianopia. Temporary achromatopsia is discussed by LAPRESLE et al. (1977). A frequent combination of symptoms is visual disturbances and giddiness, ataxia, and nausea. Meniere's disease may be closely simulated (PREIBISCH-EFFENBERGER 1970). Indeed recurrent episodes of giddiness or vertigo is the commonest single symptom of vertebrobasilar insufficiency.

Nystagmus may occur during the episode of vertigo or may persist for a period after symptoms have abated. When witnessed, the nystagmus is of central type characterised by being multidirectional and often vertical. The amplitude of the nystagmus is greater in the abducting eye. Rotation and extension of the neck associated with forcible manoeuvres of the upper limb, e.g. driving screws into the undersurface of objects may be followed by intense vertigo, lasting from one to several days and often associated with nausea or even hours of profuse vomiting.

The advent of grand mal epilepsy or of temporal lobe epilepsy may be misleading unless the history preceding the epileptic event indicates other features of transient vertebrobasilar insufficiency. Drop attacks (SHELDON 1960; SHEEHAN et al. 1960) are particularly characteristic of recurrent vertebrobasilar ischaemia and they most frequently occur in women. Momentary failure of blood supply to the reticular formation has been postulated as being responsible for these attacks (MARSHALL 1976). Turning, or extension of the neck is a frequent precipitating factor. These attacks occur without warning, the patient suddenly falling limply on to her flexed knees and hands. Consciousness is normally retained or only momentarily lost, but the patient is usually able to rise to her feet immediately. Occasionally, the old person exhibits general hypotonus and may be unable to attain the erect position until the feet are pressed against an unyielding surface, such as a wall.

Recurrent dysarthria, dysphagia or hemiplegia are encountered, but eventual progress to established hemiplegia may occur. Involvement of one side of the face and the contralateral side of the body is indicative of a brain stem lesion. Parasthesiae over the face or upper limb or transient facial weakness are occasional features. A third of patients with vertebrobasilar insufficiency have evidence of slight to moderate hearing impairment (BASSERES et al. 1974; DECROIX et al. 1975;

CARRE and HUBER 1975; LUXON 1980). Luxon found the hearing loss to be bilaterally and symmetrical in 83% of subjects. The ninth or tenth nerves may be paralysed. Occipital headache, often intense and sometimes associated with marked tenderness over the back of the scalp and upper part of the neck, may prove misleading. Akinetic mutism is a rare transient feature of vertebrobasilar insufficiency, but is not uncommon following basilar artery occlusion. Changes in level of consciousness ranging from stupour to profound coma were reported to occur in 13% of cases (LOEB and MEYER 1965).

VII. Transient Ischaemic Attacks

Transient ischaemic attacks are temporary episodes of neurological dysfunction due to vascular ischaemic events and their cardinal clinical features are represented by their brief duration, spontaneous resolution without neurological deficit and a tendency to recur. The majority of TIAs last for only minutes and less commonly for one or several hours. By agreed definition complete resolution occurs within 24 h. These attacks may result from involvement of the carotid or the vertebrobasilar territory. We are concerned only with the latter group.

The diagnostic difficulties in establishing a diagnosis of vertebrobasilar TIAs should not be underrated. The large hospital cooperative study into the frequency and characteristics of transient ischaemic attacks (DYKEN et al. 1977; SWANSON et al. 1977; HAERER et al. 1977; CALANCHINI et al. 1977; FUTTY et al. 1977; PRICE et al. 1977), indicated that the condition was erroneously diagnosed in 30% of the patients. Several factors contribute to the diagnostic difficulties: many conditions simulate TIAs, the aetiology of TIAs is multiple and attacks are frequently unwitnessed by the physician. The careful evaluation of minutiae in the historical evidence of patient or relative may form the cornerstone of diagnosis.

A combination of features indicating occipital lobe or brain stem dysfunction is highly suggestive of a vertebrobasilar TIA, but such a combination is uncommon. FUTTY et al. (1977) considered that this presentation occurred in only 0.6% of patients. Our experience is that symptoms indicating involvement of more than one focal nervous system area is frequently obscured by the elderly characteristically dwelling on the symptoms that most concern them; subsequent interviews often elicit additional diagnostic information.

Vertigo is undoubtedly by far the commonest symptom, but also the most difficult to interpret in old age. Only meticulous attention to the details associated with the onset of vertigo, the characteristics and duration of the symptoms and the presence of other apparently minor associated features either during a current or past episode can lead to diagnostic possibility or certainty of a TIA.

Transient visual field impairment; hemianopia, unilateral or bilateral visual loss; perceptual disturbances; and diplopia are common features. Dysarthria is frequently seen, but dysphagia is less common. Disorders of sensation over one or both sides of the face may be the presenting manifestation. Of considerable diagnostic value is the infrequent occurrence of hemiparesis and hemisensory disturbance on alternate sides in repetitive episodes. Drop attacks occur in about 5% of subjects. Vomiting and ataxia may occur, but are commonly associated with vertigo. Transient attacks of confusion may be difficult to identify with vertebrobasilar ischaemia in the absence of other diagnostic features. Recurrent occipital headache, which is often intense, may be associated with scalp tenderness. Syncope has been reported in 1.5% of patients with vertebrobasilar TIAs (FUTTY et al. 1977).

VIII. Subclavian Steal Syndrome

Occlusion or severe stenosis of the subclavian artery proximal to the origin of the vertebral artery may induce a reversal of blood flow in the ipsilateral-vertebral artery into the subclavian artery distal to the stenosis to provide the blood supply to the corresponding upper limb. REIVICH et al. (1961) and NORTH et al. (1962) discussed the effects of this condition of the cerebral circulation. Transient ischaemic attacks may be a clinical manifestation of this circulatory disorder, particularly following exercise-induced vasodilation of the arm. Severe occipital headache may be precipitated by exercising the arm on the affected side or pain may be localised to the ipsilateral arm. If the atheromatous process extends to involve the vertebral artery, claudication in the upper limb may be the cardinal symptom. The predominant presenting features are giddiness and visual disturbances on using the arm on the affected side, but the condition may be entirely asymptomatic. A bruit is commonly present over the subclavian artery behind the origin of the sternomastroid muscle. The blood pressure in the two arms, usually shows a systolic difference of 20–40 mm Hg pressure.

IX. Arterial Occlusion in the Vertebrobasilar Territory

The tradition that the branch vessel in which occlusion has occurred could be infallibly identified clinically is now appreciated to be unfounded. This is exemplified by the lateral medullary syndrome of Wallenberg, which was firmly attributed to obstruction of the posterior inferior cerebellar artery. It is now recognised that this syndrome is more often due to obstruction of one of the vertebral arteries (JANZEN et al. 1979). Clinical features of the lateral medullary syndrome result from infarction of the lateral aspect of the medulla and inferior surface of the cerebellum. Typically, the onset is acute with intense vertigo aggravated by attempts to sit up or to stand. Distressing vomiting is common. Dysphagia with ipsilateral paralyses of the soft palate and pharynx due to involvement of the nucleus ambiguous and nystagmus and ipsilateral inco-ordination due to cerebellar involvement are characteristic of the syndrome. Horner's syndrome and sensory loss, mainly to pain and temperature, over the face or the side of the lesion and, to a variable degree, over the trunk and limbs on the opposite side are common. Contralateral hemiplegia may complete the picture.

Occlusion of the vertebral artery may be entirely symptomless or it may give rise to a picture indistinguishable from basilar artery occlusion. CASTAIGNE et al. (1973) found autopsy evidence of infarction of the medulla or cerebellum or both in 12 out of 22 cases of vertebral artery occlusion. Crossed hemiplegia with defective postural sensibility and bilateral involvement of the bulbar cranial nerves may result from occlusion of the paramedian branches of the vertebral artery which supply the medial anterior medullary region. Regional infarction in the medullary area, pons, and midbrain may give rise to well-recognised localising clinical features.

Thrombosis of the superior cerebellar artery largely affects the superior cerebellar peduncle and the most common feature is ipsilateral cerebellar signs. With more extensive infarction, contralateral thermoanaesthesia, and analgesia, a Horner's syndrome on the side of the lesion, partial deafness and contralateral facial paresis of upper motor neurone type may be evident.

Pontine infarction is commonly associated with contralateral hemiplegia or less commonly quadriplegia. Involvement of the sixth and seventh cranial nerve fibres give rise to lateral rectus and facial paresis respectively. Lateral conjugate eye movement to the side of the lesion may be impaired. The sensory tracts subserving pain and temperature are often affected in infarction of the middle third of the pons, resulting in homolateral facial anaesthesia and contralateral hemianaesthesia. The sixth and seventh cranial nerve nuclei and the spinal root of the fifth nerve may be involved with lateral rectus and facial paresis and homolateral anaesthesia respectively. The lateral portion of the pons receives a blood supply from branches of the basilar artery and from several cerebellar arteries, and vascular lesions involving this area may give rise to impairment of coordination of movement on the affected side. The characteristic picture of involvement of the upper part of the pons results from occlusion of the superior cerebellar artery. The clinical features are variable, but are commonly represented by cerebellar signs on the infarcted side and contralateral impairment of sensation for pain and temperature. A Horner's syndrome and tremor are often present.

Infarction of the mid-brain is relatively uncommon. Some of the neurological features of mid-brain infarction, such as paralysis of vertical conjugate deviation of the eyes, are often due to basilar or superior cerebellar artery occlusion and are associated with signs of involvement of other areas of the brain stem.

X. Basilar Artery Thrombosis

Basilar artery thrombosis was for long considered an uncommon and invariably fatal condition. Where the basilar artery is thrombosed throughout its length, abrupt onset of coma, pin-point pupils and a flaccid hemiplegia with absent reflexes typify this extensive vascular catastrophe. The classic report by KUBIK and ADAMS (1946) demonstrated that a segment of the basilar artery could be thrombosed and that the clinical presentation was dependent on the precise area of basilar occlusion. BIEMOND (1951) discussed the changing clinical picture and WILLIAMS and WILSON (1962) described the features of basilar artery insufficiency. Seventy per cent of autopsy proven cases of basilar artery thrombosis have transitory premonitory ischaemic symptoms within the vertebrobasilar territory (GAUTHIER 1963). Transient vertigo, dysarthria, occulomotor or limb paresis or syncope occurred in 70% of cases.

The level of consciousness following thrombosis of the basilar artery is impaired and ranges from slight drowsiness to profound coma. The onset may be abrupt with deep coma or slowly progressive. The level of consciousness may fluctuate considerably over hours or days. Where consciousness is marginally depressed, vertigo, ataxia, vomiting, dysarthria or anarthria may be evident. Disorders of conjugate eye movements, occulomotor paresis, cortical blindness (MELAMED et al. 1974), pseudobulbar signs, hemiparesis or quadriparesis, unilateral or bilateral seventh or eighth nerve paresis may variously dominate the clinical scene. Akinetic mutism is a not uncommon manifestation of basilar artery occlusion (REUTHER and DORNDORF 1973), and is characterised by the preservation of consciousness in a patient who remains motionless, apart from his eyes following events around him. The site of damage is probably in the reticular formation in the upper brain stem.

In some patients with an acute onset it may be possible to clinically identify the site of a segmental basilar occlusion. More commonly any attempt at clinical correlation between segmental basilar occlusion or vertebral artery occlusion is rendered sterile due to anatomical or haemodynamic factors.

C. Investigations

I. Laboratory

The relevant investigations will largely depend on clinical presentation and associated features. Considerable elevation of the ESR will be commonly noted in cervical cord tumours, tumour emboli from distal primary neoplasms, multiple myeloma, giant-cell arteritis, polyarteritis nodosa, and active rheumatoid arthritis. Serological examination for syphilis may be indicated by signs other than those involving the vertebrobasilar system. Where hyperviscosity states are responsible for impaired vertebrobasilar perfusion, an immunoglobulin profile may confirm myeloma or macroglobulinaemia. Haemoglobin estimation, haematocrit value, and red cell mass determination are relevant in the diagnosis of polycythaemia. Positive blood cultures may confirm infective endocarditis, but negative cultures do not exclude the diagnosis. An elevated titre of the differential agglutination test (sheeps' red cells) may help to establish the diagnosis of rheumatoid arthritis of the cervical spine, but an isolated positive latex slide test is of little diagnostic value in old age. Elevation of the enzyme, CPK, and particularly its M-B isoenzyme, with a progressive fall to normal over the subsequent few days is of considerable diagnostic assistance in confirming a myocardial infarction whose only presenting feature may be a stroke (PATHY 1967).

Electrocardiographic evidence of a myocardial infarction or of an arrhythmia may identify the occasional cardiac basis of vertebrobasilar signs and symptoms. However, POLIAKOFF (1972) has pointed out that in basilar artery thrombosis the ECG may simulate myocardial infarction.

II. Radiology

LAWRENCE et al. (1966) showed that 83.5% of males and 80% of females had radiological evidence of cervical disc degeneration after the age of 55 and that osteoarthrosis of the cervical zygapophyseal joints become increasingly common in later life. However, this study was based only on a lateral radiograph of the cervical spine. PALLIS et al. (1954) undertook a more detailed radiological study to include anteroposterior, lateral and both oblique radiographs. A close correlation was found between the clinical picture and combinations of radiological changes.

Due to the upward and outward direction of the lateral part of the neurocentral joint, ostophytes arising from this area are likely to impinge on the vertebral artery and can be visualised in anteroposterior and oblique views. The vertebral artery may be compressed by zygapophyseal osteophytes, which are demonstrated by an oblique view, though both obliques are preferable. PARIS and YOUNG (1967) showed that an "off lateral" view demonstrates the zygapophyseal joints in profile. In the presence of posterior subluxation, the inferior articular facet can compress the vertebal artery. Erosion of bone with marginal sclerosis may result from kinking of the vertebral artery.

III. Angiography

This is not a procedure to be undertaken lightly in the older patient and the indications must be precisely defined. Diagnostic uncertainty may justify this procedure. CAPLAN and ROSENBAUM (1975) found angiography was of particular value in separating posterior fossa occlusive vascular lesions from space-occupying lesions. With the introduction of microvascular surgery, KHODAD et al. (1977) have suggested that anastomosis between the occipital artery and posterior inferior cerebellar artery may be indicated in symptomatic low vertebrobasilar artery perfusion states. Preliminary angiography is mandatory. Vertebral angiography via brachial artery catheterisation is the most suitable technique (WOOD and HILAL 1969). Simultaneous tomography with cerebral angiography permits better identification of the vertebrobasilar circulation (ROSA 1976; SARTOR 1978).

ABRAHAM et al. (1975) found that visual evoked potentials (VEPs) performed early in patients with occipital blindness following basilar artery occlusion was of prognostic rather than diagnostic value. Responses of normal shape and amplitude after monocular and binocular stimulation were followed by complete recovery of vision. Lack of VEP was a preceding sign of permanent blindness.

IV. Percutaneous Ultrasonic Doppler Technique

KANEDA et al. (1977) compared the percutaneous ultrasonic Doppler technique with angiography and found it to be a useful screening test. KELLER et al. (1976) found the use of a bidirectional continuous wave Doppler ultrasound system applied non-invasively under local anaesthetic to the oropharynx gave 82% accurate results when compared with angiography, appearing to have merit as a safe screening method.

V. Computerised Tomography

With considerable experience and under optimum conditions, computerised tomography (CT) can outline major intracerebral vessels and define aneurysmal changes. With recordings of high technical quality, small haemorrhages of 0.5–2 cm in diameter can be identified. It has value in detecting small posterior fossa tumours which may simulate vertebrobasilar arterial lesions. KINGSLEY et al. (1980) found that the CT scan was of diagnostic value if performed within 2 weeks of the ictus in clinically diagnosed infarct or a stroke in evolution, but no CT change was demonstrated in any patients with clinically diagnosed transient ischaemic attacks.

D. Management of the Vertebrobasilar Syndrome

While treatment will be dictated by the causal factors, it is appropriate to limit discussion to those conditions in which vertebrobasilar dysfunction is the cardinal issue.

I. Cervical Spondylosis

The objective is to reduce excessive or even moderate neck movement in order to prevent compression of the extracranial segment of the vertebral arteries. In the elderly a light adjustable plastic collar which can be secured by Velco fastenings is normally very satisfactory. Considerable debate exists as to the frequency and total duration that a collar should be worn. Whereas the osteophytic spurs and bony bosses cannot diminish, it is our experience that symptoms rapidly abate over 2 or 3 days, and that if the collar is worn during the day for 3 months and then only during periods of significant physical activity, most patients will obtain long periods of symptomatic relief. Co-existing postural hypotension or paroxysmal arrhythmias should receive attention. Traction and manipulation play no part in the treatment of vertebrobasilar syndrome due to cervical spondylosis. Where pain from associated radiotherapy is severe, 7–10 days of phenylbutazone in doses not exceeding 300 mg daily or indomethacine often gives rapid relief.

II. Surgery

Radiological changes compatible with possible vertebral artery compression by osteophytes is an indication for angiography if symptoms are severe. If the vertebral artery is compressed by spondylotic outgrowths, particularly in the absence of major atheromatous changes, surgical decompression should be seriously considered. P'ASZTOR (1978) has shown that division of constricting peri-arterial fibrous tissue may occasionally be required in addition to the removal of bony osteophytes and bosses.

III. Subclavian Steal Syndrome

Most often no treatment other than advice to refrain from vigorous use of the limb on the affected side is required. Where symptoms are frequent and severe, subclavian endarterectomy, or now more commonly a by-pass operation in the neck (e.g. carotid subclavian vein by-pass graft, EASTCOTT 1976), will relieve symptoms. However, brain infarction virtually never occurs in this condition in the absence of concomitant carotid artery disease. In these cases, carotid endarterectomy will prevent a stroke (FIELDS and LEMAK 1972).

IV. Vertebral Artery Stenosis

Progress to infarction is very uncommon and unlike carotid artery stenosis, preventive reconstructive surgery is rarely practical. However, where there is associated internal carotid artery stenosis in an otherwise fit person, reconstruction of the accompanying carotid stenosis may relieve major symptoms and prevent an established stroke. However, impaired mentation may be improved in patients with low perfusion rates by extracranial to intracranial by-pass (FERGUSSON and PEERLESS 1976; LUMLEY 1979). KHODAD et al. (1977) have suggested that anastomosis between occipital artery and the posterior inferior cerebellar artery may be indicated in low perfusion in the vertebrobasilar system.

V. Transient Ischemic Attacks Involving the Vertebrobasilar System

It is fundamental to any logical therapeutic approach that the criteria for diagnosis of TIA is precise. Only a transitory neurological deficit within the area of the central nervous system supplied by the vertebrobasilar vasculature, in which no residual deficit should exist after 24 h, may be considered as a TIA. Indeed, evidence of neurological impairment would commonly last minutes and rarely be detectable for more than 3 h. Any recurrent associated or precipitating factor such as cardiac arrhythmias or postural hypotension requires initial correction. Where recurrent micro-embolisation is reasonably certain and involves the internal carotid artery territory, where the risk of eventual established strokes is significantly greater than in TIAs of the vertebrobasilar system, considerable debate on the role of anticoagulation continues. This is largely due to questionable diagnostic criteria, poor trial design – particularly lack of effective randomisation between treatment and control groups, inadequate number of patients in single studies and variable assessment criteria of therapeutic effects. Many of those who recommend anticoagulation for TIAs would only advocate this regime where the transient neurological deficits are in the internal carotid artery territory. We continue to believe that anticoagulants have a valuable role in the management of confirmed recurrent TIAs in the vertebrobasilar territory. The anticoagulant preferred is Warfarin. It is important to appreciate that the dose of Warfarin at age 65 years is approximately a half of that required by young adults to achieve the same degree of anticoagulation, and by age 80 years the equivalent dose is one-quarter of that of the young adult. Treatment is continued for at least 3 years provided each patient is able to routinely attend an anticoagulant clinic which is organised to follow strict guide lines of detailed management.

VI. Drugs Affecting Platelet Aggregation

Several drugs affect platelet aggregability, but those which have been widely evaluated clinically include aspirin, sulphinpyrazone, and dipyridamole. The meticulous study by FIELDS et al. (1977) on aspirin and the large Canadian study (THE CANADIAN CO-OPERATIVE STUDY GROUP 1978), comparing four groups receiving aspirin or sulphinpyrazone, or aspirin and sulphinpyrazone, or placebo, indicated that aspirin reduces the risk of strokes after a TIA in 50% of men, but afforded no protection to women. Sulphinpyrazone was no more effective than placebo, but the combination of sulphinpyrazone and aspirin was demonstrated to be slightly more effective than aspirin alone. The optimum dose of aspirin has yet to be established. From experimental evidence, MONCADA and VANE (1978) suggests that aspirin should probably only be administered in weekly doses.

The possibility of preventing TIAs by drug therapy appears promising, but more carefully designed trials are required before definitive regimes can be advocated. It is nevertheless important that general advice should include reassurance that the frequency of TIAs may diminish with time, and that TIAs in the vertebro-basilar territory carry a generally good prognosis. Control of hypertension, weight reduction, avoidance of cigarette smoking and regular exercise are general measures which have cardinal merit.

References

Abraham FA, Melamed E, Levy S (1975) Prognostic nature of visual evoked potentials in occipital blindness following basilar artery occlusion. Appl Neurophysiol 38:126–135

Barnett HJM (1976) Pathogenesis of transient ischaemic attacks in cerebrovascular disease. In: Schierberg P (ed) Tenth Princeton Conference. Raven Press, New York, pp 1–21

Basseres F, Bonnieu A, Guerrier Y (1974) L'exploration audiovestibulaire. A propos de 48 cas de sténoses de l'artère vertenrale opérées. Cah Otorhinolaryngol 9:463–472

Battacharji SK (1965) The role of the extra-cranial and intracranial arteries in cerebral infarction. PhD thesis. University of Birmingham

Battacharji SK, Hutchinson EC, McCall AJ (1967) Stenosis and occlusion of vessels in cerebral infarction. Brit Med J 3:270–274

Bauer RB, Sheehan S, Wechsler, Meter JS (1962) Arteriographic study of sites, incidence and treatment of arteriosclerotic cerebrovascular lesions. Neurol 12:698–711

Biemond A (1951) Thrombosis of the basilar artery and the vascularisation of the brain. Brain 74:300–317

Boemke A (1951) Feingewebliche Befunde beim Bandscheibenvorfall. Arch Klm Chir 267:484–492

Brain R (1957) Order and disorder in the cerebral circulation. Lancet 2:857–862

Calanchini PR, Swanson PD, Gotshall RA et al. (1977) Co-operative study of hospital frequency and character of transient ischaemic attacks. IV. Reliability of diagnosis. JAMA 238:2029–2033

Caplan LW, Rosenbaum AE (1975) Role of cerebral angiography in vertebro-basilar occlusive diseases. J Neurol Neurosurg Psychiat 38:601–612

Cardell BS, Hanley T (1961) A fatal case of giant cell or temporal arteritis. J Path Bact 63:587–597

Carre J, Huber B (1975) A propos d'une sordité par troubles vasculaires. J Fr Otorhinolaryngol 24:621

Castaigne P, Lhermitte F, Gautier JC, Scourolle E, Derovesne C, Der Agopian P, Popa C (1973) Arterial occlusions in the vertebro-basilar system. A study of 44 patients with postmortem data. Brain 96:133–154

Cogan DC, Kunabara T, Moser H (1964) Fat emboli in the retina following angiography. Arch Opthalmol 71:308–313

Contorni L (1960) Il circolo collateral vertebro-vertebrale nella obliterazione della arteria succlavia alle due origine. Minerva Chir 15:268–275

Daseler EH, Anson BJ (1959) Surgical anatomy of the subclavian artery and its branches. Surg Gynecol Obstet 108:149–174

Davenmuehle RH, Busse EW, Newman G (1961) Physical problems of older people. J Am Geriatr Soc 9:208–217

David NJ, Klintworth GK, Friedburg SJ, Dillon M (1963) Fatal atheromatous cerebral embolism associated with bright plaques in the retinal arterioles. Report of a case. Neurol (Minneap) 13:708–713

De Bakey EM, Crawford ES (1969) Surgical treatment of innominate common carotid and subclavian artery occlusion. Chap 10. In: Gillespie A (ed) Extracranial cerebrovascular disease and its management. Butterworth JA, London

Decroix G, Vaneecloo FM, Julliot JP, Quandalle P (1975) Surdite et insuffisance vertebrobasilaire. J Fr Otorhinolaryngol 24:503–509

De Kleyn A (1939) Some remarks on vestibular nystagmus. Confinia Neurol 2:257–291

Denny-Brown D (1951) Recurrent cerebro-vascular episodes. Arch Neurol Psychiat 2:194–210

De Reuck J, Inderadjaja N, Cerevits L, Coster W, Van Der Eecker HM, Roels H (1979) Vertebro-basilar insufficiency due to tremoural emboli. Clin Neurol Neurosurg 81:53–58

Dixon AS, Beardwell C, Kay A, Wanka J, Wong YT (1966) Polymyalgia rheumatica and temporal arteriis. Ann Rheum Dis 25:203–208

Dyken ML, Conneally PM, Haerer AF et al. (1977) Co-operative study of hospital frequency of character of transient ischaemic attacks: background, organisation and clinical survey. JAMA 237:882–885

Eastcott HHG (1976) Surgical management of carotid and vertebral disease. In: Gillingham FJ, Mawdesley C, Williams AE (eds) Stroke. Churchill Livingston, London New York, pp 456–468

Fergusson CG, Peerless SJ (1976) Proceedings of a joint meeting on stroke and cerebral circulation. Dallas, Texas (not published)

Fields WS, Lemak NA (1972) Joint study of extra-cranial arterial occlusion VII subclavian steal – a review of 168 cases. JAMA 222:1139–1143

Fields WS, Bruteman ME, Wievel T (1965) Collateral circulation of the brain. Surg Sci 2:183–259

Fields WS, Lemak NA, Frankowski RF (1977) Controlled trial of aspirin in cerebral ischaemia. Stroke 8:301–316

Fisher CM (1954) Occlusion of the carotid arteries. Further experiences. Arch Neurol Psychiat 72:187–204

Fisher CM (1959) Observations on the fundus oculi in transient monocular blindness. Neurol (Minneap) 9:333–347

Fisher CM (1970) Occlusion of the vertebral arteries causing transient basilar symptoms. Arch Neurol 22:3–9

Fisher CM, Gore I, Okabe N, White PD (1965) Ather-osclerosis of the carotid and vertebral arteries. Extracranial and intracranial. J Neuropath Exp Neurol 24:455–476

Frykholm R (1951) Cervical nerve root compression resulting from disc degeneration and root cleeve compression. Acta Chir Scand Supply 160

Futty DE, Conneally PM, Dyken ML et al. (1977) Study of hospital frequency and character of transient ischaemic attacks. JAMA 238:2386–2390

Gauthier G (1963) Contribution to the study of basilar artery thrombosis. Schweiz Arch Neurol Neurochir Psychiat 91:384–411

Geissinger JD, Gruner G, Ruge D (1972) Vertebral artery occlusion by a cervical "hour glass" neurofibroma. J Neurol Neurosurg Psychiat 35:899–902

Geraud J, Bes A, Delpla M, Marc-Vergnes JP (1969) Cerebral arterial-venous oxygen differences. In: Meyer JS, Echhorn O (eds) Research on the cerebral circulation. Charles C Thomas, Springfield, Ill, p 290

Gillian LA (1959) Significant superficial anastomoses in the arterial blood supply to the human brain. J Comp Neurol 112:55–73

Haerer AF, Gotshall RA, Conneally PM et al. (1977) Co-operative study of hospital frequency and character of transient ischaemic attacks. III. Variation in treatment. JAMA 238:142–146

Hardesty WH, Roberts B, Toole JF, Royster HP (1962) Studies in vertebral artery blood flow. Surg Forum 13:482–483

Hendin AS, Margoli MT, Glickman MG (1973) Occlusion of the basilar artery in tuberculous meningitis. Neuroradiology 6:193–195

Hirsch C, Paulson S, Sylven B, Snellman O (1953) Biophysical and physiological investigations on cartilage and other mesenchymal tissues: characteriestics of human nuclei pulposi during ageing. Acta Orthop Scand 22:175–183

Hollenhorst RW (1961) Significance of bright plaques in the retinal arteries. JAMA 178:23–39

Hutchinson EC, Yates PO (1956) The cervical portion of the vertebral artery. A clinico-pathological study. Brain 70:319–331

Ivanov I, Matev M (1973) Visual phenomena in cervical spondylosis with transitory vertebro-basilar obstruction. Opthalmologia 21:26–28

Janzen RW, Götze P, Kühne D (1979) Under gas Wallenberg-Syndrom. Leitsymptom des isolierten Vertebralisverschlusses. Fortschr Neurol Psychiatr 47:123–143

Jones MW, Kaufman JC (1976) Vertebro-basilar artery insufficiency in rheumatoid atlantoaxial subluxation. J Neurol Neurosurg Psychiat 39:122–128

Jörgensen L, Torvik A (1966) Ischaemic cerebrovascular diseases in an autopsy series. Part I. Prevalence, location and predisposing factors in verified thrombo-embolic occlusions and their significance in the apthogenesis of cerebral infarction. J Neurol Sci (Amsterdam) 490–509

Kameyama M, Okinaka S (1963) Collateral circulation of the brain with special reference to atherosclerosis of the major cervical and cerebral arteries. Neurol (Minneap) 13:279–286

Kaneda H, Irvine T, Minami T, Taneda M (1977) Diagnostic reliability of the percutaneous ultrasonic Doppler technique for vertebral arterial occlusive diseases. Stroke 8:571–579

Keith TA (1977) Hypertension crises. Recognition and management. JAMA 237:1570–1577

Keller HM, Meier WE, Kumpe DA (1976) Non-invasive angiography for the diagnosis of vertebral artery disease using Doppler ultrasound (vertebral artery Doppler). Stroke 7:364–369

Kempson GE (1975) The mechanical properties of articular cartilage and their relation to matrix degeneration and age. Ann Rheum Dis (Suppl) 34:111–114

Kendall RE, Marshall J (1963) Role of hypotension in the genesis of transient focal cerebral ischaemic attacks. Brit Med J 2:344–348

Khodad CI, Singh R, Clinger CP (1977) Possible prevention of brain stem stroke by microvascular anastomosis in the vertebrobasilar system. Stroke 8:316–321

Kingsley DPE, Radue EW, Dulay EPGH (1980) Evaluation of computerised tomography in vascular lesion of the vertebrobasilar territory. J Neurol Neurosurg Psychiatry 43:193–197

Kovacs A (1955) Subluxation and deformation of the cervical apophyseal joints. Acta Radiol 43:1–16

Kubik CS, Adams RD (1946) Occlusion of the basilar artery. A clinical and pathological study. Brain 69:73–121

Kurtzke JF (1976) A population study of stroke and T.I.A. In: Gillingham FJ, Mawdesley C, Williams AE (eds) Stroke. Churchill Livingston, London New York, pp 5–21

Lapresle J, Matreau R, Annabi A (1977) Transient achromatopsia in vertebro-basilar insufficiency. J Neurol 215:155–158

Lawrence JS, De Graff R, Lain VAI (1963) Degenerative joint disease in random sample and occupational groups. In: Kellgren JH, Jeffrey MR, Ball J (eds) The epidemiology of chronic rheumatism, vol 1. Blackwell Scientific Publications, Oxford

Lawrence JS, Bremner JM, Bier F (1966) Osteroarthrosis: prevalence in the population and relationship between symptoms and X-ray changes. Ann Rheum Dis 25:1

Lhermitte F (1966) Anatomopathologie et physiopathologie des stenoses carotidienees. Rev Neurol 115:641

Loeb C, Meyer JS (1965) Strokes due to vertebro-basilar disease. Charles C Thomas, Springfield, Ill

Lumley JSP (1979) Extracranial revascularisation. Brit J Surg 66:317–323

Luxon LM (1980) Hearing loss in brain stem disorders. J Neurol Neurosurg Psychiat 43:510–515

Magaard F, Ekestrom S (1975) The influence of arm ischaemic and arm hyperanaemia on subclavian and vertebral artery blood florn in patients with occlusive disease of the subclavian artery and brachiocephalic trunk. A pre-operative study. Scand J Thorac Cardiovasc Surg 9:240–249

Maroudas A, Venn A (1977) Chemical composition and swelling of normal and osteoarthritic femoral and cartilage. II. Swelling Ann Rheum Dis 36:399–406

Marshall J (1968) The differential diagnosis of little strokes. Postgrad Med J 543–548

Marshall J (1976) The management of cerebrovascular disease, 3 rd edn. Blackwell Scientific Publications, Oxford London Edinburgh Melbourne

Marshall LF, Bruce DA, Bruno L, Longfit TW (1978) Vertebro-basilar spasm: a significant cause of neurological deficit in head injury. J Neurol 48:560–564

Martin MJ, Whisnant JP, Sayre GP (1960) Occlusive vascular disease in the extracranial cerebral circulation. Arch Neurol 3:530–538

Matsumato N, Whisnant JP, Kusland LT, Okazaki H (1973) Natural history of stroke in Rochester, Minnesota, 1955 through 1969: an extension of a previous study, 1945 through 1954. Stroke 4:20–29

McBrien DJ, Bradley RD, Ashton N (1963) The nature of retinal emboli in stenosis of the internal carotid artery. Lancet 1:697–699

McGee DA, McPhedran RS, Hoffman HJ (1962) Carotid and vertebral artery disease. A clinico-pathologic survey of 70 cases. Neurol 12:848–849

Meckel GF (1828) Mannuale di antomia generale descriptiva e patologica, vol 13. Tipografik dek Reale Albergo dei Poveri

Melamed E, Abraham FA, Levy S (1974) Cortical blindness as a manifestation of basilar artery occlusion. Eur Neurol 11:22–29

Millikan CH, Sieker RG, Whisnant JP (1960) Intermittent carotid and vertebral basilar insufficiency with polycythaemia. Neurol (Minneap) 10:188–196

Mitchell JR, Schwartz CJ (1965) Arterial disease. Blackwell Scientific Publications, Oxford

Modan B, Modan M (1968) Benign erythrocytosis. Brit J Haemat 14:375–381

Moncada S, Vane JR (1978) Unstable metabolites of arachidonic acid and their role in haemostasis and thrombosis. Brit Med Bull 34:129–135

Naritomi H, Saki F, Meyer JS (1979) Pathogenesis of transient ischaemic attacks within the vertebro-basilar arterial system. Aron Neurol 36:121–128

North RR, Fields WS, DeBakey ME, Crawford ES (1962) Brachia basilar insufficiency syndrome. Neurol 12:810–820

O'Brien MD, Mallet BL (1970) Cerebral cortex perfusion rates in dementia. J Neurol Neurosurg Psychiat 3:497–500

Obrist WD, Sokoloff L, Lassen NA, Lane MH, Butler RN, Feinberg I (1963) Relation of EEG to cerebral blood flow and metabolism in old age. Electroencephal Clin Neurophysiol 15:610–619

Ostberg G (1973) An arteritis with special reference to polymyalgia. Acta Path Microbiol Scand Suppl 237:5–58

Pallis C, Jomes AM, Spillane JD (1954) Cervical spondylosis: incidence and implications. Brain 77:274–289

Paris FA, Young AC (1967) Quoted from Young AC, Chap V. In: Wilkinson W, William M (eds) Cervical spondylosis brain. Heineman Medical Books Limited, London

P'asztor E (1978) Decompression of vertebral artery in cases of cervical spondylosis. Surg Neurol 9:371–377

Pathy MS (1967) Clinical presentation of myocardial infarction in the elderly. Brit Heart J 19:290–299

Poliakoff H (1972) Basilar artery thrombosis. Electrocardiogram simulating acute infarction. State J Med NY 72:2891–2892

Preibisch-Effenberger R (1970) Durchströmungsminderung im Arteria-Vertebralis-System als Ursache Morbus Meniere-ähnlicher Krankheitsbilder – Operative Beseitigung – 5-Jahres-Heilung. Z Laryng Rhinol Otol 49:185–196

Price TR, Gotshall RA, Poskanser DG et al. (1977) Co-operative study of hospital frequency and character of transient ischaemic attacks. VI. Patients examined during an attack. JAMA 238:1512–1513

Püschel J (1930) Beiträge zur pathologischen Anatomie und zur allgemeinen Pathologie. Beitr path Anat 84:123

Ramanul FC, Abramowicz A (1964) Changes in the brain and pail vessels in arterial border zones. A study of 13 cases. Arch Neurol (Chic) 11:40–65

Romanul FC (1970) Examination of the brain and spinal cord. In: Tedeschi CG (ed) Neuropathology in methods and diagnosis. Little, Brown and Co, Boston, pp 131–214

Ramanul FC (1976) Some anatomical and apthophysiological aspects of clinical importance in stroke. In: Gillingham FJ, Mawdesley X, Williams AE (eds) Stroke. Churchill Livingston, London New York

Reivich M, Holling HE, Roberts B, Toole JF (1961) Reversal of blood flow through the vertebral artery and its effect on cerebral circulation. New Engl J Med 265:878–885

Reuther R, Dorndorf W (1973) Ventrales Pons-Syndrome (akinetischer Mutismus) bei Verschluß der A. basilaris. Nervenarzt 44:491–494

Rosa M (1976) Angiotomographic study of the normal cerebral circulation. II. The vertebro-basilar system. Neuroadiol 10:243–249

Ross-Russel RW (1961) Observations on the retinal blood vessels in monocular blindness. Lancet 2:1422–1428

Ross-Russel RW (1963) Atheromatous retinal embolism. Lancet 2:1354–1356

Ross-Russel RW (1976) Less common varieties of cerebral arterial disease. In: Ross-Russel RW (ed) Cerebral arterial disease. Churchill Livingston, London New York, p 287

Sadoshima S, Tanaka K, Takeshita M, Hirota Y, Omae T, Katsuki S (1973) Atherosclerosis and atherosclerotic disorders in the autopsy cases of Hisayana Survey in the recent ten years. Fukuoka Acta Med 65:701–713

Sartor J (1978) Vertebralis-angiotomographic. Technik – Indikation – Leistung. Roentgenblaetter 31:371–382

Schwartz CJ, Mitchell JR (1961) Atheroma of the carotid and vertebral arterial system. Brit Med J 2:1057–1063

Sheehan S, Baver RB, Meyer JS (1960) Vertebral artery compression in cervical spondylosis. Angiographic demonstration during life of vertebral artery insufficiency due to rotation and extension of the neck. Neurol (Minneap) 10:968–986

Sheldon JH (1960) Natural history of falls in old age. Brit Med J 2:1685–1690

Siekert RG, Whisnant JP, Millikan CH (1980) Anaemia and intermittent focal cerebral arterial insufficiency. Arch Neurol 3:386–390

Silverstein A, Gilbert H, Wasserman LR (1962) Neurological complications of polythaemia. Ann Int Med 57:909–916

Swanson PD, Calanchini PR, Dyken ML et al. (1977) Co-operative study of hospital frequency and character of transient ischaemic attacks. II. Performance of angiography among six centre. JAMA 237:2202–2206

Taylor AR (1953) Mechanism and treatment of spinal cord disorders associated with cervical spondylosis. Lancet 1:717–720

The Canadian Co-operative Study Group (1978) A randomised trial of aspirin and sulfinpurazone in threatened stroke. New Engl J Med 299:53–59

Toole JF, Tucker SA (1960) Influence of the head position upon cerebral circulation. Arch Neurol 2:616–623

Toole JF (1964) Reversed vertebral-artery flow. Subclavian steel syndrome. Lancet 1:872–873

Van Der Eeken HM, Adams RD (1953) The anatomy and functional significance of the meningeal arterial anastomosis of the human brain. J Neuropath Exp Neurol 12:132–137

Van Der Zwan A (1954) Angiographic diagnosis of vertebral artery thrombosis. J Neurol Neurosurg Psychiat 17:189–190

Weightman BO (1975) In vitro fatigue testing of articular cartilage. Ann Rheum Dis (Suppl) 34:108–110

Whisnant JP (1974) Epidemiology of strokes. Emphasis on transient cerebral ischaemic attacks and hypertension. Stroke 5:68–70

Whisnant JP, Martin MJ, Sayre GP (1961) Atherosclerotic stenosis of cervical arteries. Clinical significance. Arch Neurol 5:429–432

Whisnant JP, Matsumoto N, Elveback LR (1973) Transient cerebral ischaemic attacks in a community. Rochester, Minnesota, 1955 through 1969. Mayo Clin Proc 48:194–198

Williams D (1969) Syndrome associated with carotid and vertebrobasilar insufficiency. Chap 3. In: Gillespie JA (ed) Extracranial and cerebrovascular disease and its management. Butterworths, London

Williams D, Wilson TG (1962) The diagnosis of the major and minor syndrome of basilar insufficiency. Brain 85:741–742

Willis T (1720) Opera Monia. Nevetiis J Malachinus

Wood EH, Hilal SK (1969) The radiological diagnosis of extracranial cerebrovascular disease. In: Gillespie JA (ed) Extracranial cerebrovascular disease and its management. Butterworths, London

Yates PO (1976) The pathogenesis of transient ischaemic attacks. In: Gillingham FJ, Mawdesley C, Williams AE (eds) Stroke. Churchill-Livingston, London New York, pp 178–187

Young AC, Chaper VC (1967 – 1st edition). Cervical spondylosis. In: Wilkinson M, Brain WR (eds) Early diagnosis and treatment. Heinemann, London

Zucker MB (1947) Platelet aggregation vasoconstruction as factors in haemostasis in normal thombocytopenic hepannised and hypoprothombanaemic rats. Am J Physiol 148:275–288

Cardiac Glycosides

Part 1

Experimental Pharmacology of Cardiac Glycosides

With contributions by numerous experts
Editor: K. Greeff
1981. 164 figures. XXIV, 682 pages
(Handbook of Experimental Pharmacology,
Volume 56, Part 1)
ISBN 3-540-10917-X

Part 2

Pharmacokinetics and Clinical Pharmacology of Cardiac Glycosides

With contributions by numerous experts
Editor: K. Greeff
1981. 64 figures. XXI, 394 pages
(Handbook of Experimental Pharmacology,
Volume 56, Part 2)
ISBN 3-540-10918-8

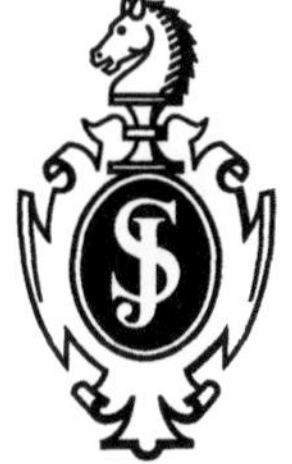

Springer-Verlag
Berlin
Heidelberg
NewYork

Digitals glycosides and their related compounds
have long been among the most important
drugs used in the treatment of various forms of
cardiac insufficiency. In this volume, leading
experts provide details concerning the modes of
action of these substances, together with information pertinent to evaluations of their pharmacological and therapeutic characteristics, in particular their interaction with other drugs, their
side-effects and their therapeutic spectra.

Psychotropic Agents

Part I

Antipsychotics and Antidepressants

Editors: G. Stille, F. Hoffmeister
With contributions by numerous experts
1980. 82 figures, 74 tables. XXIV, 734 pages
(Handbook of Experimental Pharmacology,
Volume 55, Part 1)
ISBN 3-540-09858-5

Part II

Anxiolytics, Gerontopsycho-pharmacological Agents, and Psychomotor Stimulants

Editors: F. Hoffmeister, G. Stille
With contributions by numerous experts
1981. 75 figures. XXVI, 778 pages
(Handbook of Experimental Pharmacology,
Volume 55, Part 2)
ISBN 3-540-10300-7

Part III

Alcohol and Psychotomimetics, Psychotropic Effects of Central Acting Drugs

Editors: G. Stille, F. Hoffmeister
With contributions by numerous experts
1981. 21 figures. XXVI, 508 pages
(Handbook of Experimental Pharmacology,
Volume 55, Part 3)
ISBN 3-540-10301-5

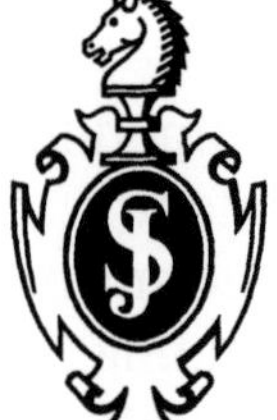

Springer-Verlag
Berlin
Heidelberg
New York